Springer Proceedings in Mathematics & Statistics

Volume 231

Springer Proceedings in Mathematics & Statistics

This book series features volumes composed of selected contributions from workshops and conferences in all areas of current research in mathematics and statistics, including operation research and optimization. In addition to an overall evaluation of the interest, scientific quality, and timeliness of each proposal at the hands of the publisher, individual contributions are all refereed to the high quality standards of leading journals in the field. Thus, this series provides the research community with well-edited, authoritative reports on developments in the most exciting areas of mathematical and statistical research today.

More information about this series at http://www.springer.com/series/10533

Jürgen Pilz · Dieter Rasch
Viatcheslav B. Melas · Karl Moder
Editors

Statistics and Simulation

IWS 8, Vienna, Austria, September 2015

Springer

Editors
Jürgen Pilz
Institute of Statistics
Alpen-Adria University of Klagenfurt
Klagenfurt
Austria

Dieter Rasch
Institute of Applied Statistics
and Computing
University of Natural Resources
and Life Sciences
Vienna
Austria

Viatcheslav B. Melas
St. Petersburg State University
St. Petersburg
Russia

Karl Moder
Institute of Applied Statistics
and Computing
University of Natural Resources
and Life Sciences
Vienna
Austria

ISSN 2194-1009 ISSN 2194-1017 (electronic)
Springer Proceedings in Mathematics & Statistics
ISBN 978-3-030-09386-0 ISBN 978-3-319-76035-3 (eBook)
https://doi.org/10.1007/978-3-319-76035-3

Mathematics Subject Classification (2010): 62XX, 68XX, 92XX

Softcover re-print of the Hardcover 1st edition 2018

Printed on acid-free paper

This Springer imprint is published by the registered company Springer International Publishing AG part of Springer Nature
The registered company address is: Gewerbestrasse 11, 6330 Cham, Switzerland

Preface

The present volume contains selected contributions given at the 8th International Workshop on Simulation held at the University of Natural Resources and Life Sciences, Vienna, Austria, September 21–25, 2015.

The conference was organized by the Center of Experimental Design of the Institute of Applied Statistics and Computing of the University of Natural Resources and Life Sciences, Vienna, in collaboration with the Department of Statistics of the Alpen-Adria University of Klagenfurt, the Department of Statistical Modelling of Saint Petersburg State University, and INFORMS Simulation Society (USA). This international conference was devoted to statistical techniques in stochastic simulation, data collection, and analysis of scientific experiments and studies representing broad areas of interest. The 1st–6th Workshops took place in St. Petersburg (Russia) in 1994, 1996, 1998, 2001, 2005, and 2009. The 7th International Workshop on Simulation took place in Rimini, May 21–24, 2013.

The conference in Vienna was held in memory of Luidmila Kopylova- Melas, the wife of Viatcheslav Melas who initiated this series of conferences. Luidmila passed away on September 21, 2013; she worked relentlessly as secretary of the whole series of our simulation workshops.

The Scientific Program Committee was chaired by Viatcheslav Melas (St. Petersburg, Russia), Dieter Rasch (Vienna, Austria), and Jürgen Pilz (Klagenfurt, Austria). We are indebted to the following members of the Scientific Program Committee for their fruitful help in organizing the sessions and making the Vienna Workshop a tremendous success: Aleksander Andronov (Latvia), Anthony Atkinson (UK), Narayanaswamy Balakrishnan (Canada), Russell Barton (USA), Michel Broniatowski (France), Ekaterina Bulinskaya (Russia), Holger Dette (Germany), Sergei Ermakov (Russia), Valerii Fedorov (USA), Nancy Flournoy (USA), Subir Ghosh (USA), Marie Hušková (Czech Republic), Jack Kleijnen (The Netherlands), Gennady Mikhailov (Russia), Simos Meintanis (Greece), Werner Müller (Austria), Valery Nevzorov (Russia), Michael Nikulin (France), Jordi

Ocania (Spain), Ingram Olkin (USA), Fortunato Pesarin (Italy), Luigi Salmaso (Italy), Rainer Schwabe (Germany), John Stufken (USA), Bruno Tuffin (France), Dariusz Ucinski (Poland), Henry Wynn (UK).

The Local Organizing Committee was led by Karl Moder (Vienna, Austria). We are thankful to the following members of this committee for their extremely helpful and efficient organizational work during the conference: Marianne Mansuri (Vienna), Beate Simma (Klagenfurt), Bernhard Spangl (Vienna), Gunter Spöck (Klagenfurt), and Albrecht Gebhardt (Klagenfurt).

The present proceedings volume consists of six parts; the first part contains four invited papers, and the remaining five parts deal with various applications of simulations.

The first of the invited papers, presented by Jack P. C. Kleijnen, gives an overview of the state of the art in the design and analysis of simulation experiments, with a special emphasis on simulation optimization in operation research. The second of the invited papers gives a review of simulation usage in the New Zealand electricity market: G. Zakeri and G. Pritchard demonstrate, in particular, how optimization of electricity consumption and reserves can be combined in an efficient way. In the third invited paper, Z. Prášková gives an overview of bootstrap changepoint testing procedures for dependent data. In the last one of the invited papers, C. Draxler and K. D. Kubinger review the present state and future challenges of power and sample size determination in psychometrics.

The contributed twenty-nine papers have been arranged in six parts dealing with different aspects of simulation in mathematical analysis, stochastic processes, statistical estimation and testing problems, clinical trials, design of experiments and in reliability and queueing theory models and applications.

The chapters in Part II (Simulation for Mathematical Modeling and Analysis) start with a contribution by T. M. Tovstik studying in detail the covariation matrix of solutions of linear algebraic system equations via the Monte Carlo method. O. N. Soboleva and E. P. Kurochkina consider large-scale simulation studies of acoustic waves in random multiscale media. H. S. Bhat, R. A. Madushani, and S. Rawat deal with parameter inference for stochastic differential equations with density tracking by quadrature. G. A. Mikhailov, N. V. Tracheva, and S. A. Ukhinov present a new Monte Carlo algorithm for the evaluation of outgoing polarized radiation.

Simulation models and their analysis for stochastic process applications played an important role at the 8th IWS. Contributions in this direction are collected in Part III of the present proceedings volume. E. Ermishkina and E. Yarovaya study the evolution and simulation of branching random walks. Y. Belopolskaya studies stochastic models for nonlinear cross-diffusion systems. N. Vollert, M. Ortner, and J. Pilz report on experiences with the application of tree-structured Gaussian process models for optimization in magnetic field shaping problems. The last three contributions in Part III deal with applications in actuarial science and stochastic finance: E. Bulinskaya and J. Gusak consider insurance models under incomplete information; Ch. Quast et al. model and compare pension systems in Austria, Chile, Slovakia, and Sweden; A. Andronov and T. Yurkina study the Markowitz portfolio problem in a particular random environment.

Part IV collects contributed chapters on the use of simulation models for statistical testing and classification problems. S. Tarima et al. report on the use of signs of residuals for testing coefficients in quantile regression. B. Darkhovsky and A. Piryatinska apply their concept of ε-complexity (based on Kolmogorov's notion of complexity) to the classification of multivariate time series and give an application to the classification of EEG data. P. Langthaler et al. analyze high-dimensional data from the spectral density curves of EEG measurements on several channels to dementia classification of patients. B. Peštová and M. Pešta use simulation studies to compare ratio and non-ratio test statistics to detect structural changes in panel data. Finally, D. Rasch and T. Yanagida report on robustness results for the two-sample triangular sequential t-test against variance heterogeneity.

Part V (Clinical Trials and Design of Experiments) starts with a contribution by N. Minois et al. on the performance of the Poisson–gamma model for patients' recruitment in clinical trials when there are pauses in the recruitments procedure. N. Savy et al. detail their views on principles and good practices for simulated clinical trials, with a focus on virtual patient generation. D. Rasch et al. report on the determination of the optimal sample size of subsamples for testing a correlation coefficient by a sequential triangular test. The last two chapters in Part V deal with experimental design issues: V. B. Melas and P. V. Shpilev give explicit solutions for determining T-optimal discriminating designs for trigonometric regression models. R. Fontana and F. Rapallo perform simulation studies on the combinatorial structure of D-optimal designs.

In the final Part VI, we have collected five contributions dealing with the role of simulations for reliability and queueing models. G. Tzavelas and P. Economou investigate the consequences of model misspecification for biased samples from the Weibull distribution. D. Kurz, H. Lewitschnig, and J. Pilz give an overview on recent advances in statistical burn-in modeling for an efficient evaluation of early life failure probabilities of semiconductor devices. K. E. Samouylov, Y. V. Gaidamaka, and E. S. Sopin describe a simplified approach to the analysis of queueing systems with additional randomness due to imperfect knowledge of the exact amount of resources released by the departure of a customer. V. Rykov and D. Kozyrev compare analytic and simulation results on the sensitivity of steady-state probabilities of a cold redundant system to the shapes of life and repair time distributions of its elements. D. Efrosinin et al. perform a reliability analysis of an aging unit with a controllable repair facility activation, using a continuous-time Markov chain model for the process of gradual aging.

It is our great pleasure to thank all authors of invited and contributed chapters for carefully preparing their manuscripts and submitting them for editorial processing of the present volume. We are indebted to our reviewers from the Scientific Program Committee for critical reading and providing constructive comments.

Finally, we are indebted to the relentless secretarial work and technical help by Beate Simma and Johannes Winkler from Alpen-Adria University of Klagenfurt and to Mrs. Veronika Rosteck from Springer International Publishing.

Klagenfurt, Austria — Jürgen Pilz
Rostock, Germany — Dieter Rasch
Vienna, Austria — Viatcheslav B. Melas
St. Petersburg, Russia — Karl Moder
September 2017

Contents

Contributors

Sandrine Andrieu INSERM UMR 1027, University of Toulouse III, Toulouse, France; Epidemiology Unit of Toulouse CHU, Toulouse, France

Alexander Andronov Transport and Telecommunication Institute, Riga, Latvia

Arne C. Bathke Paris-Lodron-University Salzburg, Salzburg, Austria

Yana Belopolskaya Saint-Petersburg State University of Architecture and Civil Engineering, St. Petersburg, Russian Federation

Harish S. Bhat University of California Merced, Merced, CA, USA

Ekaterina Bulinskaya Lomonosov Moscow State University, Moscow, Russia

Boris Darkhovsky Institute for Systems Analysis, FRC CSC RAS, Higher School of Economics, Moscow, Russia

Clemens Draxler University for Health and Life Sciences, Hall, Austria

Polychronis Economou Department of Civil Engineering, University of Patras, Rio Achaia, Greece

Dmitry Efrosinin Johannes Kepler University Linz, Linz, Austria; Institute of Control Sciences, Moscow, Russia

Ekaterina Ermishkina Department of Probability Theory, Lomonosov Moscow State University, Moscow, Russia

Mais Farkhadov Institute of Control Sciences, Moscow, Russia

Roberto Fontana Department DISMA, Politecnico di Torino, Torino, Italy

Yuliya V. Gaidamaka Peoples' Friendship University of Russia (RUDN University), Moscow, Russia; Institute of Informatics Problems, FRC CSC RAS, Moscow, Russia

Julia Gusak Lomonosov Moscow State University, Moscow, Russia

Yvonne Höller Paracelsus Medical University Salzburg, Salzburg, Austria; Department of Neurology, Christian Doppler Medical Centre and Centre of Cognitive Neuroscience, Paracelsus Medical University Salzburg, Salzburg, Austria

Zuzana Hübnerová Brno University of Technology, Brno, Czech Republic

Tatjana Jurkina Transport and Telecommunication Institute, Riga, Latvia

Jozef Kiseľák Faculty of Science, Institute of Mathematics, P.J. Šafárik University in Košice, Kosice, Slovakia

Jack P. C. Kleijnen Tilburg University, Tilburg, Netherlands

Dmitry Kozyrev Peoples' Friendship University of Russia (RUDN University), Moscow, Russian Federation; V.A. Trapeznikov Institute of Control Sciences of Russian Academy of Sciences, Moscow, Russia

Klaus D. Kubinger Division of Psychological Assessment and Applied Psychometrics, Faculty of Psychology, University of Vienna, Vienna, Austria

Ekaterina P. Kurochkina The Novosibisk State University - Baker Hughes Joint Laboratory of The Multi-Scale Geophysics and Mechanics, Novosibirsk, Russia

Daniel Kurz Department of Statistics, Alpen-Adria University of Klagenfurt, Klagenfurt, Austria

Patrick Langthaler Paris-Lodron-University Salzburg, Salzburg, Austria; Paracelsus Medical University Salzburg, Salzburg, Austria

Valérie Lauwers-Cances Epidemiology Unit, CHU Purpan, Toulouse, France

Horst Lewitschnig Infineon Technologies Austria AG, Villach, Austria

R. W. M. A. Madushani University of California Merced, Merced, CA, USA

Sébastien Marque Capionis, Paris, France; Osmose, Bordeaux, France

Viatcheslav B. Melas Department of Mathematics, St. Petersburg State University, St. Petersburg, Russia

John Meurer Institute for Health and Society, Medical College of Wisconsin, Milwaukee, WI, USA

Guillaume Mijoule University of Paris XI, Orsay, France

Gennady A. Mikhailov Institute of Computational Mathematics and Mathematical Geophysics SB RAS, Novosibirsk, Russia; Novosibirsk State University, Novosibirsk, Russia

Nathan Minois INSERM UMR 1027, University of Toulouse III, Toulouse, France

Michael Ortner CTR Carinthian Tech Research AG, Villach, Austria

Michal Pešta Faculty of Mathematics and Physics, Department of Probability and Mathematical Statistics, Charles University, Prague, Czech Republic

Barbora Peštová Department of Medical Informatics and Biostatistics, Institute of Computer Science, The Czech Academy of Sciences, Prague, Czech Republic

Jürgen Pilz Department of Statistics, Alpen-Adria University of Klagenfurt, Klagenfurt, Austria

Alexandra Piryatinska San Francisco State University, CA, USA

Rastislav Potocký Department of Applied Mathematics and Statistics, Comenius University in Bratislava, Bratislava, Slovak Republic

Geoff Pritchard Department of Statistics, University of Auckland, Auckland, New Zealand

Zuzana Prášková Faculty of Mathematics and Physics, Charles University, Prague, Czech Republic

Christian Quast Department of Applied Statistics, Johannes Kepler University, Linz, Austria

Fabio Rapallo Department DISIT, Università del Piemonte Orientale, Alessandria, Italy

Dieter Rasch University of Natural Resources and Life Sciences, Vienna, Austria

Shagun Rawat University of California Merced, Merced, CA, USA

Lisa Rein Institute for Health and Society, Medical College of Wisconsin, Milwaukee, WI, USA

Vladimir Rykov Peoples' Friendship University of Russia (RUDN University), Moscow, Russian Federation; Gubkin Russian State Oil and Gas University, Moscow, Russia

Konstantin E. Samouylov Peoples' Friendship University of Russia (RUDN University), Moscow, Russia; Institute of Informatics Problems, FRC CSC RAS, Moscow, Russia

Nicolas Savy Toulouse Institute of Mathematics, University of Toulouse III, Toulouse, France

Stéphanie Savy INSERM UMR 1027, University of Toulouse III, Toulouse, France

Berthold Schneider Institute for Biometry, Hannover Medical School, Hannover, Germany

Petr V. Shpilev Department of Mathematics, St. Petersburg State University, St. Petersburg, Russia

Olga N. Soboleva Novosibisk State Technical University, Novosibirsk, Russia; The Novosibisk State University - Baker Hughes Joint Laboratory of The Multi-Scale Geophysics and Mechanics, Novosibirsk, Russia

Eduard S. Sopin Peoples' Friendship University of Russia (RUDN University), Moscow, Russia; Institute of Informatics Problems, FRC CSC RAS, Moscow, Russia

Rodney Sparapani Institute for Health and Society, Medical College of Wisconsin, Milwaukee, WI, USA

Milan Stehlík Linz Institute of Technology and Department of Applied Statistics, Johannes Kepler University, Linz, Austria

Natalia Stepanova Altai Economics and Law Institute, Barnaul, Russia

Luboš Střelec Department of Statistics and Operation Analysis, Mendel University in Brno, Brno, Czech Republic

Janos Sztrik University of Debrecen, Debrecen, Hungary

Peter Tarassenko International Department of Management, Tomsk State University, Tomsk, Russia

Sergey Tarima Institute for Health and Society, Medical College of Wisconsin, Milwaukee, WI, USA

Tatiana M. Tovstik St. Petersburg State University, St. Petersburg, Russia

Natalya V. Tracheva Institute of Computational Mathematics and Mathematical Geophysics SB RAS, Novosibirsk, Russia; Novosibirsk State University, Novosibirsk, Russia

Bonifride Tuyishimire Institute for Health and Society, Medical College of Wisconsin, Milwaukee, WI, USA

George Tzavelas Department of Statistics and Insurance Sciences, University of Piraeus, Piraeus, Greece

Sergey A. Ukhinov Institute of Computational Mathematics and Mathematical Geophysics SB RAS, Novosibirsk State University, Novosibirsk, Russia

Vítězslav Veselý Brno University of Technology, Brno, Czech Republic

Natalie Vollert CTR Carinthian Tech Research AG, Villach, Austria; Department of Statistics, Alpen-Adria University of Klagenfurt, Klagenfurt, Austria

Takuya Yanagida University of Applied Sciences Upper Austria, Vienna, Austria; University of Vienna, Vienna, Austria

Elena Yarovaya Department of Probability Theory, Lomonosov Moscow State University, Moscow, Russia

Golbon Zakeri Department of Engineering Science, University of Auckland, Auckland, New Zealand

Part I
Invited Papers

Chapter 1
Design and Analysis of Simulation Experiments

Jack P. C. Kleijnen

Abstract This contribution summarizes the design and analysis of experiments with computerized simulation models. It focuses on two metamodel (surrogate, emulator) types, namely first-order or second-order polynomial regression, and Kriging (or Gaussian process). The metamodel type determines the design of the simulation experiment, which determines the input combinations of the simulation model. Before applying these metamodels, the analysts should screen the many inputs of a realistic simulation model; this contribution focuses on sequential bifurcation. Optimization of the simulated system may use either a sequence of first-order and second-order polynomials—so-called response surface methodology (RSM)—or Kriging models fitted through sequential designs—including efficient global optimization (EGO). Robust optimization accounts for uncertainty in some simulation inputs.

Keywords Robustness and sensitivity · Metamodel · Design · Regression
Kriging

1.1 Introduction

Simulation is used in many scientific disciplines, but we focus on statistics and engineering. Moreover, we focus on stochastic (random) simulation, but parts of our contribution are also relevant for deterministic simulation. Simulation requires several steps; see [17, p. 67]. A crucial step is the design and analysis of the experiments with the computerized simulation model. This design and analysis are "intertwined": selecting an experimental design assumes a metamodel (surrogate, emulator) for the analysis of the experimental results; e.g., changing a single factor (simulation input or parameter) at a time assumes a metamodel with non-interacting factors. We focus on the two most popular metamodel types: low-order polynomial regression and Kriging.

J. P. C. Kleijnen (✉)
Tilburg University, Postbox 90153, Tilburg, Netherlands
e-mail: kleijnen@tilburguniversity.edu

J. Pilz et al. (eds.), *Statistics and Simulation*, Springer Proceedings
in Mathematics & Statistics 231, https://doi.org/10.1007/978-3-319-76035-3_1

Mathematically, a *metamodel* is an explicit and relatively simple approximation of the input/output (I/O) function implicitly defined by the underlying simulation model. We define $w = f_{\text{sim}}(\mathbf{z}, \mathbf{r})$ where w is the random simulation output (response), f_{sim} the simulation I/O function, $\mathbf{z}$ the vector with the values of the k simulation inputs with the integer $k \geq 1$, and $\mathbf{r}$ the vector with pseudorandom numbers (PRNs) so $\mathbf{r}$ vanishes in deterministic simulation. Usually, $\mathbf{z}$ is standardized, so the resulting $\mathbf{d}$ has elements $-1 \leq d_j \leq 1$ ($j = 1, \ldots, k$). An input may be qualitative. If a qualitative input has more than two values (levels), then special care is needed; see [12, pp. 69–71].

We define $y = f_{\text{meta}}(\mathbf{x}) + e$ where y is the metamodel output, $\mathbf{x}$ the vector with (say) q metamodel inputs (explanatory variables), e the approximation (fitting) error; an example of f_{meta} is a second-order polynomial in d_j ($j = 1, \ldots, k$) so $\mathbf{x}$ has the components $d_j, d_j d_{j'}$ with $j \leq j'$, and the constant 1. Actually, a *polynomial* of any order is a *linear* regression (meta)model. Another type of metamodel is Kriging—or Gaussian process (GP)—metamodels, which are also explicit—but more complicated—models of d_j. Altogether, f_{meta} is explicit and much simpler than f_{sim}. We call f_{meta} "adequate" or "valid" if $E(e) = 0$.

We focus on simulation for *sensitivity analysis* (SA) and *optimization* of the underlying real system. Furthermore, we focus on global (not local) SA; e.g., in screening and Kriging, we use global metamodels (see Sects. 1.4 and 1.5). Nevertheless, we use local SA in response surface methodology (RSM) for optimization.

We base our survey on our book [12], which includes many Web site addresses for software and hundreds of additional references, and on our article [14]. However, compared with [14], our survey is half the length, corrects a mathematical error, and assumes familiarity with basic statistical design concepts (e.g., resolution and CCD) and basic operations research (OR) concepts (e.g., M/M/1); also see the more complicated queueing model in [23].

1.2 Basic Linear Regression and Designs

We define basic symbols and terminology used in the next sections, starting with *linear regression* (meta)models $\mathbf{y} = \mathbf{X}\boldsymbol{\beta} + \mathbf{e}$ where $\mathbf{y}$ denotes the n-dimensional vector with the dependent (explained) variable with n denoting the number of different simulated input combinations; $\mathbf{X} = (x_{i;g})$ is the $n \times q$ matrix of independent (explanatory) regression variables with $x_{i;g}$ the value of x_g in combination i ($i = 1, \ldots, n$; $g = 1, \ldots, q$), so row i of $\mathbf{X}$ is $\mathbf{x}_i = (x_{i;1}, \ldots, x_{i;q})$; $\boldsymbol{\beta}$ is the q-dimensional vector with regression parameters; $\mathbf{e}$ is the n-dimensional vector with residuals, so $\mathbf{e} = E(\mathbf{y}) - E(\mathbf{w})$ with $\mathbf{w}$ denoting the n-dimensional vector with $w_i = f_{sim}(\mathbf{z}_i, \mathbf{r}_i)$ where $\mathbf{z}_i$ denotes combination i of the k original simulation inputs that are determined by the $n \times k$ design matrix $\mathbf{D} = (d_{i;j})$, and $\mathbf{r}_i$ denotes the vector with PRNs used in combination i; row i of $\mathbf{D}$ is $\mathbf{d}_i$; x is a simple function of the original z or the standardized d.

We focus on a special case of linear regression, namely a *second-order polynomial* with k simulation inputs: $y = \beta_0 + \sum_{j=1}^{k} \beta_j x_j + \sum_{j=1}^{k} \sum_{j' \geq j}^{k} \beta_{j;j'} x_j x_{j'} + e$ with the intercept β_0, the k first-order effects β_j ($j = 1, \ldots, k$), the $k(k-1)/2$ two-factor interactions (cross products) $\beta_{j;j'}$ ($j < j'$), and the k purely quadratic effects $\beta_{j;j}$. This metamodel is nonlinear in $\mathbf{x}$, but it is linear in $\boldsymbol{\beta}$; engineers call this metamodel nonlinear, whereas statisticians call it linear.

We assume that interactions among three or more inputs are unimportant; such interactions are hard to interpret. Of course, we should check this assumption; i.e., we should "validate" the estimated metamodel.

The *least squares* (LS) estimator of $\boldsymbol{\beta}$ is $\hat{\boldsymbol{\beta}} = (\mathbf{X}'\mathbf{X})^{-1}\mathbf{X}'\mathbf{w}$. If $\mathbf{d}_i$—which determines $\mathbf{x}_i$—is simulated m_i times and m_i is a constant m, then we may replace $\mathbf{w}$ by $\overline{\mathbf{w}}$ with the n elements $\overline{w}_i = \sum_{r=1}^{m} w_{i;r}/m$ so $\mathbf{X}$ is indeed an $n \times q$ matrix. Usually, $m > 1$ in random simulation. If m_i is not a constant, then $\mathbf{x}_i$ is repeated m_i times within $\mathbf{X}$, so $\mathbf{X}$ has $\sum_{i=1}^{n} m_i$ rows and q columns.

Actually, $\hat{\boldsymbol{\beta}}$ is identical to the *maximum likelihood estimator* (MLE) if $\mathbf{e}$ is *white noise*; i.e., e_i is *normally, independently, and identically distributed* (NIID) with zero mean and constant variance σ_e^2. If the metamodel is valid, then $\sigma_e^2 = \sigma_w^2$ where σ_w^2 denotes the variance of w. The white-noise assumption implies that $\hat{\boldsymbol{\beta}}$ has the covariance matrix $\boldsymbol{\Sigma}_{\hat{\boldsymbol{\beta}}} = (\mathbf{X}'\mathbf{X})^{-1}\sigma_w^2$. Because σ_w^2 is unknown, we estimate $\sigma_w^2 = \sigma_e^2$ through the *mean squared residuals* $\text{MSR} = (\widehat{\mathbf{y}} - \mathbf{w})'(\widehat{\mathbf{y}} - \mathbf{w})/(n-q)$ where $\widehat{\mathbf{y}} = \mathbf{X}\hat{\beta}'$ and $n - q > 0$, which gives $\widehat{\boldsymbol{\Sigma}}_{\hat{\boldsymbol{\beta}}}$.

To derive *confidence intervals* (CIs) and *tests* for the individual elements of $\hat{\boldsymbol{\beta}}$, we use the estimated standard deviations $s(\widehat{\beta}_g)$ that are the square roots of $s^2(\widehat{\beta}_g)$ (estimate of $\text{Var}(\widehat{\beta}_g)$) on the main diagonal of $\widehat{\boldsymbol{\Sigma}}_{\hat{\boldsymbol{\beta}}}$. This gives the following t-statistic with $n - q$ degrees of freedom: $t_{n-q} = (\widehat{\beta}_g - \beta_g)/s(\widehat{\beta}_g)$ with $g = 1, \ldots, q$.

To select a specific design matrix $\mathbf{D}$ with $\mathbf{d}_i$ in a given experimental area, we minimize $\text{Var}(\widehat{\beta}_g)$; i.e., we select an orthogonal $\mathbf{X}$. Usually, *design of experiments* (DOE) assumes that the z_j are *standardized* (scaled) such that $-1 \leq d_{i;j} \leq 1$. If z_j has only two values in the experiment with n input combinations, then this standardization uses $d_{i;j} = (z_{i;j} - \overline{z}_j)/[(H_j - L_j)/2]$ ($i = 1, \ldots, n$; $j = 1, \ldots, k$) where L_j denotes the lower value of z_j in the experiment, H_j the higher value, $\overline{z}_j$ the average value of z_j in a *balanced* experiment with z_j observed at L_j in $n/2$ combinations. If $\mathbf{X}$ is *orthogonal*, then $\mathbf{X}'\mathbf{X} = n\mathbf{I}$ so $\boldsymbol{\Sigma}_{\hat{\boldsymbol{\beta}}} = (n\mathbf{I})^{-1}\sigma_w^2 = \mathbf{I}\sigma_w^2/n$. Hence the q estimators in $\widehat{\beta}$ are statistically independent and have the same variance. So, the $s^2(\widehat{\beta}_g)$ are constant, and we can *rank* x_g using either $\widehat{\beta}_g$ or t_{n-q} with $\beta_g = 0$ so $t_{n-q} = \widehat{\beta}_g/s(\widehat{\beta}_g)$.

Now we discuss designs of different *resolution* (R); e.g., R-III means "resolution III". Initially, we assume $m_i = 1$ ($i = 1, \ldots, n$). A *R-III or Plackett–Burman* (P–B) design gives unbiased estimators of β_j ($j = 1, \ldots, k$) if a first-order polynomial is a valid metamodel. A subclass are *fractional factorial two-level* 2_{III}^{k-p} designs with integer p such that $0 \leq p < k$ and $n = 2^{k-p} \geq 1 + k$. In a R-III design, n is a multiple of 4; e.g., $8 \leq k \leq 11$ implies $n = 12$. If $n > k + 1$, then we ignore some columns of $\mathbf{D}$. If $n = k + 1$, then $\mathbf{D}$ is *saturated*; the MSR is then undefined. To compute MSR, we may then add one or more combinations; e.g., either combinations from the 2^k

design excluding the combinations in the original saturated **D** or the combination at the *center* of the experimental area where $d_j = 0$ if d_j is quantitative, and d_j is randomly selected as -1 or 1 if d_j is qualitative with two values.

A *R-IV design* gives unbiased estimators of β_j in a first-order polynomial if *two-factor interactions* are nonzero but "higher-order" effects are zero: $\mathbf{x}_i = (1, d_{i;1}, \ldots, d_{i;k}, d_{i;1}d_{i;2}, \ldots, d_{i;k-1}d_{i;k})$. To construct a R-IV design, we apply the *foldover theorem*; i.e., we augment a R-III design **D** with its *mirror* design $-\mathbf{D}$. A R-IV design does not enable unbiased estimators of all the *individual* two-factor interactions; e.g., $k = 7$ implies $n = 2^{7-4} \times 2 = 16$ so $n < q = 1 + 7 + 21 = 29$; consequently, $\mathbf{X}'\mathbf{X}$ is singular, so the LS estimator does not exist.

A *R-V design* enables LS estimation of β_j, $\beta_{j;j'}$ with $j' > j$, and β_0 if all other effects (including $\beta_{j;j}$) are zero. Unfortunately, 2_V^{k-p} designs imply $n \gg q$. *Rechtschaffner* designs include saturated R-V designs, but they are not orthogonal; see [12, p. 62].

A *central composite design* (CCD) enables LS estimation of all the effects in a second-order polynomial if all higher-order effects are zero. A CCD consists of (i) a R-V design; (ii) the *central* combination (say) $\mathbf{0}'_k$; (iii) the $2k$ *axial* combinations, which form a *star design*; see [12, p. 63–66]. CCDs have non-orthogonal **X**, and $n \gg q$.

1.3 Assumptions Versus Practice

The *classic* statistical assumptions stipulate a single type of simulation output and white noise. A practical simulation model, however, may give *multivariate* output, and the univariate output w_i ($i = 1, \ldots, n$) may be *non-normal* with *heterogeneous* variances; w_i and $w_{i'}$ ($i, i' = 1, \ldots, n$) are correlated if the simulation uses *common random numbers* (CRN); $E(e)$ may be nonzero. In this section, we examine: (a) How realistic are the classic assumptions? (b) How can we test these assumptions? (c) Can we transform the simulation's I/O data such that the assumptions hold for the transformed data? (d) Which other statistical methods can we apply?

Multivariate Simulation Output

We assume that for r-variate simulation output with $r \geq 1$, we use r univariate linear regression metamodels, and these metamodels are polynomials of the same order (e.g., second-order):

$$\mathbf{y}^{(l)} = \mathbf{X}\beta^{(l)} + \mathbf{e}^{(l)} \text{ with } l = 1, \ldots r \tag{1.1}$$

where the various symbols are defined analogously to the univariate model (e.g., $\mathbf{y}^{(l)}$ is the dependent variable corresponding with simulation output of type l); the $\mathbf{e}^{(l)}$ have variances that may vary with l, and $e_i^{(l)}$ and $e_i^{(l')}$ ($l' = 1, \ldots, r$) are not independent. However, [21] proves that LS per output still gives the *best linear unbiased estimator* (BLUE): $\widehat{\beta}^{(l)} = (\mathbf{X}'\mathbf{X})^{-1}\mathbf{X}'\mathbf{w}^{(l)}$. We can easily obtain CIs and tests for the elements in

$\widehat{\beta}^{(l)}$, using the classic formulas. We do not know any *general* designs for multivariate output; also see [11].

Non-normality

The normality assumption often holds *asymptotically*: if the simulation run is "long," then the sample average of the autocorrelated observations is "nearly" normal. Estimated quantiles, however, may be very non-normal. The t-statistic is quite insensitive to non-normality, whereas the F-statistic is not. It seems prudent to test the normality assumption as follows.

We may use various *residual plots* and *goodness-of-fit statistics* (e.g., a chi-square statistic). A basic assumption of these statistics is that the observations are identically and independently distributed (IID). We may, therefore, obtain "many" (say, 100) replications for a specific input combination (e.g., the base scenario) if the simulation is not computationally expensive; otherwise, these statistical tests lack power and the plots are too rough.

Actually, the white noise assumption concerns e, not w. Given $m_i \geq 1$ ($i = 1, \ldots, n$) replications, we obtain $\overline{w}_i = \sum_{r=1}^{m_i} w_{i;r}/m_i$ and $\widehat{\overline{e}}_i = \widehat{y}_i - \overline{w}_i$. For simplicity of presentation, we assume $m_i = m$. If $w_{i;r}$ has a constant variance σ_w^2, then $\overline{w}_i$ also has a constant variance $\sigma_{\overline{w}}^2 = \sigma_w^2/m$. Even if $\overline{w}_i$ is independent of $\overline{w}_{i'}$ with $i \neq i'$ (no CRN), then

$$\mathbf{\Sigma}_{\widehat{\overline{\mathbf{e}}}} = [\mathbf{I} - \mathbf{X}(\mathbf{X}'\mathbf{X})^{-1}\mathbf{X}']\sigma_{\overline{w}}^2, \tag{1.2}$$

so $\widehat{\overline{e}}_i$ does not have constant variance, and $\widehat{\overline{e}}_i$ and $\widehat{\overline{e}}_{i'}$ are correlated. This complicates the interpretation of the popular plot with estimated residuals.

We may apply *normalizing transformations*; e.g., log(w) may be more normally distributed than w. Unfortunately, the metamodel now explains the behavior of the transformed output (not the original output); see [12, p. 93] and [15].

Another transformation is *jackknifing*, which may (i) give CIs for non-normal observations, or (ii) reduce bias of a given estimator. Suppose we want CIs for the q elements of $\boldsymbol{\beta}$, for non-normal w. For simplicity, we assume $m_i = m > 1$. The original LS estimator is $\hat{\boldsymbol{\beta}}$; jackknifing deletes replication r for each combination i, so

$$\widehat{\boldsymbol{\beta}}_{-r} = (\mathbf{X}'\mathbf{X})^{-1}\mathbf{X}'\overline{\mathbf{w}}_{-r} \; (r = 1, \ldots, m) \tag{1.3}$$

where $\overline{\mathbf{w}}_{-r} = (\overline{w}_{i;-r})$ with $\overline{w}_{i;-r}$ denoting the average of the $m-1$ simulation outputs excluding the output of replication r. Let us focus on β_q (last element of $\boldsymbol{\beta}$). The *pseudovalue* is

$$J_r = m\widehat{\beta}_q - (m-1)\widehat{\beta}_{q;-r}. \tag{1.4}$$

In this example, both $\widehat{\beta}_q$ and $\widehat{\beta}_{q;-r}$ are unbiased, so the m pseudovalues also remain unbiased. In general, however, possible bias is reduced by the *jackknife point estimator* $\overline{J} = \sum_{r=1}^{m} J_r/m$; an example of a biased estimator is (1.7). Jackknifing gives a CI, treating the J_r as if they were NIID. So if $t_{m-1;1-\alpha/2}$ denotes the $1-\alpha/2$ quantile of the t_{m-1}-distribution and $\widehat{\sigma}_{\overline{J}}^2$ denotes $\sum_{r=1}^{m}(J_r - \overline{J})^2/[m(m-1)]$, then the two-sided symmetric $(1-\alpha)$ CI for β_q is $\overline{J} - t_{m-1;1-\alpha/2}\widehat{\sigma}_{\overline{J}} < \beta_q < \overline{J} +$

$t_{m-1;1-\alpha/2}\widehat{\sigma_J}$. Many applications of jackknifing in simulation are given in [8] and [12, p. 95].

Another statistical method that does not assume normality is *distribution-free bootstrapping*; also see [25]. This bootstrapping may be used not only for non-normal distributions, but also for nonstandard statistics. We distinguish between the *original* w and the *bootstrapped* w^* with the usual superscript $*$ for bootstrapped observations. Standard bootstrapping assumes that the w observations are IID; indeed, $w_{i;1}, \ldots, w_{i;m}$ are IID because the m replications use non-overlapping PRN streams. We *resample with replacement* from the m original IID observations $w_{i;r}$ such that the original sample size remains m; we apply this resampling to each simulated combination, obtaining $w^*_{i;1}, \ldots, w^*_{i;m}$. This gives $\overline{\mathbf{w}}^* = (\overline{w^*_i})$, so

$$\widehat{\boldsymbol{\beta}}^* = (\mathbf{X}'\mathbf{X})^{-1}\mathbf{X}'\overline{\mathbf{w}}^*.$$

To reduce sampling variation, bootstrapping repeats this resampling B times; a typical value for this *bootstrap sample size* B is 100 or 1,000. This B gives $\widehat{\boldsymbol{\beta}}^*_b$ with $b = 1, \ldots, B$. The *percentile method* gives a non-symmetric two-sided $(1-\alpha)$ CI:

$$P(\widehat{\beta}^*_{q;(B\alpha/2)} < \beta_q < \widehat{\beta}^*_{q;(B[1-\alpha/2])}) = 1 - \alpha \tag{1.5}$$

where $\widehat{\beta}^*_{q;(B\alpha/2)}$ denotes the $\alpha/2$ quantile of the *empirical density function* (EDF) of $\widehat{\beta}^*_q$ obtained through the *order statistics* denoted by the subscript $(\cdot)$ where (for simplicity) we assume that $B\alpha/2$ is integer; an analogous definition holds for $\widehat{\beta}^*_{q;(B[1-\alpha/2])}$. We shall also mention bootstrapped CIs for quantiles, R^2, and cross-validation.

Heterogeneous Variances of Simulation Outputs

In practice, $\mathrm{Var}(w_i)$ changes as the input combination i changes. Unfortunately, $\mathrm{Var}(w_i)$ is unknown; so if $m_i > 1$, then we compute $s_i^2 = \sum_{r=1}^{m_i}(w_{i;r} - \overline{w}_i)^2/(m_i - 1)$.This s_i^2 itself has high variance (e.g., if $w_{i;r}$ is normally distributed with $\mathrm{Var}(w_{i;r}) = \sigma_i^2$, then $\mathrm{Var}(s_i^2) = 2\sigma_i^4/m_i$). To compare n estimators s_i^2, we may apply various tests; see [12, p. 101].

The transformation $\log(w)$ may be used not only to obtain Gaussian output but also to obtain constant variances. Actually, this transformation is a special case of the normalizing Box–Cox power transformation; see [12, p. 93]. Anyhow, we prefer to accept variance heterogeneity, and to adapt our analysis, as follows.

If $E(\mathbf{e}) = 0$, then $\widehat{\boldsymbol{\beta}}$ is still *unbiased*. However, $\boldsymbol{\Sigma}_{\widehat{\beta}}$ then becomes

$$\boldsymbol{\Sigma}_{\widehat{\beta}} = (\mathbf{X}'\mathbf{X})^{-1}\mathbf{X}'\boldsymbol{\Sigma}_{\overline{\mathbf{w}}}\mathbf{X}(\mathbf{X}'\mathbf{X})^{-1} \tag{1.6}$$

where $m_i = m$ so $\boldsymbol{\Sigma}_{\mathbf{w}}$ is the diagonal matrix with elements σ_i^2/m.

Alternatively, we might switch from LS to *weighted LS* (WLS), which gives $\widetilde{\boldsymbol{\beta}}$. In practice, however, $\mathrm{Var}(w_i)$ is estimated, and using s_i^2 in WLS gives *estimated WLS* (EWLS), which gives the nonlinear estimator $\widehat{\widetilde{\boldsymbol{\beta}}}$. Obviously, $\widehat{\widetilde{\boldsymbol{\beta}}}$ is non-normally distributed and may be biased, so it is difficult to derive exact CIs. Above, we have

terms; e.g., a 2^k design enables the estimation of the interactions among two or more inputs. In the discussion of (1.10), we have already mentioned the danger of overfitting. Adding more explanatory variables is called *stepwise regression*; eliminating nonsignificant variables is called *backwards elimination.*

1.4 Factor Screening: Sequential Bifurcation

Screening means searching for the really important simulation inputs among the many inputs that can be varied in a simulation experiment. *Sparsity* means that only a few inputs among these many inputs are important. Indeed, the *Pareto* principle or *20–80* rule states that only "a few" inputs (20%) are important; e.g., [12, p. 136] presents two examples, with 281 and 92 inputs, respectively; screening finds only 15 and 11 inputs to be important.

There are several types of screening designs; see [12, pp. 137–139] and [29]. We focus on designs that treat the simulation model as a *black box*: only the I/O of the simulation model is observed. We focus on *sequential bifurcation* (SB), because SB is very efficient and effective if its assumptions are satisfied. SB selects the next input combination after analyzing the preceding I/O data, so SB is indeed sequential. SB is *customized*; i.e., SB accounts for the specific simulation model.

To explain the basic SB idea, we assume *deterministic* simulation and a valid *first-order* polynomial metamodel so $\beta_{j;j'} = 0$ with $j \leq j'$. Let γ_j denote the first-order effect of z_j (original scale). SB assumes that the *sign* of γ_j is known so that we can define the low and high bounds L_j and H_j of z_j such that $\gamma_j \geq 0$. Hence, we may rank the inputs such that the most important input has $\max_j \gamma_j$; the least important input has $\min_j \gamma_j \downarrow 0$. Changing z_j from L_j to H_j makes w change by $(H_j - L_j)\gamma_j$ $= 2\beta_j$; also see [12, pp. 41–44] . SB calls z_j *important* if $2\beta_j \geq c_w$ where the users specify the threshold c_w (≥ 0).

In step 1, SB aggregates all k inputs into a single group and checks whether or not that group has an important effect. Let $w(\mathbf{L}_k)$ denote w with $\mathbf{z}_k = \mathbf{L}_k = (L_1, \ldots, L_k)'$ where $\mathbf{z}_k = (z_1, \ldots, z_k)'$; likewise, $w(\mathbf{H}_k)$ denotes w with $\mathbf{z}_k = \mathbf{H}_k = (H_1, \ldots, H_k)'$. So, SB obtains $w(\mathbf{L}_k)$ and $w(\mathbf{H}_k)$. If $\exists j : \beta_j > 0$, then $w(\mathbf{L}_k) < w(\mathbf{H}_k)$. It may happen that $\forall j : \beta_j < c_w/2$, but $w(\mathbf{H}_k) - w(\mathbf{L}_k) > c_w$; SB will discover this "false importance" in its next steps.

Assume that at least one input is important, so $w(\mathbf{H}_k) - w(\mathbf{L}_k) > c_w$. Then in step 2, SB splits the input group into two subgroups: *bifurcation.* Let k_1 and k_2 denote the size of subgroup 1 and subgroup 2 (so $k_1 + k_2 = k$). Then SB obtains $w(\mathbf{H}_{k_1})$. If $w(\mathbf{H}_{k_1}) - w(\mathbf{L}_k) < c_w$, then none of the individual inputs in subgroup 1 is important so SB *eliminates* this subgroup from further experimentation. If $w(\mathbf{H}_k) - w(\mathbf{H}_{k_1}) \geq c_w$, then one or more individual inputs in subgroup 2 may be important.

In each following step, SB splits important subgroups into smaller subgroups and eliminates unimportant subgroups. SB may find both subgroups to be important, so SB further experiments with two important subgroups in parallel. Obviously, these steps give smaller subgroups; in the final steps, SB identifies and estimates all individual inputs that are not in eliminated (unimportant) subgroups.

Assuming $\beta_j \geq 0$ ensures that the β_j within an input group do not cancel each other. In practice, the users often do know the signs of β_j. Nevertheless, if in a specific case it is hard to specify the signs of a few specific inputs, then we should not group these inputs with the other inputs (with known signs). We should treat these inputs *individually* and investigate these inputs not through SB but through a classic design. This seems safer than assuming a negligible probability of cancelation within a subgroup.

The *efficiency* of SB improves if the individual inputs are labeled such that inputs are placed in increasing order of importance. Such labeling implies that the important inputs are *clustered*; i.e., these inputs are members of the same subgroup. The efficiency further improves when placing "similar" inputs within the same subgroup; e.g., place all "transportation" inputs in the same subgroup. Anyhow, splitting a group into subgroups of *equal* size is not necessarily optimal. Practical examples of SB are given in [12, pp. 136–172].

After explaining the basics of SB, we now assume *random* simulation and a *second-order* polynomial. Moreover, if $\beta_j = 0$, then $\beta_{j;j'} = 0$ $(j \leq j')$: *heredity* assumption. SB then applies the *foldover* principle (see Sect. 1.2); i.e., SB also simulates the mirror input of the original input, to estimate β_j unbiased by $\beta_{j;j'}$. In random simulation, SB may obtain a *fixed* m (number of replications) and use the t_{m-1}-statistic for a one-sided test of $\beta_j > 0$. Or SB obtains a *random* m and uses [28]'s *sequential probability ratio test* (SPRT) with user-selected thresholds $c_{w\mathrm{U}}$ and $c_{w\mathrm{I}}$ to classify inputs with $2\beta_j \leq c_{w\mathrm{U}}$ as *unimportant*, inputs with $2\beta_j \geq c_{w\mathrm{I}}$ as *important*, and remaining inputs as *intermediate*; see [12, pp. 154–159]. In practice, simulation models have *multiple response types*; see the multiresponse SB (MSB) in [12, pp.159–172]. Note that SPRTs for testing two means (instead of group effects in SB) are given in [15].

1.5 Kriging Metamodels and Their Designs

Kriging metamodels are fitted to simulation I/O data obtained for the *global* experimental areas instead of the *local* areas in RSM.

Ordinary Kriging in Deterministic Simulation

In this subsection, we focus on ordinary Kriging (OK), which is popular in deterministic simulation. OK assumes

$$y(\mathbf{x}) = \mu + M(\mathbf{x}) \tag{1.12}$$

where μ is the constant mean $E[y(\mathbf{x})]$ and $M(\mathbf{x})$ is a stationary GP with zero mean. A GP has covariances that depend only on the distance between the input combinations $\mathbf{x}$ and $\mathbf{x}'$. We call $M(\mathbf{x})$ the *extrinsic noise*, to distinguish it from the *intrinsic noise* in stochastic simulation. Let $\mathbf{X}$ denote the $n \times k$ matrix with the n combinations $\mathbf{x}_i$ ($i = 1, \ldots, n$); in the preceding sections, we used $\mathbf{D}$, but the Kriging literature uses $\mathbf{X}$. Kriging software standardizes $\mathbf{z}_i$ to obtain $\mathbf{x}_i$ and also standardizes the simulation output w; for publications and Web sites see [12, p. 190].

OK uses the *best linear unbiased predictor* (BLUP) $\widehat{y}(\mathbf{x}_0)$ for the *new* combination $\mathbf{x}_0$:

$$\widehat{y}(\mathbf{x}_0) = \sum_{i=1}^{n} \lambda_i w_i = \boldsymbol{\lambda}'\mathbf{w}. \tag{1.13}$$

Such an "unbiased" predictor implies that if $\mathbf{x}_0 = \mathbf{x}_i$, then $\widehat{y}$ is an *exact interpolator*: $\widehat{y}(\mathbf{x}_i) = w(\mathbf{x}_i)$. This "best" predictor minimizes the *mean squared error* (MSE); because $\widehat{y}$ is unbiased, the MSE equals the variance $\mathrm{Var}[\widehat{y}(\mathbf{x}_0)]$. Altogether, the *optimal* weight vector is

$$\lambda_o' = [\boldsymbol{\sigma}_M(\mathbf{x}_0) + \mathbf{1}\frac{1 - \mathbf{1}'\boldsymbol{\Sigma}_M^{-1}\boldsymbol{\sigma}(\mathbf{x}_0)}{\mathbf{1}'\boldsymbol{\Sigma}_M^{-1}\mathbf{1}}]'\boldsymbol{\Sigma}_M^{-1} \tag{1.14}$$

where $\boldsymbol{\Sigma}_M = (\mathrm{cov}(y_i, y_{i'}))$ denotes the $n \times n$ matrix with the covariances between the metamodel's "old" outputs y_i, and $\boldsymbol{\sigma}_M(\mathbf{x}_0) = (\mathrm{cov}(y_i, y_0))$ denotes the n-dimensional vector with the covariances between y_i and the new output y_0. The weight λ_i decreases with the *distance* between $\mathbf{x}_0$ and $\mathbf{x}_i$, so $\boldsymbol{\lambda}$ is not a constant vector (unlike $\boldsymbol{\beta}$ in regression). Substitution of $\boldsymbol{\lambda}_o$ into (1.13) gives

$$\widehat{y}(\mathbf{x}_0) = \mu + \boldsymbol{\sigma}_M(\mathbf{x}_0)'\boldsymbol{\Sigma}_M^{-1}(\mathbf{w} - \mu\mathbf{1}) \tag{1.15}$$

where $\mathbf{1}$ denotes an n-dimensional vector with all elements equal to 1. Obviously, $\widehat{y}(\mathbf{x}_0)$ in (1.15) varies with $\boldsymbol{\sigma}_M(\mathbf{x}_0)$, whereas μ, $\boldsymbol{\Sigma}_M$, and $\mathbf{w}$ remain fixed.

The *gradient* $\nabla(\widehat{y})$ follows from (1.15); see [19, Eq. 2.18]. We should not confuse $\nabla(\widehat{y})$ and $\nabla(w)$; sometimes we can indeed estimate $\nabla(w)$ and use $\widehat{\nabla}(w)$ to estimate a better OK model; see [12, pp. 183–184].

Defining $\tau^2 = \mathrm{Var}(y)$ implies

$$\mathrm{MSE}\,[\widehat{y}(\mathbf{x}_0)] = \tau^2 - \boldsymbol{\sigma}_M(\mathbf{x}_0)'\boldsymbol{\Sigma}_M^{-1}\boldsymbol{\sigma}_M(\mathbf{x}_0) + \frac{[1 - \mathbf{1}'\boldsymbol{\Sigma}_M^{-1}\boldsymbol{\sigma}_M(\mathbf{x}_0)]^2}{\mathbf{1}'\boldsymbol{\Sigma}_M^{-1}\mathbf{1}}. \tag{1.16}$$

This implies $\mathrm{Var}[\widehat{y}(\mathbf{x}_0)] = 0$ if $\mathbf{x}_0 = \mathbf{x}_i$. So, $\mathrm{Var}[\widehat{y}(\mathbf{x}_0)]$ has n local minima. $\mathrm{Var}[\widehat{y}(\mathbf{x}_0)]$ has local maxima at $\mathbf{x}_0$ approximately halfway between old input combinations. Kriging gives bad extrapolations compared with interpolations (linear regression gives minimal $\mathrm{Var}[\widehat{y}(\mathbf{x}_0)]$ when $\mathbf{x}_0 = \mathbf{0}$).

Obviously, (1.14) shows that $\boldsymbol{\lambda}_o$ is a function of $\boldsymbol{\Sigma}_M$ and $\boldsymbol{\sigma}_M(\mathbf{x}_0)$ or – switching to correlations $\boldsymbol{\Omega} = \tau^{-2}\boldsymbol{\Sigma}_M$ and $\boldsymbol{\rho}(\mathbf{x}_0) = \tau^{-2}\boldsymbol{\sigma}_M(\mathbf{x}_0)$. There are several types of correlation functions, but most popular is the *Gaussian* correlation function:

$$\rho(\mathbf{h}) = \prod_{j=1}^{k} \exp\left(-\theta_j h_j^2\right) = \exp\left(-\sum_{j=1}^{k} \theta_j h_j^2\right) \tag{1.17}$$

with distance vector $\mathbf{h} = (h_j)$ where $h_j = \left|x_{g;j} - x_{g';j}\right|$ and $g, g' = 0, 1, \ldots, n$. This $\rho(\mathbf{h})$ implies that $\boldsymbol{\lambda}_o$ assigns larger weights for $\mathbf{x}_i$ closer to $\mathbf{x}_0$. Standardization of the inputs affects $\mathbf{h}$.

When estimating the *Kriging parameters* $\boldsymbol{\psi} = (\mu, \tau^2, \boldsymbol{\theta}')'$ with $\boldsymbol{\theta} = (\theta_j)$, the MLE is most popular; yet LS (L_2 norm), cross-validation, and the L_1 norm are also used; see [13]. The estimation of $\boldsymbol{\psi}$ is challenging: different values may result from different software packages or from initializing the same package with different starting values. Anyhow, we denote the estimator of $\boldsymbol{\psi}$ by $\widehat{\boldsymbol{\psi}}$. *Plugging* $\widehat{\boldsymbol{\psi}}$ into (1.15) gives $\widehat{y}(\mathbf{x}_0, \widehat{\boldsymbol{\psi}})$. This $\widehat{y}(\mathbf{x}_0, \widehat{\psi})$ is a *nonlinear* predictor. In practice, we simply *plug* $\widehat{\boldsymbol{\psi}}$ into (1.16) to obtain MSE$[\widehat{y}(\mathbf{x}_0, \widehat{\boldsymbol{\psi}})]$; moreover, we ignore possible bias of $\widehat{y}(\mathbf{x}_0)$ so $s^2\{\widehat{y}(\mathbf{x}_0)\} =$ MSE$[\widehat{y}(\mathbf{x}_0, \widehat{\boldsymbol{\psi}})]$. To compute a CI, we use $\widehat{y}(\mathbf{x}_0, \widehat{\boldsymbol{\psi}})$, $s^2\{\widehat{y}(\mathbf{x}_0)\}$, and $z_{\alpha/2}$ ($\alpha/2$ quantile of standard normal):

$$P[w(\mathbf{x}_0) \in [\widehat{y}(\mathbf{x}_0, \widehat{\boldsymbol{\psi}}) \pm z_{\alpha/2} s\{\widehat{y}(\mathbf{x}_0)\}] = 1 - \alpha. \tag{1.18}$$

Universal Kriging (UK) replaces μ in (1.12) by a low-order polynomial. UK requires the estimation of additional parameters, besides $\beta_0 = \mu$; this may explain why UK often has a higher MSE than OK has.

Designs for Deterministic Simulation

There are several design types for Kriging in deterministic simulation; e.g., [12, p. 198] mentions orthogonal array, uniform, maximum entropy, minimax, maximin, integrated mean squared prediction error, and "optimal" designs. However, the most popular design uses *Latin hypercube sampling* (LHS). LHS assumes that an adequate metamodel is more complicated than a low-order polynomial; LHS does not assume a specific type of metamodel (e.g., an OK model), but focuses on the input space formed by x_j (standardized simulation inputs). LHS results in an $n \times k$ matrix $\mathbf{X}$. There is no strict mathematical relationship between n and k, whereas DOE may use $n = 2^{k-p}$. Nevertheless, if LHS keeps n "small" and k is "large," then "space filling" LHS covers the input space so sparsely that $E(e) \neq 0$. A rule-of-thumb for LHS in Kriging is $n = 10k$; see [18].

Mathematically, LHS divides the range of x_j into n mutually exclusive and exhaustive intervals of equal probability. The LHS design is *non-collapsing*: if an input turns out to be unimportant, then each remaining input still has one observation per interval. We conjecture that the estimation of the correlation function may benefit from this non-collapsing property. Unfortunately, projections of $\mathbf{x}$ onto more than one dimension may give "bad' designs, so there are maximin LHS, nearly orthogonal, and sliced LHS designs.

Instead of LHS with its *single-shot* design, we may use *sequential* designs that are application-driven or *customized*; i.e., they account for f_{sim}. In general, sequential procedures require fewer observations than fixed-sample procedures do, because we learn about the behavior of the underlying system as we experiment with this system and collect data (also see Sect. 1.4 on SB). Kriging, however, requires extra computer time if it re-estimates $\boldsymbol{\psi}$ when new I/O data become available.

We may use sequential Kriging designs for either *SA* (so the whole experimental area is interesting) or *optimization* (only the optimum is interesting); see [12, pp. 203–206] In a sequential design, we start with a *pilot* experiment with n_0 combinations of the k inputs selected through LHS and obtain the corresponding simulation I/O data. Next we fit a Kriging model to these data. Then we may consider—but not yet simulate—$\mathbf{X}_{cand}$ which denotes a larger matrix with *candidate* combinations selected through LHS and find the "winning" candidate. In SA, this winner has $\max_{\mathbf{x}} s^2\{\widehat{y}(\mathbf{x})\}$ with $\mathbf{x} \in \mathbf{X}_{cand}$. Next we use the winner as the input to be simulated, which gives additional I/O data. We re-fit the Kriging model to the augmented I/O data (usually re-estimating $\boldsymbol{\psi}$). We stop if either the Kriging model satisfies a given goal or the computer budget is exhausted. Altogether, the design selects relatively few combinations in subareas with an approximately linear f_{sim}.

Stochastic Kriging for Random Simulation

Stochastic Kriging (SK) was developed in [1], adding the *intrinsic noise* term $\varepsilon_r(\mathbf{x}_i)$ for replication r at combination $\mathbf{x}_i$ to (1.12), which —after averaging over replications—gives

$$\overline{y}(\mathbf{x}_i) = \mu + M(\mathbf{x}_i) + \overline{\varepsilon}(\mathbf{x}_i) \tag{1.19}$$

where $\varepsilon_r(\mathbf{x}) \in N(0, \text{Var}[\varepsilon_r(\mathbf{x})])$ and $\varepsilon_r(\mathbf{x})$ is independent of $M(\mathbf{x})$. Obviously, m_i replications without CRN make $\boldsymbol{\Sigma}_{\overline{\varepsilon}}$ diagonal with main diagonal elements $\text{Var}[\varepsilon(\mathbf{x}_i)]/m_i$; CRN and $m_i = m$ give $\boldsymbol{\Sigma}_{\overline{\varepsilon}} = \boldsymbol{\Sigma}_{\varepsilon}/m$.

To estimate $\text{Var}[\varepsilon(\mathbf{x}_i)]$, SK may use s_i^2. Alternatively, SK may use another Kriging model for $\text{Var}[\varepsilon(\mathbf{x}_i)]$ (besides the Kriging model for $E[y_r(\mathbf{x}_i)]$), which may give less volatile estimates. Because s_i^2 is not normally distributed, the GP is only a rough approximation. We might also replace s_i^2 by $\log(s_i^2)$ in the Kriging model; also see [10].

SK replaces $\boldsymbol{\Sigma}_M$ in OK by $\boldsymbol{\Sigma}_M + \boldsymbol{\Sigma}_{\overline{\varepsilon}}$ and $\mathbf{w}$ by $\overline{\mathbf{w}}$, giving $\widehat{y}(\mathbf{x}_0, \widehat{\psi})$ and $s^2\{\widehat{y}(\mathbf{x}_0)\}$; see [1, Eq. 25]. SK for a *quantile* (instead of an average) is discussed in [12, p. 208].

In our discussion of (1.18), we have already mentioned the problems caused by the randomness of $\widehat{\psi}$. If $m_i \gg 1$, then we may solve this problem through *distribution-free bootstrapping*; see [12, p. 209].

Usually SK employs the same designs as OK or UK do for deterministic simulation. So, SK often uses single-shot LHS. In random simulation, however, we also need to select m_i. Above, we discussed the analogous problem in regression metamodeling; a simple rule-of-thumb is (1.8).

In sequential designs for SA, we may select $\mathbf{x}$ that gives $\max_{\mathbf{x}} s^2\{\widehat{y}(\mathbf{x})\}$. In SK, we may find this $\mathbf{x}$ through distribution-free bootstrapping. This design selects more input values in subdomains with highly nonlinear estimated I/O functions.

More Kriging: Monotonic Kriging, and Global SA

Sometimes we know that f_{sim} is *monotonic* (e.g., if the traffic rate increases, then the mean waiting time increases); see Sect. 1.4. The Kriging predictor $\widehat{y}$, however, may be *wiggling* if the sample size n is small. To make $\widehat{y}$ monotonic, we may apply *distribution-free bootstrapping* with *acceptance/rejection* explained in [12, pp. 212–216]; also see [20, 26].

So far we focused on $\widehat{y}$, but we may also measure how sensitive $\widehat{y}$—and w if $\widehat{y}$ is a valid predictor—are to the individual inputs and their interactions—assuming that $\mathbf{z}$ has a prespecified distribution. We may then apply *functional analysis of variance* (FANOVA), which decomposes σ_w^2 into fractions corresponding with individual inputs or sets of inputs; see [12, pp. 216–218].

Risk Analysis

In FANOVA, we assume a given distribution for $\mathbf{d}$ so w becomes random (even in deterministic simulation), and in risk analysis (RA)—also called uncertainty analysis—we may wish to estimate $P(w > c_1)$ with a given threshold value c_1. RA is applied in nuclear engineering, finance, water management, etc. $P(w > c_1)$ may be very small—so $w > c_1$ is called a *rare event*—but may have disastrous consequences. The uncertainty about the exact values of $\mathbf{d}$ is called *subjective* or *epistemic*, whereas the "intrinsic" uncertainty in stochastic simulation is called *objective* or *aleatory*.

SA and RA address different questions, namely "Which are the most important inputs in the simulation model?" and "What is the probability of a given (disastrous) event happening?". So, SA may identify those inputs for which the distribution in RA needs further refinement. RA and SA are also detailed in [4].

Methodologically, we propose the following method for RA aimed at estimating $P(w > c_1)$. We use a Monte Carlo method to sample $\mathbf{d}$ from its given distribution. Next we use this $\mathbf{d}$ as input into the simulation model. We run this model to transform $\mathbf{d}$ into w: *propagation of uncertainty* about the input. We repeat these steps n times to obtain the EDF of w. Finally, we use this EDF to estimate $P(w > c_1)$. This method is also known as *nested simulation*; see [8].

In *expensive* simulation, we do not run n simulation runs, but we run its *metamodel* n times. We may better estimate the true $P(w > c_1)$ through inexpensive sampling of many values from the metamodel, which is estimated from relatively few I/O values obtained from the expensive simulation model.

Uncertainty in simulation models including RA and SA is also studied by the British community *Managing uncertainty in complex models* (MUCM) and the French research group *GdR MASCOT-NUM*. For example, [6] uses Kriging to estimate the *excursion set* —which is the set of inputs that give an output that exceeds a given threshold—and quantifies uncertainties in this estimate; a sequential design may reduce this uncertainty. The volume of the excursion set is related to the *failure probability* $P(w > c_1)$. ([16] uses a first-order polynomial to estimate which combinations of uncertain inputs form the frontier that separates acceptable and unacceptable outputs; both aleatory and epistemic uncertainty are included).

RA is related to the *Bayesian* approach that assumes the parameters of the simulation model to be unknown with a given *prior* distribution. After obtaining simulation I/O data, this approach uses the Bayes theorem to compute the posterior distribution of the simulation output. *Bayesian model averaging* and *Bayesian melding* formally account—not only for the uncertainty of the input parameters—but also for the uncertainty in the form of the (simulation) model itself. In practice, however, classical frequentist RA has been applied more often than Bayesian RA; also see [24].

1.6 Simulation Optimization

Optimization of real-world systems is an important issue, especially in engineered systems as opposed to social systems Furthermore, the *uncertainty* in $\mathbf{z}$ may be important, so *robust* optimization is important.

The simplest optimization has no constraints for z_j ($j = 1, \ldots, k$) or $w^{(l)}$ ($l = 1, \ldots, r$), has no uncertain z_j, and concerns the expected value of a single output, $E(w)$. Obviously, $E(w) = p$ if $P(w = 1) = p$ and $P(w = 0) = 1 - p$. However, $E(w)$ excludes quantiles and the mode of the output distribution. Furthermore, the simplest optimization assumes continuous d_j.

There are so many optimization methods that we do not try to summarize these methods. Instead, we focus on optimization using metamodels, especially linear regression and Kriging. Metamodel-based optimization is relatively common and RSM is the most popular metamodel-based method, while Kriging is popular in theoretical publications; see [9]. Because we focus on *expensive* simulations, it is impractical to apply optimization methods such as evolutionary algorithms (EA).

A single simulation run may be computationally inexpensive—but there are extremely many input combinations. Furthermore, most simulation models have many inputs, which leads to the *curse of dimensionality*. Moreover, a single run may be expensive if we wish to estimate the steady-state mean of a queueing system with a high traffic rate. Finally, if we wish to estimate a rare event, then we may need extremely long simulation runs (unless we succeed in applying importance sampling).

Linear Regression for Optimization: RSM

RSM treats the simulation model as a *black box*. RSM is *sequential*: it uses a sequence of local experiments that is meant to lead to the optimum input combination. RSM has gained a good track record; see [12, p. 244], [17, pp. 656–679], and [22].

We assume that RSM is applied only after the important inputs and their experimental area have been identified; i.e., before RSM starts, we may need *screening* (see Sect. 1.4). However, RSM and screening are integrated in [5].

Methodologically, the goal of RSM is to minimize $E(w|\mathbf{z})$. To initialize RSM, we select a starting point; e.g., $\mathbf{z}$ is the combination currently used in practice. In the *neighborhood* of this point, we fit a first-order polynomial, assuming white noise; however, RSM allows Var(w) to change in a next step. Unfortunately, there are no general guidelines for determining the appropriate *size* of the local area in each step ([5], however, selects this size through a so-called trust region). To fit this polynomial, we use a *R-III design*. In the next steps, we *locally* fit first-order polynomials. In each of these steps, we use the *gradient* implied by the polynomial fitted in that step:

$\nabla(\widehat{y}) = \widehat{\gamma}_{-0}$ where -0 means that the intercept $\widehat{\gamma}_0$ is removed from the $(k+1)$-dimensional vector with the estimated regression parameters $\widehat{\boldsymbol{\gamma}}$. This $\nabla(\widehat{y})$ estimates the *steepest-descent* direction. We take a step in this direction, trying intuitively selected values for the step size. After a number of such steps, w will increase (instead of decrease) because the latest local first-order polynomial becomes inadequate. When this happens, we simulate the combinations of the R-III design—but now we center this design around the best combination found so far. To quantify the *adequacy* of the local polynomial, we may compute R^2. Intuitively, a first-order polynomial corresponds with a *plane* and cannot adequately represent a *valley bottom* ("mirrored" hill top) when searching to minimize $E(w|\mathbf{z})$. So, now we fit a *second-order* polynomial, using a CCD. Next we use the derivatives of this polynomial to estimate the optimum $y(\widehat{\mathbf{x}}_o)$. We may also apply *canonical analysis* to examine the shape of the optimal subregion: is it a unique minimum, a saddle point, or a ridge with stationary points? If time permits, then we may try to escape from a possible local minimum and *restart* the search from a different initial local area.

We should not eliminate inputs with *nonsignificant* effects in a local first-order polynomial: these inputs may become significant in a next local area. The selection of m_i is a moot issue (as we saw above). A higher-order polynomial is more accurate (lower bias) than a lower-order polynomial is, but may have higher variance so its MSE increases; moreover, a higher-order polynomial requires higher n.

A *scale-independent* steepest-descent direction accounting for $\mathbf{\Sigma}_{\widehat{\boldsymbol{\gamma}}}$ (covariance matrix of $\widehat{\boldsymbol{\gamma}}$) is discussed in [12, pp. 252–253]. Experimental results suggest that this direction performs better than the classic steepest-descent direction.

In practice, simulation models have *multiple* responses types. The RSM literature offers several approaches for such situations; see [11]. We focus on *generalized RSM* (GRSM) for the following *constrained nonlinear random optimization problem*:

$$\begin{aligned} &\min_{\mathbf{z}} E(w^{(1)}|\mathbf{z}) \\ E(w^{(l')}|\mathbf{z}) &\geq c_{l'} \; (l' = 2, \dots, r) \\ &L_j \leq z_j \leq H_j \text{ with } j = 1, \dots, k. \end{aligned} \tag{1.20}$$

GRSM combines RSM and interior point methods from mathematical programming (MP), avoiding creeping along the boundary of the feasible area that is determined by the constraints on the random outputs and the deterministic inputs. So, GRSM moves faster to the optimum than steepest-descent does; moreover, GRSM is scale-independent; see [12, pp. 253–258].

Obviously, it is uncertain whether the optimum estimated by GRSM is close to the true optimum. The first-order necessary optimality conditions are known as the *Karush–Kuhn–Tucker* (KKT) conditions. These conditions may be tested through parametric bootstrapping; see [12, pp. 259–266].

Kriging for Optimization

Efficient global optimization (EGO) is a well-known *sequential* method that uses Kriging; it balances *local* and *global* search (exploitation and exploration). To select

uncertainty set U. Recently, [30] derived a specific U for $\mathbf{p}$ where $\mathbf{p}$ denotes the unknown density function of $\mathbf{z}_{\text{NC}}$ that is compatible with given historical data on $\mathbf{z}_{\text{NC}}$. This type of RO develops a computationally tractable *robust counterpart* of the original problem. Compared with the output of the nominal solution in MP, RO may give better worst-case and average outputs.

Acknowledgements I thank the editors for inviting me to write a contribution for this book and W. Shi (Hubei University of Economics, Wuhan, China) for commenting on Sect. 1.4.

References

1. Ankenman, B., Nelson, B., Staum, J.: Stochastic Kriging for simulation metamodeling. Oper. Res. **58**(2), 371–382 (2010)
2. Ben-Tal, A., El Ghaoui, L., Nemirovski, A.: Robust Optimization. Princeton University Press, Princeton (2009)
3. Bischl, B., Mersmann, O., Trautmann, H., Weihs, C.: Resampling methods for meta-model validation with recommendations for evolutionary computation. Evol. Comput. **20**(2), 249–275 (2012)
4. Borgonovo, E., Plischke, E.: Sensitivity analysis: a review of recent advances. Eur. J. Oper. Res. **248**(3), 869–887 (2016)
5. Chang, K.-H., Li, M.-K., Wan, H.: Combining STRONG with screening designs for large-scale simulation optimization. IIE Trans. **46**(4), 357–373 (2014)
6. Chevalier, C., Ginsbourger, D., Bect, J., Vazquez, E., Picheny, V., Richet, Y.: Fast parallel Kriging-based stepwise uncertainty reduction with application to the identification of an excursion set. Technometrics **56**(4), 455–465 (2014)
7. Dellino, G., Kleijnen, J.P.C., Meloni, C.: Robust optimization in simulation: Taguchi and Krige combined. INFORMS J. Comput. **24**(3), 471–484 (2012)
8. Gordy, M.B., Juneja, S.: Nested simulation in portfolio risk measurement. Manag. Sci. **56**(11), 1833–1848 (2010)
9. Jalali, H., Van Nieuwenhuyse, I.: Simulation optimization in inventory replenishment: a classification. *IIE Transactions* (2015) (Accepted)
10. Kamiński, B.: A method for updating of stochastic Kriging metamodels. Eur. J. Oper. Res. **247**(3), 859–866 (2015)
11. Khuri, A.I., Mukhopadhyay, S.: Response surface methodology. Wiley Interdiscip. Rev. Comput. Stat. **2**, 128–149 (2010)
12. Kleijnen, J.P.C.: Design and Analysis of Simulation Experiments, 2nd edn. Springer, Berlin (2015)
13. Kleijnen, J.P.C.: Comment on Park et al. "Robust Kriging in computer experiments". J. Oper. Res. Soc. (2016) (in press)
14. Kleijnen, J.P.C.: Regression and Kriging metamodels with their experimental designs in simulation: a review. Eur. J. Oper. Res. **256**, 1–16 (2017)
15. Kleijnen, J.P.C., Shi, W.: Sequential probability ratio tests for nonnormal simulation responses. Tilburg University, Discussion Paper (2017)
16. Kleijnen, J.P.C., Pierreval, H., Zhang, J.: Methodology for determining the acceptability of system designs in uncertain environments. Eur. J. Oper. Res. **209**(2), 176–183 (2011)
17. Law, A.M.: Simulation Modeling and Analysis, 5th edn. McGraw-Hill, Boston (2015)
18. Loeppky, J.L., Sacks, J., Welch, W.: Choosing the sample size of a computer experiment: a practical guide. Technometrics **51**(4), 366–376 (2009)
19. Lophaven, S.N., Nielsen, H.B., Sondergaard, J.: DACE: a Matlab Kriging toolbox, version 2.0. IMM Technical University of Denmark, Kongens Lyngby (2002)

20. Maatouk, H., Bay, X.: Gaussian process emulators for computer experiments with inequality constraints (2016). arXiv:1606.01265v1
21. Markiewicz, A., Szczepańska, A.: Optimal designs in multivariate linear models. Stat. Probab. Lett. **77**, 426–430 (2007)
22. Myers, R.H., Montgomery, D.C., Anderson-Cook, C.M.: Response Surface Methodology: Process and Product Optimization Using Designed Experiments, 3rd edn. Wiley, New York (2009)
23. Naumov, V., Gaidamaka, Y., Samouylov, K., Sopin, E., Samuylov, A.: Multiserver queue with finite resources and customers of random volume. In: Moder, K., Melas, V., Pilz, J., Rasch, D. (eds.) Statistics and Simulation. Springer, Berlin (2018)
24. Nelson, B.L.: 'Some tactical problems in digital simulation' for the next 10 years. J. Simul. **10**, 2–11 (2016)
25. Praskova, Z.: Bootstrap change point for dependent data. In: Moder, K., Melas, V., Pilz, J., Rasch, D. (eds.) Statistics and Simulation. Springer, Berlin (2018)
26. Tan, M.H.Y.: Monotonic metamodels for deterministic computer experiments. Technometrics **59**(1), 1–10 (2017)
27. Vollert, N., Ortner, M., Pilz, J.: Benefits and application of tree structures in Gaussian process models to optimize magnetic field shaping problems. In: Moder, K., Melas, V., Pilz, J., Rasch, D. (eds.) Statistics and Simulation. Springer, Berlin (2018)
28. Wan, H., Ankenman, B.E., Nelson, B.L.: Improving the efficiency and efficacy of controlled sequential bifurcation for simulation factor screening. INFORMS J. Comput. **22**(3), 482–492 (2010)
29. Woods, D.C., Lewis, S.M.: Design of experiments for screening (2015). arXiv:1510.05248
30. Yanikoğlu, İ., den Hertog, D., Kleijnen, J.P.C.: Adjustable robust parameter design with unknown distributions. IIE Trans. **48**(3), 298–312 (2016)

Chapter 2
A Review of Simulation Usage in the New Zealand Electricity Market

Golbon Zakeri and Geoff Pritchard

Abstract In this chapter, we outline and review the application of simulation on the generation offer and consumption bids for the New Zealand electricity market (NZEM). We start by describing the operation of the NZEM with a particular focus on how electricity prices are calculated for each time period. The complexity of this mechanism, in conjunction with uncertainty surrounding factors such as consumption levels, motivates the use of simulation. We will then discuss simulation–optimization methods for optimal offer strategies of a generator, for a particular time period, in the NZEM. We conclude by extending our ideas and techniques to consumption bids and interruptible load reserve offers for major consumers of electricity including large manufacturers such as the steel mill.

Keywords Electricity markets · Price simulation · Demand response

2.1 Introduction to Wholesale Electricity Markets

Electricity markets have become prevalent around the world in the past two to three decades. The first example of privatization of an electric power system took place in Chile in the early 1980s. The idea behind the Chilean model was to bring rationality and transparency to the operations of the power system that would ultimately be reflected in power prices. Other rationales for the eventuation of electricity markets include better reliability and signalling appropriate levels of investment in infrastructure in the energy sector through proper pricing of this commodity. England–Wales, New Zealand, Australia, the Nord Pool, Spain and the

G. Zakeri (✉)
Department of Engineering Science, University of Auckland,
Auckland, New Zealand
e-mail: g.zakeri@auckland.ac.nz

G. Pritchard
Department of Statistics, University of Auckland, Auckland, New Zealand
e-mail: g.pritchard@auckland.ac.nz

J. Pilz et al. (eds.), *Statistics and Simulation*, Springer Proceedings
in Mathematics & Statistics 231, https://doi.org/10.1007/978-3-319-76035-3_2

Pennsylvania–Jersey–Maryland (PJM) markets are amongst the oldest electricity markets with an abundance of available data.

2.1.1 Pricing of Electricity

Arguably, proper pricing of electricity is the corner stone of the electricity market paradigm. This is a key for signalling scarcity, and it is the market signal that would drive investment decisions. While in most commodity markets the price of a good is determined through supply and demand, in the case of electricity, the physical constraints governing an electricity system also impact prices. Electricity is not a storable commodity. It is injected into a transmission grid at certain nodes of that transmission grid often referred to as grid injection points (GIPs) and flows through the grid complying with physical constraints. Electricity is withdrawn at grid exit points (GXPs) and delivered to consumers. Due to the physical constraints on the flow of electricity, in all electricity markets, the dispatch of the generation of electricity is left to an independent system operator (ISO). In most electricity markets, an additional function of the ISO is to determine the price of electricity at different nodes of the transmission network.

Typically in a wholesale electricity market, for each period of the day, each generator offers in generation quantities for each of its plants (possibly located at different GIPs), at certain prices. In its most general form, the generation offers are supply functions (also known as offer curves) denoted $p = S(q)$, where $S(q)$ is the marginal price of producing quantity q. In all electricity markets, $S(q)$ is required to be a monotone increasing function. It is important to note that these supply functions are offered by a deadline well ahead of the pertaining (market) time period; therefore, participants do not know other generator offers or a complete picture for demand.

These supply offers are collected by the ISO. The ISO estimates the demand (in the case of inflexible demands), over that period. The ISO then solves a side constrained network optimization problem where the objective is to minimize the total cost of production of electricity. The constraints of this optimization problem reflect that demand must be met at every node of the network and that physical flow constraints such as transmission line capacities and Kirchhoff's laws must be complied with. Often reactive power modelling is left out of the ISO's dispatch problem, and the problem is in fact a direct current equivalent load flow model [17, 24]. When flexible demand is offered into the market, in the form of a demand-side bid, the objective of the ISO's optimization problem becomes welfare maximization, producing system optimal amounts of generation and consumption for a time period.

A general model for the ISO's economic dispatch problem (EDP) in its simple cost-minimizing form is formulated below.

$$
\begin{array}{llll}
\text{EDP: } \textit{minimize} & \sum_i \sum_{m \in \mathcal{O}(i)} \int_0^{q_m} C_m(x)dx & & \\
\quad \textit{s.t.} & g_i(y) + \sum_{m \in \mathcal{O}(i)} q_m & = D_i, \ i \in \mathcal{N}, \ [\pi_i] & \\
& q_m \in Q_m, \quad m \in \mathcal{O}(i), & i \in \mathcal{N}, & \\
& y \in Y. & &
\end{array} \tag{2.1}
$$

We use i as the index for the nodes in the transmission grid. We use m as the index for the generators, and $\mathcal{O}(i)$ indicates the set of all generators located at node i. Generator m can supply quantity q_m, and the demand at node i is denoted by D_i. Q_m indicates the capacity of generator m. Here the components of vector x measure the dispatch of each generator, and the components of the vector y measure the flow of power in each transmission line. We denote the flow in the directed line from i to k by y_{ik}, where by convention we assume $i < k$. (A negative value of y_{ik} denotes flow in the direction from k to i.) It is required that this vector lie in the set Y, which means that each component satisfies the thermal limits on each line and satisfies loop flow constraints that are required by Kirchhoff's Law. The function $g_i(y)$ defines the amount of power arriving at node i for a given choice of y. This notation enables different loss functions to be modelled. For example, if there are no line losses, then we obtain

$$g_i(y) = \sum_{k<i} y_{ki} - \sum_{k>i} y_{ik}.$$

With quadratic losses, we obtain

$$g_i(y) = \sum_{k<i} y_{ki} - \sum_{k>i} y_{ik} - \sum_{k<i} \frac{1}{2} r_{ki} y_{ki}^2 - \sum_{k>i} \frac{1}{2} r_{ik} y_{ik}^2.$$

The price of electricity is determined as the shadow price π_i of the node balance constraints above that indicate demand must be met at all nodes. This price is the system cost of meeting one more unit of demand at node i. This method of determining the electricity price is sometimes referred to as locational marginal pricing (LMP). New Zealand and the PJM market in the USA are examples of electricity markets with LMP. It is worth noting that some wholesale electricity markets operate by assuming that demand and supply are located at the same node, and trading takes place in that one node. This means that a single price of electricity is arrived at. Nevertheless, in order to ensure that the demand is met at all nodes and that the flow complies with physical constraints, a balancing market would follow in real time where the residuals of the single node market are traded. The UK wholesale electricity market is an example of a single node market.

2.2 The New Zealand Electricity Market

Following a transition from a centralized system, to a deregulated electricity market, an immediate natural question for a generator is what supply offer function will optimize their returns. In a strictly monitored market such as the PJM, there is not much room for a generator to exercise market power. In such a market, the marginal cost of generation of electricity is relatively well known. Much of the supply is procured from thermal plants (e.g. gas and coal) with known cost of fuel or nuclear plants with a minimal marginal cost of generation. Here, it is relatively simple for a market monitor to observe the supply offers and question any offers that are significantly above the marginal cost of production.

Not all electricity markets are strictly monitored however. Markets such as Nord Pool and the New Zealand market are dominated by hydroelectric generation. While one can argue that inflows into hydro-lakes are free, there is an opportunity cost attached to using the water now or saving it for a future period. This is particularly important as the inflows are uncertain and dry periods can have disastrous consequences for the electricity system. This opportunity cost is referred to as the *value of water*. When all market participants are risk neutral, this value can be found by solving a large-scale stochastic program that minimizes the expected cost of production of electricity, using various generation sources in a coordinated fashion, over a long time horizon (e.g. a year that is divided into 52 weeks; see e.g. [18, 20]). In a real market, however, generators face various risks and it is not possible to ascertain their level of risk. Even if this information were available, it would not always be possible to solve an equivalent centralized problem to obtain the value of water [19, 23]. Hence, the New Zealand market was designed not to be a strictly regulated market. The question therefore remains, how can a generator offer supplies into this market so as to maximize their profits. The answer to this question, and a very similar question for the demand side, utilizes simulation intensely and is the topic of the remainder of the chapter.

2.2.1 The Need for Simulation: Pricing in the NZEM

While it would be highly desirable to obtain a simple analytical answer to the question of optimizing generation offers, this is not possible due to the nature of price determination. As laid out in Sect. 2.1.1, the nodal price of electricity is the value of the optimal shadow prices for the demand constraints. There is no explicit analytical form for these prices, which are clearly affected endogenously, as the firm varies their supply offer. The best way to tackle the problem of offer optimization over an electricity market is to simulate the ISO's problem and obtain prices. It is fortunate that the Electricity Authority (EA), who exercise oversight over the NZEM, has made publicly available an accurate replica of the market clearing optimization problem that is solved in New Zealand in every half hour time period. This replica is referred to as the vectorized Scheduling, Pricing and Dispatch (vSPD) that is available from the EA's web site.[1]

[1] See http://www.emi.ea.govt.nz/.

The market clearing side constrained network optimization vSPD contains over 250 nodes(GIPs and GXPs) and over 450 arcs (that form the backbone transmission network for New Zealand). The database for vSPD contains historical offer and demand information dating back to 2000. The generator offers for New Zealand are in the form of five step, step functions, where each step is referred to as a tranche. Each historical tranche of each offer is available, indicating the quantity and price pair that comprise that tranche, for each generator. Furthermore, the database contains information on the thermal capacity of the transmission lines, availability of generation units, demand data and various other necessary information for replicating any historical period. This is a rich and ideal set-up for simulation.

Another feature of the NZEM is the co-optimization of energy and reserve. Electricity markets need to be robust to failure. To that end, reserve generation is procured for every electricity market. In New Zealand, the procurement of reserves takes place in conjunction with procurement of energy. There are a number of constraints relating energy and reserves. We mention this feature of the NZEM here for completeness; however, we will refrain from dwelling on this point for the sake of simplicity. We will return to this point in Sect. 2.4 when we discuss consumption and reserve offer strategies for a major consumer of electricity.

2.3 Optimal Offers for Generation

We start this section by formulating an analytical description of the generator optimization problem under uncertainty. We will lay out a simulation–optimization approach for this problem which has been in use by generators over the NZEM. Under a number of strong assumptions, the problem of generator offer optimization can be solved analytically. Our setting is a realistic electricity market where such strong assumptions are not justified. However to place the problem in context and gain some intuition, we start with this analytically tractable case.

2.3.1 A Simplified Problem

The problem of bid–offer optimization was first approached by Klemperer and Meyer [14] who were interested in modelling an oligopoly facing uncertain demand, where each firm bids a supply function as its strategy. This is in contrast to previous models in the economics literature where firms were restricted to strategize over their quantities only (Cournot models) or their prices only (Bertrand models) and allows a firm to adapt better to an uncertain environment. Green and Newbery address the same question but in the context of the British spot market [13].

To begin, let us assume that there are only two generators supplying the market (i.e. we are dealing with a duopoly) and suppose that the offer curve of the competitor is given by $q = S(p)$. Let us also assume that the demand curve is given by $q = D(p)$, that is the market will absorb quantity q if the price is p. For their analysis, Klemperer and Meyer use the concept of the residual demand curve faced by the generator. Consider the curve given by $q = D(p) - S(p)$. This determines what quantity must be offered into the market if we desire the price to be p based on the demand curve and the competitor's offer strategy. Note that this approach makes the simplified assumption that *all transactions occur at a single node*. The inverse of this curve describes how the price is influenced by the quantity we offer and is referred to as the residual demand curve. With this information at hand, it is now easy to optimize the profits of the generator in question (see Fig. 2.1).

Recall that Klemperer and Meyer point out that supply functions allow a firm to adapt better to an uncertain environment. If there are multiple possible residual demand curves that a generator may face, the supply function response may allow selecting a point on each of these residual demand curves that would optimize the generator's profit given that that residual demand curve has realized. This is referred to as a strong supply function response (see Fig. 2.2). A number of papers construct the residual demand curve by simulating the (single node) market and explicitly building the supply function response; see e.g. [9, 10]. In [9], the residual demand curve takes on a step function form and the authors develop a nonlinear integer programming model of the generator's revenue optimization problem. They develop a combined coordinate search, branch and bound method to solve this problem. Torre et al. exploit the nature of the previous problem to develop a more efficient solution method in [10].

In a sequence of papers, Anderson and Philpott have also addressed the profit maximization problem of a price-maker generator under various assumptions. In [3], they assume that a price-maker generator knows its competitors' offer curves, but is faced with uncertain demand. They first establish the existence of a strong supply function response, for such a generator, that would be optimal for any realization of the uncertain demand. This strong supply function response is guaranteed to exist when the generation costs of the generator in question are increasing and convex,

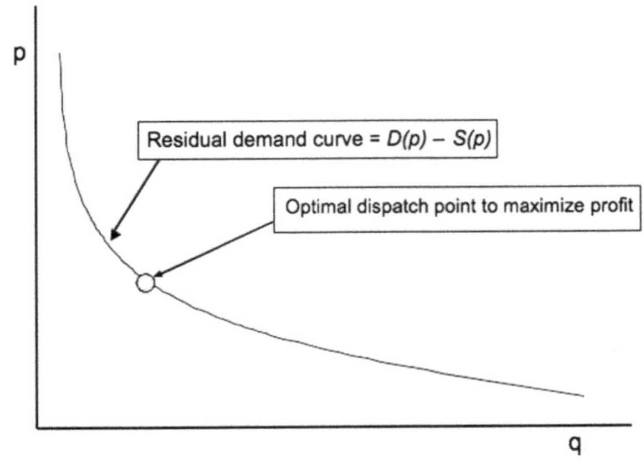

Fig. 2.1 Optimal point for a generator to get dispatched along a residual demand curve

and the competitor offers are log-concave. They discuss a procedure where the true aggregate offer stack of the competitors is approximated by a log-concave function. Note that this (aggregate) offer stack would be a step function in almost all real-world electricity markets. They construct a strong supply function response S_g, for the generator in question. Subsequently, they approximate S_g in order to comply with market rules. Finally, they provide bounds on the performance of such an offer strategy.

In [2], Anderson and Philpott generalize their model by allowing uncertainty not only in the demand but also allow the competitor offers to be unknown. They introduce the concept of a market distribution function $\psi(q, p)$ pertaining to a specific generator at a specific transmission node. They define $\psi(q, p)$ to be the probability of not being fully dispatched if the generator submits a quantity q at price p. Let $R(q, p)$ denote the or profit that the generator makes if it is dispatched q at a clearing price of p. They demonstrate that if the generator submits the curve s, and the pertinent market distribution function ψ is continuous then the expected profit of the company is given by

$$V(s) = \int_s R(q, p) d\psi(q, p).$$

They proceed to provide conditions that guarantee (local) optimality of an offer stack s that would maximize $V(s)$. To address the question of estimating the market distribution function see [4, 22].

2.3.2 *Using Simulation for the General Problem*

The work described thus far only deals with generators that are located at a single node of the market or alternatively assumes that the wholesale market is a single node market. As noted in Sect. 2.1 however, most wholesale electricity markets use locational marginal pricing where the price of electricity is different from node to

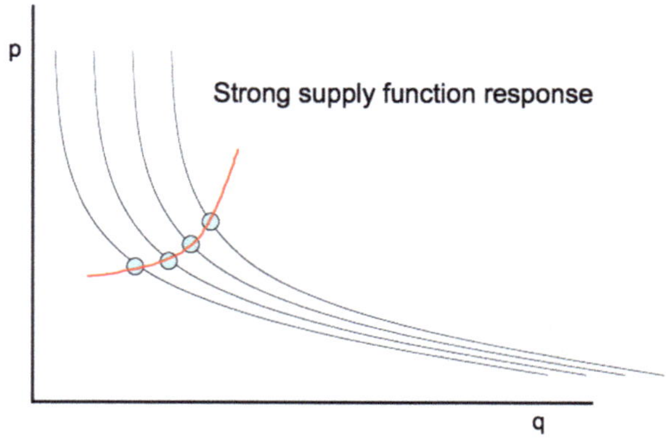

Fig. 2.2 Building a strong supply function response from a distribution of residual demand curves

node. To capture the effects of the transmission network, a generator must look at the variations in the prices from the dispatch problem EDP as a function of how it offers into the market. The revenue optimization problem is now posed as a bilevel program, or a mathematical program with equilibrium constraints (MPEC) and becomes a non-convex optimization problem.

$$\begin{array}{llll} \textit{maximize} & R(x,\pi) & & \\ \textit{s.t.} & (x,\pi) \in \textit{arg min} & \sum_i \sum_{m \in \mathscr{O}(i)} \int_0^{q_m} C_m(x)dx & \\ & \textit{s.t.} & g_i(y) + \sum_{m \in \mathscr{O}(i)} q_m & = D_i,\ i \in \mathscr{N}, \\ & & q_m \in Q_m, \quad m \in \mathscr{O}(i), & i \in \mathscr{N}, \\ & & y \in Y. & \end{array}$$

Here x denotes the vector of quantities dispatched at each node if the generator offered at that node (or is 0 if the generator in question does not own generation at a particular node), and π is the vector of electricity prices. Note that the inner optimization problem, namely the economic dispatch problem EDP can be replaced with its necessary and sufficient conditions for optimality as it is a convex problem (see e.g. Chap. 4 of [5]). In this case, the reformulation is referred to as an MPEC [16]. Furthermore, as described in Sect. 2.1, the offers submitted to the market are for a (near) future period. In particular, over the NZEM, generator offers are "locked in" two hours ahead of each time period. Therefore, generators have at best probabilistic knowledge of demand and competitor offers. The amount of randomness depends on what the generator (plant owner) is assumed to know before submitting the offer curve. Competing generators' offer curves may be modelled stochastically (if unknown) or deterministically (if known). A realistic problem is likely to contain some of each: the availability of another power plant owned by the same firm is probably known, while the availability of a wind farm is likely to be unknown. submitted very close to the time of production. We will assume that the sizes of loads require a stochastic model. The model may also include stochastic transmission line outages.

Pritchard considers this stochastic version of the above MPEC in [21]. An algorithm is developed where first the market is simulated under varying (quantity, price) offers of the generator in question. The market clearing prices faced by this generator are recorded, and a global optimization is performed that determines the best supply function offer resulting in optimal expected profits for our generator. We will proceed with detailing the steps.

We begin by subdividing the $q - p$ plane containing the offer stack, with a finite rectangular grid by considering a range of price and quantities, each subdivided into intervals. For examples, a price range may be from a \$1.00 to \$1000.00 with finer step sizes for likely prices (tens to few hundred dollars) and coarser steps further out in the range. This will restrict the class of admissible supply functions to those which follow the edges of this grid. Then there are only finitely many admissible offer stacks, each consisting of a finite sequence of horizontal or vertical line segments that are grid edges. Note that for any grid edge e, being dispatched on edge e is independent of which other edges have been included in the offer stack. Therefore,

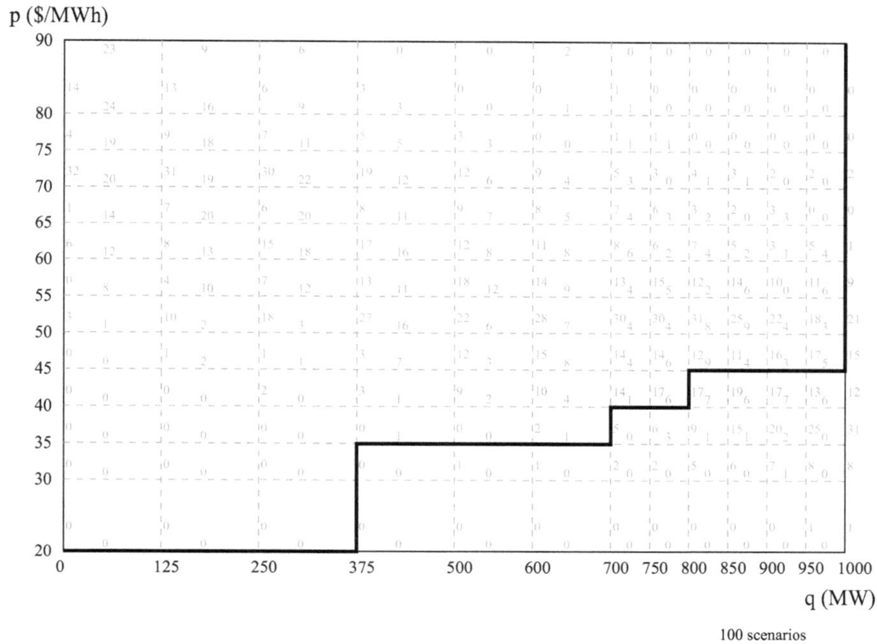

Fig. 2.3 A grid for building an optimal offer stack based on edge values using simulation

the expected payoff from any offer stack can be computed by adding the expected payoffs from the edges comprising this offer stack.

Let $V(e)$ denote the value of including edge e in the offer stack. To estimate $V(e)$ by simulation, we start with n randomly (and independently) chosen scenarios $\{\omega_1, \ldots, \omega_n\}$, where each "scenario" is a realization of the random elements of the problem (e.g. competitors' offer curves, loads, outages, etc.). Such scenarios may be extrapolated from historical information or may be based on richer ensemble forecast information. For each scenario ω_i and each edge e, we can compute the payoff $V_i(e)$ if ω_i results in a point of dispatch along e (i.e. when the offer curve includes e), or 0 if no such dispatch occurs. We can now approximate $V(e)$ by $\hat{V}(e) = \frac{1}{n}\sum_{i=1}^{n} V_i(e)$. Note that $\hat{V}(e)$ is a consistent unbiased estimator of $V(e)$. Figure 2.3 illustrates a (q, p) grid with along with frequency of dispatch attached to each edge.

To build the optimal offer stack resulting in the optimal expected profits for the generator, we can utilize dynamic programming. Due to the monotonicity constraint on any admissible offer stack, once at a vertex k of the grid, we must choose to continue right or up from that point. Therefore, the maximum expected payoff attached to a vertex k is given by

$$W(k) = \max(W_r(k), W_u(k)).$$

where

$$W_r(k) = \begin{cases} -\infty & \text{if } k \text{ is on } q = q_{max} \\ V(e_r(k)) + W(v_r(k)) & \text{otherwise.} \end{cases}$$

In the above equation, $v_r(k)$ is the vertex adjacent to k on the right and $e_r(k)$ is the edge joining these vertices. $W_u(k)$ has an analogous description involving the edge and the neighbour above k. Given that $V((q_{max}, p_{max})) = 0$, we can start at the upper right-hand corner of the (q, p) grid and utilize a Bellman recursion to determine the optimal generator stack.

2.4 Bid Optimization for Large Consumers of Electricity

Similar to generators, large consumers in an electricity market, who are exposed to spot market prices, are often able to influence the clearing price through their decisions. These users, often large industrial sites or potentially aggregated blocks of residential or commercial users who wish to actively participate in the electricity market, can carefully choose their consumption level to influence price. There is a large amount of uncertainty associated with this problem, especially for participants who bid in the co-optimized ancillary service markets. For the same reasons as outlined above in the generation case, the problem of choosing an optimal consumption level, with an associated optimal reserve offer, is too broad to undertake analytically. As an alternative, numerical simulations can be used to approach this problem. A methodology to tackle this problem numerically was presented by Cleland et al. in [8]. This methodology is similar to what has already been presented for the generation case; however, it has nuances stemming from the co-optimization of energy and reserve. We present a concise detailed version here.

2.4.1 Reserve Co-optimization

Modern markets often incorporate the provision of ancillary services (AS) into the market dispatch problem. These ancillary services such as primary, secondary and tertiary contingency reserve or regulating reserve [11, 12] are often procured differently throughout the world. New Zealand has fully co-optimized primary and secondary contingency reserve via separate markets [1]. In Spain, for example, secondary reserve is procured for both contingency and regulation purposes, but primary reserve is a non-remunerated mandatory service [15]. In New Zealand, consumers are capable of participating in the AS markets through the provision of IL, for which they are paid the spot market reserve price for the FIR (primary) and SIR (secondary) markets. This benefits the consumer (industrial site) directly through additional revenue. But also indirectly, as the provision of IL capable reserve may release spinning reserve plant back to the energy market which may alleviate constraints.

The NZEM operates under $N - 1$ reserve requirements, and sufficient reserve is procured to secure against the largest risk setter in each of New Zealand's two islands. In theory, this prevents under scheduling of reserve, in practice it can have a notable effect upon energy prices. When a risk setting asset (generator or transmission) is the marginal energy unit, the cost of securing the output from this unit (the reserve price) is incorporated into the energy price. For a marginal generator, the final energy price π is thus linked to the marginal energy, p_e, and marginal reserve, p_r, offer prices. We illustrate this through a very simple example. Let x_1 and x_2 and x_r represent the system dispatches from firms 1, 2 and reserve, respectively. Similarly, let p_1, p_2 and p_r denote the offered prices of energy and reserve by the firms, and q_1, q_2 and q_r the quantities available at the respective price. The small dispatch problem, meeting demand d in a single node network, is formulated as

$$\begin{aligned} \min \ & p_1x_1 + p_2x_2 + p_rx_r \\ \text{s/t} \quad & x_1 + x_2 = d \qquad [\pi] \\ & x_r \geq x_1 \qquad [\lambda_{r1}] \\ & x_r \geq x_2 \qquad [\lambda_{r2}] \\ & x_i \leq q_i \quad i \in \{1, 2, r\} \\ & x_i \geq 0 \quad i. \in \{1, 2, r\} \end{aligned} \tag{2.2}$$

When $c_1 + r < c_2$, and $d < q_1$, meeting a marginal unit of demand will require procurement of an extra unit of energy. Hence, $\pi = p_1 + p_r$; this is easily verified by writing the KKT conditions.

If the marginal generator is transmitted from a neighbouring reserve zone (in New Zealand, these are differentiated by the two major island land masses), then the nodal energy prices become linked via the marginal reserve price in Eq. 2.3.

$$\pi_2 = \pi_1 + p_{r,2} \tag{2.3}$$

where π_1 and π_2 denote the locational marginal prices in nodes 1 and 2, respectively.

The above two examples are very simple illustrations of the interaction of energy and reserve prices. In reality, not only does reserve have to be covered for each of the North and South islands of New Zealand, energy and reserve are also restricted through constraints that express physical limitations such as ramp rate of a turbine in the event of an emergency shortage where reserves are called upon. The joint optimization of consumption and reserve offers is therefore a significant challenge theoretically. However, it may be approached numerically through simulations. Large consumers are an inviting target for this approach due to the convergence of means (manned control rooms, real-time prices, advanced metering) and motive (profit maximization), which is often missing from smaller consumers. These consumers thus satisfy many of the conditions which are a requirement for demand elasticity [6].

2.4.2 Optimization of Consumption and Reserves

We start by determining the consumption levels for our major consumer. These are naturally derived from the plant operation modes. In order to compute consumer profits, a utility figure for electricity consumption in a designated period may be necessary; note that this figure is inputted by the user, and they are free to experiment with a range of utilities. As the operational decisions for the plant are made ahead of time, the energy offers and other consumption quantities for the period in question are uncertain. Therefore, we need to consider a distribution. To address this, the user will input a base scenario. This can be a scenario derived from historical offers, e.g. the equivalent period on the previous day or a period closely matched to hydrology or demand conditions. We develop a "rest of New Zealand" set of scenarios that are generated from randomly scaled versions of demand (in nodes other than the one in question) for the base scenario. In particular, we can use a log-normal distribution for each island and the number of these scenarios can be chosen by the user.

For each demand level, corresponding to a plant operational mode, a distribution of energy prices at the consumer (site) node is determined. The site can then use this information to determine, under uncertainty, their optimal operating level. This can be done in expectation, or with any risk measure, as the distribution of prices attached to each consumption level is provided. Prices are used as they represent the only source of permitted variability in the site profitability calculation. A graph of the price distributions, found using simulation, is presented in Fig. 2.4.

As observed in Sect. 2.4.1, there may be a significant interaction between the market clearing price of electricity and the offered reserve prices. To take full account of this and determine a combined optimal consumption and reserve offer, we require a grid containing all admissible reserve supply stacks for the site. In other words, the quantity, price plane of possible offers, is subdivided into a finite grid consisting of rectangular cells, identical to what was presented for the generator offer case. This simplifies our problem as admissible offer stacks are those which follow the edges of the cells. we now output energy (and reserve) price distributions attached to each level of consumption. However this time, the price distribution attached to each consumption level is derived from the optimal reserve offer for the corresponding consumption level, for the period. For each consumption level (drawn from plant operation mode), we simulate different market scenarios using vSPD, as before. Each simulation will record the point of dispatch on any admissible reserve offer stack confined to our reserve grid. This is effectively done by tracing out the intersections of the "reserve residual demand" on the grid (as outlined in Sect. 2.3). We are now in a position to find an optimal reserve offer stack, for this consumption level using dynamic programming. The states of this DP are the vertices of the reserve grid. It is clear that the value to go attached to the top right corner of the reserve grid is zero (no reserves above our max quantity and max price will be procured). We solve the DP using backward recursion. The actions for this DP amount to amending a vertical (moving up) or a horizontal (moving right) segment to the reserve offer stack constructed thus far. Our choices are limited to up and right moves as the stack must be increasing.

The overall approach separates the co-optimization problem into three sequential steps. The influence of each consumption level on energy and reserve prices under uncertainty is determined in phase one. In the second phase, the optimal reserve offer stack attached to each consumption level is determined using the dynamic programming, very similar to the case for generator offers. Lastly, the optimal consumption level with its associated reserve offer stack is determined through a repetition of phase one, with the optimal reserve offer level in place. Cleland et al. have reported on the effectiveness of this methodology under various performance measures on experiments that span 13 months of data. The results are outlined in [7].

2.5 Conclusions

Pricing of electricity is a complex process that relies on solving a large-side constrained network optimization problem for every time period of every market. Many decisions, such as offer strategies for generators and consumption bids for major users of electricity, ought to be made based on a good understanding of electricity

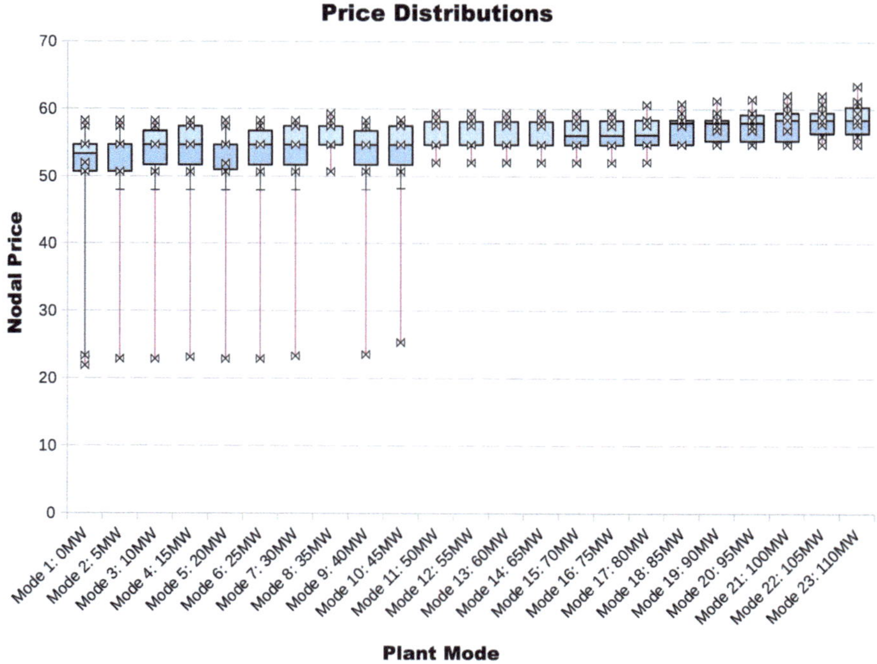

Fig. 2.4 Distribution of market clearing prices found through simulation

prices. We laid out in this chapter, two major applications of simulation–optimization over a deregulated electricity market. These applications have been developed and are in use in the NZEM.

References

1. Alvey, T., Goodwin, D., Ma, X., Streiffert, D., Sun, D.: A security-constrained bid-clearing system for the New Zealand wholesale electricity market. IEEE Trans. Power Syst. **13**(2), 340–346 (1998)
2. Anderson, E.J., Philpott, A.B.: Optimal offer construction in electricity markets. Math. Oper. Res. **27**(1), 82–100 (2002)
3. Anderson, E.J., Philpott, A.B.: Using supply functions for offering generation into an electricity market. Oper. Res. **50**(3), 477–489 (2002)
4. Anderson, E.J., Philpott, A.B.: Estimation of electricity market distribution functions. Ann. Oper. Res. **121**, 21–32 (2003)
5. Bazaraa, M., Sherali, H., Shetty, C.M.: Nonlinear Programming Theory and Algorithms. Wiley, New York (1993)
6. Borenstein, S., Jaske, M., Rosenfeld, A.: Dynamic pricing, advanced metering, and demand response in electricity markets. Center for the Study of Energy Markets (2002)
7. Cleland, N., Zakeri, G., Pritchard, G., Young, B.: a model for load consumption and reserve offers in reserve constrained electricity markets. Comput. Manag. Sci. **12**(4), 519–537 (2015)
8. Cleland, N., Zakeri, G., Pritchard, G., Young, B.: Integrating consumption and reserve strategies for large consumers in electricity markets. Lecture Notes in Economics and Mathematical Systems, vol. 682, pp. 23–30 (2016)
9. Conejo, A.J., Contreras, J., Arroyo, J.M., de la Torre, S.: Optimal response of an oligopolistic generating company to a competitive pool-based electric power market. IEEE Trans. Power Syst. **17**(2), 424–430 (2002)
10. de la Torre, S., Arroyo, J.M., Conejo, A.J., Contreras, J.: Price maker self-scheduling in a pool-based electricity market: a mixed integer LP approach. IEEE Trans. Power Syst. **17**(4), 1037–1042 (2002)
11. Ela, E., Milligan, M., Kirby, B.: Operating reserves and variable generation: a comprehensive review of current strategies, studies, and fundamental research on the impact that increased penetration of variable renewable generation has on power system operating reserves. Technical Report NREL/TP-5500-51978, NREL, NREL (2011)
12. Ellison, J.F., Tesfatsion, L.S., Loose, V.W., Byrne, R.H.: Project report: a survey of operating reserve markets in US ISO/RTO-managed electric energy regions. Sandia Natl Labs Publications. http://www.sandia.gov/ess/publications/SAND2012_1000.pdf (2012). Accessed 21 Feb 2017
13. Green, R.J., Newbery, D.M.: Competition in the british electricity spot market. J. Politi. Econ. **100**(5), 929–53 (1992)
14. Klemperer, P., Meyer, M.: Supply function equilibria in oligopoly under uncertainty. Econometrica **57**(6), 1243–1277 (1989)
15. Lobato Miguelez, E., Egido Cortes, I., Rouco Rodrguez, L., Lopez Camino, G.: An overview of ancillary services in Spain. Electr. Power Syst. Res. **78**(3), 515–523 (2008)
16. Luo, Z.Q., Pang, J.S., Ralph, D.: Mathematical Programs with Equilibrium Constraints. Cambridge University Press, Cambridge (1996)
17. Oren, S.S., Spiller, P.T., Varaiya, P., Wu, F.: Nodal prices and transmission rights: a critical appraisal. Electr. J. **8**(3), 24–35 (1995)
18. Pereira, M., Pinto, L.: Multi-stage stochastic optimization applied to energy planning. Math. Program. **52**, 359–375 (1991)

19. Philpott, A., Ferris, M., Wets, R.: Equilibrium, uncertainty and risk in hydro-thermal electricity systems. Math. Program. **157**(2), 483–513 (2016)
20. Philpott, A.B., Guan, Z.: On the convergence of stochastic dual dynamic programming and related methods. Oper. Res. Lett. **36**(4), 450–455 (2008)
21. Pritchard, G.: Optimal offering in electric power networks. Pac. J. Optim. **3**(3), 425–438 (2007)
22. Pritchard, G., Zakeri, G., Philpott, A.B.: Nonparametric estimation of market distribution functions in electricity pool markets. Math. Oper. Res. **3**(3), 621–636 (2006)
23. Ralph, D., Smeers, Y.: Risk trading and endogenous probabilities in investment equilibria. SIAM J. Optim. **25**(4), 2589–2611 (2015)
24. Schweppe, F., Caramanis, M., Tabors, R., Bohn, R.: Market Operations in Electric Power Systems. Kluwer, Boston (1988)

Chapter 3
Power and Sample Size Considerations in Psychometrics

Clemens Draxler and Klaus D. Kubinger

Abstract An overview and discussion of the latest developments regarding power and sample size determination for statistical tests of assumptions of psychometric models are given. Theoretical as well as computational issues and simulation techniques, respectively, are considered. The treatment of the topic includes maximum likelihood and least squares procedures applied in the framework of generalized linear (mixed) models. Numerical examples and comparisons of the procedures to be introduced are quoted.

Keywords Psychometrics · Power and sample size · Conditional maximum likelihood · Rasch model · Conditional tests · Analysis of variance

3.1 Introduction

The development and the application of psychometric models including techniques of estimation of model parameters and statistical tests of model assumptions have experienced a rapid growth in recent decades. Classical frequentist as well as Bayesian approaches to statistical inference have been treated and applied extensively in psychometric literature. An overview is given by, for example, Rao and Sinharay [21]. Strangely, power and sample size considerations in the classical (frequentist) sense have been neglected for a long time. Reasons may be the influence of nuisance parameters on the precision of inferential statements about the parameters of interest and the difficulty of predetermining a reasonable level of precision (e.g., the deviation from the hypothesis to be tested or the length of a confidence interval) which depends on the practical context.

C. Draxler (✉)
University for Health and Life Sciences, EWZ 1, 6060 Hall, Austria
e-mail: clemens.draxler@umit.at

K. D. Kubinger
Faculty of Psychology, University of Vienna, Liebiggasse 5, 1010 Vienna, Austria
e-mail: klaus.kubinger@univie.ac.at

J. Pilz et al. (eds.), *Statistics and Simulation*, Springer Proceedings in Mathematics & Statistics 231, https://doi.org/10.1007/978-3-319-76035-3_3

This summary chapter refers to these issues and their related problems. It reviews and discusses the latest advancements concerning power and sample size planning in psychometrics developed by [5–7] on the one hand and by [11, 12, 30] on the other hand. The treatment refers to generalized linear models [1, 14, 15] and the exponential family of probability distributions (e.g., [4]). It is concerned with both maximum likelihood and least squares approaches. Statistical tests derived from asymptotic theory are considered as well as so-called exact tests based on discrete probability distributions. Results quoted are either derived analytically or from numerical procedures. The focus lies on the Rasch model [8, 23].

3.2 Power and Sample Size in a Conditional Maximum Likelihood Framework

Draxler and Alexandrowicz [6] treat questions of sample size computations within the scope of the conditional maximum likelihood (CML) approach [3] and refer to the trinity of Wald [27], score [20, 24], and likelihood ratio tests [16, 28]. Let $f(\boldsymbol{y}, \boldsymbol{\theta}, \boldsymbol{\tau})$ denote a probability distribution (density or mass function) of the random vector $\boldsymbol{Y}$ of the natural exponential family indexed by the parameter vectors $\boldsymbol{\theta}$ and $\boldsymbol{\tau}$ taking values in natural parameter spaces Θ and T. The vector $\boldsymbol{\theta}$ is treated as the parameter of interest and $\boldsymbol{\tau}$ as a nuisance parameter vector. Denote by $\boldsymbol{T}(\boldsymbol{Y})$ a vector-valued sufficient statistic for $\boldsymbol{\tau}$ with probability distribution $g(\boldsymbol{t}, \boldsymbol{\theta}, \boldsymbol{\tau})$. Consider the sequence of independent random vectors $\boldsymbol{Y}_1, \ldots, \boldsymbol{Y}_n$, a sample of n independent observations, and their sufficient statistics $\boldsymbol{T}(\boldsymbol{Y}_1), \ldots, \boldsymbol{T}(\boldsymbol{Y}_n)$ with respective distributions $f(\boldsymbol{y}_i, \boldsymbol{\theta}, \boldsymbol{\tau}_i)$ and $g(\boldsymbol{t}_i, \boldsymbol{\theta}, \boldsymbol{\tau}_i)$, for $i = 1, \ldots, n$. Given $\boldsymbol{T}(\boldsymbol{Y}_i) = \boldsymbol{t}(\boldsymbol{y}_i)$, the conditional probability distribution $h(\boldsymbol{y}_i, \boldsymbol{\theta} \mid \boldsymbol{T}_i = \boldsymbol{t}_i) = f(\cdot)/g(\cdot)$, $g(\cdot) > 0$, does not depend on $\boldsymbol{\tau}_i$ $\forall$ i so that one obtains by

$$L(\boldsymbol{\theta}) = \sum_{i=1}^{n} \log[h(\boldsymbol{y}_i, \boldsymbol{\theta} \mid \boldsymbol{T}_i = \boldsymbol{t}_i)] \tag{3.1}$$

the logarithm of the conditional likelihood as a function of the parameter of interest $\boldsymbol{\theta}$ only and by

$$\hat{\boldsymbol{\theta}} = \arg\max_{\boldsymbol{\theta} \in \Theta} L(\boldsymbol{\theta}) \tag{3.2}$$

the CML estimate. The properties of the CML estimator are established by [3, 18] by proving a number of convergence theorems. Its asymptotic distribution is multivariate normal with mean vector $\boldsymbol{\theta}$ and covariance matrix $\boldsymbol{\Sigma}(\boldsymbol{\theta}) = \boldsymbol{I}(\boldsymbol{\theta})^{-1}$, where the Fisher information matrix is obtained by

$$\boldsymbol{I}(\boldsymbol{\theta}) = -E\left[\frac{\partial^2 L(\boldsymbol{\theta})}{\partial\boldsymbol{\theta}\partial\boldsymbol{\theta}'}\right]. \tag{3.3}$$

The latter is assumed to be positive definite. The presupposed regularity conditions generally hold for the exponential family except the following very mild condition. Roughly speaking, too many too large absolute values in the sequence of the nuisance parameters have to be excluded for the CML estimator to be (weakly) consistent. In a practical context, one will mostly be safe to assume this condition to be satisfied. Further considerations regarding power and sample size computations depend on the asymptotic properties of the CML estimator.

The precision of inferential statements about $\boldsymbol{\theta}$ and thus also power and sample size of tests of hypotheses regarding $\boldsymbol{\theta}$ obviously depend on the covariance of the estimator $\hat{\boldsymbol{\theta}}$. To attain a desired level of precision, the rate of decrease of Cov($\hat{\boldsymbol{\theta}}$) or equivalently the rate of increase of the Fisher information with increasing sample size n must be known. Unfortunately, this is not the case since the information depends on the unknown distributions of the sequence of sufficient statistics $\boldsymbol{T}_1, \ldots, \boldsymbol{T}_n$ which themselves depend on the sequence of the unknown nuisance parameters $\boldsymbol{\tau}_1,\ldots,\boldsymbol{\tau}_n$. It is an obvious consequence of the assumption that the $\boldsymbol{Y}$s need not be identically distributed. By rewriting the information matrix as

$$\boldsymbol{I}(\boldsymbol{\theta}) = -E\left[\frac{\partial^2 L(\boldsymbol{\theta})}{\partial\boldsymbol{\theta}\partial\boldsymbol{\theta}'}\right] = -\sum_{i=1}^{n} E\left\{\frac{\partial^2 \log[h(\boldsymbol{y}_i, \boldsymbol{\theta} \mid \boldsymbol{T}_i = \boldsymbol{t}_i)]}{\partial\boldsymbol{\theta}\partial\boldsymbol{\theta}'}\right\} \tag{3.4}$$

it can be seen that the information depends on the observed sequence of the sufficient statistics $\boldsymbol{T}_1 = \boldsymbol{t}_1, \ldots, \boldsymbol{T}_n = \boldsymbol{t}_n$. Since the summands on the right-hand side of (3.4), the separate pieces of information, need not be equal given different observed values of the sufficient statistics, the total information in the sample does not only depend on the total number of observations n but on the particular sequence $\boldsymbol{T}_1 = \boldsymbol{t}_1, \ldots, \boldsymbol{T}_n = \boldsymbol{t}_n$ observed. This is a problem for planning the power and sample size in experiments (before the data have been collected) since the $\boldsymbol{T}$s are random and it cannot be planned (deterministically) which values to be observed. As a consequence [6], introduce an additional assumption on the nuisance parameters so that a common distribution for the $\boldsymbol{T}$s is obtained which, besides, has another advantage. By choosing an appropriate distribution, it may be avoided to observe too many too large absolute values of the nuisance parameters meeting the requirements for the CML estimator $\hat{\boldsymbol{\theta}}$ to be consistent. Let the sequence of nuisance parameters be independent and identically distributed with probability density function $\varphi(\boldsymbol{\tau}) = \varphi(\boldsymbol{\tau}_1) = \cdots = \varphi(\boldsymbol{\tau}_n)$ so that

$$g(\boldsymbol{t}, \boldsymbol{\theta}) = \int g(\boldsymbol{t}_1, \boldsymbol{\theta}, \boldsymbol{\tau}_1)\varphi(\boldsymbol{\tau}_1)\mathrm{d}\boldsymbol{\tau}_1 = \cdots = \int g(\boldsymbol{t}_n, \boldsymbol{\theta}, \boldsymbol{\tau}_n)\varphi(\boldsymbol{\tau}_n)\mathrm{d}\boldsymbol{\tau}_n. \tag{3.5}$$

It follows for the information matrix

$$\boldsymbol{I}(\boldsymbol{\theta}) = -n\int E\left\{\frac{\partial^2 \log[h(\boldsymbol{y}_i, \boldsymbol{\theta} \mid \boldsymbol{T}_i = \boldsymbol{t}_i)]}{\partial\boldsymbol{\theta}\partial\boldsymbol{\theta}'}\right\} g(\boldsymbol{t}, \boldsymbol{\theta})\mathrm{d}\boldsymbol{t} = n\boldsymbol{H}(\boldsymbol{\theta}), \tag{3.6}$$

where the matrix $\boldsymbol{H}(\boldsymbol{\theta})$ denotes the integral in (3.6) times -1. Hence, given the assumption (3.5) and given $\boldsymbol{\theta}$, the information matrix (3.6) and $\text{Cov}(\hat{\boldsymbol{\theta}})$ are simple (one to one) functions of the sample size n.

Consider testing a class of linear hypotheses given by $\boldsymbol{J\theta} = \boldsymbol{c}$, with $\boldsymbol{c}$ as a vector of constants and $\boldsymbol{J}$ as the Jacobian matrix of the transformation $\boldsymbol{\phi}(\boldsymbol{\theta})$. The latter is assumed to be a vector-valued continuously differentiable function with lower dimensionality than $\boldsymbol{\theta}$. As is well known, the three test statistics of the trinity of testing procedures under consideration will be asymptotically equivalent if $\boldsymbol{J\theta} = \boldsymbol{c}$ is true, with common asymptotic distribution given by the central χ^2 with df = rank($\boldsymbol{J}$). If $\boldsymbol{J\theta} = \boldsymbol{c}$ does not hold asymptotic equivalence and a common distribution will only be obtained under an additional technical assumption of a sequence of alternative hypotheses (or contiguous alternative). This is a rather general result quoted by many authors. For details, the reader is referred to [6] and the references quoted therein. For computational purposes of planning the sample size, a deviation from the hypothesis to be tested must be chosen depending on practical considerations concerning the consequences of the error of the second kind of the statistical test. Provided the predetermined deviation is not too far from $\boldsymbol{J\theta} = \boldsymbol{c}$, the distributions of the test statistics are well approximated by the non-central χ^2 density with df = rank($\boldsymbol{J}$) and non-centrality parameter λ as a (quadratic) function of the chosen deviation and the sample size n (e.g., [1, 9, 10]. For the CML case and the Rasch model, results of a Monte Carlo analysis quoted by [6] hint at quite satisfying approximations of the distributions of the test statistics by the non-central χ^2 family for different levels of deviations chosen from a range of particular interest in practice. Poor approximations have only been observed in cases where the chosen deviation is tremendously large and thus unrealistic in practice. Regarding the likelihood ratio test statistic, a more extensive Monte Carlo analysis with very detailed results is provided by [2].

Let $\boldsymbol{\theta} = \boldsymbol{\theta}_1$ be a vector defining a deviation from the hypothesis to be tested so that $\boldsymbol{J\theta}_1 \neq \boldsymbol{c}$ and denote by λ_0 the particular value of the non-centrality parameter of the χ^2 distribution with df = rank($\boldsymbol{J}$) for which the β quantile equals the value of the $1 - \alpha$ quantile of the central χ^2 (with the same degrees of freedom), where α and β are the probabilities for the errors of the first and second kind of the statistical test. The sample size of the tests can be determined by replacing all random quantities (functions of the observations) in the expressions of the test statistics by their expectations evaluated at $\boldsymbol{\theta} = \boldsymbol{\theta}_1$. Then, the expectations of the test statistics are set equal to the expectation of the non-central χ^2 distribution with df = rank($\boldsymbol{J}$) and non-centrality parameter λ_0. Given $\boldsymbol{\theta} = \boldsymbol{\theta}_1$ and the assumption on the distributions of the sufficient statistics given by (3.5), the expectations of all three test statistics are one-dimensional functions of the sample size n so that the (three) equality restrictions simply have to be solved according to n. In all three cases, explicit solutions exist. Exemplarily, for the Wald test statistic W, one obtains

$$E\left\{\chi^2\left[\text{df} = \text{rank}(\boldsymbol{J}), \lambda_0\right]\right\} = E\left[W(\boldsymbol{\theta}_1)\right] \tag{3.7}$$

$$\lambda_0 + \text{rank}(\boldsymbol{J}) = (\boldsymbol{J}\boldsymbol{\theta}_1 - \boldsymbol{c})' \left[\boldsymbol{J}' n^{-1} \boldsymbol{H}(\boldsymbol{\theta}_1)^{-1} \boldsymbol{J}\right]^{-1} (\boldsymbol{J}\boldsymbol{\theta}_1 - \boldsymbol{c}) + \text{rank}(\boldsymbol{J}) \tag{3.8}$$

$$n = \text{ceil}\left\{\frac{\lambda_0}{(\boldsymbol{J}\boldsymbol{\theta}_1 - \boldsymbol{c})' \left[\boldsymbol{J}' \boldsymbol{H}(\boldsymbol{\theta}_1)^{-1} \boldsymbol{J}\right]^{-1} (\boldsymbol{J}\boldsymbol{\theta}_1 - \boldsymbol{c})}\right\}. \tag{3.9}$$

Regarding score and likelihood ratio tests, the sample size is determined on the same lines but the derivation of their expectations is slightly more complicated. For details, one is referred to [6].

3.3 Power of Pseudo-Exact or Conditional Tests of Assumptions of the Rasch Model

The following considerations are restricted to the Rasch model and are based on a Markov Chain Monte Carlo (MCMC) approach developed by [25]. Draxler and Zessin [7] discuss the power function of conditional or pseudo-exact tests which may be viewed as generalizations (multivariate and more general covariances) of Fisher's well-known exact test. The exact discrete probability distributions under the hypothesis to be tested and under a given deviation and the power function of the tests, respectively, are well approximated using the cited MCMC technique.

The Rasch model determines the discrete probability distributions of a number of persons indexed by $i = 1, \ldots, n$ to a number of items indexed by $j = 1, \ldots, k$. Let $Y_{ij} \in \{0, 1\}$ be the binary response of person i to item j and consider a $n \times k$ matrix with entries given by the binary responses of every person to every item. Given the observed values of all row sums $R_1 = r_1, \ldots, R_n = r_n$ and all column sums $C_1 = c_1, \ldots, C_k = c_k$, the conditional probability distribution of all free Bernoulli variables (binary responses) is discrete uniform and simply obtained by the reciprocal number of (possible) matrices not violating the given row and column sums of the observed matrix. The exact distribution of any suitable test statistic under the hypothesis to be tested can easily be derived from this conditional distribution. A number of practically interesting examples are quoted by [19]. The conditional distribution of a test statistic under a given deviation from the hypothesis to be tested and the power of the respective conditional test may also be derived from the uniform distribution as shown by [7]. Counting the total exact number of matrices with fixed row and column sums is a complicated problem in realistic cases with the usual numbers of persons and items. Thus, for computational purposes, the exact distributions and exact power may be sufficiently approximated by random sampling from the uniform distribution of matrices with given row and column sums which is well accomplished by the application of a MCMC approach suggested by [25].

A general expression of the power function of conditional tests may be derived as follows. Consider a generalization of the Rasch model determining the discrete probability distribution of the binary response Y_{ij}. Denote it by $P(Y_{ij} = y_{ij} \mid \boldsymbol{X} = \boldsymbol{x})$, with $\boldsymbol{X}$ as a (random) vector of covariates or a vector of any responses (of any persons to any items) other than Y_{ij} on which Y_{ij} may depend. The distribution $P(\cdot)$ is indexed by a parameter vector $\boldsymbol{\eta}$, and it is assumed that the logit of $P(\cdot)$ is linear in $\boldsymbol{\eta}$. Restricting the parameter space of $\boldsymbol{\eta}$ so that the Rasch model is obtained as a special case yields the hypothesis to be tested. Given $\boldsymbol{X} = \boldsymbol{x}$ and $\boldsymbol{\eta}$, all binary responses are assumed to be independent so that their joint probability distribution is obtained by the product over all persons and items. Let Ω denote the sample space which consists of all $n \times k$ matrices with given row and column sums. Then, it follows for the joint conditional distribution

$$P(\boldsymbol{Y} = \boldsymbol{y} \mid \boldsymbol{X} = \boldsymbol{x}, R_1 = r_1, \ldots, R_n = r_n, C_1 = c_1, \ldots, C_k = c_k) = \frac{\prod_{i=1}^{n} \prod_{j=1}^{k} P(Y_{ij} = y_{ij} \mid \boldsymbol{X} = \boldsymbol{x})}{\sum_{\Omega} \prod_{i=1}^{n} \prod_{j=1}^{k} P(Y_{ij} = y_{ij} \mid \boldsymbol{X} = \boldsymbol{x})}, \tag{3.10}$$

where $\boldsymbol{Y}$ consists of all free Bernoulli variables (binary responses). Let $C \subseteq \Omega$ be the critical region with size α of the conditional test of the hypothesis of any restriction of the parameter space of $\boldsymbol{\eta}$ yielding the Rasch model. The power function $\beta(\boldsymbol{\eta})$ of this test is then easily obtained by summation of (3.10) over all elements in C.

The denominator on the right-hand side of (3.10) is a normalizing constant. The summation has to be taken over the complete set Ω. In practice, for computational purposes, a random sample of matrices from Ω is drawn so that the summation has only to be taken over all matrices drawn. For this purpose, for instance, the R package Rasch Sampler [26] may be used. The conditional distribution of $\boldsymbol{Y}$, the size α of the critical region C, and the power function of the test can be approximated in this way. The critical region C will be most powerful at level α if it is chosen according to the fundamental lemma of [17]. Thus, it has to be composed of those $100\alpha\%$ of matrices from Ω yielding the largest values of (3.10).

An example of the parameterization of the general model which is of particular interest in practice assumes the Rasch model to hold conditionally on an additional covariate. For simplicity, consider a fixed (not random) binary covariate $x_i \in \{0, 1\}$, for instance sex. Then,

$$P(Y_{ij} = y_{ij} \mid x_i) = \frac{\exp\left[y_{ij}(\theta_i + \beta_j + \delta_j x_i)\right]}{1 + \exp(\theta_i + \beta_j + \delta_j x_i)}. \tag{3.11}$$

Factorization of the product of (3.11) over all persons and items immediately shows that the statistics $R_i = \sum_j Y_{ij}$, $C_j = \sum_i Y_{ij}$ and $T_j = \sum_i Y_{ij} x_i$ are sufficient for the parameters θ_i, β_j, and δ_j so that for the joint conditional distribution of the Ts one obtains

$$P(\boldsymbol{T} = \boldsymbol{t} \mid x_1, \ldots, x_n, R_1 = r_1, \ldots, R_n = r_n, C_1 = c_1, \ldots, C_k = c_k) = \frac{\sum_{\mathrm{T}} \exp\left(\sum_{j=1}^{k} t_j \delta_j\right)}{\sum_{\Omega} \exp\left(\sum_{j=1}^{k} t_j \delta_j\right)}, \quad (3.12)$$

with $\boldsymbol{T}' = (T_1, \ldots, T_{k-1})$. Note that one of the Ts is not free. The summation in the numerator of the right side of (3.12) has to be taken over the subset $\mathrm{T} \subseteq \Omega$ consisting of those matrices contained in Ω which satisfy $\boldsymbol{T} = \boldsymbol{t}$. The parameters $\theta_i \in \mathbb{R}$ and $\beta_j \in \mathbb{R}$ are person and item parameters which are treated as nuisance by conditioning on the observed values of their sufficient statistics, and $\delta_j \in \mathbb{R}$ is characterizing a violation of the assumption of the Rasch model of independence of the items of the covariate. Thus, δ_j is the conditional effect of item j given the covariate. For identifiability reasons, let $\delta_k = 0$ or $\sum \delta_j = 0$. Note that in this example, the θ parameters (person parameters) are nuisance parameters. This is inconsistent with the notation introduced. This is only for a notational convenience in psychometric literature (e.g., [8]).

A second example concerns a conditional test of the assumption of local independence of the responses of a person to the items. Consider the following model

$$P(Y_{i2} = y_{i2} \mid Y_{i1} = y_{i1}) \propto \exp\left[y_{i2}(\theta_i + \beta_2 + \vartheta y_{i1})\right] \quad (3.13)$$

which introduces local dependence of item 2 on item 1. The probability distributions of the binary responses of all persons to all other items (except item 2) are assumed to be given by the Rasch model. Unlike the previous example, in this case, the joint conditional distribution of all free binary responses and the power function of the conditional test of $\vartheta = 0$ is not only a function of the parameter of interest ϑ characterizing a violation of the assumption of local independence (of item 2 on item 1) but of all parameters (since the row and column sums of the matrix of responses are not sufficient for the person and item parameters). In practice, it seems to be rather difficult to choose reasonable values for all parameters of the model, in particular for the person parameters, so that the power can be computed.

Finally, a numerical example from [7] shall be presented but using different seeds for the pseudo-random number generator (so that the results will not be identical). It refers to the model given by (3.11) and (3.12), respectively, and is concerned with power computations of the conditional test of the hypothesis that all δs are equal to 0 with size $\alpha = 0.05$. Consider $n = 100$ persons and $k = 15$ items. The column sums of the observed matrix of binary responses are between 4 and 97. The row sums have large frequencies for values in the middle of the possible range and low frequencies for values near 0 and 15. For one half of the total number of respondents, the covariate takes the value 1, and for the other half, it is 0. Item 9 is chosen as the only deviating item, where item 9 is an item with a given column sum of 53 which is roughly in the middle of the possible range of values. The power is computed for different values of δ_9 deviating from 0. The R Package Rasch Sampler is used to

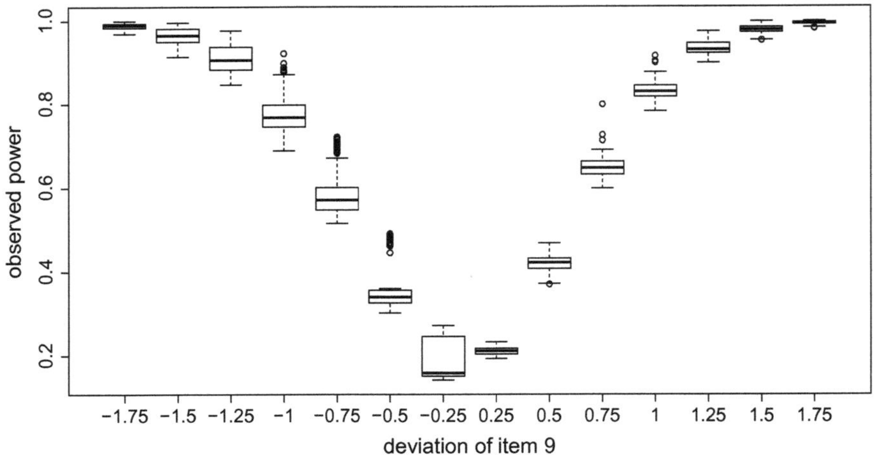

Fig. 3.1 Summaries of power computations of conditional tests of the hypothesis that all δs in (3.11) and (3.12), respectively, equal 0 considered as a function of δ_9 (deviation of item 9)

sample from Ω. For every chosen δ_9 value, 8000 matrices are drawn, and for each matrix, its conditional probability is computed using (3.12). The critical region C is chosen to consist of the 5% of matrices (400 matrices) with the largest values of (3.12). The power is computed by summation of the conditional probabilities over all matrices in *C*. This procedure is replicated 100 times to observe the precision of the approximation of the exact power. Figure 3.1 shows summaries of the results.

3.4 Linear Models and Least Squares Approach

Starting traditionally, one has to realize that most statistical tests of assumptions of the Rasch model apply test statistics which are (asymptotically) χ^2 distributed. These test statistics' degrees of freedom do not depend on the sample size but only on the number of parameters estimated. In the following, an approach is discussed where the number of degrees of freedom does depend on the sample size so that it can be used for power and sample size considerations. Kubinger, Rasch, and Yanagida [11, 12, 30] aimed for some F-distributed test statistic within the framework of analysis of variance. In general, such an approach provides a variety of procedures for power and sample size planning, whether there are one- or multi-way designs, whether there is the case of models with fixed or random effects or a mixed model, and whether the factors are crossed, nested, or mixed classified.

Since the Rasch model is a generalized linear model with logit link function, the idea of testing assumptions of the model within the framework of analysis of variance (linear models with identity link) may sound strange at first sight, but surprisingly, it works pretty well. Consider a three-way analysis of variance of the kind

$(A \succ \boldsymbol{B}) \times C$, with A as a fixed factor characterizing a covariate associated with the persons, for instance the persons′ sex, C as another fixed factor with levels given by the different items and $\boldsymbol{B}$ as a random factor with levels given by the persons (which are assumed to be drawn randomly from the population). The latter is nested within the levels of A. Hence, linear effects of the factors on the expectations of Bernoulli variables (the binary responses of persons to items) are assumed. Of interest is the hypothesis that there is no interaction effect $A \times C$. It is tested using a F test statistic obtained by dividing the mean of squares of the interaction $A \times C$ by the mean of squares of the interaction $\boldsymbol{B} \times C$ within A. Roughly speaking, providing the number of levels of A is restricted to two, this approach may be viewed as equivalent to considering the logit model given by (3.11) and testing the hypothesis that all δs (conditional effect parameters or the interaction of the covariate and the items) equal 0.

It is obvious that the probability distribution of the test statistic introduced cannot be assumed to belong to a known family of distributions, like F, since the distributions of the binary responses of persons to items cannot be of the class of normal distributions. Rasch, Rusch, Simeckova, Kubinger, Moder, and Simecek [22] provide results of a simulation study obtaining actual type I risks sometimes far exceeding the nominal level (up to five times as high). Thus, power and sample size computations have been based on numerical procedures approximating the probability distributions of the test statistic under the hypothesis to be tested as well as under a given deviation. In doing so, Kubinger, Rasch, and Yanagida [11] showed that their approach will only work if no main effect of A exists. Strictly speaking, the nominal type I risk of the statistical test of the hypothesis of no interaction $A \times C$ holds as long as no main effect of A is assumed; otherwise, the type I risk will be far too high.

3.5 Numerical Examples and Comparisons

In the following, a few numerical examples are quoted comparing the power of the χ^2 tests with the F test introduced. The size of the tests is predetermined as $\alpha = 0.05$ (nominal type I risk). The hypothesis to be tested assumes equality of the item parameters of the Rasch model between two groups of persons. The number of persons is chosen to be 300 in each of both groups, and the person parameters are drawn from the standard normal distribution. The number of items is chosen as $k = 15$. Under the hypothesis to be tested, it is assumed that the item parameters are given by -3.5, -3, -2.5, -2, -1.5, -1, -0.5, 0, 0.5, 1, 1.5, 2, 2.5, 3, and 3.5 in both groups (equality of item parameters between the groups).

The following scenarios of deviations from this hypothesis are considered. In each case, two items are considered as deviating items. The respective columns in Tables 3.1 and 3.2 quote the absolute deviations of the two deviating items from the respective values assumed under the hypothesis to be tested within both groups of persons. For example, referring to the first row and first column of Table 3.1, the parameter of item 7 is 0.1 smaller than the value under the hypothesis to be tested (so that it equals -0.6), whereas the parameter of item 9 is 0.1 larger (so that it equals

0.6) in the first group of persons. In the second group, the deviations are exactly the other way round (deviations of reversed sign). Thus, the absolute differences of the item parameters of the two items between the two groups are both 0.2 (symmetrically around the value assumed under the hypothesis to be tested).

The power for the Wald test is computed using the relations given by (3.7)–(3.9), where the distribution of each $\boldsymbol{\tau}$ (which corresponds to the person parameter in the Rasch model) is assumed to be the standard normal. The common distribution $g(\boldsymbol{t}, \boldsymbol{\theta})$ of the sufficient statistics for the $\boldsymbol{\tau}$ s is obtained using numerical integration (Gauss–Hermite). The power of the F tests is computed using simulation procedures provided by the R package pwrRasch [29]. The number of simulation runs (number of replications) is chosen to be 3600. Tables 3.1 and 3.2 show the results for all considered scenarios of deviations.

Table 3.1 Power computations for Wald and F tests referring to scenarios with deviating items 7 and 9 as well as 5 and 11

Abs. deviation of items 7 and 9	Wald test	F test	Abs. deviation of items 5 and 11	Wald test	F test
0.1	0.12	0.18 (0.07)	0.1	0.1	0.12 (0.06)
0.15	0.24	0.38 (0.07)	0.15	0.18	0.23 (0.06)
0.2	0.44	0.63 (0.07)	0.2	0.31	0.39 (0.06)
0.25	0.68	0.84 (0.06)	0.25	0.5	0.59 (0.06)
0.3	0.86	0.95 (0.07)	0.3	0.69	0.78 (0.07)
0.35	0.96	0.99 (0.07)	0.35	0.85	0.91 (0.06)
0.4	1	1 (0.06)	0.4	0.94	0.97 (0.06)
0.45	1	1 (0.06)	0.45	0.98	0.99 (0.07)

Note. The observed level of the type I risk of the F tests is quoted in parenthesis

Table 3.2 Power computations for Wald and F tests referring to scenarios with deviating items 3 and 13 as well as 1 and 15

Abs. deviation of items 3 and 13	Wald test	F test	Abs. deviation of items 1 and 15	Wald test	F test
0.1	0.08	0.08 (0.06)	0.1	0.06	0.07 (0.06)
0.15	0.11	0.1 (0.07)	0.15	0.06	0.07 (0.06)
0.2	0.18	0.13 (0.06)	0.2	0.07	0.07 (0.06)
0.25	0.27	0.2 (0.07)	0.25	0.09	0.08 (0.06)
0.3	0.4	0.28 (0.07)	0.3	0.11	0.09 (0.06)
0.35	0.54	0.39 (0.07)	0.35	0.13	0.11 (0.07)
0.4	0.68	0.52 (0.07)	0.4	0.16	0.12 (0.06)
0.45	0.8	0.66 (0.07)	0.45	0.2	0.14 (0.06)
0.5	0.89	0.8 (0.07)	0.5	0.24	0.17 (0.07)
0.55	0.95	0.89 (0.06)	0.55	0.29	0.2 (0.06)

Note. The observed level of the type I risk of the F tests is quoted in parenthesis

The main implication of the results is to be expected from theory and may be stated as follows. In terms of power, the F test performs better than the Wald test in the cases shown in Table 3.1, whereas its performance is worse in the cases shown in Table 3.2. Table 3.1 refers to examples in which the parameter values of the two deviating items are approximately in the middle of the assumed range of values matching the (assumed) mean of the distribution of person parameters. Consequently, the majority of expectations of the binary responses of persons to the respective deviating items are around 0.5, and for an expectation in a close interval around 0.5, the dependence on the assumed factors is close to linearity as is assumed in the linear modeling framework of analysis of variance. On the contrary, Table 3.2 refers to scenarios assuming the expectations of the binary responses to both deviating items to be farther from 0.5 and thus closer to the natural boundaries 0 and 1 so that the assumed linear dependence (of the expectation on the factors) is more inappropriate.

It must also be remarked that the F test seems to be biased, but the bias seems to be small. At least, this is what can be observed in the examples considered. In all scenarios, the observed type I risk is slightly larger than the nominal one as is seen by the values in parenthesis in both tables.

3.6 Discussion

In the analysis of psychometric data, one is usually confronted with nuisance parameters influencing the precision of inferential statements about parameters of interest. One way of eliminating the effect of nuisance parameters is conditioning on the observed values of their sufficient statistics and pursuing the well-known CML approach, respectively, which is, for instance, applicable for the class of Rasch models. When the data and in particular the sufficient statistics (as functions of the data) have already been observed, such an approach allows for estimating the parameters of interest and testing hypotheses about them. It is even possible to compute the power of statistical tests post hoc. Before observing the data, like in cases the sample size of an experiment is to be planned in advance, the CML approach is obviously not applicable without additional assumptions on the nuisance parameters and their sufficient statistics as discussed by [6]. Thus, one may argue that in this case CML as well as the consideration of conditional tests described in Sect. 3.3 is not suitable solutions of the problem of the influence of nuisance parameters.

Developing this thought further, one may arrive at another common approach of dealing with nuisance parameters termed as marginal maximum likelihood which is widely used for psychometric models. This approach assumes a probability distribution for the nuisance parameters since in most applications the nuisance parameters are treated as random variables anyway (since they are assumed to be drawn randomly from the population). Maydeu-Olivares and Montano [13] used the marginal maximum likelihood framework to develop procedures for power and sample size computations for a few particular statistical tests of assumptions of psychometric models.

Another point worth discussing is the problem of predetermining a deviation from the hypothesis to be tested in practice (for the computation of power and sample size, respectively). In most applications, not only one but multiple parameters are of interest and the practical meaning of a deviation from the parameter value to be tested usually differs from one parameter to the other and depends on the practical context as well. A suitable contribution on this topic is provided by [5] describing a three-step procedure facilitating the evaluation of the practical meaning of deviations from the hypothesis to be tested.

An essential difference between the conditional tests based on discrete probability distributions and all other approaches described in this summary chapter is that the conditional tests are one-sided. Hence, the power of these tests is expected to be considerably larger so that comparisons with the χ^2 and F tests (in terms of power) do not make much sense. From the practical point of view, one-sided tests may be less suitable in the context of psychometric modeling since one is usually interested in the question whether model assumptions hold or not. The directions or signs of deviations from the parameter values to be tested do not play an important role.

Finally, some comments on the utility of the F test shall be discussed. Power computations depend on Monte Carlo procedures. On the one hand, it is nice to have an R package providing the necessary numerical procedures for the approximation of the power of the tests. On the other hand, the computation of the power with the R package pwrRasch is restricted to tests of hypotheses of the following type. Regarding every single parameter of interest, exactly one value has to be chosen. That is, the item parameters have to be chosen for both groups of persons and under the hypothesis to be tested they are chosen so that they are equal between both groups (like it is described in the first two paragraphs of Sect. 3.5). Such a hypothesis is usually not the hypothesis one is interested in. Of interest is the hypothesis that the differences between the item parameters equal 0. The problem is that the power of the test does not only depend on the difference of an item parameter between the groups but also on the level on which this difference is assumed (whether it is an easy or difficult item that possibly differs between two groups) and, again, the latter is usually not of interest in an application and it will hardly ever be possible to reasonably predetermine it. Furthermore, the procedure is restricted to the Rasch model and to the question of group differences. Tests of other important assumptions of the model like local independence and equal item discriminations are excluded.

References

1. Agresti, A.: Categorical Data Analysis, 2nd edn. Wiley, New York (2002)
2. Alexandrowicz, R.W., Draxler, C.: Testing the Rasch model with the conditional likelihood ratio test: sample size requirements and bootstrap algorithms. J. Stat. Distrib. Appl. **3**, 1–25 (2016)
3. Andersen, E.B.: Asymptotic properties of conditional maximum likelihood estimators. J. R. Stat. Soc. Ser. B **32**, 283–301 (1970)

4. Barndorff-Nielsen, O.: Information and Exponential Families in Statistical Theory. Wiley, New York (1978)
5. Draxler, C.: Sample size determination for Rasch model tests. Psychometrika **75**, 708–724 (2010)
6. Draxler, C., Alexandrowicz, R.W.: Sample size determination within the scope of conditional maximum likelihood estimation with special focus on testing the Rasch model. Psychometrika **80**, 897–919 (2015)
7. Draxler, C., Zessin, J.: The power function of conditional tests of the Rasch model. Adv. Stat. Anal. **99**, 367–378 (2015)
8. Fischer, G.H., Molenaar, I.W.: Rasch Models-Foundations, Recent Developments and Applications. Springer, New York (1995)
9. Fleiss, J.L.: Statistical Methods for Rates and Proportions, 2nd edn. Wiley, New York (1981)
10. Haberman, S.J.: Tests for independence in two-way contingency tables based on canonical correlation and on linear-by-linear interaction. Ann. Stat. **9**, 1178–1186 (1981)
11. Kubinger, K.D., Rasch, D., Yanagida, T.: On designing data-sampling for Rasch model calibrating an achievement test. Psychol. Sci. Q. **51**, 370–384 (2009)
12. Kubinger, K.D., Rasch, D., Yanagida, T.: A new approach for testing the Rasch model. Educ. Res. Eval. **17**, 321–333 (2011)
13. Maydeu-Olivares, A., Montano, R.: How should we assess the fit of Rasch-type models? approximating the power of goodness-of-fit statistics in categorical data analysis. Psychometrika **78**, 116–133 (2013)
14. McCullagh, P., Nelder, J.A.: Generalized Linear Models, 2nd edn. Chapman & Hall, New York (1989)
15. Nelder, J.A., Wedderburn, R.W.M.: Generalized linear models. J. R. Stat. Soc. Ser. A **135**, 370–384 (1972)
16. Neyman, J., Pearson, E.S.: On the use and interpretation of certain test criteria for purposes of statistical inference. Biometrika **20A**, 263–294 (1928)
17. Neyman, J., Pearson, E.S.: On the problem of the most efficient tests of statistical hypotheses. Philos. Trans. R. Soc. Lond. Ser. A Contain. Pap. Math. Phys. Character **231**, 289–337 (1933)
18. Pfanzagl, J.: On the consistency of conditional maximum likelihood estimators. Ann. Inst. Stat. Math. **45**, 703–719 (1993)
19. Ponocny, I.: Nonparametric goodness-of-fit tests for the Rasch model. Psychometrika **66**, 437–460 (2001)
20. Rao, C.R.: Large sample tests of statistical hypotheses concerning several parameters with applications to problems of estimation. Proc. Camb. Philos. Soc. **44**, 50–57 (1948)
21. Rao, C.R., Sinharay, S.: Psychometrics. Handbook of Statistics, vol. 26. Elsevier, Amsterdam (2007)
22. Rasch, D., Rusch, T., Simeckova, M., Kubinger, K.D., Moder, K., Simecek, P.: Tests of additivity in mixed and fixed effect two-way ANOVA models with single sub-class numbers. Stat. Pap. **50**, 905–916 (2009)
23. Rasch, G.: Probabilistic models for some intelligence and attainment tests. Copenhagen: The Danish Institute of Education Research (1980). (Expanded Edition, 1980. Chicago: University of Chicago Press)
24. Silvey, S.D.: The Lagrangian multiplier test. Ann. Math. Stat. **30**, 389–407 (1959)
25. Verhelst, N.D.: An efficient MCMC algorithm to sample binary matrices with fixed marginals. Psychometrika **73**, 705–728 (2008)
26. Verhelst, N.D., Hatzinger, R., Mair, P.: The Rasch sampler. J. Stat. Softw. **20**, 1–14 (2007)
27. Wald, A.: Test of statistical hypotheses concerning several parameters when the number of observations is large. Trans. Am. Math. Soc. **54**, 426–482 (1943)
28. Wilks, S.S.: The large sample distribution of the likelihood ratio for testing composite hypotheses. Ann. Math. Stat. **9**, 60–62 (1938)
29. Yanagida, T., Steinfeld, J.: pwrRasch: Statistical power simulation for testing the Rasch model. R package version 0.1-2 (2015). http://CRAN.R-project.org/package=pwrRasch
30. Yanagida, T., Kubinger, K.D., Rasch, D.: Planning a study for testing the Rasch model given missing values due to the use of test-booklets. J. Appl. Meas. **16**, 432–444 (2015)

Chapter 4
Bootstrap Change Point Testing for Dependent Data

Zuzana Prášková

Abstract Critical values of change point tests in location and regression models are usually based on limit distribution of the respective test statistics under the null hypothesis. However, the limit distribution is very often a functional of some Gaussian processes depending on unknown quantities that cannot be easily estimated. In many situations, convergence to the asymptotic distribution is rather slow and the asymptotic critical values are not well applicable in small and moderate samples. It has appeared that resampling methods provide reasonable approximations for critical values of test statistics for detection changes in location and regression models. In this chapter dependent wild bootstrap procedure for testing changes in linear model with weakly dependent regressors and errors will be proposed and its validity verified. More specifically, the concept of L_p-m-approximability will be used.

Keywords Change point · Regression models · Weak dependence
Dependent wild bootstrap

4.1 Introduction

Consider model

$$Y_i = \boldsymbol{x}_i^T \boldsymbol{\beta} + \boldsymbol{x}_i^T \boldsymbol{\delta}_n I\{i > k^*\} + \varepsilon_i, \quad i = 1, \dots, n, \tag{4.1}$$

where $1 < k^* \leq n$ is an unknown change point, $\boldsymbol{x}_i = (x_{i1}, \dots, x_{id})^T$ are regressors, $\boldsymbol{\beta} = (\beta_1, \dots, \beta_d)^T$, $\boldsymbol{\delta}_n = (\delta_{1n}, \dots, \delta_{dn})^T$ are unknown parameters, and ε_i are random errors.

We want to test the null hypothesis: $H_0 : k^* = n$ against the alternative $H_1 : k^* < n$. Typical test statistics for solving the above problem are CUSUM-type test statistics that are based on functionals of cumulative sums of estimated residuals. An example

Z. Prášková (✉)
Faculty of Mathematics and Physics, Charles University,
Sokolovská 83, Prague, Czech Republic
e-mail: praskova@karlin.mff.cuni.cz

J. Pilz et al. (eds.), *Statistics and Simulation*, Springer Proceedings
in Mathematics & Statistics 231, https://doi.org/10.1007/978-3-319-76035-3_4

of such statistic is

$$T_n(h) = \sup_{0<t<1} \left\{ \frac{1}{nh^2(t)} \boldsymbol{S}^T_{\lfloor (n+1)t \rfloor} \widehat{\boldsymbol{\Sigma}}_n^{-1} \boldsymbol{S}_{\lfloor (n+1)t \rfloor} \right\} \tag{4.2}$$

where

$$\boldsymbol{S}_k = \sum_{i=1}^k \boldsymbol{x}_i \widehat{\varepsilon}_i = \sum_{i=1}^k \boldsymbol{x}_i (y_i - \boldsymbol{x}_i^T \widehat{\boldsymbol{\beta}}_n), \quad k = 1, \dots, n,$$

are cumulative sums of weighted least-squares residuals $\widehat{\varepsilon}_i = y_i - \boldsymbol{x}_i^T \widehat{\boldsymbol{\beta}}_n$, $\widehat{\boldsymbol{\beta}}_n$ is the least-squares estimator (LSE) of the parameter $\boldsymbol{\beta}$, $\widehat{\boldsymbol{\Sigma}}_n$ is an estimator of the long-run variance matrix

$$\boldsymbol{\Sigma} = \lim_{n \to \infty} \mathrm{Var}\left(\frac{1}{\sqrt{n}} \sum_{i=1}^n \boldsymbol{x}_i \varepsilon_i \right), \tag{4.3}$$

and finally, h is a positive weight function defined on $(0, 1)$. It can be shown that under quite general conditions discussed below the asymptotic distribution of this statistic under the null hypothesis is the same as the distribution of

$$\sup_{0<t<1} \left\{ \sum_{j=1}^d B_j^2(t)/h^2(t) \right\}$$

where $\{B_j(t), t \in [0,]\}$ are independent Brownian bridges. The distribution of the limiting statistics is known only for the identity function h, otherwise it should be simulated.

An alternative to the limiting distribution can be bootstrap. It is known that bootstrap procedures provide reasonable approximations for the critical values of test statistics constructed to detect changes in location and linear regression models with *independent* observations (see, e.g., Antoch et al. [2], Antoch and Hušková [1, 14], Hušková [13], Hušková and Picek [17]). What concerns dependent observations, Kirch [20] considered a location model with errors supposed to be a linear process and developed the distribution of the test based on the block random permutations of LSE-residuals. Hušková and Kirch [15, 16] considered location model with strong mixing errors and circular block bootstrap based on LSE-residuals, Hušková et al. [19], studied regression and pair bootstrap in a change point problem for an autoregressive process with i.i.d. innovations. We do not deal here with sequential procedures. For references concerning bootstrap in sequential procedures for change point detection, see, e.g., survey papers Horváth and Rice [12], Hušková and Prášková [18] or Kirch [21] respectively. Recently, Sharipov et al. [24] considered block-wise bootstrap for testing change in the mean or in the marginal distribution in a Hilbert space valued random sequences that are near epoch dependent. Bucchia and Wendler [6] used wild dependent bootstrap for testing a change in the mean of ρ-mixing Hilbert space valued random fields. Here we will consider regression model where both the regressors and errors are dependent and develop a modification of the wild dependent bootstrap procedure to approximate critical values of test statistic of type (4.2).

The chapter is further organized as follows. In the next section we formulate assumptions on the regressors and errors under which the asymptotic distribution of test statistic (4.2) holds true and summarize known results. Then we propose a wild bootstrap method and discuss its consistency. In the last section we provide some results of a numerical study.

In the sequel, we will use the following notation: $\|\cdot\|$ will denote the Euclidean norm of a vector or a matrix, and for a vector-valued random variable $\boldsymbol{X}$ we denote $\|\boldsymbol{X}\|_p = \left(\mathsf{E}\|\boldsymbol{X}\|^p\right)^{1/p}, \quad p \geq 1$, the L_p-norm of $\boldsymbol{X}$. We also assume that random variables under consideration are defined on a general probability space $(\Omega, \mathscr{A}, P)$.

4.2 Procedures with Weakly Dependent Regressors and Errors

In this section we consider model (4.1) that satisfies the following assumptions.

Assumptions on the Regressors

(A.1) For any $i \in \mathbb{Z}$, $\boldsymbol{x}_i = \boldsymbol{h}(\boldsymbol{\xi}_i, \boldsymbol{\xi}_{i-1}, \ldots)$, where $\boldsymbol{h}$ is a measurable d-dimensional function, $\{\boldsymbol{\xi}_i : i \in \mathbb{Z}\}$ is a sequence of i.i.d. random vectors (of dimension d_1, say) and $\mathsf{E}\|\boldsymbol{x}_i\|^{4+\Delta} < \infty$ for some $\Delta > 0$; $\mathsf{E}\boldsymbol{x}_i\boldsymbol{x}_i^T = \boldsymbol{C}$ is a positive definite matrix for all $i \in \mathbb{Z}$.

(A.2) For all $i \in \mathbb{Z}$,

$$\sum_{m=1}^{\infty} \|\boldsymbol{x}_i - \boldsymbol{x}_i^{(m)}\|_{2+\Delta} < \infty$$

where

$$\boldsymbol{x}_i^{(m)} = \boldsymbol{h}(\boldsymbol{\xi}_i, \boldsymbol{\xi}_{i-1}, \ldots, \boldsymbol{\xi}_{i-m+1}, \boldsymbol{\xi}_{i-m}^{(m)}, \boldsymbol{\xi}_{i-m-1}^{(m)}, \ldots),$$

$\boldsymbol{\xi}_{i-m}^{(m)}, \boldsymbol{\xi}_{i-m-1}^{(m)}, \ldots$ are i.i.d. with the same distribution as $\boldsymbol{\xi}_0$ and independent of $\{\boldsymbol{\xi}_i\}$,

(A.3) $\{\boldsymbol{x}_i\}$, $\{\varepsilon_i\}$ are independent sequences.

Assumptions on the Errors

(B.1) For any $i \in \mathbb{Z}$, $\varepsilon_i = g(\boldsymbol{\zeta}_i, \boldsymbol{\zeta}_{i-1}, \ldots)$, where g is a measurable function, $\{\boldsymbol{\zeta}_i : i \in \mathbb{Z}\}$ is a sequence of i.i.d. random vectors (of dimension r_1, say) and $\mathsf{E}\varepsilon_i = 0$, $\mathsf{E}|\varepsilon_i|^{4+\Delta} < \infty$ for some $\Delta > 0$.

(B.2) For all $i \in \mathbb{Z}$,

$$\sum_{m=1}^{\infty} |\varepsilon_i - \varepsilon_i^{(m)}|^2 < \infty$$

where

$$\varepsilon_i^{(m)} = g(\boldsymbol{\zeta}_i, \boldsymbol{\zeta}_{i-1}, \ldots, \boldsymbol{\zeta}_{i-m+1}, \boldsymbol{\zeta}_{i-m}^{(m)}, \boldsymbol{\zeta}_{i-m-1}^{(m)}, \ldots),$$

$\boldsymbol{\zeta}_{i-m}^{(m)}, \boldsymbol{\zeta}_{i-m-1}^{(m)}, \ldots$ are i.i.d., independent of $\{\boldsymbol{\zeta}_i\}$, with the same distribution as $\boldsymbol{\zeta}_0$.

Remark 1 Assumptions (A.1) and (B.1) say that the regressors and errors are one-sided Bernoulli shifts (see, e.g., Billingsley [5]) that represent a type of causal dependence, possibly non-linear, which is very often used in time series and econometrics. Assumptions (A.2) and (B.2) follow the concept of L_p-m-approximability and are motivated by the work of Hörmann and Kokoszka [10] and Berkes et al. [3]. The main idea of this concept is to approximate a sequence $\{X_n, n \in \mathbb{Z}\}$ (say) by an m-dependent process $\{X_n^{(m)}, n \in \mathbb{Z}\}$ such that for every n the sequence $\{X_n^{(m)}\}$ converges to X_n sufficiently fast as $m \to \infty$, and then obtain the limiting behaviour of the original process from the corresponding results for m-dependent sequences. This type of weak dependence include linear processes with i.i.d. innovations, NED processes (near epoch dependence) over i.i.d., non-linear sequences generated from i.i.d. innovations, augmented GARCH sequences and many others (see works by Hörmann and Kokoszka [10] and Berkes et al. [3] in which also relations to the strong mixing property and other types of weak dependence are discussed. Using m-dependent approximations also motivated us to consider dependent wild bootstrap procedure, see Sect. 4.3.

Remark 2 Let us note that the sequences $\{\boldsymbol{x}_i : i \in \mathbb{Z}\}$ and $\{\varepsilon_i : i \in \mathbb{Z}\}$ are strictly stationary and ergodic, and $\boldsymbol{x}_i$ and $\boldsymbol{x}_i^{(m)}$ are equally distributed for every $i \in \mathbb{Z}$. Similarly, ε_i and $\varepsilon_i^{(m)}$ are equally distributed for every $i \in \mathbb{Z}$. Moreover, under Assumptions (A.1)–(A.3) and (B.1)–(B.2), according to Lemma 2.1 and Theorem 4.2 in Hörmann and Kokoszka [10], $\{\boldsymbol{x}_i \varepsilon_i : i \in \mathbb{Z}\}$ is a centered L_p-m-approximable sequence, and the infinite sum in (4.3) converges (coordinate-wise) absolutely.

We will use the weight function

$$h(t) = [t(1-t)]^\gamma, \ 0 \le \gamma < \frac{1}{2}, \ t \in (0, 1) \tag{4.4}$$

that is sensitive w.r.t. contiguous alternatives (Csörgő and Horváth, [8], Chap. 3). We could allow for more general weight functions h discussed in this reference but in order to avoid technicalities we confine ourselves to functions h as in (4.4). Now we summarize known results on asymptotic distribution of test statistic (4.2).

Theorem 1 *Let us consider model* (4.1) *and suppose that Assumptions (A.1)–(A.3) and (B.1)–(B.2) are satisfied. Let the long-run variance $\boldsymbol{\Sigma}$ as defined in* (4.3) *be positive definite and $\widehat{\boldsymbol{\Sigma}}_n$ be an estimator of $\boldsymbol{\Sigma}$ such that, as $n \to \infty$,*

$$\widehat{\boldsymbol{\Sigma}}_n - \boldsymbol{\Sigma} = o_p(1). \tag{4.5}$$

If we assume that $h(t)$ satisfies (4.4) *then, under H_0, as $n \to \infty$,*

$$T_n(h) \xrightarrow{\mathscr{D}} \sup_{0<t<1} \left\{ \sum_{j=1}^{d} B_j^2(t)/h^2(t) \right\} \tag{4.6}$$

where $\{B_j(t), t \in [0, 1]\}$, $j = 1, \ldots, d$, *are independent Brownian bridges and* $\xrightarrow{\mathscr{D}}$ *denotes the convergence in distribution.*

Proof The proof follows as a special case of Theorem 2.1 in Prášková and Chochola [22] where general $M-$ estimators are used. □

Large values of the statistic $T_n(h)$ indicate that the null hypothesis is violated. In the next we will consider kernel estimators of $\boldsymbol{\Sigma}$ defined by

$$\widehat{\boldsymbol{\Sigma}}_n = \sum_{|k| \le q(n)} \omega(k/q(n)) \widehat{\boldsymbol{\Gamma}}_k \tag{4.7}$$

where

$$\widehat{\boldsymbol{\Gamma}}_k = \begin{cases} \frac{1}{n} \sum_{j=1}^{n-k} \boldsymbol{x}_j \boldsymbol{x}_{j+k}^T \widehat{\varepsilon}_j \widehat{\varepsilon}_{j+k}, & k \ge 0 \\ \widehat{\boldsymbol{\Gamma}}_{-k}^T, & k < 0 \end{cases} \tag{4.8}$$

and ω is a kernel function that be specified below.

Theorem 2 *Let Assumptions (A.1)–(A.3) and (B.1)–(B.2) be satisfied. Let* $\widehat{\boldsymbol{\Sigma}}_n$ *be the estimator of* $\boldsymbol{\Sigma}$ *as given in (4.7) with kernel that satisfies the assumptions*

(i) $\omega(0) = 1$,
(ii) ω *is a symmetric and Lipschitz function,*
(iii) ω *has a bounded support,*
(iv) *the Fourier transform of* ω *is also Lipschitz and integrable.*

Let $q(n) \to \infty$ *and* $q(n)/n^{1/2} \to 0$ *as* $n \to \infty$. *Then, under* H_0,

$$\widehat{\boldsymbol{\Sigma}}_n = \boldsymbol{\Sigma} + o_p(1). \tag{4.9}$$

Proof See Theorem 2.2 in Prášková and Chochola [22]. □

It can be shown that the Bartlett kernel

$$\omega(x) = (1 - |x|) I\{|x| \le 1\} \tag{4.10}$$

satisfies conditions of Theorem 2. In the next we will consider estimators with this kernel.

Theorem 3 *Let us consider model* (4.1) *with* $\boldsymbol{\delta}_n = \boldsymbol{\delta} n^{-1/2}$, $\boldsymbol{\delta} \ne \boldsymbol{0}$ *and* $k_n^* = \lfloor n\tau \rfloor$, $0 < \tau < 1$. *Let Assumptions (A.1)–(A.3) and (B.1)–(B.2) be satisfied and* $\boldsymbol{\Sigma}$ *be positive definite. Let* $\widehat{\boldsymbol{\Sigma}}_n$ *be a kernel estimator of* $\boldsymbol{\Sigma}$ *that satisfies Theorem 2. Then, as* $n \to \infty$,

$$T_n(h) \xrightarrow{\mathcal{D}} \sup_{0<t<1} \left\{ (\boldsymbol{B}(t) + \boldsymbol{s}(t,\tau))^T (\boldsymbol{B}(t) + \boldsymbol{s}(t,\tau))/h^2(t) \right\} \tag{4.11}$$

where $h(t)$ *is given in* (4.4) *and* $\boldsymbol{B}(t) = (B_j(t), j = 1, \ldots, d)^T$, $\{B_j(t), t \in [0, 1]\}$ *are independent Brownian bridges, and*

$$\boldsymbol{s}(t,\tau) = f(t,\tau)\boldsymbol{\Sigma}^{-1/2}\boldsymbol{C}\boldsymbol{\delta}$$

with

$$f(t,\tau) = \begin{cases} t(1-\tau), & 0 < t \le \tau < 1, \\ \tau(1-t), & 0 < \tau \le t < 1. \end{cases}$$

Proof The proof is a modification of the proof of Theorem 3 in Prášková and Chochola [22]. □

4.3 Dependent Wild Bootstrap

The dependent wild bootstrap (Shao, [23], also dependent multiplier bootstrap, Bücher and Kojadinovic [7]) generalizes the wild bootstrap by Wu [25] to dependent observations with the aim to mimic their dependency structure. Here we propose using the wild bootstrap to CUSUM statistics and their functionals as given in (4.2).

First notice that under H_0, the cumulative sums $\boldsymbol{S}_k$ can be written in the form

$$\boldsymbol{S}_k = \sum_{i=1}^{k} \boldsymbol{x}_i \widehat{\varepsilon}_i = \sum_{i=1}^{k} \boldsymbol{x}_i \varepsilon_i - \boldsymbol{C}_k \boldsymbol{C}_n^{-1} \sum_{i=1}^{n} \boldsymbol{x}_i \varepsilon_i, \qquad \boldsymbol{C}_k = \sum_{i=1}^{k} \boldsymbol{x}_i \boldsymbol{x}_i^T. \tag{4.12}$$

For given observations $y_i, \boldsymbol{x}_i, i = 1, \ldots, n$, we propose to replace dependent errors ε_i in $\boldsymbol{S}_k$ by bootstrap errors ε_i^* defined by $\varepsilon_i^* = \widehat{\varepsilon}_i Z_i$, where $\widehat{\varepsilon}_i$ are the LSE residuals and $Z_i = Z_{i,n}$ are random variables that satisfy the conditions below. We get the bootstrap cumulative sums $\boldsymbol{S}_k^*$. To obtain a bootstrap statistic $T_n^*(h)$ we also need to find a proper bootstrap estimator of the long-run variance $\boldsymbol{\Sigma}$.

Assumptions on Bootstrap Errors

(C.1) For every $n \in \mathbb{N}$, $\{Z_{i,n} : i \in \mathbb{N}\}$ is strictly stationary and independent of $\boldsymbol{x}_i$, $\varepsilon_i, i = 1, \ldots, n$.

(C.2) $\mathsf{E}Z_{i,n} = 0$ and $\sup_n \mathsf{E}|Z_{in}|^{2+\nu} < \infty$ for a $\nu > 0$.

(C.3) $\mathsf{Var}Z_{i,n} = 1$, $\mathsf{Cov}(Z_{i,n}, Z_{j,n}) = \omega((i-j)/q_n)$, $i, j = 1, \ldots, n$, $n = 1, 2, \ldots$, where $\omega(0) = 1, \omega(x) = 0, |x| > 1$.

(C.4) $Z_{i,n}$ are q_n - dependent, such that $q_n \to \infty$ as $n \to \infty$ and $q_n = o(n^{\Delta/(2+\Delta)})$.

Obviously, $\varepsilon_i^* = \varepsilon_{i,n}^*$ also depends on n. With the superscript * we will further denote probability and moments related to bootstrap, i.e., conditionally on $\boldsymbol{x}_i, \varepsilon_i, i = 1, \ldots, n$. Then we have

$$\mathsf{E}^*\varepsilon_i^* = \mathsf{E}\widehat{\varepsilon}_i Z_{i,n}|(\boldsymbol{x}_i, \varepsilon_i, i = 1, \ldots, n) = 0, \quad \mathsf{Cov}^*(\varepsilon_t^*, \varepsilon_s{}^*) = \widehat{\varepsilon}_t\widehat{\varepsilon}_s\omega((t-s)/q_n)) \tag{4.13}$$

Next theorem gives us properties of bootstrap variance estimators.

Theorem 4 *Let* $\boldsymbol{\Sigma}$ *be as given in* (4.3). *Let* $\widehat{\boldsymbol{\Sigma}}_n$ *be the estimator of* $\boldsymbol{\Sigma}$ *defined in* (4.7) *with Bartlett kernel* (4.10). *Denote*

$$\boldsymbol{\Sigma}_n^* = Var^* \frac{1}{\sqrt{n}} \sum_{i=1}^{n} \boldsymbol{x}_i \varepsilon_i Z_{i,n} \tag{4.14}$$

$$\widehat{\boldsymbol{\Sigma}}_n^* = Var^* \frac{1}{\sqrt{n}} \sum_{i=1}^{n} \boldsymbol{x}_i \widehat{\varepsilon}_i Z_{i,n} \tag{4.15}$$

and

$$\widetilde{\boldsymbol{\Sigma}}_n = \sum_{|k| \le q(n)} \omega(k/q(n)) \widetilde{\boldsymbol{\Gamma}}_k \tag{4.16}$$

where

$$\widetilde{\boldsymbol{\Gamma}}_k = \begin{cases} \frac{1}{n}\sum_{j=1}^{n-k} \boldsymbol{x}_j \boldsymbol{x}_{j+k}^T \varepsilon_j \varepsilon_{j+k}, & k \ge 0 \\ \widetilde{\boldsymbol{\Gamma}}_{-k}^T, & k < 0. \end{cases} \tag{4.17}$$

Then, under Assumptions (A.1)–(A.3), (B.1)–(B.2), (C.1)–(C.4), with ω *given by* (4.10) *and* $q_n = q(n)$, *as* $n \to \infty$,

$$\boldsymbol{\Sigma}_n^* = \widetilde{\boldsymbol{\Sigma}}_n \tag{4.18}$$

$$\widehat{\boldsymbol{\Sigma}}_n^* = \widehat{\boldsymbol{\Sigma}}_n \tag{4.19}$$

$$\boldsymbol{\Sigma}_n^* = \boldsymbol{\Sigma} + o_p(1) \tag{4.20}$$

$$\widehat{\boldsymbol{\Sigma}}_n^* = \boldsymbol{\Sigma} + O_p(q_n n^{-1/2}) + o_p(1). \tag{4.21}$$

Proof The assertions (4.18) and (4.19) follow from (4.13) by direct computations. Assertion (4.20) is a consequence of the fact that $\{\boldsymbol{x}_i\varepsilon_i\}$ is L_p-m-approximable (see Remark 2) and Theorem 16.6 in [11], (4.21) follows from (4.19) and the proof of Theorem 2.2 in [22]. □

Remark 3 Convergence in (4.21) holds both under the null hypothesis and the contiguous alternatives considered in Theorem 3.

The bootstrap statistic is

$$T_n^*(h) = \max_{1 \le k \le n} \frac{1}{nh^2(k/n)} \boldsymbol{S}_k^{*T} \widehat{\boldsymbol{\Sigma}}_n^{*-1} \boldsymbol{S}_k^* \tag{4.22}$$

Now, let us consider the bootstrap version of the cumulative sums S_k. From (4.12), if we replace errors ε_i by their bootstrap counterparts ε_i^* we get, under H_0

$$
\begin{aligned}
S_k^* &= \sum_{i=1}^{k} \boldsymbol{x}_i \varepsilon_i^* - \boldsymbol{C}_k \boldsymbol{C}_n^{-1} \sum_{i=1}^{n} \boldsymbol{x}_i \varepsilon_i^* \\
&= \sum_{i=1}^{k} \boldsymbol{x}_i \varepsilon_i Z_{i,n} - \boldsymbol{C}_k \boldsymbol{C}_n^{-1} \sum_{i=1}^{n} \boldsymbol{x}_i \varepsilon_i Z_{i,n} + \left[\sum_{i=1}^{k} \boldsymbol{x}_i \boldsymbol{x}_i^T Z_{i,n} - \boldsymbol{C}_k \boldsymbol{C}_n^{-1} \sum_{i=1}^{n} \boldsymbol{x}_i \boldsymbol{x}_i^T Z_{i,n} \right] (\widehat{\boldsymbol{\beta}} - \boldsymbol{\beta})
\end{aligned}
\tag{4.23}
$$

where $\widehat{\boldsymbol{\beta}}$ is the LSE of $\boldsymbol{\beta}$. Under H_1 the expression for S_k^* is more complicated. The following theorem which is a kind of conditional functional central limit theorem with respect to probability measure P^*, i.e., conditionally on given $\boldsymbol{x}_i, \varepsilon_i, i = 1 \ldots, n$, is a crucial step in proving the consistency of the bootstrap procedure.

Theorem 5 *Let Assumptions (A.1)–(A.3), (B.1)–(B.2), (C.1)–(C.4) hold true and assume also that, as $n \to \infty$,*

$$
\widetilde{\boldsymbol{\Sigma}}_n \to \boldsymbol{\Sigma} \ almost \ surely \ [P] \tag{4.24}
$$

and $\boldsymbol{\Sigma}$ is finite and positive definite. Consider process

$$
\boldsymbol{Y}_n(t) = \frac{1}{\sqrt{n}} \boldsymbol{\Sigma}_n^{*-\frac{1}{2}} \sum_{i=1}^{\lfloor nt \rfloor} \boldsymbol{x}_i \varepsilon_i Z_{i,n}, \quad t \in [0, 1]. \tag{4.25}
$$

Then, as $n \to \infty$,

$$
\{\boldsymbol{Y}_n(t), t \in [0, 1]\} \stackrel{*}{\Rightarrow} \{\boldsymbol{W}_d(t), t \in [0, 1]\} \ almost \ surely \ [P] \tag{4.26}
$$

where $\{\boldsymbol{W}_d(t), t \in [0, 1]\}$ is a standard d-dimensional Wiener process on $[0, 1]$ *and $\stackrel{*}{\Rightarrow}$ means the weak convergence with respect to P^*.*

Proof We will start with a one-dimensional process $\{\boldsymbol{\lambda}^T \boldsymbol{Y}_n(t), t \in [0, 1]\}$ for any vector $\boldsymbol{\lambda}$ such that $\boldsymbol{\lambda}^T \boldsymbol{\lambda} = 1$. To make the proof more readable, let us introduce the following notation: Put

$$
\boldsymbol{V}_n = \frac{1}{\sqrt{n}} \boldsymbol{\Sigma}_n^{*-\frac{1}{2}}, \quad n = 1, 2, \ldots \tag{4.27}
$$

$$
\boldsymbol{H}_{i,n} = \boldsymbol{V}_n \boldsymbol{x}_i \varepsilon_i Z_{i,n}, \quad i = 1, 2, \ldots, n = 1, 2, \ldots \tag{4.28}
$$

$$
h_{i,n} = \boldsymbol{\lambda}^T \boldsymbol{H}_{i,n}, \quad \boldsymbol{\lambda}^T \boldsymbol{\lambda} = 1, \tag{4.29}
$$

$$
c_{i,n} = |\boldsymbol{\lambda}^T \boldsymbol{V}_n \boldsymbol{x}_i \varepsilon_i| \tag{4.30}
$$

Consider $\sigma-$fields $\mathscr{F}_{j,n}^k = \sigma\{Z_{j,n}, Z_{j+1,n}, \ldots, Z_{j+k,n}\}$, $j, k = 1, \ldots, n = 1, \ldots$ It can be shown that given $\boldsymbol{x}_i, \varepsilon_i$ the array $\{h_{i,n}\}$ is near epoch dependent (NED) with respect to $\{Z_{i,n}\}$ (for a definition see, e.g., Chap. 17 in [9]). Indeed, due to Assumptions C.1–C.4, we have

$$\mathsf{E}^*\|h_{i,n}\|^2 \leq \|\boldsymbol{\lambda}^T \boldsymbol{V}_n\|^2 \|\boldsymbol{x}_i\varepsilon_i\|^2 < \infty$$

which holds almost surely [P] due to the remaining assumptions of the theorem. Further,

$$\|h_{i,n} - \mathsf{E}^* h_{i,n}|\mathscr{F}_{i-m,n}^{i+m}\|_2 = [\mathsf{E}^*|h_{i,n} - \mathsf{E}^* h_{i,n}|\mathscr{F}_{i-m,n}^{i+m}|^2]^{1/2} = 0 \leq c_{in}\psi_m \quad (4.31)$$

which holds for any sequence of nonnegative numbers $\psi_k \searrow 0$ and $c_{i,n} > 0$. Thus we can put $c_{i,n} = |\boldsymbol{\lambda}^T \boldsymbol{V}_n \boldsymbol{x}_i \varepsilon_i|$. Since $\{Z_{i,n}\}$ is supposed to be q_n-dependent and thus strong mixing of any size, we can apply Theorem 29.6 in [9] to the array $\{h_{i,n}\}$ and prove that conditionally on $\boldsymbol{x}_i, \varepsilon_i, i = 1, \ldots, n$, the univariate process $\{\boldsymbol{\lambda}^T \boldsymbol{Y}_n(t), t \in [0, 1]\}$ converges weakly to a standard Wiener process $\{W_t, t \in [0, 1]\}$ almost surely [P]. For this we need to verify that conditions (a)–(f) in Theorem 29.6 in [9] with $k_n(t) = \lfloor nt \rfloor$ are satisfied almost surely [P].

Condition (a) holds true since

$$\mathsf{E}^* h_{i,n} = \boldsymbol{\lambda}^T \boldsymbol{V}_n \boldsymbol{x}_i \varepsilon_i \mathsf{E}^* Z_{i,n} = \boldsymbol{\lambda}^T \boldsymbol{V}_n \boldsymbol{x}_i \varepsilon_i \mathsf{E} Z_{i,n} = 0$$

almost surely [P]. Coefficients ψ_k can be chosen such that $\psi_k = \frac{1}{k^\gamma}$ for $\gamma > \gamma_0 = 1$. Moreover, we can assume that $\{Z_{i,n}\}$ is strong mixing of size $\frac{-r}{r-2}$ with $r > 2$. Then the assumption (c) is satisfied. For assumption (b) we have

$$\sup_n \sup_i \|h_{i,n}/c_{i,n}\|_r = \sup_n \sup_i [\mathsf{E}^*|Z_{i,n}|^r]^{1/r} = \sup_n [\mathsf{E}|Z_{i,n}|^r]^{1/r} < \infty$$

for any $r > 2$ which follows from Assumptions (C.1)–(C.2). For condition (d) we have

$$\frac{1}{a} \sum_{i=\lfloor nt \rfloor+1}^{\lfloor n(t+a) \rfloor} c_{i,n}^2 \leq \|\boldsymbol{\lambda}^T \boldsymbol{\Sigma}_n^*\|^2 \frac{1}{n} \cdot \frac{1}{a} \sum_{i=\lfloor nt \rfloor+1}^{\lfloor n(t+a) \rfloor} \|\boldsymbol{x}_i \varepsilon_i\|^2. \quad (4.32)$$

Sequences $\{\boldsymbol{x}_i\}$ and $\{\varepsilon_i\}$ are strictly stationary and ergodic which follows from Assumptions (A.1), (A.3) and (B.1) and so is $\{\|\boldsymbol{x}_i\varepsilon_i\|^2\}$. Hence, as $n \to \infty$,

$$\frac{1}{n} \sum_{i=1}^{n} \|\boldsymbol{x}_i \varepsilon_i\|^2 \to M \quad almost\ surely\ [P]$$

where $M = \mathsf{E}\|\boldsymbol{x}_i\varepsilon_i\|^2 < \infty$. From here,

$$\frac{1}{n} \cdot \frac{1}{a} \sum_{i=\lfloor nt \rfloor+1}^{\lfloor n(t+a) \rfloor} \|\boldsymbol{x}_i \varepsilon_i\|^2 = \frac{1}{a} \left[\frac{1}{n} \sum_{i=1}^{\lfloor n(t+a) \rfloor} (\|\boldsymbol{x}_i \varepsilon_i\|^2 - M) - \frac{1}{n} \sum_{i=1}^{\lfloor nt \rfloor} (\|\boldsymbol{x}_i \varepsilon_i\|^2 - M) \right]$$
$$+ \frac{1}{an} M(\lfloor n(t+a) \rfloor - \lfloor nt \rfloor) \to M$$

which holds uniformly in t and a as $n \to \infty$ and almost surely [P]. Since we assume (4.24), we can conclude that on a set of probability 1

$$\sup_{t\in[0,1],a\in(0,1-t)} \limsup_{n\to\infty} \frac{1}{a} \sum_{i=\lfloor nt\rfloor}^{\lfloor n(t+a)\rfloor} c_{i,n}^2 < \infty$$

which is condition (d) of Theorem 29.6 in [9]. What concerns condition (f), we have

$$\begin{aligned}
\mathsf{E}^*\left(\sum_{i=1}^{\lfloor nt\rfloor} h_{i,n}\right)^2 &= \mathsf{E}^*\left(\boldsymbol{\lambda}^T \boldsymbol{V}_n \sum_{i=1}^{\lfloor nt\rfloor} \boldsymbol{x}_i \varepsilon_i Z_{i,n}\right)^2 = \boldsymbol{\lambda}^T \boldsymbol{V}_n \mathsf{Var}^*\left(\sum_{i=1}^{\lfloor nt\rfloor} \boldsymbol{x}_i \varepsilon_i Z_{i,n}\right) \boldsymbol{V}_n \boldsymbol{\lambda} \\
&= \boldsymbol{\lambda}^T \boldsymbol{\Sigma}_n^{*-1/2} \mathsf{Var}^*\left(\frac{1}{\lfloor nt\rfloor} \sum_{i=1}^{\lfloor nt\rfloor} \boldsymbol{x}_i \varepsilon_i Z_{i,n}\right) \boldsymbol{\Sigma}_n^{*-1/2} \boldsymbol{\lambda} \frac{\lfloor nt\rfloor}{n} \\
&= \boldsymbol{\lambda}^T \boldsymbol{\Sigma}_n^{*-1/2} \boldsymbol{\Sigma}_{\lfloor nt\rfloor}^{*} \boldsymbol{\Sigma}_n^{*-1/2} \boldsymbol{\lambda} \frac{\lfloor nt\rfloor}{n} \to t
\end{aligned}$$

almost surely [P] due to (4.18) and (4.24). Hence, condition (f) is verified. With the choice $\gamma_0 = 1$ in assumption (c), assumption (e) can be omitted, see a remark on p. 482 in [9].

Thus, we have verified conditions of Theorem 29.6 in [9] and we can conclude that, as $n \to \infty$

$$\left\{\boldsymbol{\lambda}^T \frac{1}{\sqrt{n}} \boldsymbol{\Sigma}_n^{*-\frac{1}{2}} \sum_{i=1}^{\lfloor nt\rfloor} \boldsymbol{x}_i \varepsilon_i Z_{i,n}, \quad t \in [0,1]\right\} \stackrel{P^*}{\Rightarrow} \{W(t), t \in [0,1]\} \textit{ almost surely } [P] \tag{4.33}$$

for any vector $\boldsymbol{\lambda}$, $\boldsymbol{\lambda}^T\boldsymbol{\lambda} = 1$. Now, according to the Cramér–Wold device and Theorems 29.16 and 26.23 in [9], we get

$$\{\boldsymbol{Y}_n(t), t \in [0,1]\} \stackrel{*}{\Rightarrow} \{\boldsymbol{W}_d(t), t \in [0,1]\} \textit{ almost surely } [P]. \tag{4.34}$$

□

Remark 4 Condition (4.24) of almost sure convergence of the Bartlett estimator of the long-run variance matrix $\boldsymbol{\Sigma}$ needs some stronger conditions like cumulant assumptions and additional conditions on the kernel bandwidth q_n. For a univariate case and four-order stationary sequence the result was obtained by Berkes et al. [4]. In our case we should modify conditions (A.2) and (B.2) to L_4-m-approximable random variables, consider a component-wise cumulant equivalent condition like (16.23) in [11] and choose kernel function with the bandwidth of order $O(n/(\log n)^4)$ but we will not go into details.

Since the stationarity and ergodicity of $\{\boldsymbol{x}_i\}$ imply

$$\sup_{0\le t\le 1} (\boldsymbol{C}_{\lfloor nt\rfloor}\boldsymbol{C}_n^{-1} - t\boldsymbol{I}_d) \to 0 \; almost \; surely \; [P] \tag{4.35}$$

where $\boldsymbol{I}_d$ is the unit matrix, we immediately get

$$\{\boldsymbol{Y}_n(t) - \boldsymbol{C}_{\lfloor nt\rfloor}\boldsymbol{C}_n^{-1}\boldsymbol{Y}_n(1), t \in [0,1]\} \overset{*}{\Rightarrow} \{\boldsymbol{B}_d(t), t \in [0,1]\} \; almost \; surely \; [P] \tag{4.36}$$

where $\{\boldsymbol{B}_d(t), t \in [0,1]\}$ is a standard $d-$dimensional Brownian bridge. The consistency of the method will be proved if we show that

$$T_n^*(h) \overset{\mathscr{D}^*}{\to} \sup_{t\in[0,1]} \sum_{j=1}^{d} B_j^2(t)/h^2(t) \tag{4.37}$$

almost surely [P] (or in probability). For simplicity, we will further consider $h(t) = 1$, only. We also need the following result.

Theorem 6 *Under assumptions of Theorem 5, as* $n \to \infty$,

$$\max_{1\le k\le n} \left\| \sum_{i=1}^{k} \boldsymbol{V}_n \boldsymbol{x}_i \boldsymbol{x}_i^T (\widehat{\boldsymbol{\beta}} - \boldsymbol{\beta}) Z_{i,n} \right\| \overset{P^*}{\to} 0 \;\; almost \; surely \; [P] \tag{4.38}$$

where $\boldsymbol{V}_n$ *is defined in* (4.27).

Proof It can be shown that given $\boldsymbol{x}_i, \varepsilon_i, i = 1\ldots n$, for any $\boldsymbol{\lambda}$ such that $\boldsymbol{\lambda}^T\boldsymbol{\lambda} = 1$, the array $\{\boldsymbol{\lambda}^T \boldsymbol{V}_n \boldsymbol{x}_i \boldsymbol{x}_i^T (\widehat{\boldsymbol{\beta}} - \boldsymbol{\beta}) Z_{i,n}\}$ is an L_2 mixingal (for a definition, see, e.g., Chap. 16 in [9]) with respect to the filtration $\mathscr{F}_{j,n} = \sigma\{Z_{j,n}, Z_{j-1,n}\ldots\}$ where we can choose $c_{i,n} = |\boldsymbol{\lambda}^T \boldsymbol{V}_n \boldsymbol{x}_i \boldsymbol{x}_i^T (\widehat{\boldsymbol{\beta}} - \beta)|$ and

$$\psi_k = \begin{cases} 1, & k \le q_n \\ \frac{1}{k}, & k > q_n. \end{cases} \tag{4.39}$$

With this choice of ψ_k, it can be easily shown that condition (16.41) in [9] is satisfied. Then, according to Corollary 16.10 in [9],

$$\mathsf{E}^* \left(\max_{1\le k\le n} \sum_{i=1}^{k} \boldsymbol{\lambda}^T \boldsymbol{V}_n \boldsymbol{x}_i \boldsymbol{x}_i^T (\widehat{\boldsymbol{\beta}} - \boldsymbol{\beta}) Z_{i,n} \right)^2 \le K \sum_{i=1}^{n} c_{i,n}^2 \tag{4.40}$$

for a positive constant K. Further, when we use (4.27),

$$\sum_{i=1}^{n} c_{i,n}^2 \le \boldsymbol{\lambda}^T \boldsymbol{\Sigma}_n^{*-1} \boldsymbol{\lambda} (\widehat{\boldsymbol{\beta}} - \boldsymbol{\beta})^T \frac{1}{n} \sum_{i=1}^{n} (\boldsymbol{x}_i \boldsymbol{x}_i^T)(\boldsymbol{x}_i \boldsymbol{x}_i^T)(\widehat{\boldsymbol{\beta}} - \boldsymbol{\beta}). \tag{4.41}$$

Table 4.1 Asymptotic, simulated and dependent wild bootstrap quantiles of distribution of (4.2), $\boldsymbol{x}_i = (1, \xi_i)$, $\xi_i \sim \mathcal{N}(0,1)$, $\varepsilon_i \sim AR(1)$ with the parameter ρ, $n = 250$

Quantiles	δ	90%	95%	99%
Asymptotic		2.1080	2.5036	3.3621
$\rho = 0.3$				
Simulated	(0, 0)	2.0604	2.4139	3.2456
Bootstrap	(0, 0)	1.9363	2.2329	2.8990
	(0.25, 0.25)	2.0088	2.3140	2.9731
	(0.5, 0.5)	2.2187	2.5736	3.2827
$\rho = 0.5$				
Simulated	(0, 0)	2.2670	2.6534	3.4631
Bootstrap	(0, 0)	1.9858	2.3059	2.9615
	(0.25, 0.25)	2.0862	2.4022	3.0988
	(0.5, 0.5)	2.2436	2.5788	3.2634

From the stationarity and ergodicity of $\{\boldsymbol{x}_i\}$ and Assumption (A.1) we get that $\frac{1}{n}\sum_{i=1}^{n}(\boldsymbol{x}_i\boldsymbol{x}_i^T)(\boldsymbol{x}_i\boldsymbol{x}_i^T) = O(1)$ almost surely [P] and from assumption (4.24) $\boldsymbol{\lambda}^T\boldsymbol{\Sigma}_n^{*-1}\boldsymbol{\lambda} = O(1)$ almost surely [P]. Next, $(\widehat{\boldsymbol{\beta}} - \boldsymbol{\beta}) = o(1)$ almost surely [P], which again follows from the ergodicity and stationarity and Assumption (B.1). The latter results hold true both under the null hypothesis and conditions of Theorem 3. Hence, we can conclude that the right-hand side of (4.40) converges to 0 almost surely [P]. We conclude the proof by using the Markov inequality. □

Using this result and (4.35) we get

$$\max_{1\le k\le n}\left\|\boldsymbol{V}_n\left(\sum_{i=1}^{k}\boldsymbol{x}_i\boldsymbol{x}_i^T Z_{i,n} - \boldsymbol{C}^k\boldsymbol{C}_n^{-1}\sum_{i=1}^{n}\boldsymbol{x}_i\boldsymbol{x}_i^T Z_{i,n}\right)(\widehat{\boldsymbol{\beta}} - \boldsymbol{\beta})\right\| \xrightarrow{P^*} 0 \quad almost\ surely\ [P] \tag{4.42}$$

and combining it with (4.36) and (4.23) we get

$$\sup_{0\le t\le 1}\frac{1}{n}\boldsymbol{S}_{\lfloor nt\rfloor}^{*T}\boldsymbol{\Sigma}_n^{*-1}\boldsymbol{S}_{\lfloor nt\rfloor}^{*} \xrightarrow{\mathscr{D}^*} \sup_{0\le t\le 1}\sum_{j=1}^{d}B_j^2(t)\ almost\ surely\ [P]. \tag{4.43}$$

Since

$$\mathsf{E}^*\|\boldsymbol{\Sigma}_n^* - \widehat{\boldsymbol{\Sigma}}_n^*\| = \|\boldsymbol{\Sigma}_n^* - \widehat{\boldsymbol{\Sigma}}_n^*\| \to 0$$

in P-probability due to Theorem 4, we can replace $\boldsymbol{\Sigma}_n^*$ by $\widehat{\boldsymbol{\Sigma}}_n^*$ in (4.43) from which we conclude that (4.37) holds in probability. This gives the consistency of the method. We have proved this asymptotic result under the null hypothesis but the result (4.37) is true under local alternatives considered in Theorem 3. The proofs are more complicated and not presented here.

Table 4.2 Asymptotic, simulated and dependent wild bootstrap quantiles of distribution of (4.2), $\boldsymbol{x}_i \sim \mathcal{N}_2(\mathbf{0}, \boldsymbol{V})$, $\varepsilon_i \sim AR(1)$ with the parameter ρ, $n = 250$.

Quantiles	δ	90%	95%	99%
Asymptotic		2.1080	2.5036	3.3621
$\rho = 0.3$				
Simulated	(0, 0)	1.8955	2.1969	2.8832
Bootstrap	(0, 0)	1.9189	2.2235	2.8514
	(0.25, 0.25)	2.0152	2.3279	2.9737
	(0.5, 0.5)	2.3812	2.7713	3.5455
$\rho = 0.5$				
Simulated	(0, 0)	1.8979	2.2323	2.9130
Bootstrap	(0, 0)	1.8041	2.0885	2.6841
	(0.25, 0.25)	1.9858	2.2880	2.9200
	(0.5, 0.5)	2.3111	2.6815	3.4183

Table 4.3 Empirical level of rejection of H_0 based on asymptotic and bootstrap critical values, nominal level $\alpha = 0.05$, $\boldsymbol{x}_i = (1, \xi_i)$, $\xi_i \sim \mathcal{N}(0, 1)$, $\varepsilon_i \sim AR(1)$ with the parameter ρ, $n = 250$

Asymptotic			Bootstrap		
$\rho = 0.3$			$\rho = 0.3$		
δ	(0,0)	0.0458	δ	(0,0)	0.0732
	(0.25,0.25)	0.3892		(0.25,0.25)	0.4644
	(0.5,0.5)	0.9638		(0.5,0.5)	0.9550
$\rho = 0.5$			$\rho = 0.5$		
δ	(0,0)	0.0716	δ	(0,0)	0.0834
	(0.25,0.25)	0.3316		(0.25,0.25)	0.3654
	(0.5,0.5)	0.8840		(0.5,0.5)	0.8688

Table 4.4 DWB: Empirical level of rejection of H_0 based on asymptotic and bootstrap critical values, nominal level $\alpha = 0.05$, $\boldsymbol{x}_i =\sim \mathcal{N}_2(\mathbf{0}, \boldsymbol{V})$, $\varepsilon_i \sim AR(1)$ with the parameter ρ, $n = 250$

Asymptotic			Bootstrap		
$\rho = 0.3$			$\rho = 0.3$		
δ	(0,0)	0.0306	δ	(0,0)	0.0484
	(0.25,0.25)	0.8440		(0.25,0.25)	0.8742
	(0.5,0.5)	1.0000		(0.5,0.5)	1.0000
$\rho = 0.5$			$\rho = 0.5$		
δ	(0,0)	0.0238	δ	(0,0)	0.0690
	(0.25,0.25)	0.7538		(0.25,0.25)	0.8238
	(0.5,0.5)	1.0000		(0.5,0.5)	0.9996

4.4 Simulations

In this section we present results of a short simulation study. In the simulation experiment we have simulated model (4.1) both under the null hypothesis ($\boldsymbol{\delta} = \mathbf{0}$) and alternatives ($\boldsymbol{\delta} \neq \mathbf{0}$) for various values of vector $\boldsymbol{\delta}$. For regressors we have chosen either the vectors $\boldsymbol{x}_i = (1, \xi_i)^T$ with $\xi_i \sim \mathcal{N}(0, 1)$ or the vectors $\boldsymbol{x}_i \sim \mathcal{N}_2(\mathbf{0}, \boldsymbol{V})$, with the variance matrix

$$\boldsymbol{V} = \begin{pmatrix} 5/4, 1 \\ 1, 5/4 \end{pmatrix}.$$

The errors ε_i were generated as an AR(1) process with the autoregressive parameter ρ and standard normal innovations, and vector $\boldsymbol{\beta}$ was chosen to be $\boldsymbol{\beta} = (1, 1)^T$. The bootstrap variables were generated to satisfy a moving average MA($q - 1$) process,

$$Z_i = Z_{i,n} = (\eta_i + \cdots + \eta_{i-q})/\sqrt{q}$$

with η_i to be i.i.d. random variables distributed as $\mathcal{N}(0, 1)$ and $q = q_n$ was an integer between $n^{1/4}$ and $n^{1/3}$. Size of sample was either $n = 100, 250, 625$. Test statistic (4.2) was computed for function $h(t) = 1$. Quantiles of the asymptotic distribution were taken from [22] and compared with empirical quantiles computed by 5,000 Monte Carlo experiments and with quantiles obtained by dependent wild bootstrap procedure based on 500 bootstrap samples and for 500 repetitions, see Tables 4.1, 4.2 where the results for $n = 250$ are presented. It can be seen that the bootstrap quantiles are close to the true (based on Monte Carlo method) values in almost all cases. It Tables 4.3, 4.4 we compare the power of the asymptotic and bootstrap test which demonstrate that dependent wild bootstrap performs well. Change point k^* was chosen to be $k^* = \lfloor n/2 \rfloor$ and we used 5,000 Monte Carlo experiments. Sample size $n = 250$ used here can be considered mild due to computational complexity necessary to estimate the long-run variance matrix.

Acknowledgements Research supported by the Czech Science Foundation project GA15-09663S.

References

1. Antoch, J., Hušková, M.: Permutation tests for change point analysis. Stat. Probab. Lett. **53**, 37–46 (2001)
2. Antoch, J., Hušková, M., Veraverbeke, N.: Change-point problem and bootstrap. J. Nonparametric Stat. **5**, 123–144 (1995)
3. Berkes, I., Hörmann, S., Schauer, J.: Split invariance principles for stationary processes. Ann. Probab. **39**, 2441–2473 (2011)
4. Berkes, I., Horváth, L., Kokoszka, P., Shao, Q.M.: Almost sure convergence of the Bartlett estimator. Period. Math. Hung. **51**, 11–25 (2005)
5. Billingsley, P.: Convergence of Probability Measures. Wiley, New York (1968)
6. Bucchia B., Wendler, M.: Change-point detection and bootstrap for Hilbert space valued random fields (2015). arXiv: 1511.02609v1

7. Bücher, A., Kojadinovic, I.: Dependent multiplier bootstrap for non-degenerate $U-$statistics under mixing conditions with applications. J. Stat. Plann. Inference **170**, 83–105 (2016)
8. Csörgő, M., Horváth, L.: Limit Theorems in Change-point Analysis. Wiley, Chichester (1997)
9. Davidson, J.: Stochastic Limit Theory. Oxford University Press, New York (1994)
10. Hörmann, S., Kokoszka, P.: Weakly dependent functional data. Ann. Stat. **38**, 1845–1884 (2010)
11. Horváth, L., Kokoszka, P.: Inference for Functional Data with Applications. Springer, New York (2012)
12. Horváth, L., Rice, G.: Extensions of some classical methods in change point analysis. Test **23**, 219–255 (2014)
13. Hušková, M.: Permutation principle and bootstrap in change point analysis. In: Asymptotic Methods in Stochastics. Fields Institute Communications, vol. 44, pp. 273–291 (2004)
14. Hušková, M., Antoch, J.: Detection of structural changes in regression. Tatra Mt. Math. Publ. **26**, 201–215 (2003)
15. Hušková, M., Kirch, C.: Bootstrapping confidence intervals for the change point of time series. J. Time Ser. Anal. **29**, 947–972 (2008)
16. Hušková, M., Kirch, C.: A note on studentized confidence intervals for the change-point. Comput. Stat. **25**, 269–289 (2010)
17. Hušková, M., Picek, J.: Bootstrap in detection of changes in linear regression. Sankhya **67**, 200–226 (2005)
18. Hušková, M., Prášková, Z.: Comments on extensions of some classical methods in change point analysis. Test **23**, 265–269 (2014)
19. Hušková, M., Kirch, C., Prášková, Z., Steinebach, J.: On detection of changes in autoregressive time series II: resampling procedures. J. Stat. Plann. Inference **138**, 1697–1721 (2008)
20. Kirch, C.: Block permutation principles for the change analysis of dependent data. J. Stat. Plann. Inference **137**, 2453–2474 (2007)
21. Kirch, C.: Comments on extensions of some classical methods in change point analysis. Test **23**, 270–275 (2014)
22. Prášková, Z., Chochola, O.: M-procedures for detection of a change under weak dependence. J. Stat. Plann. Inference **149**, 60–76 (2014)
23. Shao, X.: The dependent wild bootstrap. J. Am. Stat. Assoc. **105**, 218–235 (2010)
24. Sharipov, O., Tewes, J., Wendler, M.: Sequential block bootstrap in a Hilbert space with application to change point analysis (2014). arXiv: 1412.0446v1
25. Wu, C.F.J.: Jackknife, bootstrap and other resampling methods in regression analysis. Ann. Stat. **14**, 1261–1295 (1986)

Part II
Simulation for Mathematical Modeling and Analysis

Chapter 5
The Covariation Matrix of Solution of a Linear Algebraic System by the Monte Carlo Method

Tatiana M. Tovstik

Abstract A linear algebraic system is solved by the Monte Carlo method generating a vector stochastic series. The expectation of a stochastic series coincides with the Neumann series presenting the solution of a linear algebraic system. An analytical form of the covariation matrix of this series is obtained, and this matrix is used to estimate the exactness of the system solution. The sufficient conditions for the boundedness of the covariation matrix are found. From these conditions, it follows the stochastic stability of the algorithm using the Monte Carlo method. The number of iterations is found, which provides for the given exactness of solution with the large enough probability. The numerical examples for systems of the order 3 and of the order 100 are presented.

Keywords Linear algebraic system · Monte Carlo method
Covariation matrix of solution

5.1 Introduction

In [1], a solution of a linear algebraic system is build by the Monte Carlo method in combination with ideas of simulation of Gibbs's fields [2], the corresponding algorithm being given. In the present chapter, which continues the studies of [1], an analytical form of the covariation matrix of a stochastic vector solution series is obtained. This matrix is used to estimate the exactness of the approximate solution. Sufficient conditions for the boundedness of the covariation matrix are found.

As a rule, using the Monte Carlo method for solving a linear algebraic system involves the calculation of one component vector solution or of a scalar product of the vector solution and a given vector [3]. Following [4, 5], in the present chapter the entire vector solution is estimated. In [4, 5], the Monte Carlo algorithms are given allowing one to put forward a solution under restrictions more weak than those for the standard Monte Carlo method.

T. M. Tovstik (✉)
St. Petersburg State University, Universitetsraya nab. 7/9, St. Petersburg 199340, Russia
e-mail: peter.tovstik@mail.ru

J. Pilz et al. (eds.), *Statistics and Simulation*, Springer Proceedings
in Mathematics & Statistics 231, https://doi.org/10.1007/978-3-319-76035-3_5

In [6], the Monte Carlo algorithm is presented to simulate a random vector. The expectation of the successive approximation coincides with the corresponding results, as obtained by Zeidel's method.

5.2 The Monte Carlo Method of Solution

Let

$$\mathbf{X} = \mathbf{A} \cdot \mathbf{X} + \mathbf{f}, \tag{5.1}$$

be a system of linear algebraic equations, where $\mathbf{A} = [\, A_{ij} \,]_{i,j=1,n}$ is a square matrix, and $\mathbf{X} = (x_1, \ldots, x_n)^T$ and $\mathbf{f} = (f_1, \ldots, f_n)^T$ are n-vectors.

We assume that $\|\mathbf{A}\|_m \, \|\mathbf{A}\|_l < 1$, where

$$\|\mathbf{A}\| = \|\mathbf{A}\|_m = \max_{1 \le i \le n} \sum_{k=1}^{n} |A_{ik}| < 1, \quad \|\mathbf{A}\|_l = \max_{1 \le j \le n} \sum_{k=1}^{n} |A_{kj}|$$

are the m- and l-norms of a matrix $\mathbf{A}$, respectively.

If $\|\mathbf{A}\|_m < 1$, then the solution $\bar{\mathbf{X}}$ of Eq. (5.1) may be represented as the Neumann series

$$\bar{\mathbf{X}} = \sum_{k=0}^{\infty} \mathbf{A}^k \cdot \mathbf{f}, \tag{5.2}$$

where $\mathbf{f}$ is a vector of initial approximation.

We introduce the stochastic series

$$\hat{\zeta} = \zeta^{(0)} + \zeta^{(1)} + \cdots + \zeta^{(m)} + \ldots \tag{5.3}$$

in which $\zeta^{(0)} = \mathbf{f}$, and the successive vectors $\zeta^{(m)}$, $m = 1, 2, \ldots,$ are simulated so that $\mathbf{E}\zeta^{(m)} = A^m \cdot \mathbf{f}$. We also introduce the stochastic matrix $\mathbf{P}$ connected with the matrix $\mathbf{A}$:

$$\mathbf{P} = [\, p_{ij} \,], \qquad p_{ij} = |A_{ij}| / \sum_{k=1}^{n} |A_{ik}| \ge 0, \quad 1 \le i, j \le n. \tag{5.4}$$

It is clear that $p_{ij} > 0$ if $A_{ij} \ne 0$, and $\sum_{j=1}^{n} p_{ij} = 1$, $1 \le i \le n$.

We successively simulate the vectors $\zeta^{(m)}$, $m \ge 1$ by as follows. Given each m and for all i $(i = 1, \ldots, n)$, we accidentally choose a number i_m according to the distribution

1	2	$\ldots$	n
p_{i1}	p_{i2}	$\ldots$	p_{in}

Next, we find the components of the vector $\zeta^{(m)}$,

$$\zeta_i^{(m)} = \frac{A_{ii_m}}{p_{ii_m}} \zeta_{i_m}^{(m-1)}, \tag{5.5}$$

and obtain the components $\hat{\zeta}_i$ in the series (5.3),

$$\hat{\zeta}_i = f_i + \sum_{m=1}^{\infty} \frac{A_{ii_m}}{p_{ii_m}} \cdots \frac{A_{i_2 i_1}}{p_{i_2 i_1}} f_{i_1}. \tag{5.6}$$

From Eq. (5.5) with given $\zeta^{(m-1)}$, it follows that the conditional expectation $\zeta_i^{(m)}$ is equal

$$\mathbf{E}(\zeta_i^{(m)} | \zeta^{(m-1)}) = \sum_{j=1}^{n} A_{ij} \zeta_j^{(m-1)}.$$

Therefore, $\mathbf{E}(\zeta^{(m)}) = \mathbf{A} \cdot \mathbf{E}(\zeta^{(m-1)})$. We have $\mathbf{E}(\zeta^{(0)}) = \zeta^{(0)} = \mathbf{f}$, and hence $\mathbf{E}(\zeta^{(m)}) = \mathbf{A}^m \cdot \mathbf{f}$, $m = 1, 2, \ldots$ The Neumann series converges; therefore, $\mathbf{E}(\hat{\zeta}) = \bar{\mathbf{X}}$.

It is possible to estimate the solution of system (5.1) in the form (5.2) by an averaging N samples of the random vectors

$$\hat{\zeta}^M = \mathbf{f} + \sum_{m=1}^{M} \zeta^{(m)}, \tag{5.7}$$

namely

$$\bar{\mathbf{X}} \approx \bar{\hat{\zeta}}^{MN} = \frac{1}{N} \sum_{s=1}^{N} (\hat{\zeta}^M)_s, \tag{5.8}$$

where $(\hat{\zeta}^M)_s$ is the sth sample.

Let $\mathbf{R} = [\, R_{ij} \,]$ be the covariation matrix of the random vector $\hat{\zeta}$ (see (5.3)):

$$\mathbf{R} = \mathbf{E}\left((\hat{\zeta} - \mathbf{E}\hat{\zeta}) \cdot (\hat{\zeta} - \mathbf{E}\hat{\zeta})^T \right). \tag{5.9}$$

The variance $\mathbf{D}\zeta_i^{(m)}$ of the ith component of the vector $\zeta^{(m)}$ is as follows:

$$\mathbf{D}\zeta_i^{(m)} = d_i^{(m)} = {\sum}' \frac{A_{ii_m}^2}{p_{ii_m}} \frac{A_{i_m i_{m-1}}^2}{p_{i_m i_{m-1}}} \cdots \frac{A_{i_2 i_1}^2}{p_{i_2 i_1}} f_{i_1}^2 - \left({\sum}' A_{ii_m} A_{i_m i_{m-1}} \cdots A_{i_2 i_1} f_{i_1} \right)^2. \tag{5.10}$$

Introduce designations Throughout the symbol $\sum'$, we denote a summation which is carried out for all indexes with sub-indexes $i_k,\ j_\ell$ in the range $1 \le i_k,\ j_\ell \le n$. For example, in (5.10)

$$\sum{}' = \sum_{i_1, i_2, \ldots, i_m = 1}^{n} . \tag{5.11}$$

Throughout the symbol $\sum_G'$, we denote a summation for all indexes with sub-indexes at which the additional restriction G is imposed.

We next consider the nth order diagonal matrices $\mathbf{D}^{(m)}$ and $\mathbf{D}$ with entries

$$d_i^{(m)} = \left(\mathbf{D}^{(m)}\right)_{ii} \quad \text{and} \quad d_i = \sum_{m=1}^{\infty} d_i^{(m)}, \tag{5.12}$$

respectively.

For any matrix $\mathbf{C} = [C_{ij}]$, we write $(\mathbf{C})_{ij} = C_{ij}$.

The symbol $\{\mathbf{C}\}$ will denote the diagonal matrix with entries coinciding with the diagonal entries of a matrix $\mathbf{C}$.

We shall consider the following matrices

$$\bar{\mathbf{A}} = \sum_{m=1}^{\infty} \mathbf{A}^m, \quad \mathbf{B} = [\, B_{ij} \,] = [\, A_{ij}^2 \,],$$

$$\mathbf{H}(1) = \sum_{m=1}^{\infty} \mathbf{A}^m \cdot \mathbf{D} \cdot (\mathbf{A}^m)^T, \quad \mathbf{H}(t) = \sum_{m=1}^{\infty} \mathbf{A}^m \cdot \{\mathbf{H}(t-1)\} \cdot (\mathbf{A}^m)^T, \quad t = 2, 3 \ldots$$

$$\tilde{\mathbf{H}} = \sum_{t=1}^{\infty} (-1)^{t+1} \mathbf{H}(t), \tag{5.13}$$

where ^{T} denotes transposition.

We shall also need the following matrix norms:

$$d = \|\mathbf{D}\| = \max_i d_i, \quad \mu = \|\mathbf{A}\|_m, \quad \nu = \|\mathbf{A}\|_l, \quad \beta = \mu \cdot \nu, \quad \gamma = \|\mathbf{B}\|. \tag{5.14}$$

5.3 Sufficient Conditions for the Convergence of the Series $\tilde{\mathbf{H}}$

The norm of a diagonal matrix $\mathbf{D}$ with entries (5.12) is as given by $d = \|\mathbf{D}\| = \max_i \left((\bar{\mathbf{Z}})_i - \sum_{m=1}^{\infty} ((\mathbf{A}^m \cdot \mathbf{f})_i)^2\right)$. Here, $\bar{\mathbf{Z}} = \sum_{m=0}^{\infty} \chi^m \cdot \mathbf{g}$ is the Neumann series for the system of linear algebraic equations $\mathbf{Z} = \chi \cdot \mathbf{Z} + \mathbf{g}$ with the matrix $\chi = [\, \chi_{ij} \,] = [\, A_{ij}^2 / p_{ij} \,]$ and the vector $\mathbf{g}$ with components $g_i = f_i^2$. If the entries of the matrix $\mathbf{P}$ are given by Eq. (5.4), then $\|\chi\| = \|\mathbf{A}\|^2 < 1$, and the series $\bar{\mathbf{Z}}$ converges.

Therefore, the boundedness of the norm $\mathbf{D}$ is secured by the convergence of the series $\sum_{m=1}^{\infty}(\mathbf{A}^m \cdot \mathbf{f})^2$, which follows from the convergence of series (5.2).

Remark 1 If the entries of the matrix $\mathbf{P}$ differ from (5.4), then additionally the condition $\|\chi\| < 1$ is to be fulfilled.

Sufficient conditions for the series (5.13) to converge are given in the following.

Theorem 5.1 *If the norms of matrices* $\mathbf{A}$ *and* $\mathbf{B}$ *satisfy the inequalities*

$$\mu = \|\mathbf{A}\|_m < 1, \quad \beta = \|\mathbf{A}\|_m \cdot \|\mathbf{A}\|_l < 1, \quad \gamma + \mu^2 = \|\mathbf{B}\| + \|\mathbf{A}\|^2 < 1, \tag{5.15}$$

then the series (5.13) converges and the norm of the matrix $\tilde{\mathbf{H}}$ *is bounded,*

$$\|\tilde{\mathbf{H}}\| \leq d \frac{\beta}{1-\beta} \frac{\gamma}{1-\gamma-\mu^2}. \tag{5.16}$$

Proof We estimate the norm of the matrix $\mathbf{H}(1) = \sum_{m=1}^{\infty} \mathbf{A}^m \cdot \mathbf{D} \cdot (\mathbf{A}^m)^T$. In the notation (5.14), if $\beta < 1$, then

$$\|\mathbf{H}(1)\| \leq \sum_{k=1}^{\infty} (\|\mathbf{A}\|)^k \|\mathbf{D}\|_m (\|\mathbf{A}^T\|)^k = d \sum_{k=1}^{\infty} \beta^k = d \frac{\beta}{1-\beta}.$$

Let $\mathbf{D}(t) = \{\mathbf{H}(t)\}$ be the diagonal matrix with entries $d_i(t) = \{\mathbf{H}(t)\}_i$. We consider its norm $\|\mathbf{D}(t)\|_m = \max_i |d_i(t)|$. The diagonal matrix $\{\mathbf{H}(1)\}$ reads as

$$\{\mathbf{H}(1)\} = \{\mathbf{A} \cdot \mathbf{D} \cdot \mathbf{A}^T\} + \{\mathbf{A}^2 \cdot \mathbf{D} \cdot (\mathbf{A}^2)^T\} + \ldots$$

It is easy to verify that $\{\mathbf{A} \cdot \mathbf{D} \cdot \mathbf{A}^T\}_i = \sum_{k=1}^{n} A_{ik}^2 d_k$, and, as a result,

$$d_i(1) = \sum_{t=1}^{\infty} \sum_{k=1}^{n} ((A^t)_{ik})^2 d_k = \tag{5.17}$$

$$\sum_{k=1}^{n} A_{ik}^2 d_k + \sum_{t=2}^{\infty} \sum{}' A_{ij_1} A_{j_1,j_2} \cdots A_{j_{t-2}j_{t-1}} \sum{}' A_{ii_1} A_{i_1,i_2} \cdots A_{i_{t-2}i_{t-1}} \sum_{k=1}^{n} A_{j_{t-1}k} A_{i_{t-1}k} d_k.$$

We have $|\sum_{k=1}^{n} A_{j_{t-1}k} A_{i_{t-1}k} d_k| \leq d\gamma$, and hence, $|d_i(1)| \leq d\gamma(1 + \sum_{t=2}^{\infty} \mu^{2(t-1)})$, the norm of matrix $\{\mathbf{H}(1)\}$ satisfies the inequality $\|\{\mathbf{H}(1)\}\| = \|\mathbf{D}(1)\| \leq d\gamma/(1-\mu^2)$. Next, we have $\mathbf{H}(t) = \sum_{t=1}^{\infty} \mathbf{A}^m \cdot \mathbf{D}(t-1) \cdot (\mathbf{A}^m)^T$ at $t \geq 2$, and hence,

$$\|\mathbf{D}(t)\| = \|\{\mathbf{H}(t)\}\| \leq \|\mathbf{D}(t-1)\| \tfrac{\gamma}{1-\mu^2} = d\left(\tfrac{\gamma}{1-\mu^2}\right)^t,$$

$$\|\mathbf{H}(t)\| \leq \|\mathbf{D}(t-1)\| \tfrac{\beta}{1-\beta} \leq \tfrac{d\beta}{1-\beta}\left(\tfrac{\gamma}{1-\mu^2}\right)^t.$$

Now it is possible to estimate the norm of the matrix $\tilde{\mathbf{H}}$ under the assumption that $\gamma/(1-\mu^2) < 1$. Namely,

$$\|\tilde{\mathbf{H}}\| \le \sum_{t=1}^{\infty} \|\mathbf{H}(t)\| \le \frac{d\beta}{1-\beta} \sum_{t=1}^{\infty} \left(\frac{\gamma}{1-\mu^2}\right)^t = \frac{d\beta}{1-\beta} \frac{\gamma}{1-\gamma-\mu^2}.$$

Therefore, if the norms of the matrices **A** and **B** satisfy inequalities (5.15), then according to inequality (5.16) the norm of the matrix $\tilde{\mathbf{H}}$ is bounded. □

From (5.17), it follows that $d_i(1) \ge 0$, and the algorithm for calculation $d_i(t)$ gives that $d_i(t) \ge 0$ for $t \ge 1, i = 1, \dots n$, and therefore, $\|\mathbf{D}(t)\| = \max_i d_i(t)$.

5.4 The Covariation Matrix R of the Vector $\hat{\zeta}$

We denote the covariation of components $\zeta_i^{(m)}$ and $\zeta_j^{(s)}$ of the vectors $\zeta^{(m)}$ and $\zeta^{(s)}$ as: $K_{ij}^{(m,s)} = \mathbf{Cov}(\zeta_i^{(m)}, \zeta_j^{(s)})$. Now the variance R_{ii} of the ith component of the vector $\hat{\zeta}$ in Eq. (5.9) and the covariation R_{ij} of its components $\hat{\zeta}_i$ and $\hat{\zeta}_j$ read as

$$\begin{aligned} R_{ii} &= \mathbf{E}\Big(\sum_{m=1}^{\infty} \zeta_i^{(m)}\Big)^2 - \Big(\mathbf{E}\sum_{m=1}^{\infty} \zeta_i^{(m)}\Big)^2 = \sum_{m=1}^{\infty} d_i^{(m)} + 2\sum_{m=1}^{\infty}\sum_{s=1}^{\infty} K_{ii}^{(m,m+s)}, \\ R_{ij} &= \sum_{m=1}^{\infty} K_{ij}^{(m,m)} + \sum_{m=1}^{\infty}\sum_{s=1}^{\infty} K_{ij}^{(m,m+s)} + \sum_{m=1}^{\infty}\sum_{s=1}^{\infty} K_{ij}^{(m+s,m)}, \quad i \ne j, \end{aligned} \tag{5.18}$$

In [1], the following formulas for the covariations $K_{ij}^{(m,s)}$ in Eq. (5.18) are obtained:

$$\begin{aligned} K_{ii}^{(m,m)} &= d_i^{(m)}, \quad K_{ii}^{(m,m+s)} = K_{ii}^{(m+s,m)} = \sum{}' A_{ii_{m+s}} \cdots A_{i_{m+2}i_{m+1}} J_{i_{m+1}i}^{(m)}, \\ K_{ij}^{(m,m)} &= \sum_{i_m, j_m = 1}^{n} A_{ii_m} A_{jj_m} J_{i_m j_m}^{(m-1)}, \quad i \ne j, \\ K_{ij}^{(m,m+s)} &= K_{ji}^{(m+s,m)} = \sum{}' A_{jj_{m+s}} \cdots A_{j_{m+2}j_{m+1}} J_{j_{m+1}i}^{(m)}, \quad i \ne j. \end{aligned} \tag{5.19}$$

Here,

$$\begin{aligned} & J_{i_2,j_2}^{(1)} = \delta_{i_2,j_2} d_{i_2}^{(1)}, \\ & J_{j_{m+1}i_{m+1}}^{(m)} = \delta_{j_{m+1},i_{m+1}} d_{j_{m+1}}^{(m)} + \\ & \sum_{\ell=0}^{m-2} \sum{}' \prod_{t=0}^{\ell} (1-\delta_{j_{m+1-t},i_{m+1-t}}) A_{j_{m+1-t}j_{m-t}} A_{i_{m+1-t}i_{m-t}} \delta_{j_{m-t},i_{m-t}} d_{j_{m-t}}^{(m-t-1)}, \end{aligned} \tag{5.20}$$

where $m > 1$, $\delta_{i,j}$ is the Kronecker delta.

Theorem 5.2 *The components of the covariation matrix* $\mathbf{R} = [\,R_{ij}\,]$ *of the vector* $\hat{\zeta}$ *in Eq. (5.6), which estimates the solution of system (5.1), are as follows:*

$$R_{ii} = d_i + 2(\bar{\mathbf{A}})_{ii}d_i - 2(\bar{\mathbf{A}})_{ii}(\tilde{H})_{ii} + 2(\bar{\mathbf{A}}\cdot\tilde{\mathbf{H}})_{ii}. \tag{5.21}$$

$$R_{ij} = (\tilde{\mathbf{H}})_{ij} + (\bar{\mathbf{A}})_{ij}d_j + (\bar{\mathbf{A}})_{ji}d_i - (\bar{\mathbf{A}})_{ij}(\tilde{\mathbf{H}})_{jj} - (\bar{\mathbf{A}})_{ji}(\tilde{\mathbf{H}})_{ii} + (\bar{\mathbf{A}}\cdot\tilde{\mathbf{H}})_{ij} + (\bar{\mathbf{A}}\cdot\tilde{\mathbf{H}})_{ji}. \tag{5.22}$$

For the boundedness of the covariations R_{ij} *it is necessary that the norms of the matrices* **A** *and* **B** *satisfy the first two inequalities (5.15) (see Theorem 5.1), and it is sufficient that all inequalities (5.15) be fulfilled.*

Proof To prove the theorem, we calculate the sums of series on the right of Eqs. (5.18)–(5.20) and find the explicit expressions for R_{ii} and R_{ij}. At first, we prove the equality (5.21). The components

$$\zeta_i^{(m)} = \frac{A_{ii_m}}{p_{ii_m}}\cdots\frac{A_{i_2i_1}}{p_{i_2i_1}}f_{i_1},\quad \zeta_i^{(s+m)} = \frac{A_{ij_{m+s}}}{p_{ij_{m+s}}}\cdots\frac{A_{j_{m+1}j_m}}{p_{j_{m+1}j_m}}\cdots\frac{A_{j_2j_1}}{p_{j_2j_1}}f_{j_1},\quad s\ge 1, \tag{5.23}$$

depend on the random states $i_1,\ldots,i_m$ and $j_1,\ldots,j_{m+s}$.

If $j_{m+1}\ne i$ and $i_\ell \ne j_\ell$ for all ℓ, $1\le \ell\le m$, then the components $\zeta_i^{(m)}$ and $\zeta_i^{(s+m)}$ are independent and their covariation is zero:

$$\mathbf{Cov}((\zeta_i^{(m)},\zeta_i^{(s+m)})\mid\ j_{m+1}\ne i,\ \ i_\ell\ne j_\ell,\ \ 1\le\ell\le m) = 0.$$

We introduce the expansion

$$K_{ii}^{(m,m+s)} = \sum_{k=1}^{m} J(i,m,s,k) \tag{5.24}$$

and study three cases $k=m$, $k=m-1$, and $1\le k\le m-2$ as follows

$$k=m:\ \ J(i,m,s,m) = \mathbf{Cov}\left((\zeta_i^{(m)},\zeta_i^{(s+m)})\,\middle|\ j_{m+1}=i\right) = \sum{}' A_{ij_{m+s}}A_{j_{m+s}j_{m+s-1}}\cdots A_{j_{m+2}i}d_i^{(m)}, \tag{5.25}$$

$$k=m-1:\ \ J(i,m,s,m-1) = \sum_{G(m-1)}{}' I(i,m,s,m-1) = \mathbf{Cov}\left((\zeta_i^{(m)},\zeta_i^{(s+m)})\,\middle|\ j_{m+1}\ne i,\, j_m = i_m\right), \tag{5.26}$$

with $G(m-1)=\{j_{m+1}\ne i\}$ (see the Definition 1 for $\sum'$ and $\sum'_{G(m-1)}$ with the restriction $G(m-1)$),

$$1 \le k \le m-2: \quad J(i,m,s,k) = \sum_{G(k)}{}' I(i,m,s,k) = \\ \mathbf{Cov}\left((\zeta_i^{(m)}, \zeta_i^{(s+m)})\Big| \, i_{k+1}=j_{k+1},\; j_{m+1}\ne i,\; i_\ell \ne j_\ell,\; m \ge \ell \ge k+2\right) \tag{5.27}$$

with $G(k) = \{j_{m+1} \ne i,\; j_\ell \ne i_\ell,\; k+2 \le \ell \le m\}$.

In Eqs. (5.26) and (5.27) (for $k \le m-1$)

$$I(i,m,s,k) = A_{ij_{m+s}} A_{j_{m+s}j_{m+s-1}} \cdots A_{j_{m+1}j_m} \cdots A_{j_{k+2}j_{k+1}} A_{ii_m} A_{i_m i_{m-1}} \cdots A_{i_{k+2}j_{k+1}} d_{j_{k+1}}^{(k)}.$$

Equation (5.25) can be written as

$$J(i,m,s,m) = (\mathbf{A}^s)_{ii} d_i^{(m)}. \tag{5.28}$$

Summation the both sides of Eq. (5.28) in s and m according to Eq. (5.18) gives

$$\sum_{s=1}^{\infty}\sum_{m=1}^{\infty} J(i,m,s,m) = (\bar{\mathbf{A}})_{ii} d_i, \tag{5.29}$$

where $\bar{\mathbf{A}}$ is given in Eq. (5.13).

The remaining summands in Eq. (5.24) according Eqs. (5.26), (5.27) for $1 \le k \le m-1$ have the form:

$$J(i,m,s,k) = \sum_{G(k)}{}' I(i,m,s,k). \tag{5.30}$$

Now we analyse the summation area on the right of Eq. (5.30). Let Ω be the summation area without any restrictions on the summation indexes $\sum_\Omega = \sum'$ (see (5.11) in the Definition 1 of $\sum'$).

We denote by Ω_{m+1} the summation area with one restriction $j_{m+1} = i$, namely $\sum'_{\Omega_{m+1}} = \sum'_{j_{m+1}=i}$, then $G(m-1) = \overline{\Omega}_{m+1} = \Omega - \Omega_{m+1}$.

We denote by Ω_r and $\overline{\Omega}_r$ the summation areas

$$\sum_{\Omega_r}{}' = \sum_{j_r=i_r}{}', \qquad \sum_{\overline{\Omega}_r}{}' = \sum_{j_r\ne i_r}{}', \qquad \Omega = \Omega_r + \overline{\Omega}_r.$$

In these designations for $1 \le k \le m-1$

$$G(k) = \bigcap_{r=k+2}^{m+1} \overline{\Omega}_r = \Omega + \sum_{t=1}^{m-k} (-1)^t S(t), \\ S(t) = \bigcup_{\ell=1}^{K(t)} \Omega^{t,\ell}, \qquad \Omega^{t,\ell} = \bigcap_{j=1}^{t} \Omega_{r_j^\ell}, \qquad K(t) = C_{m-k}^t. \tag{5.31}$$

Here $S(t)$ is the range of summation consisting of the union of all intersections of t separate areas Ω_j, $k+2 \le j \le m+1$. The range $S(t)$ appears if $m > t+1$. It is possible to choose t numbers from $m-k$ by $K(t) = C^{\,t}_{m-k}$ variants. We enumerate them and let the ℓth variant be r^ℓ_j, $1 \le \ell \le K(t)$. Without loss of generality, we assume that $r^\ell_1 < r^\ell_2 < \cdots < r^\ell_t$.

Remark 2 Delivering Eq. (5.31), we many times use the well-known relation: Let U be a persistent reliable event, and let events $V_1 \in U$, $V_2 \in U$, then $\overline{V_1}\,\overline{V_2} = U - V_1 - V_2 + V_1 V_2$.

We write $S(t)$ as the sum of two areas $S(t) = S(t)' + S(t)''$, where the $S(t)''$ does not contain Ω_{m+1}. We have

$$\begin{aligned} S(t)' &= \Omega_{m+1} \bigcup_{\ell=1}^{K'} \bigcap_{j=1}^{t-1} \Omega_{r^\ell_j}, \quad K' = C^{\,t-1}_{m-k-1}, \quad k+2 \le r^\ell_j \le m, \\ S(t)'' &= \bigcup_{\ell=1}^{K''} \bigcap_{j=1}^{t} \Omega_{r^\ell_j}, \quad K'' = C^{\,t}_{m-k-1}, \quad k+2 \le r^\ell_j \le m. \end{aligned} \tag{5.32}$$

It is possible to find the sum (5.28) by using summations in the ranges Ω_r according to the right-hand side of Eq. (5.31).

Let us find the sums of values $I(i, m, s, k)$ in the ranges Ω and Ω_r and denote them short as $I = I(i, m, s, k)$.

We have at the summation in the range Ω

$$\sum_{\Omega} I = \sum{}' I = (\mathbf{A}^{s+m-k} \cdot \mathbf{D}^{(k)} \cdot \mathbf{A}^{(m-k)T})_{ii},$$

$$\sum_{s=1}^{\infty} \sum_{m=2}^{\infty} \sum_{k=1}^{m-1} \sum_{\Omega} I = \sum_{s=1}^{\infty} \sum_{k=1}^{\infty} \sum_{m=k+1}^{\infty} \sum_{\Omega} I = \sum_{j=1}^{\infty} (\bar{\mathbf{A}} \cdot \mathbf{A}^j \cdot \mathbf{D} \cdot \mathbf{A}^{jT})_{ii} = (\bar{\mathbf{A}} \cdot \mathbf{H}(1))_{ii}.$$

The summation in the range Ω_{m+1} is carried out under the restriction $j_{m+1} = i$. Changing j_{m+1} by i we get

$$\sum{}'_{\Omega_{m+1}} I = \sum{}' A_{i j_{m+s}} \cdots A_{j_{m+2} i} A_{i j_m} A_{j_m j_{m-1}} \cdots A_{j_{k+2} j_{k+1}} A_{i i_m} A_{i_m i_{m-1}} \cdots A_{i_{k+2} j_{k+1}} d^{(k)}_{j_{k+1}} = (\mathbf{A}^s)_{ii} (\mathbf{A}^{m-k} \cdot \mathbf{D}^{(k)} \cdot \mathbf{A}^{(m-k)T})_{ii}.$$

The further summation in s, m, k according to Eq. (5.13) gives

$$\sum_{s=1}^{\infty} \sum_{m=2}^{\infty} \sum_{k=1}^{m-1} \sum{}'_{\Omega_{m+1}} I = (\bar{\mathbf{A}})_{ii} (\mathbf{H}(1))_{ii}.$$

The summation in the range Ω_r with $k+2 \le r \le m$ and $m \ge 3$ gives

$$\sum_{\Omega_r}{}' I = \sum{}' A_{ij_{m+s}} \cdots A_{j_{k+2}j_{k+1}} A_{ii_m} A_{i_m i_{m-1}} \cdots A_{i_{r+1}j_r} A_{j_r i_{r-1}} \cdots A_{i_{k+2}j_{k+1}} d^{(k)}_{j_{k+1}} =$$
$$(\mathbf{A}^s \cdot \mathbf{A}^{m-r+1} \cdot \{\mathbf{A}^{r-k-1} \cdot \mathbf{D}^{(k)} \cdot \mathbf{A}^{(r-k-1)T}\} \cdot \mathbf{A}^{(m-r+1)T})_{ii}.$$

After changing the order of summation, we get

$$\sum_{s=1}^{\infty}\sum_{m=3}^{\infty}\sum_{k=1}^{m-1}\sum_{r=k+2}^{m}\sum_{\Omega_r}{}' I = \sum_{k=1}^{\infty}\sum_{p=1}^{\infty}\sum_{j=1}^{\infty}(\bar{\mathbf{A}} \cdot \mathbf{A}^p \cdot \{\mathbf{A}^j \cdot \mathbf{D}^{(k)} \cdot \mathbf{A}^{jT}\} \cdot \mathbf{A}^{pT})_{ii} = (\bar{\mathbf{A}} \cdot \mathbf{H}(2))_{ii}.$$

If $k+2 \le r_1 < r_2 \le m$, then the summation of values $I(i, m, s, k)$ in the range $\Omega_{12} = \Omega_{r_1} \bigcap \Omega_{r_2}$ gives

$$\sum_{\Omega_{12}}{}' I = (\mathbf{A}^s \cdot \mathbf{A}^{m-r_2+1} \cdot \{\mathbf{A}^{r_2-r_1} \cdot \{\mathbf{A}^{r_1-k-1} \cdot \mathbf{D}^{(k)} \cdot \mathbf{A}^{(r_1-k-1)T}\} \cdot \mathbf{A}^{(r_2-r_1)T}\} \cdot \mathbf{A}^{(m-r_2+1)T})_{ii},$$

and, if $k+2 \le r_1 \le m$, the summation in the range $\Omega_{r_1} \bigcap \Omega_{r_{m+1}}$ gives

$$\sum_{\Omega_{r_1} \bigcap \Omega_{m+1}} I = (\mathbf{A}^s)_{ii} \left(\mathbf{A}^{m-r_1+1} \cdot \{\mathbf{A}^{r_1-k-1} \cdot \mathbf{D}^{(k)} \cdot \mathbf{A}^{(r_1-k-1)T}\} \cdot \mathbf{A}^{(m-r_1+1)T}\right)_{ii}.$$

Therefore, $\sum{}'_{S(2)} I$ corresponds to the relation

$$\sum_{S(2)}{}' I = \sum_{j_1=1}^{m-k-1} (\mathbf{A}^s)_{ii} \left(\mathbf{A}^{j_1} \cdot \{\mathbf{A}^{m-k-j_1} \cdot \mathbf{D}^{(k)} \cdot \mathbf{A}^{(m-k-j_1)T}\} \cdot \mathbf{A}^{j_1T}\right)_{ii} +$$
$$\sum_{j_1=1}^{L_1}\sum_{j_2=1}^{L_2} \left(\mathbf{A}^s \cdot \mathbf{A}^{j_1} \cdot \{\mathbf{A}^{j_2} \cdot \{\mathbf{A}^{m-k-j_1-j_2} \cdot \mathbf{D}^{(k)} \cdot \mathbf{A}^{(m-k-j_1-j_2)T}\} \cdot \mathbf{A}^{j_2T}\} \cdot \mathbf{A}^{j_1T}\right)_{ii}.$$

with $L_1 = m-k-2,\ L_2 = m-k-j_1-1$.

For the following summations in s, m, k, we obtain

$$\sum_{s=1}^{\infty}\sum_{m=4}^{\infty}\sum_{k=1}^{m-1}\sum_{\mathbf{S}(2)}{}' I = (\bar{\mathbf{A}})_{ii}(\mathbf{H}(2))_{ii} + (\bar{\mathbf{A}} \cdot \mathbf{H}(3))_{ii}.$$

Remark 3 All the summations of values $I(i, m, s, k)$ in the ranges consisting of any intersections of Ω_r, $k+2 \le r \le m+1$ lead to expressions, in which between each bold braces there is a matrix $\mathbf{A}$ at least in the first power.

The cases $t = 1$ and $t = 2$ with one or two restrictions are already examined. In the general case $t > 2$ we find, at first, $\sum'_{S(t)''} I$, where $S(t)''$ is given by Eq. (5.32), in which the numbers r_j^ℓ are ordered $k+2 \le r_1^\ell < r_2^\ell < \cdots < r_t^\ell \le m$. We have $S(t)'' = \bigcap_{j=1}^{t} \Omega^\ell_{r_j}$, and further,

$$\sum_{S(t)''}{}' I =$$

$$\left(\mathbf{A}^s \mathbf{A}^{m-r_t^\ell+1}\{\mathbf{A}^{r_t^\ell - r_{t-1}^\ell}\{\cdots\{\mathbf{A}^{r_1^\ell-k-1}\mathbf{D}^{(k)}\mathbf{A}^{(r_1^\ell-k-1)T}\}\cdots\}\mathbf{A}^{(r_t^\ell-r_{t-1}^\ell)T}\}\mathbf{A}^{(m-r_t^\ell+1)T}\right)_{ii},$$

$$\sum_{s=1}^{\infty}\sum_{m=t+2}^{\infty}\sum_{k=1}^{m-1}\sum_{S(t)''}{}' I = (\bar{\mathbf{A}}\cdot\mathbf{H}(t+1))_{ii}, \quad t \geq 2.$$

Taking into account Eqs. (5.31) and (5.32), we conclude that

$$\sum_{s=1}^{\infty}\sum_{m=t+2}^{\infty}\sum_{k=1}^{m-1}\sum_{S(t)}{}' I = (\bar{\mathbf{A}})_{ii}\cdot\mathbf{H}(t)_{ii} + (\bar{\mathbf{A}}\cdot\mathbf{H}(t+1))_{ii}, \quad t \geq 2. \tag{5.33}$$

The covariations R_{ii} according Eq. (5.18) contain the value d_i (see Eq. (5.12)), the summand $(\bar{\mathbf{A}})_{ii}d_i$ (see Eq. (5.29)), and a summation in t with due account of the alternation of signs in Eqs. (5.31), (5.33)

$$R_{ii} = d_i + 2\left(\bar{\mathbf{A}}\right)_{ii} d_i + 2\left(\bar{\mathbf{A}}\right)_{ii}\left(\sum_{t=1}^{\infty}(-1)^t\mathbf{H}(t)\right)_{ii} + 2\left(\bar{\mathbf{A}}\cdot\sum_{t=1}^{\infty}(-1)^{t+1}\mathbf{H}(t)\right)_{ii}. \tag{5.34}$$

In the notation (5.13) Eq. (5.34) coincides with Eq. (5.21).

Now we calculate the cross-covariations R_{ij}. The covariation $K_{ij}^{(m,m+s)}$ is equal to the covariation of random values (5.23) and $\zeta_j^{(s+m)} = \frac{A_{jj_{m+s}}}{p_{jj_{m+s}}}\cdots\frac{A_{j_{m+1}j_m}}{p_{j_{m+1}i_m}}\cdots\frac{A_{j_2j_1}}{p_{j_2j_1}}f_{j_1}$.

The covariation $K_{ij}^{(m,m+s)}$ can be calculated by the third formula in (5.19). The summation of $K_{ij}^{(m,m+s)}$ in m and s gives

$$\sum_{s=1}^{\infty}\sum_{m=1}^{\infty}K_{ij}^{(m,m+s)} = (\bar{\mathbf{A}})_{ji}d_i - (\bar{\mathbf{A}})_{ji}(\tilde{\mathbf{H}})_{ii} + (\bar{\mathbf{A}}\cdot\tilde{\mathbf{H}})_{ji}. \tag{5.35}$$

From Eq. (5.19), it follows $K_{ij}^{(m,m+s)} = K_{ji}^{(m+s,m)}$; therefore,

$$\sum_{s=1}^{\infty}\sum_{m=1}^{\infty}K_{ij}^{(m+s,m)} = (\bar{\mathbf{A}})_{ij}d_j - (\bar{\mathbf{A}})_{ij}(\tilde{\mathbf{H}})_{jj} + (\bar{\mathbf{A}}\cdot\tilde{\mathbf{H}})_{ij}.$$

To finish calculation R_{ij} by Eq. (5.18), it is necessary to find $K_{ij}^{(m,m)} = K_{ji}^{(m,m)}$. With $m = 1$, the covariation $K_{ij}^{(1,1)} = 0$, and with $m \geq 2$, we have

$$K_{ji}^{(m,m)} = \sum{}' A_{jj_m} A_{ij_m} d_{j_m}^{(m-1)} +$$

$$\sum_{k=1}^{m-2} \sum_{G_1(k)}{}' A_{jj_m} A_{j_m j_{m-1}} \cdots A_{j_{k+2} j_{k+1}} A_{ii_m} A_{i_m i_{m-1}} \cdots A_{i_{k+2} j_{k+1}} d_{j_{k+1}}^{(k)} \qquad (5.36)$$

with the restriction (see Definition 1) $G_1(k) = \{i_\ell \neq j_\ell,\ k+2 \leq \ell \leq m\}$.

The way of calculation $K_{ji}^{(m,m)}$ by Eq. (5.36) is the same as the calculation $K_{ii}^{(m,m+s)}$ by Eqs. (5.27), (5.28). But here $s = 0$, and therefore, $S(t) = S(t)''$ for the range of summation, and as a result in Eq. (5.35), the first two summands are absent, and in the third summand, the matrix $\bar{\mathbf{A}}$ is to be replaced by the unit matrix. Finally,

$$\sum_{m=1}^{\infty} K_{ji}^{(m,m)} = (\tilde{\mathbf{H}})_{ji}. \qquad (5.37)$$

Taking into account Eqs. (5.35) and (5.37), and using the symmetry of the matrix $\tilde{\mathbf{H}}$, we verify that Eq. (5.17) leads to Eq. (5.22). This proves Theorem 2. □

5.5 Estimate of the Number of Iterations *M*

To solve Eq. (5.1) by the Monte Carlo method, the stochastic series (5.3) is constructed. By using Theorems 1 and 2, the stochastic properties of this series are investigated in the case of the infinite number of summands. Now we study the random value (5.7), which contains the $(M+1)$ first summands. Here, M is the number of iterations. Also, we consider the average value (5.8) as a result of N imitation averaging.

The expectation $\mathbf{E}(\hat{\zeta}^M)$ coincides with the corresponding partial sum of the Neumann series. It is important to estimate M. In [7], for $\|\mathbf{A}\|_m = \mu$ the estimate

$$|X_i - \mathbf{E}(\hat{\zeta}_i^M)| \leq \frac{\mu^{M+1}}{1-\mu} \|\mathbf{f}\|, \quad X_i^{(0)} = f_i, \quad i = 1, \ldots, n \qquad (5.38)$$

is obtained. We set $\sigma_i(M) = \sqrt{\mathbf{D}(\hat{\zeta}_i^M)}, \quad 1 \leq i \leq n, \sigma(M) = \max_i \sigma_i(M)$.

Now, according to the central limit theorem [8] with probability α close to 1 (for example, $\alpha = 0.95$ for $x_\alpha = 1.96$), the inequality (5.38) leads to an estimate

$$\left| \frac{1}{N} \sum_{s=1}^{N} \zeta_i^M(s) - X_i \right| \leq \frac{\sigma(M)(x_\alpha + h)}{\sqrt{N}}, \quad 1 \leq i \leq n, \quad \text{with} \quad \frac{\sigma(\mathrm{M})\mathrm{h}}{\sqrt{\mathrm{N}}} \approx \frac{\mu^{(\mathrm{M}+1)}}{1-\mu} \|\mathbf{f}\|. \qquad (5.39)$$

The number M of iterations for the given $h \approx 1$ is to be chosen from Eq. (5.39).

The value $\sigma(M)$ is unknown. If the norms of the matrix $\mathbf{A}$ and the vector $\mathbf{f}$ are less than 1, then $\sigma(M) \approx O(1)$.

5.6 Numerical Examples

Example 1 Let the matrix $\mathbf{A}$ and the vector $\mathbf{f}$ in the system (5.1) be

$$\mathbf{A} = \begin{pmatrix} 0.5 & -0.3 & 0.1 \\ -0.25 & 0.3 & -0.3 \\ 0.2 & -0.2 & 0.4 \end{pmatrix}, \qquad \mathbf{f} = \begin{pmatrix} 0.4 \\ -0.5 \\ 0.6 \end{pmatrix}.$$

The norms of matrices are $\mu = \|\mathbf{A}\|_m = 0.9,\ \ \nu = \|\mathbf{A}\|_l = 0.95, \gamma = \|\mathbf{B}\| = 0.15$, therefore the conditions of Theorem 5.1 are fulfiled.

The covariation matrix $\mathbf{R}$ with the components (5.21) and (5.22) is as follows (see Theorem 5.2):

$$\mathbf{R} = \begin{pmatrix} 2.01701 & -1.11503 & 1.01365 \\ -1.11503 & 1.29587 & -0.61386 \\ 1.01365 & -0.61386 & 0.96000 \end{pmatrix}.$$

The exact solution of system (5.1) is given by $\mathbf{X} = (1.44329, -0.52062, 1.65464)^T$.

Here, we give the maximal absolute differences between the exact solution $\mathbf{X}$ and its sampling estimation $\bar{\hat{\xi}}^{\mathbf{MN}}$, and also the differences between the components of the matrix $\mathbf{R}$ and the components of the sampling covariation matrix $\hat{\mathbf{R}}^{MN}$:

$$N = 10^6,\ M = 80 : \max_i |X_i - \bar{\hat{\xi}}_i^{MN}| \le 0.00059,\ \ \max_{ij} |\hat{R}_{ij}^{MN} - R_{ij}| \le 0.00383,$$
$$N = 10^8,\ M = 80 : \max_i |X_i - \bar{\hat{\xi}}_i^{MN}| \le 0.00016,\ \ \max_{ij} |\hat{R}_{ij}^{MN} - R_{ij}| \le 0.00024.$$

The errors decrease simultaneously as the number N of imitations increases.

Example 2 Consider system (5.1) of dimension $n = 100$. We form the vector $\mathbf{f}$ and the matrix $\mathbf{A}$ by simulating random numbers uniformly distributed in (0, 1). We change a sign at some components of matrix $\mathbf{A}$. Next, we transform the components of vector $\mathbf{f}$ and matrix $\mathbf{A}$, so that the norms (5.14) are as follows:

$$\mu = 0.9, \quad \nu = 1.0155, \quad \gamma = 0.0118, \quad \|\mathbf{f}\| = 0.9951.$$

The results of simulation with $N = 10^6,\ M = 80$ are given by

$$\max_i |X_i - \bar{\hat{\xi}}_i^{MN}| \le 0.0024, \qquad \max_{ij} |\hat{R}_{ij}^{MN} - R_{ij}| \le 0.0054.$$

These examples support the correctness of the formulas obtained above.

5.7 Conclusions

An algorithm for approximate solution of a system of linear algebraic equations by the Monte Carlo method in combination with the ideas of Gibbs and Metropolis of fields simulation is presented. The explicit expressions for components of the covariation matrix of a stochastic vector are obtained to estimate the solution of the system. The sufficient conditions, for which the components of the covariation matrix are finite, are found. The obtained relations allow us to find the variance of the inner product of the vector solution and the given vector.

Acknowledgements The work is supported by Russian Foundation of Basic Researches, grant 14.01.00271a.

References

1. Tovstik, T.M.: On the solution of systems of linear algebraic equations by Gibbs's method. Vestn St.Peterburg Univ.: Math. **44**(4), 317–323 (2011)
2. Winkler, G.: Image analysis, Random Fields and Dynamic Monte Carlo Methods: A Mathematical Introduction. Springer, Berlin (1995)
3. Ermakov, S.M.: Monte Carlo Method and Close Problems, 327 p. Nauka, Moscow (1971). [In Russian]
4. Belyaeva, A.A., Ermakov, S.M.: On the Monte Carlo method with remembering of the intermediate results. Vestn. St.Petersburg Univ. Ser. 1 **3**, 8–11 (1996)
5. Dmitriev, A.V., Ermakov, S.M.: Monte Carlo and method asynchronic iterations. Vestn. St.Petersburg Univ. **44**(4), 517–528 (2011)
6. Tovstik T.M., Volosenko K.S.: Monte Carlo algorithm for a solution of a system linear algebraic eqetions by the Zeidel method. In: Proceedings of the Conference on Actual Problems of Computational and Applied Mathematics, Novosibirsk (2015). ISBN 978-5-9905347-2-8. [In Russian]
7. Demidovich, B.P., Maron, I.A.: Foundations of Computation Mathematic, 664 p. Nauka, Moscow (1970). [In Russian]
8. Feller, W.: An Introduction to Prabability Theory and its Applications. Willey, Chapman & Hall, Limited, New York, London (1957)

Chapter 6
Large-Scale Simulation of Acoustic Waves in Random Multiscale Media

Olga N. Soboleva and Ekaterina P. Kurochkina

Abstract The effective coefficients in the problem of the acoustic wave propagation have been calculated for a multiscale 3D medium by using a subgrid modeling approach. The density and the elastic stiffness have been represented by the Kolmogorov multiplicative cascades with a log-normal probability distribution. The wavelength is assumed to be large as compared with the scale of heterogeneities of the medium. We consider the regime in which the waves propagate over a distance of the typical wavelength in source. If a medium is assumed to satisfy the improved Kolmogorov similarity hypothesis, the term for the effective coefficient of the elastic stiffness coincides with the Landau-Lifshitz-Matheron formula. The theoretical results are compared with the results of a direct 3D numerical simulation.

Keywords Propagation of acoustic waves · Subgrid modeling
Multiplicative cascades

6.1 Introduction

The numerical solution of the wave propagation problem in a medium with variations of parameters on all the scales requires high computer costs. The small-scale heterogeneities are taken into account with the help of effective parameters or additional terms in wave equations like the Frenkel–Biot models [1]. There are three different wave propagation regimes (waves in a smoothly varying body, coda waves, and a homogenized part of a wave field) depending on the ratio of wave field characteristic scale to the one of the heterogeneities. It is very difficult to find a clear spatial scale

O. N. Soboleva (✉)
Novosibisk State Technical University,
Prospekt K. Marksa, 20, Novosibirsk, Russia 630073
e-mail: olgasob@gmail.com; olga@nmsf.sscc.ru

O. N. Soboleva · E. P. Kurochkina
The Novosibisk State University - Baker Hughes Joint Laboratory
of The Multi-Scale Geophysics and Mechanics, Novosibirsk 90, Russia
e-mail: e.p.kurochkina@gmail.com

J. Pilz et al. (eds.), *Statistics and Simulation*, Springer Proceedings
in Mathematics & Statistics 231, https://doi.org/10.1007/978-3-319-76035-3_6

delimitation, to catch wave field properties in each of these regimes. The two-scale homogenization approaches are well known in the solid mechanics community. An example of a two-scale approach for the dynamic case can be found in [2, 3]. The spatial geometry of small-scale heterogeneities is not exactly known. It is customary to assume these parameters to be random fields. However, it is difficult to measure higher-order statistical moments for the geophysical parameters. At best, only the mean values and the second-order correlation functions are known. Hence, effective solutions cannot be constructed using only the conventional perturbation theory with a high accuracy. In [4], the analytical results are discussed and proved in detail for the waves propagation in randomly layered media. The authors obtain the analytical results and illustrate them with numerical simulations for three regimes of separation of scales of the wave propagation in a 1D case. It has been shown that the irregularity of elastic parameters, density, permeability, porosity increases as the scale of measurements decreases for some natural media [5, 6]. Many natural media are "scale regular" in the sense that they can be described by multifractals and hierarchical cascade models with non-Gaussian distributions [6]. In this chapter, using this fact we apply the subgrid modeling method to hierarchical cascade models of media with non-Gaussian distributions of parameters. We study propagation of acoustic waves in the media, in which heterogeneities are represented by the spatial distribution of the local acoustic parameters that have essential variations of all scales from a finite interval at each spatial point. The density of a medium and its elastic stiffness is approximated by a multiplicative cascade with log-normal joint probability distribution functions. The wavelength essentially exceeds a maximum scale of heterogeneity. If a medium is assumed to satisfy the improved Kolmogorov similarity hypothesis [7], the effective coefficients coincide with the Landau-Lifshitz-Matheron formula. The derived formulas for 3D media are verified by the direct numerical modeling. For numerical testing, we consider the regime, in which the wave propagates over a distance that is of the same order as the typical wavelength of a source.

6.2 The Model and Governing Equation

The propagation of acoustic waves in a heterogeneous medium is described by the equation

$$\rho(\mathbf{x}) \frac{\partial^2 u(\mathbf{x}, t)}{\partial t^2} - \frac{\partial}{\partial x_i}\left(\lambda(\mathbf{x}) \frac{\partial}{\partial x_i} u(\mathbf{x}, t)\right) = F(\mathbf{x}, t), \tag{6.1}$$

where $\mathbf{x}$ is the vector of spatial coordinates, $F(\mathbf{x}, t)$ is the source with the dominant frequency ω_0 and the pulse width ω_1. The wavelength is assumed to be large as compared with the maximum scale of the heterogeneities L. For the approximation of the coefficients $\rho(\mathbf{x})$, $\lambda(\mathbf{x})$, we use the approach described in [8]. Let, for example, the field $\lambda(\mathbf{x})$ be known. This means that the field is measured on a small scale l_0 at each point $\mathbf{x}$, $\lambda_{l_0}(\mathbf{x}) = \lambda(\mathbf{x})$. Following Kolmogorov [7], let us consider a dimensionless field ψ, which is equal to the ratio of two fields obtained by smoothing the field $\lambda(\mathbf{x})_{l_0}$ at two different scales l, l'. Let $\lambda_l(\mathbf{x})$ denotes the parameter $\lambda_{l_0}(\mathbf{x})$ smoothed at the scale l. Then $\psi(\mathbf{x}, l, l') = \lambda(\mathbf{x})_{l'}/\lambda(\mathbf{x})_l$, $l' < l$. Expanding the field ψ to a power series in $(l - l')$ and retaining first-order terms of the series, at $l' \to l$, we obtain the equation $\frac{\partial \ln \lambda_l(\mathbf{x})}{\partial \ln l} = \varphi(\mathbf{x}, l)$, where $\varphi(\mathbf{x}, l') = (\partial \psi(\mathbf{x}, l', l'y)/\partial y)\,|_{y=1}$. The small-scale fluctuations of the field φ are observed only in the interval (l_0, L). The solution of the equation is

$$\lambda_{l_0}(\mathbf{x}) = \lambda_0 \exp\left(-\int_{l_0}^{L} \varphi(\mathbf{x}, l_1)\frac{dl_1}{l_1}\right), \tag{6.2}$$

where λ_0 is the constant. The field φ determines the statistical properties of the elastic stiffness. According to the central limit theorem for sums of independent random variables if the variance of $\varphi(\mathbf{x}, l)$ is finite, the integral in (6.2) tends to a field with a normal distribution as the ratio L/l_0 increases. It is assumed that the field $\varphi(\mathbf{x}, l)$ is statistically homogeneous with a normal distribution. The density coefficient $\rho(\mathbf{x})$ is constructed by analogy with the elastic stiffness coefficient:

$$\rho_{l_0}(\mathbf{x}) = \rho_0 \exp\left(-\int_{l_0}^{L} \chi(\mathbf{x}, l_1)\frac{dl_1}{l_1}\right). \tag{6.3}$$

The fluctuations of the fields $\varphi(\mathbf{x}, l)$, $\chi(\mathbf{x}, l)$ are considered to be statistically independent on two different scales:

$$< \varphi(\mathbf{x}, l)\varphi(\mathbf{y}, l') > - < \varphi(\mathbf{x}, l) >< \varphi(\mathbf{y}, l') >= \Phi^{\varphi\varphi}(\mathbf{x} - \mathbf{y}, l, l')\delta\left(\ln l - \ln l'\right),$$
$$< \varphi(\mathbf{x}, l)\chi(\mathbf{y}, l') > - < \varphi(\mathbf{x}, l) >< \chi(\mathbf{y}, l') >= \Phi^{\varphi\chi}(\mathbf{x} - \mathbf{y}, l, l')\delta\left(\ln l - \ln l'\right),$$

where $\langle\rangle$ means statistical averaging. To derive subgrid formulas to calculate effective coefficients, this assumption may be ignored. However, this assumption is important for the numerical simulation of the field ρ, λ. If the fields are statistically invariant to the scale transform, the following equality is valid for any positive K: $\Phi^{\varphi\varphi}(\mathbf{x} - \mathbf{y}, l) = \Phi^{\varphi\varphi}(K(\mathbf{x} - \mathbf{y}), Kl)$, $\Phi^{\chi\chi}(\mathbf{x} - \mathbf{y}, l) = \Phi^{\chi\chi}(K(\mathbf{x} - \mathbf{y}), Kl)$. For simplicity, we use the same notation Φ in the right side. When $\mathbf{x} = \mathbf{y}$, the functions $\Phi^{\varphi\varphi}$, $\Phi^{\chi\chi}$ are equal to the constants $\Phi_0^{\varphi\varphi}$, $\Phi_0^{\chi\chi}$, $\Phi_0^{\varphi\chi}$. The estimation of correlation functions from (6.2), (6.3) have been obtained in [8], for $r < L$:

$$< \lambda_{l_0}(\mathbf{x})\lambda_{l_0}(\mathbf{x} + \mathbf{r}) >\simeq C\,(r/L)^{-\Phi_0^{\varphi\varphi}},$$

where $C = \lambda_0^2\,(L/l_0)^{-2\langle\varphi\rangle}\,e^{-\Phi_0^{\varphi\varphi}\gamma}$, $\gamma = 0.57722$ is the Euler constant. For $r \gg L$, we have $< \lambda_{l_0}(\mathbf{x})\lambda_{l_0}(\mathbf{x} + \mathbf{r}) >\to \lambda_0^2$.

Further, we consider the correlation functions $\Phi^{\varphi\varphi}$, $\Phi^{\varphi\chi}$, $\Phi^{\chi\chi}$ as rapidly decreasing functions with correlation radii that are much smaller than the wavelength. The double correlation radii determine the length of correlated fluctuations of parameters. In order to take into account the fluctuations of the parameters, one must have a measurement scale to be three times less than the minimum correlation radius. The parameters ρ, λ are cross-correlated

6.3 Subgrid Modeling

The density and the elastic stiffness $\rho(\mathbf{x}) = \rho_{l_0}(\mathbf{x})$, $\lambda(\mathbf{x}) = \lambda_{l_0}(\mathbf{x})$ are divided into two components with respect to the scale l. The large-scale (ongrid) components $\lambda(\mathbf{x}, l)$, $\rho(\mathbf{x}, l)$ are obtained, respectively, by the statistical averaging over all $\varphi(\mathbf{x}, l_1)$ and $\chi(x, l_1)$ with $l_0 < l_1 < l, l - l_0 = dl$, where dl is small. The small-scale (subgrid) components are equal to $\rho'(\mathbf{x}) = \rho(\mathbf{x}) - \rho(\mathbf{x}, l)$, $\lambda'(\mathbf{x}) = \lambda(\mathbf{x}) - \lambda(x, l)$. Applying (6.2), (6.3) yields the formulas:

$$\rho(\mathbf{x}, l) = \rho_0 \exp\left[-\int_l^L \chi(\mathbf{x}, l_1)\frac{dl_1}{l_1}\right]\left\langle \exp\left[-\int_{l_0}^l \chi(\mathbf{x}, l_1)\frac{dl_1}{l_1}\right]\right\rangle,$$
$$\lambda(\mathbf{x}, l) = \lambda_0 \exp\left[-\int_l^L \varphi(\mathbf{x}, l_1)\frac{dl_1}{l_1}\right]\left\langle \exp\left[-\int_{l_0}^l \varphi(\mathbf{x}, l_1)\frac{dl_1}{l_1}\right]\right\rangle. \tag{6.4}$$

From formulas (6.4) with second order of accuracy in dl/l follows

$$\rho(\mathbf{x}, l) = \rho_l(\mathbf{x}),\ \lambda(\mathbf{x}, l) \simeq \left[1 - \langle\varphi\rangle \frac{dl}{l} + \frac{1}{2}\Phi^{\varphi\varphi}(0, l)\frac{dl}{l}\right]\lambda_l(\mathbf{x})$$
$$\langle\lambda'(\mathbf{x})\lambda'(\mathbf{x}')\rangle \simeq \Phi^{\varphi\varphi}(\mathbf{x}-\mathbf{x}', l)\,\lambda(\mathbf{x}, l)^2\frac{dl}{l},\ \langle\rho'(\mathbf{x})\rho'(\mathbf{x}')\rangle \simeq \Phi^{\chi\chi}(\mathbf{x}-\mathbf{x}', l)\,\rho(\mathbf{x}, l)^2\frac{dl}{l},$$
$$\langle\rho'(\mathbf{x})\lambda'(\mathbf{x}')\rangle \simeq \Phi^{\chi\varphi}(\mathbf{x}-\mathbf{x}', l)\,\rho(\mathbf{x}, l)\,\lambda(\mathbf{x}, l)\frac{dl}{l}. \tag{6.5}$$

Let us consider the temporal Fourier transform of Eq. (6.1)

$$\omega^2\rho(\mathbf{x})\,u(\omega, \mathbf{x}) + \frac{\partial}{\partial x_i}\left(\lambda(\mathbf{x})\frac{\partial}{\partial x_i}u(\omega, \mathbf{x})\right) = -F(\omega, \mathbf{x}). \tag{6.6}$$

The large-scale (ongrid) component of the displacement $u(\omega, \mathbf{x}, l)$ is obtained by averaging the solutions to Eq. (6.6), in which the large-scale components of the density $\rho(\mathbf{x}, l)$ and the elastic stiffness $\lambda(\mathbf{x}, l)$ are fixed and the small components $\rho'(\mathbf{x})$, $\lambda'(\mathbf{x})$ are random variables. The subgrid component of the displacement is equal to $u'(\omega, \mathbf{x}) = u(\omega, \mathbf{x}) - u(\omega, \mathbf{x}, l)$. Substituting the relations for $u(\omega, \mathbf{x})$ and $\rho(\mathbf{x})$, $\lambda(\mathbf{x})$ into Eq. (6.6) and averaging over small-scale components, we have

$$\omega^2\rho(\mathbf{x}, l)\,u(\omega, \mathbf{x}, l) + \omega^2\langle\rho'(\mathbf{x})\,u'(\mathbf{x})\rangle + \frac{\partial}{\partial x_i}\left(\lambda(\mathbf{x}, l)\frac{\partial}{\partial x_i}u(\omega, \mathbf{x}, l)\right)$$
$$+\frac{\partial}{\partial x_i}\left\langle\lambda'(\mathbf{x})\frac{\partial}{\partial x_i}u'(\mathbf{x})\right\rangle = -F(\omega, \mathbf{x}). \tag{6.7}$$

The subgrid terms $S_1 = \omega^2 \left\langle \rho'(\mathbf{x})\, u'(\mathbf{x}) \right\rangle$, $S_2 = \left\langle \lambda'(\mathbf{x}) \frac{\partial}{\partial x_i} u'(\mathbf{x}) \right\rangle$ in Eq. (6.7) are unknown. These terms cannot be neglected without preliminary estimation. The form of these terms in (6.7) determines a subgrid model. The subgrid terms are estimated using perturbation theory. Subtracting Eq. (6.7) from Eq. (6.6) and taking into account only the first-order terms, the reduced equation for the subgrid displacement $u'(\mathbf{x})$ is given by

$$\omega^2 \rho(\mathbf{x}, l)\, u'(\mathbf{x}) + \lambda(\mathbf{x}, l) \frac{\partial^2 u'(\mathbf{x})}{\partial x_i^2} = -\omega^2 \rho'(\mathbf{x})\, u(\omega, \mathbf{x}, l) - \frac{\partial}{\partial x_i} \lambda'(\mathbf{x}) \frac{\partial u(\omega, \mathbf{x}, l)}{\partial x_i}. \tag{6.8}$$

The variable $u(\omega, \mathbf{x}, l)$ in the right-hand side of (6.8) is assumed to be known. For the fields, in which a small variation in the scale causes significant fluctuations of the field as it is (this is typical of fractal fields) possible to consider $\lambda(\mathbf{x}, l)$, $\rho(\mathbf{x}, l)$, $u(\mathbf{x}, l)$ and their derivatives varying slower than $\lambda(\mathbf{x})'$, $\rho(\mathbf{x})'$, u' and their derivatives. If the first derivatives $\frac{\partial}{\partial x_j} u'(\omega, \mathbf{x})$ and $\frac{\partial}{\partial x_j} u(\omega, \mathbf{x}, l)$ are of the same order, the subgrid term $\left\langle \lambda'(\mathbf{x}) \frac{\partial}{\partial x_j} u'(\omega, \mathbf{x}) \right\rangle$ is small as compared to $\left(\lambda(\mathbf{x}, l) \frac{\partial}{\partial x_j} u(\omega, \mathbf{x}, l) \right)$ because $\lambda'(\mathbf{x})$ is small. Then, it is the well-solvable problem with smooth coefficients. The solution of Eq. (6.8) takes the form

$$u'(\mathbf{x}) = \frac{1}{\lambda(\mathbf{x}, l)} \int_{-\infty}^{\infty} G(r) \left(\frac{\partial}{\partial x'_j} \lambda'(\mathbf{x}') \frac{\partial u(\omega, \mathbf{x}', l)}{\partial x'_j} + \omega^2 \rho'(\mathbf{x}')\, u(\omega, \mathbf{x}', l) \right) d\mathbf{x}', \tag{6.9}$$

where $r = \left| \mathbf{x} - \mathbf{x}' \right|$, $G(r)$ is the Green function of Eq. (6.8) if the coefficients $\lambda(\mathbf{x}, l)$, $\rho(\mathbf{x}, l)$ are assumed to be constants in according to the method of "frozen coefficients." Substituting this solution in the subgrid terms gives

$$S_1 = \left\langle \frac{\omega^2 \rho'(\mathbf{x})}{\lambda(\mathbf{x}, l)} \int_{-\infty}^{\infty} G(r) \left(\frac{\partial}{\partial x'_j} \lambda'(\mathbf{x}') \frac{\partial}{\partial x'_j} u(\omega, \mathbf{x}', l) + \omega^2 \rho'(\mathbf{x}')\, u(\omega, \mathbf{x}', l) \right) d\mathbf{x}' \right\rangle$$
$$S_2 = \left\langle \lambda'(\mathbf{x}) \frac{\partial}{\partial x_i} \frac{1}{\lambda(\mathbf{x}, l)} \int_{-\infty}^{\infty} G(r) \left(\frac{\partial}{\partial x'_j} \lambda'(\mathbf{x}') \frac{\partial}{\partial x'_j} u(\omega, \mathbf{x}', l) + \omega^2 \rho'(\mathbf{x}')\, u(\omega, \mathbf{x}', l) \right) d\mathbf{x}' \right\rangle. \tag{6.10}$$

Again, treating the terms with lower derivatives of the large-scale field $u(\mathbf{x}, l)$, $\lambda(\mathbf{x}, l)$, $\rho(\mathbf{x}, l)$ as constants in the integrand and taking into account $\frac{\partial}{\partial x_i} r = -\frac{\partial}{\partial x'_i} r$, using (6.5) one can write down

$$S_1 = \int_{-\infty}^{\infty} G(r) \frac{\partial}{\partial x'_j} \Phi^{\chi\varphi} \left(\mathbf{x} - \mathbf{x}', l \right) d\mathbf{x}' \frac{dl}{l} \omega^2 \rho(\mathbf{x}, l) \frac{\partial}{\partial x_j} u\left(\omega, \mathbf{x}', l \right)$$
$$+ \frac{\omega^2 \rho(\mathbf{x}, l)}{\lambda(\mathbf{x}, l)} \int_{-\infty}^{\infty} G(r)\, \Phi^{\chi\chi} \left(\mathbf{x} - \mathbf{x}', l \right) d\mathbf{x}' \frac{dl}{l} \omega^2 \rho(\mathbf{x}, l)\, u(\omega, \mathbf{x}, l)$$

$$S_2 = \int_{-\infty}^{\infty} \frac{\partial^2 G(r)}{\partial x_i' \partial x_j'} \Phi^{\varphi\varphi}\left(\mathbf{x}-\mathbf{x}', l\right) d\mathbf{x}' \frac{dl}{l} \lambda(\mathbf{x}, l) \frac{\partial}{\partial x_j'} u(\omega, \mathbf{x}, l)$$

$$- \int_{-\infty}^{\infty} \frac{\partial G(r)}{\partial x_i'} \Phi^{\chi\varphi}\left(\mathbf{x}-\mathbf{x}', l\right) d\mathbf{x}' \frac{dl}{l} \omega^2 \rho(\mathbf{x}, l) u(\omega, \mathbf{x}, l) \tag{6.11}$$

In isotropic media, the correlation functions depend only on $r = \left|\mathbf{x}-\mathbf{x}'\right|$. These functions and the Green function are the even functions, but the partial derivatives of G, Φ with respect to x_i or x_j are the odd functions. Hence, the integrals on the first and last lines of (6.11) are equal to zero. For $i = j$, we apply the formula $\frac{\partial^2 G(r)}{\partial^2 x_i'} = -\frac{1}{D}\left(\frac{\omega^2 \rho(\mathbf{x},l)}{\lambda(\mathbf{x},l)} G(r, l) + \delta\left(\mathbf{x}-\mathbf{x}'\right)\right)$, where D is the dimension of space. If $i \neq j$, the integrals in (6.11) are equal to zero. Now, we come to:

$$S_1 = -\frac{\omega^2 \rho(\mathbf{x}, l)}{\lambda(\mathbf{x}, l)} \int_{-\infty}^{\infty} G(r) \Phi^{\chi\chi}(r, l)\, d\mathbf{x}' \frac{dl}{l} \omega^2 \rho(\mathbf{x}, l) u(\omega, \mathbf{x}, l),$$

$$S_2 = -\frac{1}{D} \frac{\omega^2 \rho(\mathbf{x}, l)}{\lambda(\mathbf{x}, l)} \int_{-\infty}^{\infty} G(r, l) \Phi^{\varphi\varphi}(r, l)\, d\mathbf{x}' \frac{dl}{l} \lambda(\mathbf{x}, l) \frac{\partial}{\partial x_i'} u(\omega, \mathbf{x}, l)$$

$$-\frac{1}{D} \Phi^{\varphi\varphi}(0, l) \frac{dl}{l} \lambda(\mathbf{x}, l) \frac{\partial}{\partial x_i'} u(\omega, \mathbf{x}, l). \tag{6.12}$$

The correlation radii of ρ, λ are much smaller than the wavelength, since the maximum scale of inhomogeneities L much smaller than the wavelength. So, the integrals in (6.12) are of second order in L. If the following inequalities hold, $\Phi^{\varphi\varphi}(0, l) L^2 \omega^2 \rho(\mathbf{x}, l) / \lambda(\mathbf{x}, l) \ll 1, \Phi^{\chi\chi}(0, l) L^2 \omega_1^2 \rho(\mathbf{x}, l) / \lambda(\mathbf{x}, l) \ll 1$, the integral terms in (6.12) may be discarded. Hence, obtain

$$\omega^2 \left\langle \rho' u' \right\rangle \simeq 0, \quad \left\langle \lambda'(\mathbf{x}) \frac{\partial}{\partial x_i} u'(\mathbf{x}) \right\rangle \simeq -\frac{1}{D} \Phi^{\varphi\varphi}(0, l) \frac{dl}{l} \lambda(\mathbf{x}, l) \frac{\partial}{\partial x_i'} u(\omega, \mathbf{x}, l). \tag{6.13}$$

Substituting the formulas from (6.5) and (6.13) in the ongrid Eq. (6.7) gives

$$\omega^2 \rho(\mathbf{x}, l) u(\omega, \mathbf{x}, l) + \frac{\partial}{\partial x_i}\left[\lambda_{l0} \exp\left(-\int_l^L \varphi(\mathbf{x}, l_1) \frac{dl_1}{l_1}\right) \frac{\partial}{\partial x_i} u(\omega, \mathbf{x}, l)\right] = -F(\omega, \mathbf{x}), \tag{6.14}$$

where λ_{l0} satisfies the equation with the second order of accuracy in (dl/l)

$$\lambda_{0l} = \left(1 - \langle\varphi\rangle \frac{dl}{l} + \frac{D-2}{2D} \Phi^{\varphi\varphi}(0, l) \frac{dl}{l}\right) \lambda_0.$$

As $dl \to 0$, the effective equation for λ_{0l}, ρ_{0l} becomes

$$\rho_{0l} = \rho_0, \quad \frac{d\ln\lambda_{0l}}{d\ln l} = \frac{D-2}{2D}\Phi^{\varphi\varphi}(0,l) - \langle\varphi\rangle, \quad \lambda_{0l_0} = \lambda_0. \tag{6.15}$$

In the scale-invariant media, the solution of equation (6.15) has a simple form and coincides with the Landau-Lifshitz-Matheron formula:

$$\rho_{0l} = \rho_0, \quad \lambda_{0l} = \lambda_0\left(\frac{l}{l_0}\right)^{\frac{D-2}{2D}\Phi_0^{\varphi\varphi} - \langle\varphi\rangle} = K_G \exp\left(\frac{D-2}{2D} * \sigma_0^2\right), \tag{6.16}$$

where $K_G = \lambda_0 \exp\left(-\langle\varphi\rangle(\ln l - \ln l_0)\right)$ is the geometrical mean of $\lambda_l(\mathbf{x})$, $\sigma_0^2 = \Phi_0^{\varphi\varphi}\ln(l/l_0)$. By virtue of formulas (6.15) in isotropic case, the form of the correlation functions has no effect on the effective coefficients.

6.3.1 The Anisotropic Case

In the anisotropic case, the study of the problem in question requires the knowledge of the form of correlation functions. To determine the form of correlation functions, one must measure the physical parameter at a large number of points and in different intervals. Such regular measurements are time-consuming and expensive and seldom available in scientific papers. One of the main difficulties in solving geophysical tasks is to extract an undisturbed core. Nevertheless, correlation functions of some parameters are obtained, for example, in the paper [4]. To get an idea of the influence of the form of correlation functions on the effective coefficients for the wave equation, some correlation functions for 3D are considered in the case, when the coefficient λ is isotropic at any point, but the correlation function of the field λ is anisotropic. Real geophysical media have often anisotropy of such a kind because of the layering. Such a medium is composed of many isotropic blocks close to a parallelepiped with a random λ. The mass density is constant, and the medium is stratified so that λ by the coordinates x_1, x_3 has the correlation radius greater than the correlation radius by the coordinate x_2. Let us assume $l_1 = \alpha_1 l$ to be the scale by the coordinates x_1, x_3, $l_2 = \alpha_2 l$ is the scale by the coordinate x_2, $\alpha_1 < \alpha_2$. The same scales by the coordinate x_1, x_3 are assumed to avoid cumbersome calculations and numerical calculations of elliptic integrals for the 3D correlation functions. We calculate effective coefficients from (6.11) for the two correlation functions and constant mass density:

$$\Phi_1^{\varphi\varphi}\left(\mathbf{x}-\mathbf{x}',l\right)=\Phi_0^{\varphi\varphi}e^{\left[-\frac{\alpha_1^2}{l^2}\left((x_1'-x_1)^2+(x_3'-x_3)^2\right)-\frac{\alpha_2^2}{l^2}(x_2'-x_2)^2\right]}, \tag{6.17}$$

$$\Phi_2^{\varphi\varphi}\left(\mathbf{x}-\mathbf{x}',l\right)=\Phi_0^{\varphi\varphi}f_1\times f_2\times f_3 \tag{6.18}$$

$$f_i=\left(\frac{2l\sin\left(\frac{\alpha_i\pi\left(x_i-x_i'\right)}{2l}\right)}{\alpha_i\pi\left(x_i-x_i'\right)}\right)^2,\ i=1,3,\ f_2=\left(\frac{2l\sin\left(\frac{\alpha_2\pi\left(x_2-x_2'\right)}{2l}\right)}{\alpha_2\pi\left(x_2-x_2'\right)}\right)^2.$$

Additionally, we consider the widely used approximation of the correlation function:

$$\Phi_3^{\varphi\varphi}\left(\mathbf{x}-\mathbf{x}',l\right)=\begin{cases}\Phi_0^{\varphi\varphi}(l),\ \alpha_i\left|x_i-x_i'\right|\le l,\\ 0,\qquad \alpha_i\left|x_i-x_i'\right|>l\end{cases}. \tag{6.19}$$

In this case, the expression for the effective coefficients, which correctly describes the expectation of the displacement, takes the following form:

$$\frac{d\ln\lambda_{0l}^{im}}{d\ln l}=\frac{\Phi_0^{\varphi\varphi}}{2}+\eta_{m1}-\langle\varphi\rangle,\ i=1,3,\ \frac{d\ln\lambda_{0l}^{2m}}{d\ln l}=\frac{\Phi_0^{\varphi\varphi}}{2}+\eta_{m2}-\langle\varphi\rangle, \tag{6.20}$$

where $\lambda_{0l}^{i}(\mathbf{x})$ is the effective coefficient in Eq. (6.1), and m is number of the correlation function. The coefficients η are given by For $\alpha_2<\alpha_1$, we have

$$\eta_{11}=-\frac{1}{2}\Phi_0^{\varphi\varphi}\frac{\alpha_1^2}{\left(\alpha_1^2-\alpha_2^2\right)}\left(\frac{\alpha_2}{\sqrt{\alpha_1^2-\alpha_2^2}}\arctan\sqrt{\frac{\alpha_1^2-\alpha_2^2}{\alpha_2^2}}-\frac{\alpha_2^2}{\alpha_1^2}\right),\ i=1,3$$

$$\eta_{12}=-\Phi_0^{\varphi\varphi}\frac{\alpha_1^2}{\alpha_1^2-\alpha_2^2}\left[1-\frac{\alpha_2}{\sqrt{\alpha_1^2-\alpha_2^2}}\arctan\left(\sqrt{\frac{\alpha_1^2-\alpha_2^2}{\alpha_2^2}}\right)\right],\ i=2 \tag{6.21}$$

For $\alpha_2>\alpha_1$:

$$\eta_{11}=\frac{1}{2}\frac{\alpha_1^2}{\left(\alpha_2^2-\alpha_1^2\right)}\Phi_0^{\varphi\varphi}\left(\frac{\alpha_2}{2\sqrt{\alpha_2^2-\alpha_1^2}}\ln\frac{\alpha_2+\sqrt{\alpha_2^2-\alpha_1^2}}{\alpha_2-\sqrt{\alpha_2^2-\alpha_1^2}}-\frac{\alpha_2^2}{\alpha_1^2}\right),\ i=1,3,$$

$$\eta_{12}=\frac{\alpha_1^2}{\left(\alpha_2^2-\alpha_1^2\right)}\Phi_0^{\varphi\varphi}\left[1-\frac{\alpha_2}{2\sqrt{\alpha_2^2-\alpha_1^2}}\ln\frac{\alpha_2+\sqrt{\alpha_2^2-\alpha_1^2}}{\alpha_2-\sqrt{\alpha_2^2-\alpha_1^2}}\right],\ i=2. \tag{6.22}$$

The coefficient η_{22} is equal to

Table 6.1 Comparison of coefficients η_{m1} for different correlation functions $\Phi_m^{\varphi\varphi}$

$\frac{\alpha_1}{\alpha_2}$	0.01	0.05	0.1	0.25	1.0	4.0	10	20	100
η_{11}	0.500	0.497	0.489	0.462	0.333	0.148	0.069	0.037	0.008
η_{21}	0.500	0.498	0.493	0.470	0.333	0.130	0.057	0.029	0.006
η_{31}	0.500	0.499	0.496	0.481	0.333	0.110	0.045	0.025	0.004

$$\eta_{22} = \Phi_0^{\varphi\varphi}\left[1 - \frac{\pi\alpha_2}{2\alpha_1}(I_{11} + I_{12}) + \frac{\alpha_2}{\alpha_1}(I_{21} + I_{22})\right], \ \psi^* = \arctan\left(\frac{\alpha_1}{\alpha_2}\right),$$

$$I_{11} = \frac{1}{3}\left(\frac{\sin\psi^*}{2\cos^2\psi^*} + \frac{1}{2}\ln\left|\tan\left(\frac{\pi}{4} + \frac{\psi^*}{2}\right)\right|\right), \ I_{12} = \frac{\alpha_1^2}{3\alpha_2^3}\left(\frac{\cos\psi^*}{2\sin^2\psi^*} - \frac{1}{2}\ln\left|\tan\left(\frac{\psi^*}{2}\right)\right|\right),$$

$$I_{21} = -\frac{\alpha_1}{6\alpha_2} + \frac{1}{3}\int_0^{\psi^*}\arctan\left(\frac{1}{\cos\psi}\right)\frac{d\psi}{\cos^3\psi} + \frac{1}{6}\int_0^{\psi^*}\ln\left(1 + \frac{1}{\cos^2\psi}\right)d\psi,$$

$$I_{22} = -\frac{\alpha_1}{6\alpha_2} + \frac{\alpha_1^3}{3\alpha_2^3}\int_{\psi^*}^{\pi/2}\arctan\left(\frac{\alpha_1}{\alpha_2\sin\psi}\right)\frac{d\psi}{\cos^3\psi} + \frac{1}{6}\int_{\psi^*}^{\pi/2}\ln\left(1 + \frac{\alpha_1^2}{\alpha_2^2\sin^2\psi}\right)d\psi.$$

the coefficients η_{31}, η_{32} are equal to

$$\eta_{31} = -2\Phi_0^{\varphi\varphi}\arctan\left(\alpha_2/\left(\sqrt{2\alpha_1^2 + \alpha_2^2}\right)\right)/\pi$$

$$\eta_{32} = -2\Phi_0^{\varphi\varphi}\arctan\left(\alpha_1^2/\left(\alpha_2\sqrt{2\alpha_1^2 + \alpha_2^2}\right)\right)/\pi.$$

Table 6.1 shows the degree of a difference between the coefficients for the correlation functions, $\Phi_0^{\varphi\varphi} = 1$. It is easy to see that the results of calculations for all the formulas are quite close to each other, except for the interval, where the coefficients η_{mi} are small and where is important only the order of magnitude. Hence, effective coefficients depend on the ratio between the correlation radii along the coordinate axes and slightly depend on the form of the correlation functions.

It is easy to see that the results of calculations for all the formulas are quite close to each other, except for the interval, where the coefficients η_{mi} are small and where is important only the order of magnitude. Hence, effective coefficients depend on the ratio between the correlation radii along the coordinate axes and slightly depend on the form of the correlation functions.

6.4 Numerical Verification of the Above Obtained Formulas

We have carried out the numerical simulation of the 3D problem by solving Eq. (6.1), using the finite-difference method with second-order discretization with a respect to

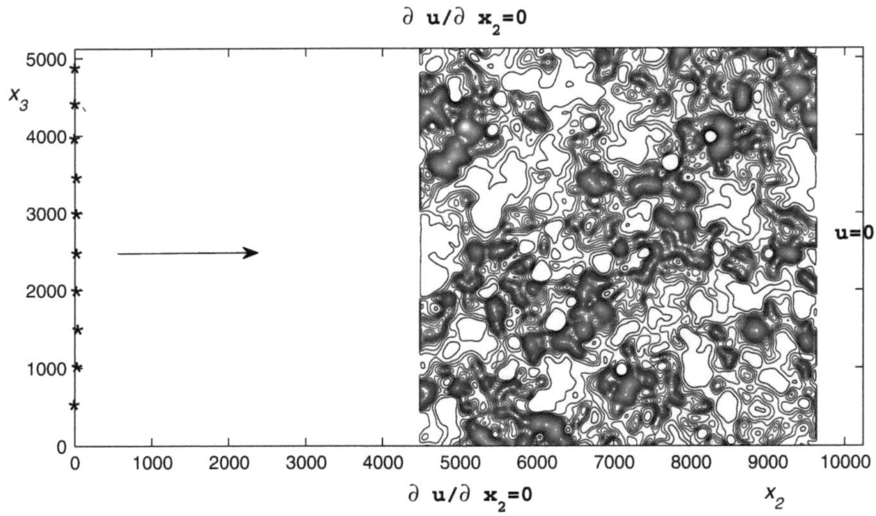

Fig. 6.1 Geometry of the domain of integration in cross section $x_1 = 128\,\mathrm{h}$. The arrow shows the main direction of wave propagation, and stars show location of wave sources

temporal and the spatial variables. We used $512 \times 1024 \times 512$ grids (where x_2 is the main direction of wave propagation). The domain of integration is separated into three subdomains.

In the subdomains $0 < x_1 \le 512\,\mathrm{h}$, $0 < x_2 \le 450\,\mathrm{h}$, $0 < x_3 \le 512\,\mathrm{h}$ and $0 < x_1 \le 512\,\mathrm{h}$, $962\,\mathrm{h} < x_2 \le 1024\,\mathrm{h}$, $0 < x_3 \le 512\,\mathrm{h}$, the coefficients ρ, λ are equal to $\rho = \rho_0 = 2000\,\mathrm{kg/m^3}$, $\lambda = \lambda_0 = 1.8 * 10^{10}\mathrm{Pa}$. On the plane boundaries $x_1 \times x_2$ at $x_3 = 0$, $x_1 \times x_2$ at $x_3 = 512\,\mathrm{h}$ and $x_2 \times x_3$ at $x_1 = 0$, $x_2 \times x_3$, $x_1 = 512\,\mathrm{h}$, the partial derivatives $\partial u\,(t, \mathbf{x})\,/\partial x_2$ are equal to zero; on the plane boundary $x_1 \times x_3$ at $x_2 = 1024\,\mathrm{h}$, the displacement u is equal to zero. In the subdomain $0 < x_1 \le 512\,\mathrm{h}$, $450\,\mathrm{h} < x_2 \le 962\,\mathrm{h}$, $0 < x_3 \le 512\,\mathrm{h}$, the spatial distributions of ρ, λ are simulated by the multiplicative cascades (6.2), (6.3), in which the integrals are approximated by the sums. Figure 6.1 shows geometry of the domain of integration in cross section $x_1 = 128\,\mathrm{h}$. The arrow shows the main direction of wave propagation, and stars show location of wave sources. The following pulse wave source is used for numerical simulation:

$$f(t) = \left(1 - 2\pi^2\,(t_0 - t)^2\right)\exp\left(-\pi^2\,(t_0 - t)^2\right),$$

where $t_0 = 0.8$, the dominant frequency is 1 Hz. In Fig. 6.2, *6.3*, the averaged numerical solution are compared with the solution of the effective equation and the solution obtained with the mean value of the coefficients ρ, λ. in the subdomain $0 < x_1 \le 512\,\mathrm{h}$, $450\,\mathrm{h} < x_2 < 962\,\mathrm{h}$, $0 < x_3 \le 512\,\mathrm{h}$. Line 1 is the result obtained for $\rho = \rho_0$, $\lambda = \lambda_0$; line 2 is the result obtained by the effective equation; line 3 is the result of numerical modeling with λ calculated by formula (6.2), $\rho = \rho_0$; line 4 is the result of numerical modeling for ρ and λ calculated by formulas (6.2), (6.3)

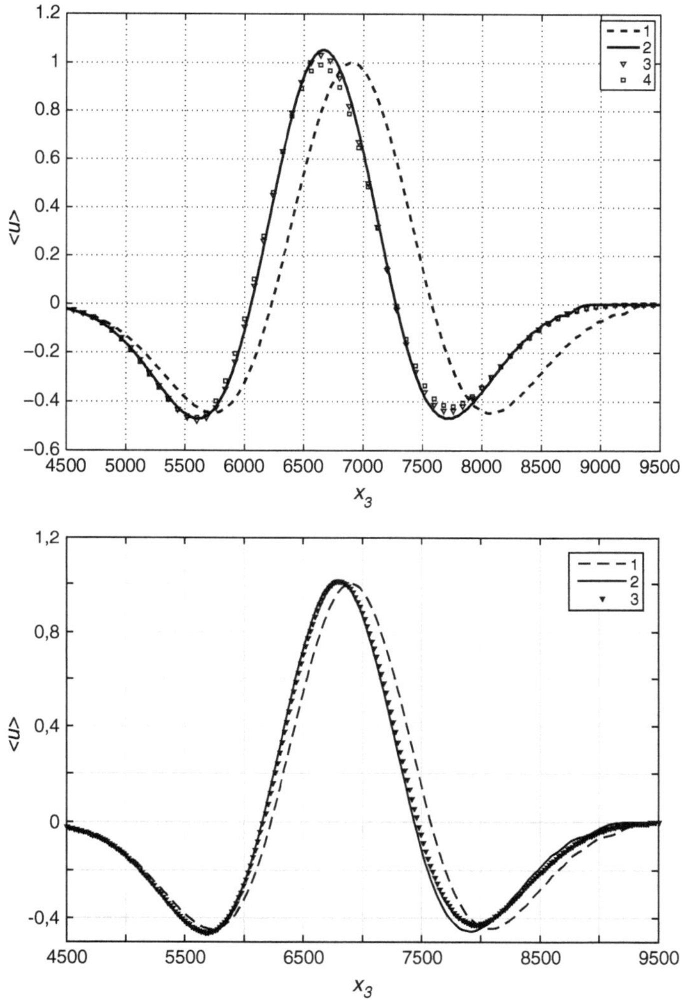

Fig. 6.2 Average of the displacement, the wave propagates along the axis x_3, $t = 3.1$ s

with the coefficient of correlation $\nu = 0.9$ In the first graph of *Fig.* 6.2: the isotropic case for the three scales $l_j = 8\,\text{h}, 16\,\text{h}, 32\,\text{h}$; $\Phi_0^{\varphi\varphi} = 0.3$, $\varphi_0 = 0.15$. In the second graph, the anisotropic case for the two scales 1/64, 1/32 of the wavelength along the axes x_1, x_2, 1/16, 1/8 of the wavelength along the axes x_3 with $\Phi_0^{\varphi\varphi} = 0.45$, $\varphi_0 = 0.225$. In *Fig.* 6.3: the anisotropic case for the two scales 1/16, 1/8 of the wavelength along the axes x_1, x_2, 1/64, 1/32 of the wavelength along the axes x_3. In the first graph of *Fig.* 6.3, the parameters $\Phi_0^{\varphi\varphi}$, φ_0 are equal to 0.45, 0.225, in the second graph $\Phi_0^{\varphi\varphi} = 0.6$, $\varphi_0 = 0.3$. We combine the spatial averaging over the planes (x_1, x_2) for each value of x_3 with ensemble averaging. The results were averaged over 45 realizations.

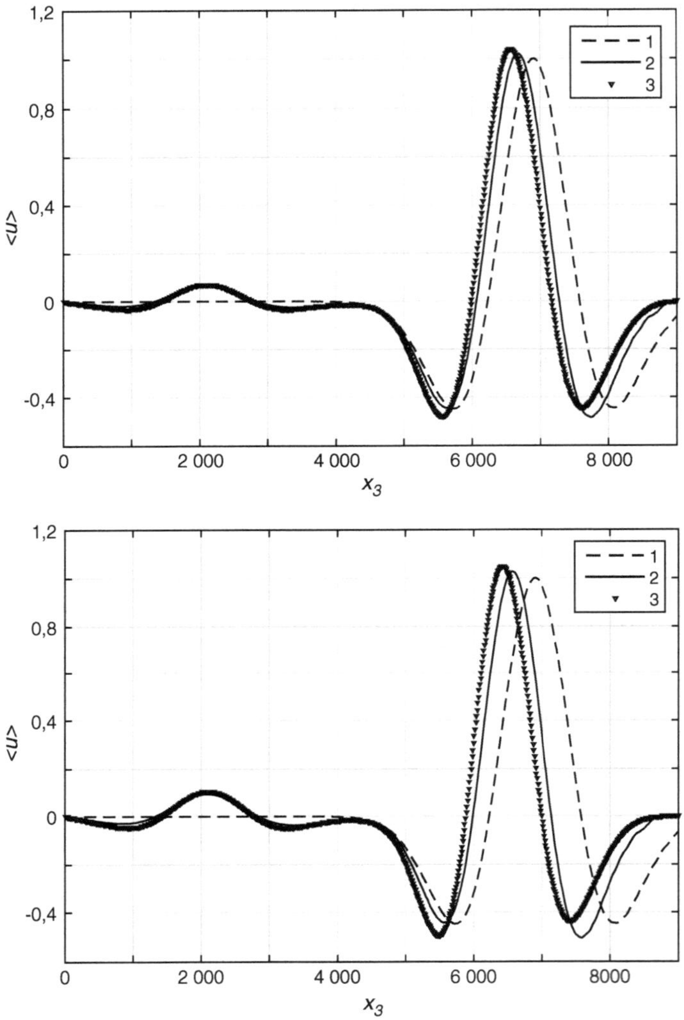

Fig. 6.3 Average of the displacement, the wave propagates along the axis x_3, $t = 3.1$ s

6.5 Conclusion

We have presented the effective coefficients for the wave equation if its parameters are described by extremely irregular small-scale fields that are close to multifractals. The multifractals can be obtained if a minimum scale l_0 in formulas (6.2), (6.3) tends to zero. The proof of multifractality of cascades is given in [9, 10]. The derivatives of these coefficients grow rapidly and become huge with the increasing number of layers in cascades. Hence, to solve equations numerically is very difficult. This may not be possible for modern computers. The coefficients smoothing algorithm is needed for such media. The smoothing algorithm is proposed. To approximate the medium, we started from the modified Kolmogorov theory in terms of the ratios of smoothed fields. As a minimum scale is not equal to zero and any singularities are absent, we use only the theory of differential equations and the theory of stochastic processes. The theoretical approach does not require an exact scale invariance of the medium. It has been shown that the small-scale heterogeneities affect the acoustic wave propagation in the first order of the scale of heterogeneities. Since the wavelength is much larger than the scale of variations of the medium, the wave cannot probe the small scales efficiently. The fluctuations of the medium tend to be averaged by low sensitivity of the wave at these scales and effective coefficients do not depend on the form of the correlation functions. The numerical testing was carried out at the scales for which the problem can be numerically solved. The wave propagates over a distance that is of the same order as the typical wavelength of a source. The numerical verification illustrates the efficiency of the approach proposed.

The numerical testing illustrates the efficiency of the approach proposed when the scales of heterogeneities are much less than the size of the wavelength.

Acknowledgements The work was supported by the RFBR N15-01-01458.

References

1. Imomnazarov, Kh., Mikhailov A.A.: Application of a spectral method for numerical modeling of propagation of seismic waves in porous media for dissipative case. Sib. Zh. Vychisl. Mat. **17**, 139–147 (2014)
2. Capdeville, Y., Guillot, L., Marigo, J.J.: Second order homogenization of the elastic wave equation for non-periodic layered media. Geophys. J. Int. **170**, 823–838 (2007)
3. Shelukhin, V., Igor, Yeltsov I., Paranichev, I.: The electrokinetic cross-coupling coefficient: two-scale homogenization approach. World J. Mech. **1**, 127–136 (2011)
4. Fouque, J.-P., Garnnier, J., Papanicolaou, G., Solna, K.: Wave Propagation and Time Reversal in Randomly Reversal in Randomly Layered Media. Stochastic Modelling and Applied Probability, vol. 56. Springer, Berlin (2007)
5. Sahimi, M.: Flow phenomena in rocks: from continuum models, to fractals, percolation, cellular automata, and simulated annealing. Rev Mod. Phys. **65**, 1393–1534 (1993)
6. Koohi lai, Z., Vasheghani, F.S., Jafari, G.R.: Non-Gaussianity effect of petrophysical quantities by using q-entropy and multi fractal random walk. Phys. A. **392** 3039–3044 (2013)
7. Kolmogorov, A.N.: A refinement of previous hypotheses concerning the local structure of turbulence in a viscous incompressible fluid at high Reynolds number. J. Fluid Mech. **13**, 82–85 (1962)
8. Kuz'min, G.A., Soboleva, O.N.: Subgrid modeling of filtration in porous self-similar media. App. Mech. Tech. Phys. **43**, 583–592 (2002)
9. Molchan, G.M.: Turbulent cascades: limitations and a statistical test of the lognormal hypothesis. Phys. Fluids **9**(8), 2387–2396 (1997)
10. Molchan, G.M.: Scaling exponents and multifractal dimensions for independed random cascades. Commun. Math. Phys. **179**, 681–702 (1996)

Chapter 7
Parameter Inference for Stochastic Differential Equations with Density Tracking by Quadrature

Harish S. Bhat, R. W. M. A. Madushani and Shagun Rawat

Abstract We derive and experimentally test an algorithm for maximum likelihood estimation of parameters in stochastic differential equations (SDEs). Our innovation is to efficiently compute the transition densities that form the log likelihood and its gradient, and to then couple these computations with quasi-Newton optimization methods to obtain maximum likelihood estimates. We compute transition densities by applying quadrature to the Chapman–Kolmogorov equation associated with a time discretization of the original SDE. To study the properties of our algorithm, we run a series of tests involving both linear and nonlinear SDE. We show that our algorithm is capable of accurate inference, and that its performance depends in a logical way on problem and algorithm parameters.

Keywords Stochastic differential equations · Parameter inference
Maximum likelihood estimation

7.1 Introduction

Consider the stochastic differential equation (SDE)

$$dX_t = f(X_t; \theta)dt + g(X_t; \theta)dW_t \tag{7.1}$$

where X_t is a scalar stochastic process, $\theta \in \mathbb{R}^N$ is a vector of parameters and W_t is standard Brownian motion. Here f and g are referred to, respectively, as the drift and diffusion functions. Suppose we have collected data $\mathbf{x} = x_0, x_1, \ldots, x_M$. Each

H. S. Bhat (✉) · R. W. M. A. Madushani · S. Rawat
University of California Merced, 5200 N. Lake Rd., Merced, CA, USA
e-mail: hbhat@ucmerced.edu

R. W. M. A. Madushani
e-mail: rmadushani@ucmerced.edu

S. Rawat
e-mail: srawat2@ucmerced.edu

J. Pilz et al. (eds.), *Statistics and Simulation*, Springer Proceedings
in Mathematics & Statistics 231, https://doi.org/10.1007/978-3-319-76035-3_7

x_j is a vector of ν samples of X_{t_j}. In this chapter, we take $t_j = j\Delta t$ for some fixed $\Delta t > 0$. Based on this data, we would like to infer θ.

One way to carry out this inference is through numerical maximization of the likelihood function. For the actual SDE, the exact likelihood $p(\mathbf{x}|\theta)$ can only be computed in very special cases, i.e. when we can solve analytically for the transition density of (7.1). Therefore, prior work has focused on approximating the exact likelihood, through analytical and/or numerical methods.

For a thorough review of past work on this problem, see [9, 10, 16]. Here we focus on past work that is particularly helpful to understand our approach. Consider the transition density $p_{X_{t_{j+1}}}(x_{j+1}|X_{t_j} = x_j, \theta)$ of a process that evolves according to the SDE (7.1), starting from $X_{t_j} = x_j$ and ending at $X_{t_{j+1}} = x_{j+1}$. Let $p(x, t)$ denote the density function of X_t. Then, one approach to approximating the transition density is to numerically solve the forward Kolmogorov (or Fokker–Planck) equation with the initial condition $p(x, 0) = \delta(x - x_j)$ up to time $T = t_{j+1} - t_j = \Delta t$.

Our approach is similar in that we also numerically track the density $p(x, t)$ without sampling. However, instead of numerically solving a partial differential equation, we track the density by applying quadrature to the Chapman–Kolmogorov equation associated with a time discretization of the SDE (7.1). We describe this density tracking by quadrature (DTQ) method in Sect. 7.2. Note that in [3], we have established conditions under which the densities computed by DTQ converge in L^1 to the true density of the SDE, as temporal and spatial grid spacings tend to zero.

Other methods similar to ours are those of [14, 15]. In these methods, one also starts with the Chapman–Kolmogorov equation for the Euler–Maruyama scheme applied to (7.1). However, instead of evaluating the resulting integrals by deterministic quadrature, Pedersen and Santa-Clara evaluate the integrals by Monte Carlo methods. These methods involve generating numerical sample paths of the SDE at times in between the observation times. This approach is problematic unless one generates sample paths conditional on both the initial condition $X_{t_j} = x_j$ and the final condition $X_{t_{j+1}} = x_{j+1}$.

The work of [1] shares our goal of computing an accurate approximation of the exact transition density and resulting likelihood function. Instead of applying quadrature, Aït-Sahalia expands the transition density in a Gram–Charlier series and then computes the expansion coefficients up to a certain order.

In the present chapter, we are primarily interested in developing properties of our algorithm, to establish a set of examples in which the algorithm succeeds. We reserve for future work a detailed comparison of our algorithm against existing approaches for inference in stochastic differential equation models.

The chapter is structured as follows: in Sect. 7.2, we give detailed derivations of temporally and spatially discretized versions of the log likelihood and its gradient. We carry out the derivations for the cases where the data consists of either one or multiple sample path(s). After deriving the algorithms, we conduct numerical tests to study their performance when both model and algorithm parameters are varied. The results of these tests are described in Sect. 7.3. In Sect. 7.4, we discuss the implications of these results and how they will inform future work.

7.2 Methods

We begin by deriving our method and algorithm in the case where $\mathbf{x}$ represents a scalar time series. This corresponds to the case where $\nu = 1$, and the data consists of only one time-discretized sample path of (7.1). Subsequently, we show how to generalize this derivation to the case where there are $\nu > 1$ sample paths.

Derivation for One Sample Path. Fix h, the internal time step, to be a small fraction of Δt, i.e. $h = \Delta t / F$ where $F \in \mathbb{Z}$ and $F \geq 2$. Let $\{Z_j\}$ denote an i.i.d. family of Gaussian random variables with mean 0 and variance 1. Then, the Euler–Maruyama discretization of (7.1) is

$$\widetilde{X}_{j+1/F} = \widetilde{X}_j + f(\widetilde{X}_j; \theta)h + g(\widetilde{X}_j; \theta)h^{1/2} Z_{j+1/F}. \tag{7.2}$$

When the index j is an integer, the random variable $\widetilde{X}_j$ is intended to approximate X_{t_j}. When the index j is not an integer, $\widetilde{X}_j$ represents a random variable that *interpolates in time* between the random variables that have been sampled to give us our data. We are now in a position to compute the likelihood. Let us specify our notation. If $A_1, \ldots, A_N$ is a collection of random variables, then $p_{A_1,\ldots,A_N}(z_1, \ldots, z_N)$ denotes the joint probability density function of $A_1, \ldots, A_N$. Conditional densities will be denoted similarly. Then the likelihood we seek to compute, the quantity we wrote as $p(\mathbf{x}|\theta)$ above, can be more accurately written as $p_{X_{t_M},\ldots,X_{t_0}}(x_M, \ldots, x_0|\theta)$. First, let us use the fact that the SDE (7.1) is an Ito diffusion and therefore satisfies the strong Markov property [8]. This enables us to define the log likelihood:

$$\mathscr{L}(\theta) = \log p_{X_{t_M},\ldots,X_{t_0}}(x_M, \ldots, x_0|\theta) = \sum_{j=0}^{M-1} \log p_{X_{t_{j+1}}}(x_{j+1}|X_{t_j} = x_j, \theta). \tag{7.3}$$

On the right-hand side, we have omitted the term $\log p_{X_0}(x_0|\theta)$. Under the assumption that x_0 is independent of θ, this term equals $\log p_{X_0}(x_0)$ and therefore plays no role in maximizing $\mathscr{L}(\theta)$. Now we introduce our first approximation: $p_{X_{t_j}} \approx p_{\widetilde{X}_j}$. The idea is to approximate the density of X_{t_j} by the density of $\widetilde{X}_j$. We can do the same for conditional densities, i.e. $p_{X_{t_{j+1}}}(x_{j+1}|X_{t_j} = x_j, \theta) \approx p_{\widetilde{X}_{j+1}}(x_{j+1}|\widetilde{X}_j = x_j, \theta)$. Convergence theory for the Euler–Maruyama method indicates that this approximation incurs an $O(h)$ error in the L^1 norm—see [2]. With this approximation,

$$\log p_{X_{t_M},\ldots,X_{t_0}}(x_M, \ldots, x_0|\theta) \approx \sum_{j=0}^{M-1} \log p_{\widetilde{X}_{j+1}}(x_{j+1}|\widetilde{X}_j = x_j, \theta).$$

Now we can use the density tracking by quadrature (DTQ) method to evaluate each transition density in the sum: the idea is to use quadrature to gradually evolve the density forward from time t_j to time t_{j+1}. To begin the derivation, we introduce interpolating random variables and then apply the Markov property recursively:

$$p_{\widetilde{X}_{j+1}}(x_{j+1}|\widetilde{X}_j = x_j, \theta) = \int\limits_{x_{j+(F-1)/F}} \cdots \int\limits_{x_{j+1/F}} \underbrace{dx_{j+(F-1)/F} \cdots dx_{j+1/F}}_{d\mathbf{x}}$$

$$p_{\widetilde{X}_{j+1}, \widetilde{X}_{j+(F-1)/F}, \ldots, \widetilde{X}_{j+1/F}}(x_{j+1}, x_{j+(F-1)/F}, \ldots, x_{j+1/F}|\widetilde{X}_j = x_j, \theta)$$

$$= \int \cdots \int d\mathbf{x} \prod_{i=1}^{F} p_{\widetilde{X}_{j+i/F}}(x_{j+i/F}|\widetilde{X}_{j+(i-1)/F} = x_{j+(i-1)/F}, \theta) \tag{7.4}$$

The last equation is the Chapman–Kolmogorov equation for the Markov chain given by (7.2). Now let $G_\theta^h(x, y)$ be the probability density function of a Gaussian random variable with mean $y + f(y; \theta)h$ and variance $g(y; \theta)^2 h$, evaluated at x. Then the crucial observation is that, for each $i \in \{1, \ldots, F\}$,

$$p_{\widetilde{X}_{j+i/F}}(x_{j+i/F}|\widetilde{X}_{j+(i-1)/F} = x_{j+(i-1)/F}, \theta) = G_\theta^h(x_{j+i/F}, x_{j+(i-1)/F}). \tag{7.5}$$

This follows from (7.2). With this observation, (7.4) simplifies to:

$$p_{\widetilde{X}_{j+1}}(x_{j+1}|\widetilde{X}_j = x_j, \theta) = \int\limits_{x_{j+(F-1)/F}} G_\theta^h(x_{j+1}, x_{j+(F-1)/F}) \int\limits_{x_{j+(F-2)/F}} \cdots$$

$$\left[\int\limits_{x_{j+1/F}} G_\theta^h(x_{j+2/F}, x_{j+1/F}) G_\theta^h(x_{j+1/F}, x_j) dx_{j+1/F} \right] dx_{j+2/F} \cdots dx_{j+(F-1)/F} \tag{7.6}$$

Our next approximation is to evaluate the integrals by quadrature. We introduce the spatial grid spacing $k > 0$. We will use superscripts to denote spatial grid locations, so that, for instance, $x_{j+1}^a = ak$ for all $a \in \mathbb{Z}$. Then, repeatedly applying the trapezoidal rule on the real line, we obtain

$$p_{\widetilde{X}_{j+1}}(x_{j+1}|\widetilde{X}_j = x_j, \theta) \approx k \sum_{a_{F-1}} G_\theta^h(x_{j+1}, x_{j+(F-1)/F}^{a_{F-1}})$$

$$k \sum_{a_{F-2}} G_\theta^h(x_{j+(F-1)/F}^{a_{F-1}}, x_{j+(F-2)/F}^{a_{F-2}}) \cdots k \sum_{a_1} G_\theta^h(x_{j+2/F}^{a_2}, x_{j+1/F}^{a_1}) G_\theta^h(x_{j+1/F}^{a_1}, x_j)$$

In practice, we evaluate these sums on a finite subset of $\mathbb{Z}$; this is justified by the Gaussian decay of each G_θ^h. We think of $kG_\theta^h(x_{j+2/F}^{a_2}, x_{j+1/F}^{a_1})$ as the (a_2, a_1) element of a matrix K. In this way, the above formula reduces to repeated matrix-vector multiplication. Specifically, let us define the a_1th element of the vector $\hat{p}_{j+1/F}$ by $\hat{p}_{j+1/F}^{a_1} = G_\theta^h(x_{j+1/F}^{a_1}, x_j)$. Then, multiplication by the matrix K corresponds to stepping forward in time by h; i.e. $\hat{p}_{j+2/F} = K\hat{p}_{j+1/F}$ and $\hat{p}_{j+(F-1)/F} = K^{F-2}\hat{p}_{j+1/F}$. Finally, noting that x_{j+1} is a known data point, let us define the a_{F-1}th element of the vector Γ_{F-1} by $\Gamma_{F-1}^{a_{F-1}} = kG_\theta^h(x_{j+1}, x_{j+(F-1)/F}^{a_{F-1}})$. Then we have

$$p_{\widetilde{X}_{j+1}}(x_{j+1}|\widetilde{X}_j = x_j, \theta) \approx \left[\Gamma_{F-1}\right]^T K^{F-2} \hat{p}_{j+1/F}, \tag{7.7}$$

where ^{T} denotes transpose. We insert this computation into (7.3) to obtain

$$\mathscr{L}(\theta) \approx \sum_{j=0}^{M-1} \log \left[\Gamma_{F-1}\right]^T K^{F-2} \hat{p}_{j+1/F}. \tag{7.8}$$

Gradient. Next, we compute the gradient of the log likelihood with respect to θ. This gradient is important for numerical optimization. We start with

$$\begin{aligned}\frac{\partial}{\partial \theta_\ell}\mathscr{L}(\theta) &= \frac{\partial}{\partial \theta_\ell} \log p_{X_{t_M},\ldots,X_{t_0}}(x_M, \ldots, x_0|\theta) \\ &\approx \sum_{j=0}^{M-1} \frac{1}{p_{\widetilde{X}_{j+1}}(x_{j+1}|\widetilde{X}_j = x_j, \theta)} \frac{\partial}{\partial \theta_\ell} p_{\widetilde{X}_{j+1}}(x_{j+1}|\widetilde{X}_j = x_j, \theta). \end{aligned} \tag{7.9}$$

The remaining derivative looks like this:

$$\begin{aligned}&\frac{\partial}{\partial \theta_\ell} p_{\widetilde{X}_{j+1}}(x_{j+1}|\widetilde{X}_j = x_j, \theta) \\ &= \int\limits_{x_{j+(F-1)/F}} \cdots \int\limits_{x_{j+1/F}} \sum_{r=0}^{F-1} \left\{ \frac{\partial}{\partial \theta_\ell} p_{\widetilde{X}_{j+(r+1)/F}}(x_{j+(r+1)/F}|\widetilde{X}_{j+r/F} = x_{j+r/F}, \theta) \right. \\ &\left. \prod_{\substack{s \neq r \\ s=0,\ldots,F-1}} p_{\widetilde{X}_{j+(s+1)/F}}(x_{j+(s+1)/F}|\widetilde{X}_{j+s/F} = x_{j+s/F}, \theta) \right\} dx_{j+(F-1)/F} \cdots dx_{j+1/F}\end{aligned}$$

Let us derive an algorithm to compute this quantity. First, we peel off the $r = F - 1$ term in the sum to write:

$$\begin{aligned}&\frac{\partial}{\partial \theta_\ell} p_{\widetilde{X}_{j+1}}(x_{j+1}|\widetilde{X}_j = x_j, \theta) \\ &= \int\limits_{x_{j+(F-1)/F}} \cdots \int\limits_{x_{j+1/F}} \left\{ \frac{\partial}{\partial \theta_\ell} p_{\widetilde{X}_{j+1}}(x_{j+1}|\widetilde{X}_{j+(F-1)/F} = x_{j+(F-1)/F}, \theta) \right. \\ &\qquad \left. \prod_{s=0,\ldots,F-2} p_{\widetilde{X}_{j+(s+1)/F}}(x_{j+(s+1)/F}|\widetilde{X}_{j+s/F} = x_{j+s/F}, \theta) \right\} \\ &\qquad + \left[p_{\widetilde{X}_{j+1}}(x_{j+1}|\widetilde{X}_{j+(F-1)/F} = x_{j+(F-1)/F}, \theta) \right. \\ &\qquad \times \sum_{r=0}^{F-2} \left(\frac{\partial}{\partial \theta_\ell} p_{\widetilde{X}_{j+(r+1)/F}}(x_{j+(r+1)/F}|\widetilde{X}_{j+r/F} = x_{j+r/F}, \theta) \right.\end{aligned}$$

$$\prod_{\substack{s \neq r \\ s=0,\ldots,F-2}} p_{\widetilde{X}_{j+(s+1)/F}}(x_{j+(s+1)/F} | \widetilde{X}_{j+s/F} = x_{j+s/F}, \theta)\Bigg)\Bigg] \, dx_{j+(F-1)/F} \cdots dx_{j+1/F}$$

Again, we can use the definition of G together with the crucial observation described above to simplify the above expression to:

$$\frac{\partial}{\partial \theta_\ell} p_{\widetilde{X}_{j+1}}(x_{j+1} | \widetilde{X}_j = x_j, \theta)$$
$$= \int_{x_{j+(F-1)/F}} \cdots \int_{x_{j+1/F}} \left\{ \frac{\partial}{\partial \theta_\ell} G^h_\theta(x_{j+1}, x_{j+(F-1)/F}) \prod_{s=0,\ldots,F-2} G^h_\theta(x_{j+(s+1)/F}, x_{j+s/F}) \right\}$$
$$+ \Bigg[G^h_\theta(x_{j+1}, x_{j+(F-1)/F}) \sum_{r=0}^{F-2} \Bigg(\frac{\partial}{\partial \theta_\ell} G^h_\theta(x_{j+(r+1)/F}, x_{j+r/F})$$
$$\prod_{\substack{s \neq r \\ s=0,\ldots,F-2}} G^h_\theta(x_{j+(s+1)/F}, x_{j+s/F}) \Bigg) \Bigg] \, dx_{j+(F-1)/F} \cdots dx_{j+1/F}$$

We discretize in space, again using the trapezoidal rule repeatedly:

$$\frac{\partial}{\partial \theta_\ell} p_{\widetilde{X}_{j+1}}(x_{j+1} | \widetilde{X}_j = x_j, \theta)$$
$$\approx k^{F-1} \sum_{a_{F-1}} \cdots \sum_{a_1} \left\{ \frac{\partial}{\partial \theta_\ell} G^h_\theta(x_{j+1}, x^{a_{F-1}}_{j+(F-1)/F}) \prod_{s=0,\ldots,F-2} G^h_\theta(x^{a_{s+1}}_{j+(s+1)/F}, x^{a_s}_{j+s/F}) \right\}$$
$$+ \Bigg[G^h_\theta(x_{j+1}, x^{a_{F-1}}_{j+(F-1)/F})$$
$$\sum_{r=0}^{F-2} \Bigg(\frac{\partial}{\partial \theta_\ell} G^h_\theta(x^{a_{r+1}}_{j+(r+1)/F}, x^{a_r}_{j+r/F}) \prod_{\substack{s \neq r \\ s=0,\ldots,F-2}} G^h_\theta(x^{a_{s+1}}_{j+(s+1)/F}, x^{a_s}_{j+s/F}) \Bigg) \Bigg]$$

In the above expression and in what follows, any instance of $x_j^{a_0}$ should be interpreted as simply x_j. Now let us push all summations over $a_1, \ldots, a_{F_2}$ inside to obtain

$$\frac{\partial}{\partial \theta_\ell} p_{\widetilde{X}_{j+1}}(x_{j+1} | \widetilde{X}_j = x_j, \theta) \approx k \sum_{a_{F-1}} \Bigg\{ \frac{\partial}{\partial \theta_\ell} G^h_\theta(x_{j+1}, x^{a_{F-1}}_{j+(F-1)/F})$$
$$\Bigg(k^{F-2} \sum_{a_{F-2}} \cdots \sum_{a_1} \prod_{s=0,\ldots,F-2} G^h_\theta(x^{a_{s+1}}_{j+(s+1)/F}, x^{a_s}_{j+s/F}) \Bigg) \Bigg\}$$
$$+ \Bigg[G^h_\theta(x_{j+1}, x^{a_{F-1}}_{j+(F-1)/F}) k^{F-2} \sum_{a_{F-2}} \cdots \sum_{a_1} \sum_{r=0}^{F-2} \Bigg(\frac{\partial}{\partial \theta_\ell} G^h_\theta(x^{a_{r+1}}_{j+(r+1)/F}, x^{a_r}_{j+r/F})$$
$$\prod_{\substack{s \neq r \\ s=0,\ldots,F-2}} G^h_\theta(x^{a_{s+1}}_{j+(s+1)/F}, x^{a_s}_{j+s/F}) \Bigg) \Bigg]$$

Now note that by our previous definitions, we have that

$$k^{F-2}\sum_{a_{F-2}}\cdots\sum_{a_1}\prod_{s=0,\ldots,F-2} G_\theta^h(x_{j+(s+1)/F}^{a_{s+1}}, x_{j+s/F}^{a_s}) = K^{F-2}\hat{p}_{j+1/F} = \hat{p}_{j+(F-1)/F}.$$

Analogously, let us define the a_{F-1}th element of the vector $\hat{q}_{j+(F-1)/F,\ell}$ by

$$\hat{q}_{j+(F-1)/F,\ell}^{a_{F-1}} = k^{F-2}\sum_{a_{F-2}}\cdots\sum_{a_1}$$
$$\sum_{r=0}^{F-2}\left(\frac{\partial}{\partial\theta_\ell}G_\theta^h(x_{j+(r+1)/F}^{a_{r+1}}, x_{j+r/F}^{a_r})\prod_{\substack{s\neq r\\ s=0,\ldots,F-2}} G_\theta^h(x_{j+(s+1)/F}^{a_{s+1}}, x_{j+s/F}^{a_s})\right). \quad (7.10)$$

Let $\Gamma_{F-1,\ell}^{a_{F-1}} = k\frac{\partial}{\partial\theta_\ell}G_\theta^h(x_{j+1}, x_{j+(F-1)/F}^{a_{F-1}})$ define the a_{F-1}th element of the vector $\Gamma_{F-1,\ell}$. Using this together with our old definition of Γ_{F-1}, we have

$$\frac{\partial}{\partial\theta_\ell}p_{\widetilde{X}_{j+1}}(x_{j+1}|\widetilde{X}_j = x_j, \theta) \approx \left[\Gamma_{F-1,\ell}\right]^T \hat{p}_{j+(F-1)/F} + \left[\Gamma_{F-1}\right]^T \hat{q}_{j+(F-1)/F,\ell}.$$

Now let $K_\ell^{a_{r+1},a_r} = k\frac{\partial}{\partial\theta_\ell}G_\theta^h(x_{j+(r+1)/F}^{a_{r+1}}, x_{j+r/F}^{a_r})$ define the (a_{r+1}, a_r) element of the matrix K_ℓ. Then, let us return to (7.10). Peeling off the $r = F-2$ term,

$$\hat{q}_{j+(F-1)/F,\ell} = K_\ell\hat{p}_{j+(F-2)/F} + K\hat{q}_{j+(F-2)/F,\ell},$$

where $\hat{q}_{j+(F-2)/F,\ell}$ is defined analogously to $\hat{q}_{j+(F-1)/F,\ell}$, simply decrementing F by 1 on the right-hand side. It is clear that after a finite number of such manipulations, we will reach the $r = 0$ term. In this case, the product term will be empty (and hence equal 1), leaving us with only the derivative with respect to θ_ℓ of $G_\theta^h(x_{j+1/F}^{a_1}, x_j)$. In this way, we may derive the following algorithm:

1. We begin with $\hat{q}_{j+1/F,\ell}^{a_1} = \frac{\partial}{\partial\theta_\ell}G_\theta^h(x_{j+1/F}^{a_1}, x_j)$.
2. We then iteratively define, for $r = 1, \ldots, F-2$,

$$\hat{q}_{j+(r+1)/F,\ell} = K_\ell\hat{p}_{j+r/F} + K\hat{q}_{j+r/F,\ell}. \quad (7.11)$$

3. We finish with:

$$\frac{\partial}{\partial\theta_\ell}p_{\widetilde{X}_{j+1}}(x_{j+1}|\widetilde{X}_j = x_j, \theta) \approx \left[\Gamma_{F-1,\ell}\right]^T \hat{p}_{j+(F-1)/F} + \left[\Gamma_{F-1}\right]^T \hat{q}_{j+(F-1)/F,\ell}.$$

Combining this with (7.7) and (7.9), we obtain

$$\frac{\partial}{\partial \theta_\ell} \mathscr{L}(\theta) \approx \sum_{j=0}^{M-1} \frac{\left[\Gamma_{F-1,\ell}\right]^T \hat{p}_{j+(F-1)/F} + \left[\Gamma_{F-1}\right]^T \hat{q}_{j+(F-1)/F,\ell}}{\left[\Gamma_{F-1}\right]^T K^{F-2} \hat{p}_{j+1/F}}. \tag{7.12}$$

Derivation for Many Sample Paths. We revisit (7.6) and write

$$p_{\widetilde{X}_{j+1/F}}(x_{j+1/F} | \widetilde{X}_j = x_j, \theta) = G_\theta^h(x_{j+1/F}, x_j) = \int_y G_\theta^h(x_{j+1/F}, y) \delta(y - x_j) \, dy. \tag{7.13}$$

The term on the right-hand side can be interpreted as evolving the initial density $p_{\widetilde{X}_j}(y) = \delta(y - x_j)$ forward by h units of time. We note that conditioning on $\widetilde{X}_j = x_j$ on the left-hand side leads to a Dirac delta initial density on the right-hand side. This will be an important ingredient in the algorithm that follows.

Now let us reinterpret $\mathbf{x} = x_0, x_1, \ldots, x_M$ as a sequence of vector-valued observations. For each $s = 1, 2, \ldots, \nu$, the sequence $x_0^s, x_1^s, \ldots, x_M^s$ is a scalar time series. With these changes, the derivation of the log likelihood from (7.3) to (7.4) holds without any changes. The only real change is that (7.5) only holds for $i \in \{2, \ldots, F\}$. When $i = 1$, the quantity that must be computed is:

$$p_{\widetilde{X}_{j+1/F}}(x_{j+1/F} | \widetilde{X}_j = x_j, \theta), \tag{7.14}$$

where we have many samples $\{x_j^s\}_{s=1}^{\nu}$ of the random variable $\widetilde{X}_j$. When $\nu > 1$, these samples can be used to estimate the density of $\widetilde{X}_j$ as follows:

$$p_{\widetilde{X}_j}(y) \approx \frac{1}{\nu} \sum_{r=1}^{\nu} \delta(y - x_j^s). \tag{7.15}$$

This approximation is a density estimate that corresponds to the spatial derivative of the empirical cumulative distribution function of the samples. By logic analogous to (7.13) and the above discussion, we can then evaluate (7.14) by

$$p_{\widetilde{X}_{j+1/F}}(x_{j+1/F} | \widetilde{X}_j = x_j, \theta) = \int_y G_\theta^h(x_{j+1/F}, y) p_{\widetilde{X}_j}(y) dy \approx \frac{1}{\nu} \sum_{r=1}^{\nu} G_\theta^h(x_{j+1/F}, x_j^s). \tag{7.16}$$

We make the approximation (7.15) so that the density along each sample path evolves with the same initial condition. Without such an approximation, the calculation (7.8) would have to be repeated ν times.

The calculation of the likelihood proceeds as in (7.4) with $G_\theta^h(x_{j+1/F}, x_j)$ replaced by (7.16). We now redefine $\hat{p}_{j+1/F}$ such that its a_1th element is (7.16) evaluated at $x_{j+1/F} = x_{j+1/F}^{a_1}$. We redefine Γ_{F-1} to be a matrix whose (a_F, a_{F-1}) entry is given by $\Gamma_{F-1}^{a_F, a_{F-1}} = k G_\theta^h(x_{j+1}^{a_F}, x_{j+(F-1)/F}^{a_{F_1}})$. With these definitions, (7.7) becomes

$$p_{\widetilde{X}_{j+1}}(x_{j+1}|\widetilde{X}_j = x_j, \theta) \approx \prod_{a_F=1}^{\nu} \left(\left[\Gamma_{F-1} \right]^T K^{F-2} \hat{p}_{j+1/F} \right)_{a_F}, \tag{7.17}$$

where $(w)_s$ denotes the sth component of the vector w. Similarly, (7.8) becomes

$$\mathscr{L}(\theta) \approx \sum_{j=0}^{M-1} \sum_{a_F=1}^{\nu} \log \left(\left[\Gamma_{F-1} \right]^T K^{F-2} \hat{p}_{j+1/F} \right)_{a_F}. \tag{7.18}$$

Gradient. The derivation of the gradient of $\mathscr{L}(\theta)$ proceeds just as before with $G_\theta^h(x_{j+1/F}, x_j)$ replaced by (7.16). The only changes required in the algorithm are, first, to redefine $\hat{q}^{a_1}_{j+1/F,\ell} = \frac{1}{\nu} \sum_{r=1}^{\nu} \frac{\partial}{\partial \theta_\ell} G_\theta^h(x_{j+1/F}, x_j^s)$, and second, to redefine $\Gamma_{F-1,\ell}$ as a matrix whose (a_F, a_{F-1}) entry is $\Gamma^{a_F, a_{F-1}}_{F-1,\ell} = k \frac{\partial}{\partial \theta_\ell} G_\theta^h(x^{a_F}_{j+1}, x^{a_{F-1}}_{j+(F-1)/F})$. With these changes, the gradient becomes

$$\frac{\partial}{\partial \theta_\ell} \mathscr{L}(\theta) \approx \sum_{j=0}^{M-1} \sum_{a_F=1}^{\nu} \frac{\left(\left[\Gamma_{F-1,\ell} \right]^T \hat{p}_{j+(F-1)/F} + \left[\Gamma_{F-1} \right]^T \hat{q}_{j+(F-1)/F,\ell} \right)_{a_F}}{\left(\left[\Gamma_{F-1} \right]^T K^{F-2} \hat{p}_{j+1/F} \right)_{a_F}}, \tag{7.19}$$

where $\hat{q}$ is computed using (7.11) just as before.

Inference. The procedure for carrying out inference is now straightforward. We use the algorithms derived above to compute the objective function, $J(\theta) = -\mathscr{L}(\theta)$ and its gradient. We pass J and its gradient to a numerical optimization package, NLopt [11]. We specify an initial condition and instruct NLopt to use one of its methods (typically the low-storage BFGS algorithm [12, 13]) to numerically minimize J. We use $\hat{\theta}$ to denote the minimizer of $J(\theta)$; $\hat{\theta}$ is our maximum likelihood estimate of θ. All implementations are coded in *R*. We call algorithms from NLopt using **nloptr** [18].

7.3 Results

We now present numerical tests of our algorithm in three cases. For each case, we generate multiple sample paths using a specified SDE with known parameters. We use θ to denote the true parameter vector. Using the data thus generated, we then use our method to produce $\hat{\theta}$, our maximum likelihood estimate of the parameter vector. In the first two scenarios, the SDE we use for generating data coincides with the SDE used for inference. In the third scenario, we use a generic polynomial SDE for inference—this SDE includes as a special case the SDE used for generating data.

Table 7.1 Results for Case 1. Using either 300 or 100 sample paths produced by Euler–Maruyama simulation with time step $\xi = 10^{-4}$, we study the effect of reducing h, the internal DTQ time step

Estimated $\hat{\theta}$	Iterations	h	Paths	RMS error
(1.020, 0, 1.404)	31	0.05	300	0.6597
(1.041, 0, 1.430)	30	0.02	300	0.6916
(1.048, 0, 1.438)	34	0.01	300	0.7028
(1.052, 0, 1.443)	34	0.005	300	0.7084
(1.054, 0, 1.445)	35	0.002	300	0.7119
(0.671, 0, 1.143)	31	0.01	100	0.2238
(0.673, 0, 1.146)	28	0.005	100	0.2264
(0.674, 0, 1.147)	26	0.002	100	0.2284

To test the performance of the algorithm, we generate the data using the Euler–Maruyama approximation of the SDE. We step forward in time, starting from t_0 to a final time point $T > 0$. We use a step size of ξ, where $\xi = 10^{-4}$ unless specified otherwise. We retain the samples only at times $t = m\Delta t$ from $m = 0$ to $m = M$, where $M\Delta t = T$. For consistency during comparisons, we set $t_0 = 0$, $T = 25$, and $\Delta t = 1$.

Case 1: Linear SDE (Ornstein–Uhlenbeck process). We consider the SDE for the Ornstein–Uhlenbeck process with linear drift and constant diffusion terms.

$$dX_t = \theta_1(\theta_2 - X_t)dt + \theta_3 dW_t \tag{7.20}$$

For the first set of experiments, the true parameter vector is $\theta = (0.5, 0, 1)$. We start the optimizer with an initial condition $\theta_0 = (1, 2, 0.5)$. We study how well we are able to infer the parameters as a function of DTQ's internal time step h and the number of sample paths. For this set of experiments, the spatial grid spacing k is set to $k = h^{0.75}$. In Table 7.1, we summarize this information together with the RMS (root-mean-square) error between the estimated and true parameter values. This is equivalent to the 2-norm error, $\|\theta - \hat{\theta}\|_2$. We also record the number of iterations required for the optimizer to converge to the minimizer of the objective function, the negative log likelihood.

The method is not as sensitive to h as one might expect. Instead, what we find is that the error decreases when we decrease the number of sample paths. When we use only 100 sample paths, we obtain a qualitatively reasonable solution for all three components of θ, with θ_2 in particular identified up to machine precision.

To explore whether the above findings were peculiar to the way we generated the data, we conducted another series of tests starting with a true parameter vector of $\theta = (0.5, 0.9, 1)$. The results are displayed in Table 7.2. This time, when we use the Euler–Maruyama method to generate data, we use an internal time step of $\xi = 10^{-6}$, retaining all other parameters described above. For the inference, we give the optimizer an initial guess of $\theta_0 = (1, 0.5, 0.5)$. We again set the spatial grid spacing to $k = h^{0.75}$ and record the RMS error.

Table 7.2 Results for Case 1. Using either 300 or 100 sample paths produced by Euler–Maruyama simulation with time step $\xi = 10^{-6}$, we study the effect of reducing h, DTQ's internal time step

Estimated $\hat{\theta}$	Iterations	h	Paths	RMS error
(0.361, 0.968, 0.836)	39	0.050	50	0.2254
(0.362, 0.968, 0.839)	46	0.020	50	0.2226
(0.362, 0.968, 0.840)	42	0.010	50	0.2219
(0.362, 0.968, 0.841)	28	0.005	50	0.2212
(0.463, 0.885, 0.966)	45	0.050	300	0.05244
(0.466, 0.886, 0.973)	22	0.020	300	0.04561
(0.467, 0.886, 0.975)	22	0.010	300	0.04370
(0.468, 0.886, 0.976)	26	0.005	300	0.04237
(0.468, 0.886, 0.976)	20	0.002	300	0.04237

The results from Table 7.2 show that if we increase the number of sample paths from 50 to 300, the error decreases dramatically. This leads us to our view that, for the present version of DTQ, the quality of the data is important. When we decrease the Euler–Maruyama time step from $\xi = 10^{-4}$ to $\xi = 10^{-6}$, we gain roughly one extra decimal place of accuracy in the sample paths. This leads DTQ towards higher-quality estimates of the parameters in the Ornstein–Uhlenbeck model (7.20).

The performance of DTQ should increase as the number of sample paths increases. In this regard, we believe the results from Table 7.1 are an artefact of how the data was generated. We will see confirmation of this in the results below on a nonlinear SDE model.

Additionally, we note that Table 7.2 confirms that DTQ's results are relatively insensitive to decreasing h, the internal time step of DTQ. Note that the data set we use for the experiments is collected at intervals of $\Delta t = 1$. We have found, in practice, that the choice $h = \Delta t/20$ is sufficient for inference. This is consistent with the results of [14], who chooses $h \approx \Delta t/25$.

Case 2: Nonlinear SDE (Double Well Potential). As our second example, we consider the following SDE with a nonlinear drift and constant diffusion term:

$$dX_t = \theta_1 X_t(\theta_2 - X_t^2)dt + \theta_3 dW_t \tag{7.21}$$

In Table 7.3, we show the results of an initial set of tests. In these tests, we vary both the true parameter vector θ and the initial guess θ_0 that is given to the optimizer. For these tests, the data consists of 100 sample paths and the DTQ grid spacing is given by $k = h^{0.75}$. Note that even when θ_0 is far from θ, the estimated parameters $\hat{\theta}$ are close to θ. This trend holds for different values of θ. In fact, DTQ's RMS errors are quite low for all tests involving the nonlinear model (7.21).

Next, in Table 7.4, we study the effect of decreasing DTQ's internal time step, h, when all other problem/algorithm parameters are kept fixed. For these tests, we set $\theta = (1, 4, 0.5)$, $\theta_0 = (2, 2, 1)$, and $k = h^{0.75}$. The data consists of 100 sample paths.

Table 7.3 Results for Case 2. We study a collection of problems involving different true θ values and different initial guesses θ_0

True θ	Initial θ_0	Estimated $\hat{\theta}$	Iterations	h	RMS Error
(0.2, 1, 0.5)	(1, 1, 1)	(0.162, 0.886, 0.488)	37	0.05	0.06901
(0.4, 1, 0.5)	(1, 1, 1)	(0.629, 1.023, 0.618)	24	0.05	0.14965
(1, 4, 0.5)	(0.5, 0.5, 0.5)	(0.928, 3.990, 0.467)	50	0.01	0.04568
(1, 4, 0.5)	(2, 2, 1)	(0.925, 3.990, 0.430)	48	0.01	0.05935
(1, 4, 0.5)	(8, 8, 2)	(0.928, 3.990, 0.467)	47	0.01	0.04571

Table 7.4 Results for Case 2. We study the effect of decreasing h, keeping all other parameters fixed

Estimated $\hat{\theta}$	Iterations	h	RMS error
(0.925046, 3.990012, 0.430020)	37	0.05	0.05948
(0.925311, 3.990029, 0.430068)	48	0.01	0.05935
(0.926930, 3.990418, 0.471400)	48	0.005	0.04563
(0.925808, 3.990464, 0.473724)	41	0.002	0.04577
(0.925433, 3.990480, 0.474493)	31	0.001	0.04583

The results show that it is possible to slightly reduce the RMS error by decreasing h, the internal time step. Based on these results, we see that there is no disadvantage incurred by using our method with $h = 0.05$; at this internal time step, the method runs very quickly in R.

In Table 7.5, we run a series of tests where each test is repeated twice, once with the spatial grid spacing set to $k = h^{0.75}$ and again with $k = h$. For these tests, we generate data with $\theta = (1, 4, 0.5)$. If we examine the first two rows of Table 7.5, what we see is that decreasing the spatial grid spacing has a significant, beneficial effect on the RMS error. What has happened here is that we have given the optimizer an initial guess where the third element of θ_0 is 0.1, a relatively small value. If we go back to the SDE (7.21), we see that this third element of θ_0 corresponds to the diffusion coefficient. When the diffusion coefficient is small, the Gaussian kernel G_θ^h becomes very narrow. This necessitates a finer spatial grid in order to resolve the kernel well enough to perform accurate quadrature. For the final four rows of Table 7.5, the third element of θ_0 is 1 and we do not observe as significant a reduction in RMS error when we refine the spatial grid.

Finally, in Table 7.6, we study the effect of increasing the number of Euler–Maruyama sample paths in the data set that we feed into the inference algorithm. We keep all other algorithm and problem parameters fixed, with $\theta = (1, 4, 0.5)$, $\theta_0 = (2, 2, 1)$, $h = 0.01$ and $k = h^{0.75}$. The results show a steady improvement in the estimated $\hat{\theta}$ as the number of sample paths increase. The last row of Table 7.6 contains our best result for this inference problem with an RMS error less than 0.01.

Table 7.5 Results for Case 2. We compare spatial grid laws $k = h^{0.75}$ and $k = h$

Initial θ_0	Estimated $\hat{\theta}$	Iterations	k	Paths	RMS error
(0.5, 0.5, 0.1)	(0.100, 4.024, 0.100)	39	$h^{0.75}$	100	0.5688
(0.5, 0.5, 0.1)	(1.035, 3.993, 0.499)	43	h	100	0.0205
(2, 2, 1)	(0.925, 3.990, 0.430)	48	$h^{0.75}$	100	0.0593
(2, 2, 1)	(0.955, 3.995, 0.481)	35	h	100	0.0283
(2, 2, 1)	(1.035, 3.993, 0.499)	75	$h^{0.75}$	300	0.0206
(2, 2, 1)	(1.022, 4.008, 0.497)	32	h	300	0.0138

Table 7.6 Results for Case 2. We examine the effect of increasing the number of sample paths in the data set, keeping all other parameters fixed

Estimated $\hat{\theta}$	Iterations	Paths	RMS error
(0.776, 4.060, 0.424)	100	2	0.1408
(0.899, 3.992, 0.510)	27	10	0.0583
(0.833, 4.018, 0.440)	35	50	0.1030
(0.925, 3.990, 0.430)	48	100	0.0593
(0.901, 4.007, 0.464)	33	200	0.0609
(1.035, 3.993, 0.499)	75	300	0.0206
(1.107, 3.994, 0.513)	43	400	0.0624
(0.988, 3.999, 0.489)	33	1000	0.0094

Case 3: Generic Polynomial Drift and Diffusion Functions. For our third example, we reuse (7.21) to generate simulated data, but we use a more general model for the drift function, a generic cubic polynomial. In other words, for the purposes of inference, we use the SDE model

$$dX_t = (\theta_0 + \theta_1 X_t + \theta_2 X_t^2 + \theta_3 X_t^3)dt + \theta_4 dW_t. \qquad (7.22)$$

We infer the parameters $\theta = (\theta_0, \theta_1, \theta_2, \theta_3, \theta_4)$ in the SDE (7.22) from the observations generated using the SDE (7.21) to see if we recover the correct form of the drift function. Ideally, DTQ will infer that θ_0 and θ_2 in (7.22) are zero.

In Table 7.7, we display our results for three values of h, the internal time step. We generate our data by simulating 100 sample paths of (7.21) with $\theta_1 = 0.2, \theta_2 = 4$ and $\theta_3 = 0.4$. Note that in terms of the inference model (7.22), this corresponds to $\theta = (0, 0.8, 0, -0.2, 0.4)$. For the initial guess, we use $\theta_0 = (0, 0, 0, 0, 0.5)$. In this particular set of tests, instead of using the BFGS algorithm described above, we use NLopt's method of moving asymptotes (MMA) algorithm [17].

Overall, DTQ correctly identifies the qualitative form of the model. That is, we find that the first and third components of $\hat{\theta}$ are close to zero, and the remaining components of $\hat{\theta}$ are also close to their true values.

Table 7.7 Results for Case 3. We perform inference using model (7.22), which has a higher-dimensional parameter space than (7.21), the model used to generate the data

Estimated $\hat{\theta}$	Iterations	h	RMS error
(0.014, 0.619, −0.003, −0.154, 0.357)	69	0.005	0.0859
(0.014, 0.867, −0.003, −0.217, 0.424)	57	0.002	0.0334
(0.012, 0.766, −0.003, −0.192, 0.408)	89	0.001	0.0168

7.4 Discussion and Conclusion

In this chapter, we have both derived and experimentally studied a new algorithm for parameter inference in stochastic differential equation models. The crux of the algorithm is to use quadrature to compute the transition densities required for the both the log likelihood function and its gradient.

The results in Sect. 7.3 clearly demonstrate several conditions under which DTQ performs well. In particular, we find empirical evidence justifying the approximations made in Sect. 7.2—especially (7.15) and (7.16), which have not been justified in prior theoretical work. Once the internal time step h is sufficiently small, further reduction of h does not significantly improve the quality of the inferred $\hat{\theta}$. We do find that certain algorithm parameters, such as the spatial grid spacing k, do need to be adjusted to handle scenarios such as very small diffusion coefficients.

We have seen that the primary challenge to be addressed is that the present version of DTQ, in order to produce highly accurate results, requires high-quality data. In future work, we will continue ongoing efforts to overcome this obstacle, including an adjoint method to evaluate the gradient $\nabla_\theta \mathscr{L}(\theta)$ [4] and measurement models that enable filtering of noisy observations [6]. Other improvements to the method we seek to explore include implementing core parts of the algorithm in C++ [5], allowing for time-dependent drift and diffusion coefficients [7], and also allowing for data that is not equispaced in time [6].

Acknowledgements This work was partly supported by a grant from the Committee on Research at UC Merced.

References

1. Aït-Sahalia, Y.: Maximum likelihood estimation of discretely sampled diffusions: a closed-form approximation approach. Econometrica **70**(1), 223–262 (2002)
2. Bally, V., Talay, D.: The law of the Euler scheme for stochastic differential equations. II. Convergence rate of the density. Monte Carlo Methods Appl. **2**(2), 93–128 (1996)
3. Bhat, H.S., Madushani, R.W.M.A.: Density tracking by quadrature for stochastic differential equations (2016). https://arxiv.org/abs/1610.09572. Accessed 22 July 2017

4. Bhat, H.S., Madushani, R.W.M.A.: Nonparametric adjoint-based inference for stochastic differential equations. In: 2016 IEEE International Conference on Data Science and Advanced Analytics (DSAA), pp. 798–807 (2016)
5. Bhat, H.S., Madushani, R.W.M.A., Rawat, S.: Rdtq: density tracking by quadrature (2016). http://cran.r-project.org/package=Rdtq. Accessed 22 July 2017 (R package version 0.1)
6. Bhat, H.S., Madushani, R.W.M.A., Rawat, S.: Scalable SDE filtering and inference with Apache Spark. Proc. Mach. Learn. Res. **53**, 18–34 (2016)
7. Bhat, H.S., Madushani, R.W.M.A., Rawat, S.: Bayesian inference of stochastic pursuit models from basketball tracking data. In: Bayesian Statistics in Action: BAYSM 2016, Florence, Italy, June 19–21, pp. 127–137. Springer, Berlin (2017)
8. Bhattacharya, R.N., Waymire, E.C.: Stochastic Processes with Applications. Society for Industrial and Applied Mathematics (SIAM), Philadelphia (2009)
9. Fuchs, C.: Inference for Diffusion Processes: With Applications in Life Sciences. Springer, Berlin (2013)
10. Iacus, S.M.: Simulation and Inference for Stochastic Differential Equations: With R Examples. Springer Series in Statistics. Springer, New York (2009)
11. Johnson, S.G.: The NLopt nonlinear-optimization package (2016). http://ab-initio.mit.edu/nlopt. Accessed 22 July 2017
12. Nocedal, J.: Updating quasi-Newton matrices with limited storage. Math. Comput. **35**, 773–782 (1980)
13. Nocedal, J., Liu, D.C.: On the limited memory BFGS method for large scale optimization. Math. Program. **45**(3), 503–528 (1989)
14. Pedersen, A.R.: A new approach to maximum likelihood estimation for stochastic differential equations based on discrete observations. Scand. J. Stat. **22**(1), 55–71 (1995)
15. Santa-Clara, P.: Simulated likelihood estimation of diffusions with an application to the short term interest rate. Working Paper 12-97, UCLA Anderson School of Management (1997)
16. Sørensen, H.: Parametric inference for diffusion processes observed at discrete points in time: a survey. Int. Stat. Rev. **72**(3), 337–354 (2004)
17. Svanberg, K.: A class of globally convergent optimization methods based on conservative convex separable approximations. SIAM J. Optim. **12**(2), 555–573 (2002)
18. Ypma, J.: NLoptr: R interface to NLopt (2014). http://cran.r-project.org/web/packages/nloptr/. Accessed 22 July 2017

Chapter 8
New Monte Carlo Algorithm for Evaluation of Outgoing Polarized Radiation

Gennady A. Mikhailov, Natalya V. Tracheva and Sergey A. Ukhinov

Abstract This chapter is devoted to the discussion of a distinctive Monte Carlo method for evaluation of angular distribution of outgoing polarized radiation. The algorithm in consideration is based on the modification of N. N. Chentsov method for unknown probability density evaluation via the orthonormal polynomial expansion. A polarization was introduced into a mathematical model of radiation transfer with use of four-dimensional vector of Stokes parameters. Corresponding weighted Monte Carlo algorithm was constructed. Using this method and precise computer simulation, the angular distribution of outgoing radiation was investigated. Special attention was given to the value of polarization impact in the mathematical model of radiation. Algorithm in consideration allows us precisely estimate even a small effect of polarization as well as a deviation of the calculated angular distribution from the Lambertian one.

Keywords Statistical modeling · Radiation transfer · Polarization
Stokes vector · Orthogonal expansion · Jacobi polynomials

8.1 Introduction

The measuring and modelling of the angular distribution of outgoing and backscattered radiation are of a great importance to characterizing the properties of the medium and have been used in many study areas. It is well known that Monte Carlo method can be very efficient in case of the problems which are reducible to evaluation of not very large series of functionals. Thus, the method of N. N. Chentsov

G. A. Mikhailov · N. V. Tracheva (✉) · S. A. Ukhinov
Institute of Computational Mathematics and Mathematical Geophysics SB RAS,
prospect Akademika Lavrentjeva 6, Novosibirsk 630090, Russia
e-mail: tnv@osmf.sscc.ru

G. A. Mikhailov · N. V. Tracheva · S. A. Ukhinov
Novosibirsk State University, Pirogova str. 2, Novosibirsk 630090, Russia

J. Pilz et al. (eds.), *Statistics and Simulation*, Springer Proceedings
in Mathematics & Statistics 231, https://doi.org/10.1007/978-3-319-76035-3_8

(see, e.g., [1]) of randomized orthogonal expansion for estimating of an unknown probability density is particularly useful in application to the problem of angular distribution of outgoing polarized radiation evaluation. This method is based on the decomposition of desired probability density in terms of a system of a standard function that is orthonormal with weight. Note that coefficients of expansion are mathematical expectations of weighted random values of that standard functions.

In this chapter, we consider modification of N. N. Chentsov method based on effective factorization of desired probability density. This modification can essentially reduce the number of expansion terms in the case of evaluation of an angular distribution of scattered by media radiation. Thus, we can efficiently compare densities of probability for varied problem settings.

Using this modification, we reveal the significant effect of polarization on the angular distribution mentioned above. Moreover, we managed to evaluate numerically a deviation of this angular distribution from the Lambertian one.

8.2 Mathematical Model of Polarized Light Propagation and the Problem Statement

Let us consider polarized radiation transfer in the scattering and absorbing medium. In order to include polarization in the mathematical radiative model, we use the widespread and convenient method that was proposed by Stokes in 1852 [2]. Four parameters with the dimension of intensity are introduced in the radiation model. In different combination, they determine collectionwise the intensity, degree of polarization, polarization plane, and degree of ellipticity of radiation. In what follows, we consider the corresponding components of the Stokes vector function of light intensity:

$$\boldsymbol{\Phi}(\mathbf{r}, \omega) = \left(\Phi^{(1)}(\mathbf{r}, \omega), \Phi^{(2)}(\mathbf{r}, \omega), \Phi^{(3)}(\mathbf{r}, \omega), \Phi^{(4)}(\mathbf{r}, \omega)\right)^T.$$

Here, $\mathbf{r}$ is a point of R^3 space, and $\omega = (a, b, c)$ is a unit direction vector aligned with the run of the particle $(a^2 + b^2 + c^2 = 1)$.

Consider stationary integro-differential vector equation of polarized radiation transfer:

$$\omega \nabla \boldsymbol{\Phi}(\mathbf{r}, \omega) + \sigma(\mathbf{r})\boldsymbol{\Phi}(\mathbf{r}, \omega) = \int_{\Omega} \sigma_s(\mathbf{r}) P(\omega', \omega, \mathbf{r})\boldsymbol{\Phi}(\mathbf{r}, \omega')\, d\omega' + \mathbf{I_0}(\mathbf{r}, \omega). \tag{8.1}$$

Here, $\boldsymbol{\Phi}(\mathbf{r}, \omega)$ is the vector function of radiation intensity at $\mathbf{r}$ point in ω direction; σ_s is the scattering coefficient, $\sigma = \sigma_s + \sigma_c$ is the extinction coefficient, σ_c is the absorbtion coefficient;

$$P(\omega', \omega, \mathbf{r}) = L(\pi - i_2)R(\omega', \omega, \mathbf{r})L(-i_1),$$

$R(\omega', \omega, \mathbf{r})$ is the scattering phase matrix, $L(i)$ is the rotation matrix:

$$L(i) = \begin{bmatrix} 1 & 0 & 0 & 0 \\ 0 & \cos 2i & \sin 2i & 0 \\ 0 & -\sin 2i & \cos 2i & 0 \\ 0 & 0 & 0 & 1 \end{bmatrix},$$

i_1 is the angle between the plane ω', s and the scattering plane ω', ω; i_2 is the angle between the scattering plane ω', ω and the plane ω, s; and s is a vector of the local spherical system of coordinates [3]; $\mathbf{I_0}$ is the vector function of radiation source distribution density.

For an anisotropic medium, all 16 components of the scattering matrix $R(\omega', \omega, \mathbf{r})$ are generally different. For an isotropic medium, the scattering matrix simplifies to

$$R(\omega', \omega, \mathbf{r}) = \begin{bmatrix} r_{11} & r_{12} & 0 & 0 \\ r_{21} & r_{22} & 0 & 0 \\ 0 & 0 & r_{33} & r_{34} \\ 0 & 0 & -r_{43} & r_{44} \end{bmatrix}, r_{ij} \equiv r_{ij}(\mu, \mathbf{r}).$$

If the scattering particles are homogeneous spheres, then $r_{11} = r_{22}$, $r_{12} = r_{21}$, $r_{33} = r_{44}$, $r_{34} = r_{43}$. The matrix R is normalized so that $\int_{-1}^{1} r_{11}(\mu)\, d\mu = 1$.

To solve the scalar analog of Eq. (8.1) we construct a Markov chain of "collisions" separated by "free paths" which have inhomogeneous exponential distribution with coefficient $\sigma(r)$, $r \in R^3$. We assume that $\sigma \equiv \sigma_c > 0$ outside the medium, in order to normalize the free path distribution. The distribution of a direction ω after scattering is determined by an indicatrix $\mathrm{w}(\omega', \omega) = \frac{1}{2\pi} g(\omega'\omega)$ (see, e.g., [3]). We simulate the trajectory of this chain with a computer and calculate statistical estimations for desired functionals. Note that in the scalar model, $\Phi^{(2)}(\mathbf{r}, \omega) = \Phi^{(3)}(\mathbf{r}, \omega) = \Phi^{(4)}(\mathbf{r}, \omega) = 0$ (see, e.g., [3]). To take into account polarization, we associate with each particle the Stokes vector $\boldsymbol{\Phi}(\mathbf{r}, \omega)$ and the scattering indicatrix is replaced by the scattering matrix.

New photon's direction ω after scattering is defined by the scattering angle θ and the azimuthal angle φ. The cosine μ of the angle θ is simulated according to the r_{11}, i.e., according to the scattering phase function. The angle $\varphi \in (0, 2\pi)$ is assumed to be isotropic and is equal to that between the planes ω', s and ω, ω' measured counterclockwise when viewed against the incident ray ω'. Thus, the azimuthal angle is equal to i_1. After the new direction was chosen, i_1 and i_2 can be found using spherical trigonometry formulas.

The procedure for updating the Stokes vector after scattering includes the formulas

$$\begin{aligned}
\Phi^{(1)}(\mathbf{r}, \omega) &= r_{11} \cdot \Phi^{(1)}(\mathbf{r}, \omega') + r_{12} \cdot A, \\
\Phi^{(2)}(\mathbf{r}, \omega) &= (r_{21}\Phi^{(1)}(\mathbf{r}, \omega') + Ar_{22}) \cos 2i_2 - \\
&\quad - (r_{33}B - r_{34}V(\mathbf{r}, \omega')) \sin 2i_2, \\
\Phi^{(3)}(\mathbf{r}, \omega) &= (r_{21}\Phi^{(1)}(\mathbf{r}, \omega') + Ar_{22}) \sin 2i_2 + \\
&\quad + (r_{33}B - r_{34}V(\mathbf{r}, \omega')) \cos 2i_2, \\
\Phi^{(4)}(\mathbf{r}, \omega) &= r_{43}B + r_{44}\Phi^{(4)}(\mathbf{r}, \omega'),
\end{aligned}$$

where

$$\begin{aligned}
A &= \Phi^{(2)}(\mathbf{r}, \omega') \cos 2i_1 - \Phi^{(3)}(\mathbf{r}, \omega') \sin 2i_1, \\
B &= \Phi^{(2)}(\mathbf{r}, \omega') \sin 2i_1 + \Phi^{(3)}(\mathbf{r}, \omega') \cos 2i_1.
\end{aligned}$$

The simplest phenomenological Markov model of polarized radiative transfer arises when the medium is assumed to be isotropic. The only difference from the standard scalar model is that the scattering phase function is replaced with a scattering matrix, which transforms the Stokes vector associated with a given photon at a scattering point [3].

Simulation of random trajectories of a physical process of radiation transfer is a direct Monte Carlo simulation without weights. Variances of Monte Carlo estimates, in this case, are finite. However, introducing Stokes vector includes adding matrix weight into the radiation transfer model. In this concern, we use general matrix-weighted algorithms for solving systems of integral equations in the theory of radiation with polarization transfer, which were constructed and preliminarily studied in (see, [4]).

For definiteness, we consider transport of particles through a plane layer $0 < z < H$ from a source located on the boundary $z = 0$ and directed along Oz axis.

Of practical importance is the numerical study of the intensity $\Phi(\mu, H)$ of transmitted radiation, where $\mu = \omega_z$. It is known (see, e.g., [3]) that $\Phi(\mu, H) = F(\mu, H)/2\pi\mu$; moreover, in the scalar case, $F(\mu, H)$ is the distribution density of the particles escaping from the layer with respect to cosine μ. We use the notations

$$P_H = \int_0^1 F(x, H)\, dx, \quad f(x) \equiv f(x, H) = P_H^{-1} F(x, H), \quad \varphi(x) = f(x)/x \,.$$

This chapter is devoted to the numerical investigation of the angular distribution of the intensity of transmitted radiation, i.e., the function

$$f(x, H)/x, \;\; 0 < x < 1,$$

in order to analyze the variation of this function under the growth of H and under the introduction of polarization in the mathematical radiation model as specified above.

8.3 A Modification of N. N. Chentsov Method for an Unknown Probability Density Evaluation in Application to the Problem of Evaluation of an Angular Distribution of the Radiation Scattered by Media

The method of an unknown probability density $f(x)$ evaluation, suggested by Chentsov [1], is based on the expansion in terms of the system of functions $\psi_i(x)$, orthonormal with weight $p(x)$:

$$f(x) = \sum_{n=0}^{\infty} a_i \psi_i(x), \quad \int_{-\infty}^{+\infty} p(x)\psi_i(x)\psi_j(x)\,dx = \begin{cases} 1, & i = j \\ 0, & i \neq j, \end{cases} \tag{8.2}$$

with

$$a_i = \int_{-\infty}^{+\infty} p(x)\psi_i(x) f(x)\,dx = E\big[p(\xi)\psi_i(\xi)\big], \tag{8.3}$$

where ξ - is a random variable distributed with the density $f(x)$.

This relation gives us opportunity to statistically evaluate coefficients a_i. In other words, we can obtain orthonormal randomized expansion of the density $f(x)$ using the sample of ξ values.

For this purpose, we use suggested by Mikhailov [5] modification of this algorithm based on the following representation of the function $f(x)$

$$f(x) = p(x)\sum_{i=0}^{\infty} a_i \psi_i(x), \quad a_i = \int_{-\infty}^{+\infty} f(x)\psi_i(x)\,dx = E\psi_i(\xi).$$

It is well known (see, e.g., [6]) that for a large H and a weak absorption of particles in the medium, the density $f(x)$ is close to the Lambert density $f_0(x) = 2x$. Therefore, since $\varphi(x) = f(x)/x$, it is expedient to set $p(x) = x$.

For a system $\psi_i(x)$ of orthonormal over interval (0, 1) with weight x functions, let us consider a special case of the Jacobi polynomials $P_n^{(\alpha,\beta)}(y)$, orthogonal with weight $(1-y)^\alpha(1+y)^\beta$ over $(-1, 1)$ (see, e.g., [7]). Setting $\alpha = 0$, $\beta = 1$, making the change of variables $y = 2x - 1$, and the normalization of polynomials give us the following explicit form for functions $\psi_i(x)$:

$$\psi_i(x) = \sqrt{2i+2}\sum_{k=0}^{i} \frac{(-1)^k\,(2i+1-k)!}{(i-k)!\,k!\,(i+1-k)!}\,x^{i-k}.$$

We use the following notation: N is the size of a sample of random trajectories of particles, and N_H is a random number of particles that have reached the boundary $z = H$.

According to the (8.2) equality, a random estimate of the function is constructed as the following

$$\varphi(x, H) \approx \sum_{i=0}^{n} a_i \psi_i(x) = \varphi_n(x) \approx \tilde{\varphi}_n(x) = \sum_{i=0}^{n} \alpha_i \psi_i(x),$$

where $\alpha_i = \sum_{j=0}^{N_H} Q_j \psi_i(\mu_j) / \sum_{j=0}^{N_H} Q_j$ and Q_j is the weight of a jth particle, escaping from the layer in the direction μ_j (i.e., the first component of the Stokes vector).

In scalar case, we can, evidently, get $\alpha_i = N_H^{-1} \sum_{j=0}^{N_H} \psi_i(\mu_j)$.

Moreover, apparently, the following expressions hold true (see [8]):

$$\mathrm{E}\alpha_i = a_i + O(N^{-1}),$$

and

$$\mathrm{E}\tilde{\varphi}_n(x) = \varphi_n(x) + O(N^{-1}) \text{ and } \int_0^1 x\tilde{\varphi}_n(x)\,dx = \int_0^1 x\alpha_0\psi_0(x)\,dx = \int_0^1 2x\,dx = 1.$$

According to [8] variance $D\alpha_i$ asymptotically with $N \to \infty$ equals to

$$\mathrm{D}\alpha_i = \frac{1}{N}\frac{\mathrm{D}_N\xi_i - 2\dfrac{\mathrm{E}_N\xi_i}{\mathrm{E}_N\xi_P}\mathrm{cov}_N(\xi_P, \xi_i) + \left(\dfrac{\mathrm{E}_N\xi_i}{\mathrm{E}_N\xi_P}\right)^2 \mathrm{D}_N\xi_P}{(\mathrm{E}_N\xi_P)^2} + o(N^{-1}),$$

where

$$\mathrm{E}_N\xi_P = \frac{1}{N}\sum_{j=0}^{N_H} Q_j, \quad \mathrm{D}_N\xi_P = \frac{1}{N}\sum_{j=0}^{N_H} Q_j^2 - (\mathrm{E}_N\xi_P)^2,$$

$$\mathrm{E}_N\xi_i = \frac{1}{N}\sum_{j=0}^{N_H} Q_j\psi_i(\mu_j), \quad \mathrm{D}_N\xi_i = \frac{1}{N}\sum_{j=0}^{N_H}(Q_j\psi_i(\mu_j))^2 - (\mathrm{E}_N\xi_i)^2,$$

$$\mathrm{cov}_N(\xi_P, \xi_i) = \frac{1}{N}\sum_{j=0}^{N_H} Q_j^2\psi_i(\mu_j) - \mathrm{E}_N\xi_P\, \mathrm{E}_N\xi_i.$$

Here, by characters E_N, D_N, cov_N, the statistical estimations of corresponding moments are denoted, and $\xi_P = Q$, $\xi_i = Q\psi_i(\mu)$, $E\xi_P = P_H$, $E\xi_i = \int_0^1 F(\mu, H)$ $\psi_i(\mu)\, d\mu$ holds true.

8.4 Numerical Results and Discussion

In our numerical calculations, we use the well-known matrix of molecular (Rayleigh) scattering (see, e.g., [3]) and the matrix of aerosol scattering, calculated according to the Mie theory for an aerosol medium with the following parameters (see, e.g., [9]): The refractive index of particles is $n = 1.331 - i1.3 \times 10^{-4}$ (water); the size distribution of particles is lognormal with density $f(r) = \frac{1}{r}\exp(-\frac{1}{2\sigma_g^2}\ln^2(\frac{r}{r_g}))$, $r \in (0, 10\,\text{mkm})$, $r_g = 0.12$ mkm, $\sigma_g = 0.5$; and the radiation wave length is 0.65 mkm. The mean cosine of the scattering angle for that matrix of scattering is $\mu_0 = 0.7292$.

The influence of polarization on the integral flow P_H of radiation transmitted through a layer and on the expansion coefficients a_i in (8.3) was numerically investigated. Precise calculations, with 10^{10} trajectories simulated, showed that, for layers of optical thickness between $H = 2$ and $H = 20$, the influence of polarization on P_H increases with the increase of the layer thickness.

Tables 8.1 and 8.2 show statistically significant estimates of the relative (with respect to P_H in case without polarization) differences of fluxes Δ_{P_H} with and without account of polarization, as well as their standard deviations $\sigma_N(\Delta_{P_H})$. As shown, the impact of the polarization on the integral flux equals to 0.03% for aerosol media and to 4.3% for molecular media, depending on the layer thickness.

Tables 8.3 and 8.4 give the values of the relative difference $\Delta\alpha_i$ of estimates of the coefficients α_i with and without account of polarization, as well as estimates of the corresponding standard deviations $\sigma_N(\Delta\alpha_i)$. For the layer H = 20, the influence of the polarization on the coefficients α_i turned out to be statistically insignificant in consequence of insufficient size of sample.

Tables 8.5 and 8.6 give statistically significant estimates of the coefficients a_i for $H = 2, 5, 10$. Since these estimates rapidly decrease and the relative error of the

Table 8.1 Polarization effect on flux P_H. Aerosol scattering

H	Δ_{P_H}	$\sigma_N(\Delta_{P_H})$	P_H
2	-8.3×10^{-5}	5.4×10^{-7}	0.69596
5	1.3×10^{-4}	1.7×10^{-6}	0.60416
10	2.5×10^{-4}	4.8×10^{-6}	0.41314
20	2.9×10^{-4}	1.6×10^{-5}	0.25008

Table 8.2 Polarization effect on flux P_H. Molecular scattering

H	Δ_{P_H}	$\sigma_N(\Delta_{P_H})$	P_H
1	−0.0010257	8.8×10^{-6}	0.29165
2	−0.0022453	1.9×10^{-5}	0.34846
3	−0.0028396	5.2×10^{-5}	0.32906
5	−0.0021608	4.3×10^{-4}	0.25557
10	0.0426098	8.1×10^{-3}	0.14755

Table 8.3 Polarization effect on coefficients α_i ($\alpha_0 \equiv a_0 = \sqrt{2}$). Aerosol scattering

i	H = 2		H = 5		H = 10	
	$\Delta\alpha_i$	$\sigma_N(\Delta\alpha_i)$	$\Delta\alpha_i$	$\sigma_N(\Delta\alpha_i)$	$\Delta\alpha_i$	$\sigma_N(\Delta\alpha_i)$
1	8.5×10^{-3}	4.1×10^{-5}	7.9×10^{-3}	9.4×10^{-5}	2.0×10^{-3}	2.3×10^{-4}
2	5.8×10^{-3}	9.8×10^{-5}	3.6×10^{-2}	9.0×10^{-4}	2.3×10^{-2}	6.8×10^{-3}
3	-1.3×10^{-3}	1.7×10^{-4}	5.3×10^{-3}	1.1×10^{-3}	5.7×10^{-3}	1.6×10^{-2}

Table 8.4 Polarization effect on coefficients α_i ($\alpha_0 \equiv a_0 = \sqrt{2}$). Molecular scattering

i	H = 2		H = 3		H = 5	
	$\Delta\alpha_i$	$\sigma_N(\Delta\alpha_i)$	$\Delta\alpha_i$	$\sigma_N(\Delta\alpha_i)$	$\Delta\alpha_i$	$\sigma_N(\Delta\alpha_i)$
1	0.46	9.4×10^{-4}	0.17	1.2×10^{-3}	0.05	9.1×10^{-3}
2	0.40	2.3×10^{-3}	0.42	6.6×10^{-3}	0.37	0.13
3	−0.22	1.4×10^{-2}	4.52	1.48	2.33	3.02
4	−0.28	6.9×10^{-2}	−0.39	0.27	0.69	2.45

Table 8.5 The expansion coefficients α_i without account of polarization. Aerosol scattering

H	2	5	10
α_0	1.4142	1.4142	1.4142
α_1	0.5302	0.3287	0.2841
α_2	0.2380	0.0355	−0.0097
α_3	0.1402	0.0302	0.0041
α_4	0.0638	0.0120	-6.0×10^{-4}
α_5	0.0334	0.0065	6.8×10^{-4}
α_6	0.0181	0.0029	-1.3×10^{-4}
α_7	0.0103	0.0018	1.7×10^{-4}
α_8	0.0052	8.0×10^{-4}	6.0×10^{-5}
α_9	0.0024	4.5×10^{-4}	8.5×10^{-5}

Table 8.6 Expansion coefficients α_i without account of polarization. Molecular scattering

H	1	2	3	5	10
α_0	1.4142	1.4142	1.4142	1.4142	1.4142
α_1	−0.0322	0.1258	0.1996	0.2533	0.2681
α_2	−0.0334	−0.0498	−0.0352	−0.0135	−0.0045
α_3	0.0273	0.0081	-1.6×10^{-4}	-7.4×10^{-4}	0.0016
α_4	−0.0083	0.0016	9.2×10^{-4}	-8.5×10^{-4}	-7.9×10^{-4}
α_5	2.1×10^{-4}	4.5×10^{-4}	6.8×10^{-4}	5.1×10^{-4}	2.7×10^{-4}
α_6	1.2×10^{-3}	4.2×10^{-4}	-1.3×10^{-4}	-1.4×10^{-4}	-1.4×10^{-4}
α_7	-6.7×10^{-4}	1.6×10^{-4}	1.7×10^{-4}	8.6×10^{-5}	1.4×10^{-4}
α_8	6.2×10^{-5}	-4.8×10^{-5}	6.0×10^{-5}	-6.6×10^{-5}	-5.3×10^{-5}
α_9	1.9×10^{-4}	2.9×10^{-5}	8.5×10^{-5}	5.8×10^{-5}	1.1×10^{-5}

Table 8.7 Error $\bar{\Delta}_n = \|\tilde{\varphi}_n - \tilde{\varphi}_9\|^2$ estimation. Aerosol scattering

H	2	5	10	20
$\bar{\Delta}_0$	0.36	0.11	0.08	0.08
$\bar{\Delta}_1$	8.2×10^{-2}	2.4×10^{-3}	1.1×10^{-4}	1.4×10^{-4}
$\bar{\Delta}_2$	2.5×10^{-2}	1.1×10^{-3}	1.8×10^{-5}	1.2×10^{-5}
$\bar{\Delta}_3$	5.7×10^{-3}	1.9×10^{-4}	8.9×10^{-7}	1.4×10^{-6}
$\bar{\Delta}_4$	1.6×10^{-3}	5.5×10^{-5}	5.2×10^{-7}	2.8×10^{-7}
$\bar{\Delta}_5$	4.7×10^{-4}	1.2×10^{-5}	5.8×10^{-8}	7.8×10^{-8}

Table 8.8 Error $\bar{\Delta}_n = \|\tilde{\varphi}_n - \tilde{\varphi}_9\|^2$ estimation. Molecular scattering

H	2	3	5	10
$\bar{\Delta}_0$	0.02	0.04	0.06	0.07
$\bar{\Delta}_1$	2.5×10^{-3}	1.2×10^{-3}	1.8×10^{-4}	2.4×10^{-5}
$\bar{\Delta}_2$	6.9×10^{-5}	1.3×10^{-6}	1.6×10^{-6}	3.3×10^{-6}
$\bar{\Delta}_3$	3.3×10^{-6}	1.3×10^{-6}	1.0×10^{-6}	7.4×10^{-7}
$\bar{\Delta}_4$	7.7×10^{-7}	4.1×10^{-7}	2.9×10^{-7}	1.2×10^{-7}
$\bar{\Delta}_5$	2.0×10^{-7}	2.1×10^{-7}	3.5×10^{-8}	4.3×10^{-8}

estimates $\Delta\alpha_i$ with respect to i rapidly increases, we used only $\alpha_0, \alpha_1, \alpha_2$, and α_3 for the analysis of the influence of polarization on the function φ.

For same reason, to construct estimators $\bar{\Delta}_n$ of mean square errors (with weight x) $\|\tilde{\varphi}_n - \varphi\|^2$, $n = 0, \ldots, 5$ without polarization, an approximation $\varphi \approx \tilde{\varphi}_9$ was used. Tables 8.7 and 8.8 show that values $\bar{\Delta}_n$, as well as values α_i with polarization, decrease approximately in geometric progression.

The obtained numerical results witness that radiation, escaping the layer, differs from Lambert radiation, for which $a_i = 0$ when $i > 0$, that is shown in Fig. 8.1.

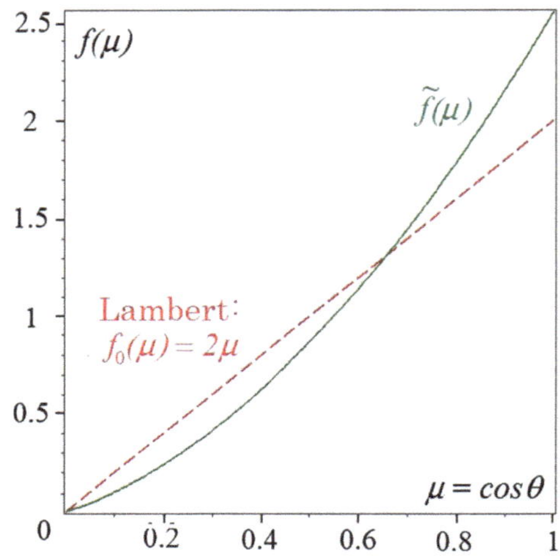

Fig. 8.1 Estimate of the angular distribution density of the radiation going out the optically thick layer ($\tau = 20$) compared to the Lambertian one

Estimates of the corresponding standard deviations are the elements of the first row in Tables 8.7 and 8.8. The maximum difference in the intensity of the radiation for $H = 10$ and $H = 20$ is attained at $x = 0$ and amount to about 64%. In case, when we take into account only the coefficients α_0 and α_1, this difference equals to 57%.

Analytical and numerical study performed in [4] showed that if photons are weakly absorbed, then the variance of the estimate of the intensity of polarized radiation may be infinite. In our work, we ensured the finiteness of variance by constraining the first component of the Stokes vector, which had virtually no effect on the final estimates.

8.5 Conclusion

In this work, a modification of N. N. Chentsov method for the unknown probability density evaluation via the orthonormal randomized polynomial expansion was constructed and discussed in application to the problems of atmospheric optics.

Suggested method was used to analyze the angular characteristics of scattered by media radiation in cases when polarization effect was ignored (scalar theory) and was taken into account (vector case).

Results from this study show that polarization has a statistically significant impact on the integral flux P_H of the radiation passed through the layer and on the coefficients of expansion α_i of the function of angular distribution of this radiation. Moreover, calculations show that polarization effect increases with the increase of the layer thickness.

The above-presented results show that the absolute values of estimates of coefficients α_i are rapidly decreasing. It gives us opportunity to use less (to be exact, two) terms of expansion in the density of distribution analysis.

Obtained numerical results show, as well, that going out of the layer radiation differs from the Lambertian one. Difference between these two types of radiation as great as 64% was observed for the angular radiation distribution in case of $H = 20$. It was observed that it grows with a decrease in optical thicknesses of the layer.

Note that suggested method is particularly suitable for detailed analysis of various radiation characteristics. Certain other polarized radiation parameters are planning on to be studied with proposed method. Specifically, the degree of polarization is one of the subjects of high priority.

Finally, we should mention that besides parallelization possibility of the proposed Monte Carlo algorithm, it allows us to calculate various function expansions simultaneously on the same trajectories with the wide range of the layer optical thicknesses at the same time.

Acknowledgements This work was partially supported by the Russian Foundation for Basic Research (no. 15-01-00894 a, no. 16-31-00123 mol_a, no. 17-01-00823 a) and the Presidium of Russian Academy of Science (program I.33II).

References

1. Chentsov, N.N.: Statistical Decision Rules and Optimal Inference. Nauka, Moscow (1987). (In Russian)
2. Chandrasekhar, S.: Radiative Transfer. Dover Publications, New York (1960)
3. Marchuk, G.I., Mikhailov, G.A., Nazaraliev, M.A., et al.: Monte Carlo Methods in Atmospheric Optics. Nauka, Novosibirsk (1976); Springer, Heidelberg (1980)
4. Mikhailov, G.A., Ukhinov, S.A., Chimaeva, A.S.: Variance of a standard vector Monte Carlo estimate in the theory of polarized radiative transfer. Comp. Math. Math. Phys. **46**(11), 2006–2019 (2006)
5. Mikhailov, G.A.: Problems of the Theory of Monte Carlo Methods. Nauka, Novosibirsk (1974). (In Russian)
6. Davison, B.: Neutron Transport Theory. Clarendon Press, Oxford (1957)
7. Krylov, V.I.: Approximate Evaluation of Integrals. Nauka, Moscow (1967). (In Russian)
8. Mikhailov, G.A., Tracheva, N.V., Ukhinov, S.A.: A new Monte Carlo algorithm for estimation the angular distribution of scattered polarized radiation based on orthogonal expansion. Dokl. Math. **92**(2), 572–576 (2015)
9. Mikhailov, G.A., Tracheva, N.V., Ukhinov, S.A.: Time asymptotics of the intensity of polarized radiation. Russ. J. Numer. Anal. Math. Model. **22**(5), 487–503 (2007)

Part III
Simulation for Stochastic Processes and Their Applications

Chapter 9
Simulation of Stochastic Processes with Generation and Transport of Particles

Ekaterina Ermishkina and Elena Yarovaya

Abstract In modeling of a cell population evolution, the key characteristics are the existence of several sources where cells can proliferate their copies or die, and migration of cells over an environment. One of the study aims is to obtain the threshold value of a parameter which separates different types of the cell proliferation process at the sources. Continuous-time branching random walks on multidimensional lattices with a few sources of branching can be used for modeling of a cell population dynamics. For example, active growth of the cancer cellular population in the frame of branching random walk models may be explained by the excess of the threshold value. Branching random walks is an appropriate tool to describe such processes in terms of generation and transport of particles. The effect of phase transitions on the asymptotic behavior of a particle population in the frame of branching random walks was studied analytically in detail by many authors. Simulation of branching random walks is applied for numerical estimation of a threshold value of the parameter on limited time intervals. Obtained results are used to define strategies that may delay a cell population progression to some extent. The work may be treated as the first step to the simulation of branching random walks. We assume that the process started by the initial particle which walks on the lattice until it reaches one of the sources where its behavior changes, and new copies may appear. All particles behave independently of each other and of their history. We present an approach to simulation of the mean number of particles over the lattice and in every point of the lattice. Simulation of the process is based on a well-known algorithm of queue data structures and the Monte Carlo method.

Keywords Branching processes · Random walks · Branching random walks Simulation · The Monte Carlo method

---

E. Ermishkina · E. Yarovaya (✉)
Department of Probability Theory, Lomonosov Moscow State University,
Leninskie Gory, Main Building, Moscow, Russia
e-mail: yarovaya@mech.math.msu.su

E. Ermishkina
e-mail: k.ermishkina@gmail.com

J. Pilz et al. (eds.), *Statistics and Simulation*, Springer Proceedings
in Mathematics & Statistics 231, https://doi.org/10.1007/978-3-319-76035-3_9

9.1 Introduction

The processes with generation and transport of particles on a d-dimensional lattice $\mathbf{Z}^d$, $d \geq 1$, are usually called *branching random walks* (BRWs). It is convenient to describe such processes in terms of birth, death, and walks of particles on $\mathbf{Z}^d$. Recent investigations, see, e.g., [12], have demonstrated that continuous-time BRWs on $\mathbf{Z}^d$ give an important example of stochastic processes whose evolution depends on the structure of an environment and the spatial dynamics.

We assume that the structure of an environment is defined by the offspring reproduction law at a finite number of particle generation centers situated on $\mathbf{Z}^d$ and called *branching sources*. The spatial dynamics of particles is considered under different assumptions about underlying random walks: simple symmetric, symmetric, or non-symmetric.

Continuous-time BRWs on $\mathbf{Z}^d$ with a few centers of branching, introduced in [11], can be used, e.g., for modeling of a cell population dynamics. In modeling of a cell population evolution, the key characteristic is the existence of one or several sources where cells can proliferate their copies or die, and migration of cells over an environment. Based on such characteristics, we can apply a continuous-time BRW to study the evolution of a cell population with migration and division of cells. Probabilistic approach to study proliferation and migration dichotomy in tumor cell invasion based on models of random walks or branching processes is used by many authors, see, e.g., [4, 7] and bibliography therein. Self-reproducibility of the cancer cells is a specific feature of such systems. In virtue of it, a branching process may represent tumor cell proliferation at the source. The environment where the transport of cells takes place is a multidimensional lattice, e.g., $\mathbf{Z}^3$. The points of the lattice are compartments. The migration of cancer tumor cells is described by a random walk on this lattice, and the processes of metastasis are described by BRWs with several sources. Cancer cells are assumed to be found at every compartment, but proliferation takes place only at the sources. One of the main problems is to estimate a threshold value of model parameter which separates different types of the cell proliferation process at the sources and above which cell proliferation has active growth. For example, simulation of the tumorigenesis can be roughly determined in terms of a cell population evolution by the following rules:

- the underlying random walks is simple,
- at the moment τ_1 of the first reaction in a source, the cell is duplicated $P \to P + P$, where both copies independently start moving from the point $x(\tau_1)$ with the same law,
- intensities of the sources are equal.

In the frame of BRW models, the exponential growth of the cellular population may occur when the intensity of the source β surpasses the critical value β_c, see [10], so the situation of weakly supercritical BRWs for which $\beta \downarrow \beta_c$ considered in [13] has a keen interest for the study of cell evolution. The effect of phase transitions on the asymptotic behavior of a particle population in BRWs was studied analytically in detail by many authors, see, e.g., [1, 8, 9, 12] and the bibliography therein. We assume that the initial particle walks on the lattice until it reaches the source where its behavior changes. Newborn particles behave independently of each other and of their history

In the present work, simulation of BRWs is applied for numerical estimation of a threshold value of the parameter on limited time intervals. Obtained results are used to define strategies that may delay a particle population progression to some extent.

The work may be treated as the first step to the simulation of BRWs. We present an approach to simulation of the mean number of particles over the lattice and at every lattice point. Simulation of the process is based on queue data structures, see, e.g., [2], and the Monte Carlo method described, e.g., in [5]. This approach allows to simulate BRWs with sources of different intensities and random walks with jumps not only to neighbor lattice points.

The structure of the chapter is as follows: In Sect. 9.2, the evolution of particle system in BRWs is carried out in accordance with the four rules used for constructing the algorithm for the BRW simulation. Some necessary theoretical results for an interpretation of the simulation are given.

In Sect. 9.3, the algorithm of the simulation is introduced. The results of the simulation are presented for a simple symmetric BRW with one source of branching. In a simple symmetric BRW, a particle can move only to one of $2d$ neighbor points on d-dimensional lattice with equal intensities, see for detail [9]. As it was explained above, this case is important to study the cell evolution dynamics. Then, the simulation is extended to the case of a few sources of equal intensities, and the effect of space configuration of the sources on the behavior of the mean numbers of particles is demonstrated, see analytical investigations of the model in [13, 14]. In conclusion, a more general BRWs with a finite number of sources of different intensities and random walks with jumps not only to neighbor lattice points with finite variance of jumps considered in [12] are simulated.

9.2 Evolution of Branching Random Walks

An informal description of BRWs on $\mathbf{Z}^d$, $d \geq 1$, is rather simple. The population of individuals is initiated at time $t = 0$ by a single particle at a point $x \in \mathbf{Z}^d$. Being outside of the sources, the particle performs a continuous-time random walk on $\mathbf{Z}^d$ until reaching one of the sources. At a source, it spends an exponentially distributed time and then either jumps to a point $y \in \mathbf{Z}^d$ (distinct from the source) or dies producing just before the death a random number of offsprings. The newborn particles behave independently and stochastically in the same way as the parent individual.

We will be mainly interested in describing the evolution of particles on $\mathbf{Z}^d$ in terms of the local number of particles $\boldsymbol{n(t, x, y)}$ at a point $\boldsymbol{y \in \mathbf{Z}^d}$ and the total number $n(t, x) = \sum_{y \in \mathbf{Z}^d} \boldsymbol{n(t, x, y)}$ over the lattice; their moments $m_k(t, x, y)$ $:= E_x n^k(t, x, y)$ and $m_k(t, x) := E_x n^k(t, x)$, $k \in \mathbf{N}$, where E_x denotes the mathematical expectation under the conditions $n(0, x, y) = \delta_y(x)$ or $n(0, x) \equiv 1$, respectively.

Now, we describe the evolution of particles in BRWs with a few branching sources in more detail. In [1, 8, 9], the models of a BRW with the single source were introduced and thoroughly investigated. In the present work, we will be interested in the modeling of a more general situation, when under consideration a BRW may have 'branching sources' $\{z_1, \dots, z_r\}$, several points $\{y_1, \dots, y_m\}$ at which the symmetry of walk may be broken, and several points $\{x_1, \dots, x_k\}$ at which both branching and 'non-symmetric walk' may happen. It will be supposed that the sets $\{x_i\}$, $\{y_j\}$, and $\{z_s\}$ are pairwise non-intersecting, see for detail [11, 12].

The evolution of a particle in such a BRW is performed in accordance with the following four rules:

1. Being outside of the set $\{x_i\} \cup \{y_j\} \cup \{z_s\}$, say at a point x, the particle may perform a random walk specified by an infinite matrix $A = (a(x, y))_{x,y \in \mathbf{Z}^d}$ of transition intensities: $a(x, y) \geq 0$ for $x \neq y$, $a(x, x) < 0$; $a(x, y) = a(y, x) = a(0, y - x) = a(y - x)$ and $\sum_z a(z) = 0$. More precisely, in this case the particle stays at the point x a random time distributed in accordance with the exponential law with parameter $|a(0, 0)|$ and then jumps to a point $y \neq x$ with the probability $a(x, y)/|a(0, 0)|$;
2. Being at some point $x \in \{y_j\}$, say at a point $x = y_j$, the particle also performs a random walk. But this time symmetry of the walk is assumed to be broken by a factor $1 + \chi_j$, $\chi_j > -1$, which changes the y_jth row $\{a(y_j, y)\}_{y \in \mathbf{Z}^d}$ of the matrix of the transition intensities in the following way: $\{(1 + \chi_k)a(y_j, y)\}_{y \in \mathbf{Z}^d}$.
In this case, the time which the particle spends at the point $x = y_j$ is distributed in accordance with the exponential law given by parameter $(1 + \chi_j)|a(0, 0)|$, and then, the particle jumps to a point $y \neq y_j$ with the probability $a(y_j, y)/|a(0, 0)|$. In fact, this case differs from the case 1 only by the distribution of time which the particle spends at the point $x = y_j$. Since in this case the behavior at the point $x = y_j$ does not obey the symmetric walk law, the points $x \in \{y_j\}$ are called in [11, 12] *pseudo-sources*;
3. Being at a point $x \in \{z_s\}$, say at a point $x = z_s$, the particle performs a symmetric random walk or branching. The branching in this case is performed in accordance with the Bienayme–Galton–Watson process specified by the infinitesimal generation function $f_s(u) := \sum_{n=0}^{\infty} b_{s,n} u^n$, where $b_{s,n} \geq 0$ for $n \neq 1$, $b_{s,1} < 0$, and $\sum_n b_{s,n} = 0$. We assume that $\beta_{s,r} := f_s^{(r)}(1) < \infty$, $r \in \mathbf{N}$, and denote $\beta_s := \beta_{s,1}$. So, in this case the behavior of the particle is assumed as follows: First, it stays at the point x a random time distributed in accordance with the exponential law $e^{(a(0,0)+b_{s,1})t}$ and then either jumps to a point $y \neq x$ with the probability $a(x, y)/|a(0, 0) + b_{s,1}|$ or generates $n \neq 1$ offsprings with the probability $b_{s,n}/|a(0, 0) + b_{s,1}|$. Notice that in the case $n = 0$ the particle is 'died';
4. The last case is when the particle is positioned at a point $x = x_i \in \{x_i\}$. This case is the combination of the cases 2 and 3. Here, the particle may jump to a point $y \neq x$ with the intensity which is factored by $1 + \zeta_i$ with $\zeta_i > -1$, as in the case 2, or performs branching, as in the case 3. The branching obeys

the Bienayme–Galton–Watson process with the infinitesimal generation function $\bar{f}_i(u) := \sum_{n=0}^{\infty} \bar{b}_{i,n} u^n$, where $\bar{b}_{i,n} \geq 0$ for $n \neq 1$, $\bar{b}_{i,1} < 0$ and $\sum_n \bar{b}_{i,n} = 0$. We assume that $\eta_{i,r} := \bar{f}_i^{(r)}(1) < \infty$, $r \in \mathbf{N}$, and denote $\eta_i := \eta_{i,1}$.
More precisely, we will assume that the particle first spends at the point $x = x_i$ a random time distributed in accordance with the exponential law determined by the parameter $|(1 + \zeta_i)a(0, 0) + \bar{b}_{i,1}|$, and then, it either jumps to a point $y \neq x = x_i$ with the probability

$$\frac{(1 + \zeta_i)a(x_i, y)}{|(1 + \zeta_i)a(0, 0) + \bar{b}_{i,1}|},$$

or generates $n \neq 1$ offsprings with the probability

$$\frac{\bar{b}_{s,n}}{|(1 + \zeta_i)a(0, 0) + \bar{b}_{i,1}|}.$$

A description of the BRW with several sources and pseudo-sources, given above, is convenient for numerical modeling which in theoretical investigation of the process the following 'infinitesimal' description in terms of evolution equations in Banach spaces is preferable.

As was shown, e.g., in [11, 12], the evolution of transition probabilities in this case can be also described by the following differential equations

$$\frac{dp}{dt} = \mathscr{A} p + \sum_{i=1}^{k} \zeta_i \Delta_{x_i} \mathscr{A} p + \sum_{j=1}^{m} \chi_j \Delta_{y_j} \mathscr{A} p, \quad p(0) = \delta_y, \tag{9.1}$$

where $\mathscr{A} : l^q(\mathbf{Z}^d) \to l^q(\mathbf{Z}^d)$, $q \in [1, \infty]$, is the symmetric operator generated by the matrix A of transition intensities and acting by the formula

$$(\mathscr{A} u)(z) := \sum_{z' \in \mathbf{Z}^d} a(z - z')u(z'),$$

$\Delta_x = \delta_x \delta_x^T$, $\delta_x = \delta_x(\cdot)$ denotes the column vector on the lattice which is equal to 1 at the point x and to zero at the other points. At the same time, the mean numbers of particles $m_1(t) = m_1(t, \cdot, y)$ at point $y \in \mathbf{Z}^d$ satisfy

$$\frac{dm_1}{dt} = \mathscr{H} m_1, \quad m_1(0) = \delta_y, \tag{9.2}$$

where

$$\mathscr{H} = \mathscr{A} + \left(\sum_{s=1}^{r} \beta_s \Delta_{z_s} \right) + \left(\sum_{i=1}^{k} \zeta_i \Delta_{x_i} \mathscr{A} + \sum_{i=1}^{k} \eta_i \Delta_{x_i} \right) + \left(\sum_{j=1}^{m} \chi_j \Delta_{y_j} \mathscr{A} \right). \tag{9.3}$$

In (9.2), (9.3), the linear operator $\mathscr{A}$ describes the symmetric walk outside of sources (case 1 in the above description). The second term in (9.3) corresponds to the branching sources where the walk is symmetric (case 2 in the above description), while the third term corresponds to the branching sources where the symmetry of walk is broken (case 3 in the above description). At last, the fourth term corresponds to the points (pseudo-sources) where the symmetry of walk is broken but there are no branching (case 4 in the above description).

Asymptotic behavior of solutions of Eq. (9.2) is determined by the spectrum of linear operators in the right-hand sides of the corresponding equations [3]. A detailed spectral analysis of the operator Y has been carried out in [11, 12].

The presence of leading positive eigenvalues in the spectrum of the evolutionary operator implies an exponential growth of the number of particles at arbitrary lattice point, as well as on the entire lattice. Therefore, the previous studies, see, e.g., [1, 8, 9] and bibliography therein, were usually limited to finding only the leading eigenvalue. At the same time for the spatiotemporal analysis considered, e.g., in [6], the information about whether the positive eigenvalue is unique, or if it is not unique then how it is located with respect to other eigenvalues, can be significant in the analysis of the behavior of BRWs. In connection with this, it was found [13, 14] that the number of positive eigenvalues of the discrete spectrum of the evolutionary operator and their multiplicity depends not only on the intensity of the sources but also on the spatial configuration of the sources.

In the BRWs with finitely many sources of equal intensity $\beta := \beta_1 = \beta_{1,1}$ studied in [13, 14], there arise multipoint perturbations of the symmetric random walk operator $\mathscr{A}$, which have the form

$$\mathscr{H}_\beta = \mathscr{A} + \beta \sum_{i=1}^{N} \Delta_{x_i}, \tag{9.4}$$

where $x_i \in \mathbf{Z}^d$. The perturbation $\beta \sum_{i=1}^{N} \Delta_{x_i}$ of the operator $\mathscr{A}$ can result in the appearance of positive eigenvalues of the operator $\mathscr{H}_\beta$, the number of positive eigenvalues of which does not exceed N (the number of terms in the sum) counting multiplicity.

As was shown, e.g., in [1, 9], the evolution of $m_1(t,x,y)$ and $m_1(t,x)$ for a symmetric BRW with the one branching source generated by operator (9.4) in the form

$$\mathscr{H}_\beta = \mathscr{A} + \beta \Delta_{x_1} \tag{9.5}$$

dramatically changes when the parameter β traverses some value β_c called critical, where $\beta_c = (-\phi(\theta))^{-1}$ and $\phi(\theta) = \sum_{z\in\mathbf{Z}^d} a(z)e^{i(z,\theta}$, $\theta \in [-\pi,\pi]^d$.

In a case of a finite variance of random walk jumps, i.e., if $\sum_{z\in\mathbf{Z}^d} a(z)|z|^2 < \infty$, where $|\cdot|$ is the Euclidean norm of a vector z, then $\beta_c = 0$ for $d = 1$ and $d = 2$, and $\beta_c > 0$ for $d \geq 3$. The exhaustive classification of the limit behavior (up to a scalar factor) of the local mean number of particles at the source $u(t)$ and the total mean number of particles $\nu(t)$ is represented in Table 9.1, where λ is the positive eigenvalue of the operator (9.5). Note that for the situation of simple random walk the operator $\mathscr{A}$ has the form of difference Laplacian: $\varkappa\Delta$, with a diffusion parameter $\varkappa$, see, e.g., [6].

9.3 Simulation of Branching Random Walks

Description 1–4 from Sect. 9.2 is well suited for algorithm design.

9.3.1 Algorithm

We will describe the state of a BRW under simulation as a set of triplets (x, t_1, t_2). Each of triplets corresponds to a single particle staying at the point $x \in \mathbf{Z}^d$ on the time interval $[t_1, t_2)$ getting at the point x at the moment t_1 and 'performing the evolution' at the moment t_2. By the 'evolution,' we mean either a jump to another point or birth of offsprings, or death of the particle. During the simulation, the triplet under consideration will be removed from the list of triplets and be replaced by one or several new triplets corresponding to a new state of the particle system arising as a result of the given 'evolution.'

Initialization. First, we choose the finite sets of points $\{x_i\}_{i=1}^k$, $\{y_j\}_{j=1}^m$ and $\{z_s\}_{s=1}^r$ and specify all the necessary quantities determining the matrix of transition intensities A and the infinitesimal generating functions $f_s(u)$ with $s = 1, 2, \dots, r$ and $\bar{f}_i(u)$ with $i = 1, 2, \dots, k$. Fix also the quantities $\chi_j > -1$, $\zeta_i > -1$ and calculate $\beta_s = \beta_{s,1} = f_s'(1)$ and $\eta_i = \eta_{i,1} = \bar{f}_i'(1)$ for the corresponding sets of indices i, j, s. We also specify the length of the interval $[0, T_{MAX}]$ on which simulation will be conducted.

At last, we fix an 'initial point' x where, at the initial time $t = t_1 = 0$, stays a single particle. Then, with the help of a random number generator, we calculate the time t_2 in accordance with the distribution law and placement of the point x, see cases 1–4 in Sect. 9.2. So, we get the 'initial' triplet (x, t_1, t_2).

Step of algorithm. At this step, we have a set of triplets (x, t_1, t_2) 'waiting' for their processing. We choose an arbitrary triplet $X = (x, t_1, t_2)$ from this set and calculate the 'evolution' of the corresponding particle at the moment $t = t_2$ in accordance with the placement of the point x, see cases 1–4 above. As a result, we obtain either a new particle at a point $y \neq x$ or a set of new particles (offsprings) at the point x.

For the position x_{new} of each newly generated particle we first determine a 'non-complete' triplet $(x_{new}, t_{1,new}, \cdot)$ where $t_{1,new} = t_2$. Then, with the help of a random number generator, we calculate time $t_{2,new}$ until which the particle will stay at the point x_{new}, in accordance with the corresponding distribution law and placement of the point x, see cases 1–4.

Finally, we add all newly generated triplets $(x_{new}, t_{1,new}, t_{2,new})$ to the list of all triplets in the system, whereas the triplet X is removed from the list.

Termination. The algorithm stops when all the t_1 values for all the triplets in the system exceed the specified time interval T_{MAX}.

Collecting of data. After the termination of the algorithm, following the Monte Carlo method, we repeat simulation with the same parameters (but with different runs of a random number generators) several times to collect needed number of data samples (simulations) which would be sufficient for statistical data treatment. After collection of all the data, we start evaluation of the characteristics of the BRW under consideration.

9.3.2 Implementation

Our algorithm is naturally randomized as its behavior is determined by both the input BRW characteristics and the values produced by random number generators. We assume that we have at our disposal a random number generator and we use two types of random number generators which produce values according to an exponential distribution and to a discrete distribution. The random number generator

$$\mathit{DISCR}((a_1, w_1), \dots, (a_n, w_n)), \quad w_i \geq 0,\ i = 1, 2 \dots, n,$$

produces a value a_i with the probability $P(a_i) = \frac{w_i}{\sum_{k=1}^{n} w_k}$, and the random number generator

$$\mathit{EXP}(a), \quad a > 0,$$

returns a floating point value according to the exponential distribution with parameter a.

As was said, the particle can perform a random walk or branching that we will process in two consecutive steps: First, we choose a type of evolution, and then, we emulate chosen an action. The behavior of the functions that have coordinates x of processed particle as the argument depends on whether the point x belongs to one of the sets $\{x_i\}$, $\{y_j\}$, or $\{z_s\}$ or does not belong to any of them.

TYPE_OF_EVOLUTION(x)
if $x \in \{z_s\}$ **then**
  return $\mathit{DISCR}\left(\left(\text{“walk”}, \frac{a(x,y)}{|a(0,0)+b_{s,1}|}\right), \left(\text{“branching”}, \frac{|b_{s,1}|}{a(x,y)|a(0,0)+b_{s,1}|}\right)\right)$
else if $x \in \{x_i\}$ **then**
  return $\mathit{DISCR}\left(\left(\text{“walk”}, \frac{(1+\zeta_i)a(x_i,y)}{|(1+\zeta_i)a(0,0)+\bar{b}_{i,1}|}\right), \left(\text{“branching”}, \frac{|\bar{b}_{i,1}|}{|(1+\zeta_i)a(0,0)+\bar{b}_{i,1}|}\right)\right)$
else
  return “walk”
end if

The probability with which a particle jumps from the point x to a point y, under the condition of jumping, is equal to $a(x, y)/|a(0, 0)| = a(0, y - x)/|a(0, 0)|$ for all lattice points. So we can determine the function $JUMP(x)$ that returns the point at which the particle jumps from the point x:

$JUMP(x)$
return $x + DISCR\left(\left\{\left(y, \frac{a(0,y)}{|a(0,0)|}\right) \,\middle|\, y \in \mathbf{Z}^d,\ y \neq 0\right\}\right)$,

where we assume that the points x and y are summarized as appropriate vectors.

In the case of branching (i.e., when $x \in \{z_s\} \cup \{x_i\}$), we obtain the number of offsprings, generated by a particle at the point x, by calling the following function:

$OFFSPRINGS\_NUMBER(x)$
if $x = z_s \in \{z_s\}$ **then**
  return $DISCR(\{(n, b_{s,n}) \mid n \neq 1\})$
else if $x = x_i \in \{x_i\}$ **then**
  return $DISCR(\{(n, \bar{b}_{s,n}) \mid n \neq 1\})$
end if

For any new triplet $(x, t_1, \cdot)$, the moment of 'evolution' t_2 is obtained as a sum of t_1 and the sojourn time spending by the particle at the point x.

$SOJOURN\_TIME(x)$
if $x = y_j \in \{y_j\}$ **then**
  return $EXP((1 + \chi_j)|a(0,0)|)$
else if $x = z_s \in \{z_s\}$ **then**
  return $EXP(|(a(0,0) + b_{s,1})|)$
else if $x = x_i \in \{x_i\}$ **then**
  return $EXP(|(1 + \zeta_i)a(0,0) + \bar{b}_{i,1}|)$
else
  return $EXP(|a(0,0)|)$
end if

We define the *system state* as a set of all triplets $Q = \{q = (x, t_1, t_2)\}$. We use *queue* data type for Q realization as it supports required operation: add element, demonstrate that some element belongs to the collection, and erase it from collection. Initially, the system state consists of only one particle located at the point $x \in \mathbf{Z}^d$. The simulation of one BRW realization on the time interval $[0, T_{MAX}]$ looks as follows:

$Q = \{(x, 0, SOJOURN\_TIME(x))\}$
while $Q \neq \emptyset$ **do**
  $q = (x, t_1, t_2) \in Q$
  $Q = Q \setminus \{q\}$
  if $t_2 > T_{MAX}$ **then**
    break
  end if
  if $TYPE\_OF\_EVOLUTION(x) =$ "*walk*" **then**
    $y = JUMP(x)$
    $q' = (y, t_2, t_2 + SOJOURN\_TIME(y))$

```
            Q = Q ∪ {q'}
            MEMORIZE_DATA(q')
        else
            for i = 1 to OFFSPRINGS_NUMBER(x) do
                q' = (x, t2, t2 + SOJOURN_TIME(x))
                Q = Q ∪ {q'}
                MEMORIZE_DATA(q')
            end for
        end if
    end while
```

The function *MEMORIZE_DATA* collects data for its further processing (e.g., to evaluate the total and the local number of particles). To obtain statistically significant data, the algorithm of BRW modeling must be called *ITERATION_NUMBER* times, where *ITERATION_NUMBER* is chosen from statistical considerations. It may be convenient to divide the given time interval $[0; T_{MAX}]$ into K equal smaller parts and to memorize not the exact time t but the order number of smaller interval that contains time t.

9.3.3 *Results of Simulation*

For demonstrating the proposed algorithm, we considered three types of models: The first one is in which there is only one source located at zero, the second one is in which there are three sources of equal intensities located at the vertices of a simplex, and the third one is the model which has two sources of non-equal intensities. All the simulations presented in this section were made with the number of the Monte Carlo trials equal to 1000.

As it was mentioned in Sect. 9.1, the tumorogenesis, the process in which a cell can be duplicated, may be treated as a kind of simple symmetric BRWs with the branching sources of the type $\{z_s\}$, whose infinitesimal generating functions are the same, that is $f_s(u) = -\beta u + \beta u^2$, where the parameter $\beta = f_1'(1)$ varies. We simulated a BRW on $\mathbf{Z}^3$ with only one source of the type $\{z_s\}$ located at the lattice point $z_1 = (0, 0, 0)$. The matrix A of transition intensities with the elements $a(x, y) = \frac{1}{2}$ for $|x - y| = 1$, $a(x, x) = -d$, and $a(x, y) = 0$ in other cases generates the difference Laplacian of the form $\frac{1}{2}\Delta$. We put $T_{MAX} = 1000$. Figure 9.1 illustrates, for different values of the parameter β, the behavior of the total number of particles $m_1(t, 0)$. As is seen from these plots, under the given conditions, the critical value is as follows: $\beta_c \approx 1.978$. The plots are in a good agreement with the theoretical results presented in Table 9.1.

In Fig. 9.2, the local mean number of particles $m_1(t, 0, 0)$ is plotted for the same situation. Again, the related plots are in a good agreement with the theoretical results, see Table 9.1. The simulation results in Figs. 9.1 and 9.2 demonstrate that a minor excess of $\beta \approx 2.040$ over $\beta_c \approx 1.978$ leads to a significant distinction in behavior of $m_1(t, 0)$, or $m_1(t, 0, 0)$, from their behavior in the case $\beta = \beta_c$.

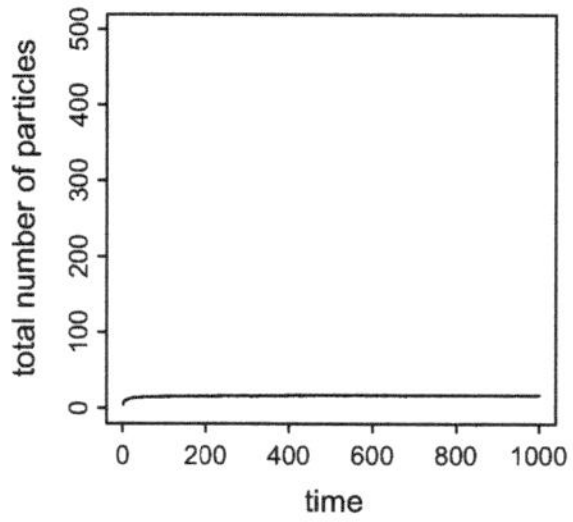

(a) $\beta = 1.7$

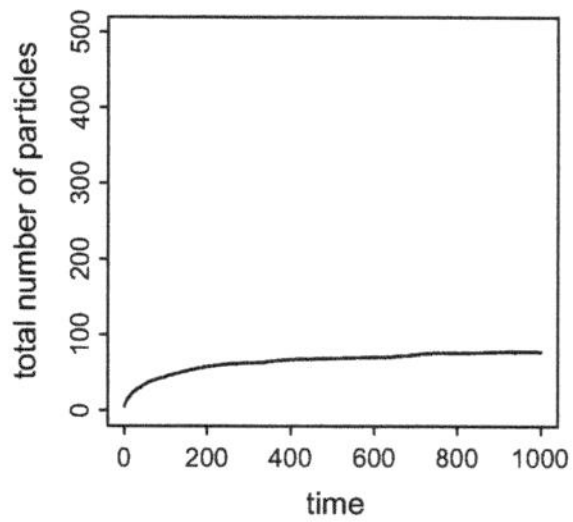

(b) $\beta = 1.978$

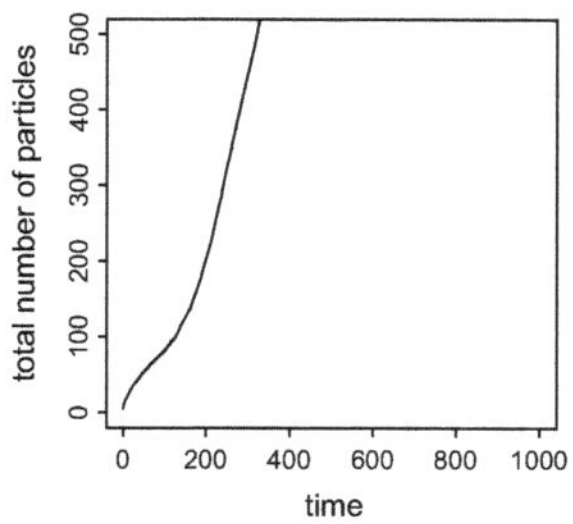

(c) $\beta = 2.04$

Fig. 9.1 Total number of particles for BRW on $\mathbf{Z}^3$ with one source for different values of β

Table 9.1 Limit behavior of the local and total mean number of particles for one source

Branching process at the source	Random walk	Branching random walk	$u(t)$	$v(t)$
Supercritical $\beta > 0$	Recurrent $d = 1, 2$, $\beta_c = 0$	Supercritical $\beta > \beta_c$	$e^{\lambda t}$	$e^{\lambda t}$
Supercritical $\beta > 0$	Transient $d \geq 3$, $\beta_c > 0$	Supercritical $\beta > \beta_c$	$e^{\lambda t}$	$e^{\lambda t}$
Supercritical $\beta > 0$	Transient $d = 3$, $\beta_c > 0$	Critical $\beta = \beta_c$	$1/\sqrt{t}$	$\sqrt{t}$
Supercritical $\beta > 0$	Transient $d = 4$, $\beta_c > 0$	Critical $\beta = \beta_c$	$1/\ln t$	$t/\ln t$
Supercritical $\beta > 0$	Transient $d \geq 5$, $\beta_c > 0$	Critical $\beta = \beta_c$	1	t
Supercritical $\beta > 0$	Transient $d \geq 3$, $\beta_c > 0$	Subcritical $\beta_c > \beta > 0$	$t^{-d/2}$	1
Critical $\beta = 0$	Recurrent $d = 1$, $\beta_c = 0$	Critical $\beta = \beta_c$	$1/\sqrt{t}$	1
Critical $\beta = 0$	Recurrent $d = 2$, $\beta_c = 0$	Critical $\beta = \beta_c$	$1/t$	1
Critical $\beta = 0$	Transient $d \geq 3$, $\beta_c > 0$	Subcritical $\beta_c > \beta = 0$	$t^{-d/2}$	1
Subcritical $\beta < 0$	Recurrent $d = 1$, $\beta_c = 0$	Subcritical $\beta < \beta_c$	$t^{-3/2}$	$1/\sqrt{t}$
Subcritical $\beta < 0$	Recurrent $d = 2$, $\beta_c = 0$	Subcritical $\beta < \beta_c$	$(t \ln^2 t)^{-1}$	$1/\ln t$
Subcritical $\beta < 0$	Transient $d \geq 3$, $\beta_c > 0$	Subcritical $\beta < \beta_c$	$t^{-d/2}$	1

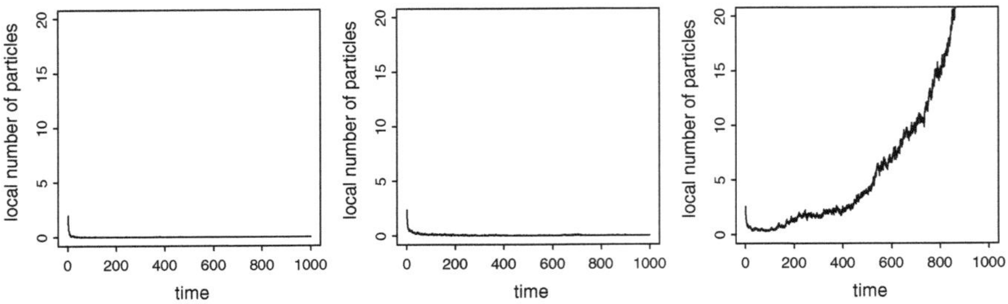

(a) $\beta = 1.7$ (b) $\beta = 1.978$ (c) $\beta = 2.04$

Fig. 9.2 Local number of particles at a source for BRW on $\mathbf{Z}^3$ with one source for different values of β

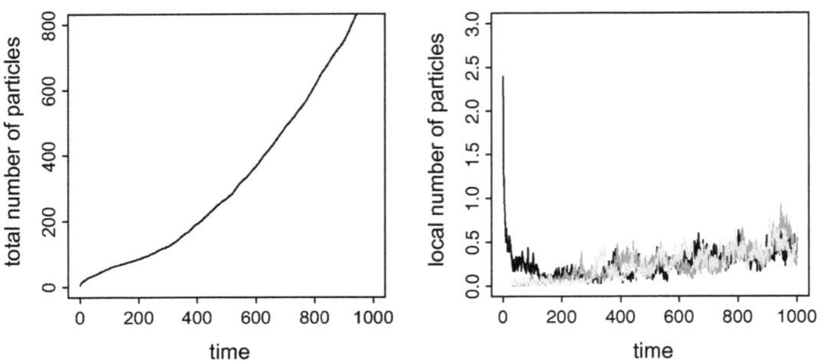

(a) Total number of particles (b) Local number of particles in sources

Fig. 9.3 BRW on $\mathbf{Z}^3$ with three sources with equal intensity 1.97839 at the points (10, 0, 0), (0, 10, 0), and (0, 0, 10)

After that, we simulated the BRW on $\mathbf{Z}^3$ for the case of three branching sources of the type $\{z_s\}_{s=1}^r$ located at the points $z_1 = (10, 0, 0)$, $z_2 = (0, 10, 0)$ and $z_3 = (0, 0, 10)$. The infinitesimal generating function $f_s(u)$ with $s = 1, 2, 3$ for every source is of the form $f_s(u) = 0.4 - (0.4 + \beta + 0.2)u + \beta u^2 + 0.2u^3$, i.e. every particle can die without offsprings or reproduce two or three offsprings. The matrix of transition intensities A in this case is the same as before, and $T_{MAX} = 1000$. The results of simulation for $m_1(t, z_1)$ are represented in Fig. 9.3a, and for $m_1(t, z_1, z_1)$, $m_1(t, z_1, z_2)$, $m_1(t, z_1, z_3)$ the corresponding results are represented in Fig. 9.3b.

We also simulated the similar system which differs from the previous one only by the location of the sources: $z_1 = (100, 0, 0)$, $z_2 = (0, 100, 0)$, and $z_3 = (0, 0, 100)$ in order to compare the behavior of these two systems.

Figures 9.3 and 9.4 show that increasing of the distance between the vertices of the simplex located on $\mathbf{Z}^d$, $d \geq 3$, leads to decreasing of the rate of growth of the mean of total and local numbers of particles. For example, Fig. 9.4 shows that the behavior of the local number of particles in one of the sources is exactly the same as the behavior of the local number of particles in Fig. 9.5, while in the remaining two sources the

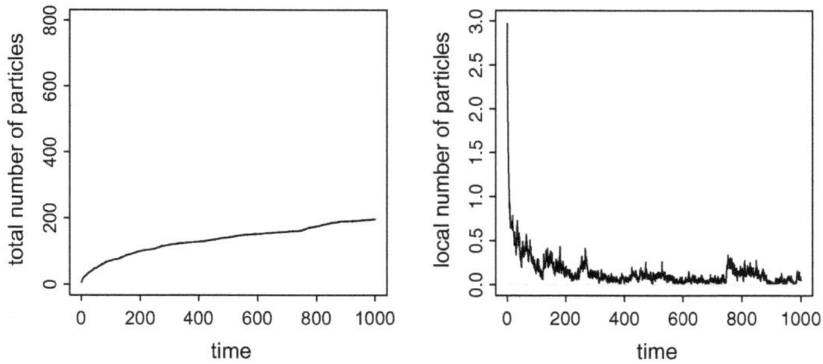

(a) Total number of particles

(b) Local number of particles in sources

Fig. 9.4 BRW on $\mathbf{Z}^3$ with three sources with equal intensity 1.97839 at the points (100, 0, 0), (0, 100, 0), and (0, 0, 100)

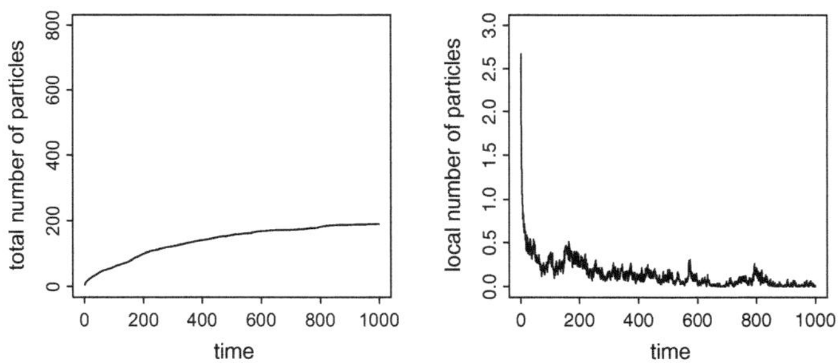

(a) Total number of particles

(b) Local number of particles in source

Fig. 9.5 BRW on $\mathbf{Z}^3$ with one source of intensity 1.97839

local number of particles is identically zero. This effect is explained by the transient property of a random walk on $\mathbf{Z}^d$, $d \geq 3$, and confirms the fact that the particles, within a finite time, do not have time to reach distant sources. Thus, the behavior of the mean number of particles is determined by the intensity of the source, at which the particle can get during the specified time. So, in this case when the distance between the vertices of the simplex grows, the total mean number of particles behaves similar to the case of single source with equal infinitesimal generating function presented in Fig. 9.5. From Fig. 9.4, it is seen that BRW did not reach any sources except the initial point, so it can be treated as a system with one source.

Finally, we simulated the BRW on $\mathbf{Z}^2$ with the matrix of transition intensities A and two branching sources located at the points $z_1 = (0, 0)$ and $z_2 = (1, 1)$ with the different infinitesimal generating functions $f_{z_1}(u) = 0.75(u^2 - u)$ and $f_{z_2}(u) = 0.5(1 - u)$. In this case, $T_{MAX} = 8000$. In Fig. 9.6, one may observe the exponential growth of both the total $m_1(t, z_1)$ and local numbers of particles $m_1(t, z_1, z_1)$ and $m_1(t, z_1, z_2)$ at the sources. However, the number of particles $m_1(t, z_1, z_1)$

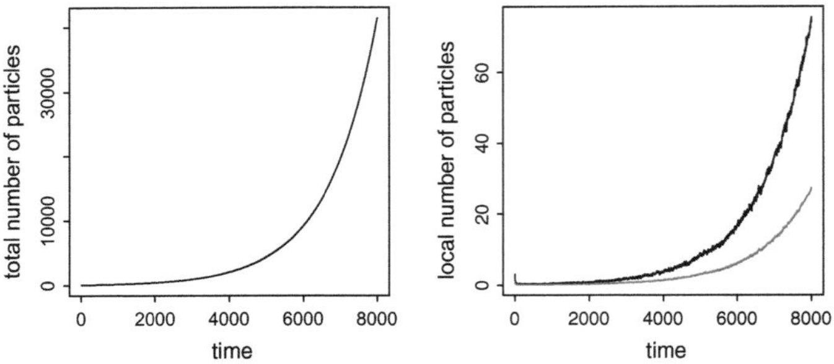

(a) Total number of particles (b) Local number of particles in sources

Fig. 9.6 BRW on $\mathbf{Z}^2$ with two sources of different intensities at the points $z_1 = (0, 0)$ and $z_2 = (1, 1)$

substantially differs from $m_1(t, z_1, z_2)$. Since the rate of growth of the curves in Fig. 9.6 is lower than in Figs. 9.1, 9.2, 9.3, 9.4, and 9.5, it is much harder to evaluate, on short time intervals, the behavior of the particle system.

The simulation results demonstrate that, in the frame of BRWs, the influence of phase transitions, with respect to the parameters of BRWs, on the asymptotic behavior of the mean numbers of a particle population may be observed on limited time intervals. Obtained results may be potentially used to define strategies for choosing the parameters of a BRW which allow to obtain a 'desired' behavior of the system. In particular, these results can be used to define strategies to delay a cell population progression to some extent.

Acknowledgements This study was performed at Lomonosov Moscow State University and at Steklov Mathematical Institute of Russian Academy of Sciences. The work was supported by the Russian Science Foundation, project no. 14-21-00162.

References

1. Albeverio, S., Bogachev, L.V., Yarovaya, E.B.: Asymptotics of branching symmetric random walk on the lattice with a single source. C. R. Acad. Sci. Paris Sér. I Math. **326**(8), 975–980 (1998). https://doi.org/10.1016/S0764-4442(98)80125-0
2. Cormen, T.H., Leiserson, C.E., Rivest, R.L., Stein, C.: Introduction to Algorithms, 3rd edn. MIT Press, Cambridge (2009)
3. Daletski, Y.L., Krein, M.G.: Ustoichivost reshenii differentsialnykh uravnenii v banakhovom prostranstve. Izdat. Nonlinear Analysis and its Applications Series. "Nauka", Moscow (1970) (in Russian)
4. Fedotov, S., Iomin, A.: Probabilistic approach to a proliferation and migration dichotomy in tumor cell invasion. Phys. Rev. E **77**(3), 031,911, 10 (2008). https://doi.org/10.1103/PhysRevE.77.031911
5. Fishman, G.S.: Monte Carlo: Concepts, Algorithms, and Applications. Springer Series in Operations Research. Springer, New York (1996)

6. Molchanov, S.A., Yarovaya, E.B.: The population structure inside the propagation front of a branching random walk with a finite number of particle generation centers. Dokl. Akad. Nauk **447**(3), 265–268 (2012). https://doi.org/10.1134/S1064562412060178
7. Thalhauser, C.J., Lowengrub, J.S., Stupack, D., Komarova, N.L.: Selection in spatial stochastic models of cancer: migration as a key modulator of fitness. Biol. Direct **5**(21), 1–17 (2010). https://doi.org/10.1186/1745-6150-5-21
8. Vatutin, V.A., Topchiĭ, V.A., Yarovaya, E.B.: Catalytic branching random walks and queueing systems with a random number of independent servers. Theory Probab. Math. Stat. **69**, 1–15 (2003)
9. Yarovaya, E.B.: Branching random walks in a heterogeneous environment. Center of Applied Investigations of the Faculty of Mechanics and Mathematics of the Moscow State University, Moscow (2007) (In Russian)
10. Yarovaya, E.B.: Criteria for the exponential growth of the number of particles in models of branching random walks. Teor. Veroyatn. Primen. **55**(4), 705–731 (2010). https://doi.org/10.1137/S0040585X97985091
11. Yarovaya, E.B.: Spectral properties of evolutionary operators in branching random walk models. Math. Notes **92**(1), 115–131 (2012)
12. Yarovaya, E.B.: Branching random walks with several sources. Math. Popul. Stud. **20**(1), 14–26 (2013)
13. Yarovaya, E.B.: The structure of the positive discrete spectrum of the evolution operator arising in branching random walks. Dokl. Math. **92**(1), 507–510 (2015). https://doi.org/10.1134/S1064562415040316
14. Yarovaya, E.: Positive discrete spectrum of the evolutionary operator of supercritical branching walks with heavy tails. Methodol. Comput. Appl. Probab. 1–17 (2016). https://doi.org/10.1007/s11009-016-9492-9

Chapter 10
Stochastic Models for Nonlinear Cross-Diffusion Systems

Yana Belopolskaya

Abstract Under a priori assumptions concerning existence and uniqueness of the Cauchy problem solution for a system of quasilinear parabolic equations with cross-diffusion, we treat the PDE system as an analogue of systems of forward Kolmogorov equations for some unknown stochastic processes and derive expressions for their generators. This allows to construct a stochastic representation of the required solution. We prove that introducing stochastic test function we can check that the stochastic system gives rise to the required generalized solution of the original PDE system. Next, we derive a closed stochastic system which can be treated as a stochastic counterpart of the Cauchy problem for a parabolic system with cross-diffusion.

Keywords Stochastic flow · Cross-diffusion · PDE generalized solution
Probabilistic representation

10.1 Probabilistic Approach to Generalized Solutions of Nonlinear Parabolic Systems

Parabolic systems with self-diffusion and cross-diffusion terms arise as mathematical model of various physical, chemical, and biological phenomena. In particular, many biological problems can be written as reaction–diffusion systems

$$\frac{\partial u}{\partial t} = div(F(u)\nabla u) + f(u), \quad x \in R^d, t > 0,$$

where $u = (u^1, \dots, u^{d_1}) \in R^{d_1}$ and u^m, $m = 1, \dots, d_1$, are type m particle densities. Here

$$[F(u)\nabla u]_i^m = \sum_{j=1}^{d}\sum_{l=1}^{d_1} F_{ij}^{ml}(u)\nabla_j u^l$$

Y. Belopolskaya (✉)
Saint-Petersburg State University of Architecture and Civil Engineering,
St. Petersburg 190005, Russian Federation
e-mail: yana@yb1569.spb.edu

J. Pilz et al. (eds.), *Statistics and Simulation*, Springer Proceedings
in Mathematics & Statistics 231, https://doi.org/10.1007/978-3-319-76035-3_10

is a particle flux, and $f(u) \in R^{d_1}$ is a reaction term. In the case when the tensor F_{ij}^{ml} is diagonal in upper indices and moreover $F_{ij}^{ml} \equiv F_{ij} > 0$, the probabilistic approach to constructing generalized solutions of the above Cauchy problem was developed in papers [1, 2] based on the Kunita theory of stochastic flows [3–5]. Unfortunately, one cannot apply these results immediately to a nondiagonal case. Here, we show how one can overcome the obstacles arising in the latter case.

For the sake of simplicity, we specify our construction to the case $div[F(u)\nabla u]_m = \Delta(u^m g(u))$, $m = 1, 2$ which corresponds to a model of population dynamics suggested by Shigesada, Kawasaki, Teramoto [6], provided $g(u) = u^1 + u^2$.

Consider the Cauchy problem

$$\frac{\partial u^m}{\partial t} = \Delta(u^m[u^1 + u^2]) + c_u^m u^m, \quad u^m(0, x) = u_0^m(x), \; m = 1, 2, \tag{10.1}$$

where

$$c_u^m = c_m - c_{m1}u^1 - c_{m2}u^2.$$

This system was investigated in a number of papers (see [7, 8] and references there) where existence and uniqueness theorems were established and some properties of generalized solutions were studied.

Our aim is to construct a probabilistic representation of a generalized solution to the Cauchy problem in terms of averages over trajectories of some diffusion processes.

Note that probabilistic approach to nonlinear PDEs and systems as a rule consists of three steps. At the first step under an a priori assumption that there exists a unique required solution of the Cauchy problem for the original PDE, one has to construct stochastic processes which allow to derive a stochastic representation of this solution. At the second step, one needs to obtain a closed system of stochastic relations to define stochastic processes that take part in the construction of the constructed probabilistic representation. At the final third step, one has to verify that solution of the stochastic system exists and possesses properties that allow to construct the required solution of the original Cauchy problem.

Below, we give constructions that implement the first two steps. The third step will be studied elsewhere.

A probabilistic background of parabolic systems with cross-diffusion is justified for example by the fact that one can formally derive such a system from a master equation for a random walk on a lattice in the diffusion limit with transition rates which depend linearly on the species densities [9]. They can be also deduced as the limit equations of an interacting particle system modeled by stochastic differential equations with interaction forces which depend linearly on the corresponding stochastic processes [10, 11].

We propose here an alternative construction of a probabilistic counterpart to this system. Actually, we construct stochastic processes such that a generalized solution of (10.1) admits a stochastic representation via averaging over trajectories of these processes. To this end, we derive a closed system of stochastic equations which describes these processes.

Let us start with a definition of a generalized solution to (10.1). To this end, we need a number of functional spaces.

Denote by H^k the set of all real functions h defined on R^d such that h and all distributional derivatives $\nabla^\alpha h$ of order $|\alpha| = \sum_{j=1}^{k} \alpha_j \le k$, where $k = 0, 1, 2, \ldots$, belong to $L^2(R^d)$. It is a Hilbert space with the norm

$$\|h\|_k = \left(\sum_{|\alpha| \le k} \int_{R^d} \|\nabla^\alpha h(x)\|^2 dx \right)^{\frac{1}{2}}.$$

We denote by H^{-k} the dual space with the norm $\|u\|_{-k} = sup_{\|h\|_k \le 1} |\langle\langle u, h \rangle\rangle|$, where $\langle\langle u, h \rangle\rangle = \int_{R^d} u(x)h(x)dx$. We use this notation for a scalar product in H^k as well.

Let $C^k(R^d)$ denote the space of k times differentiable functions and $C_0^k(R^d)$ be the space of k differentiable functions with compact supports.

Definition 10.1 A pair of functions u^m, $m = 1, 2$ is called a generalized solution of (10.1) if it has the following properties:

(i) $u^1, u^2 \in L^\infty((0, \infty); L^\infty(R^d))$ and $u^1, u^2 \ge 0$ a.e. in $(0, \infty) \times R^d$;
(ii) $u^m \in L^2_{loc}((0, \infty) \times R^d)$, $\nabla u^m \in L^2_{loc}((0, \infty) \times R^d)$;
(iii) for any test function $h \in C_0^\infty(R^d)$.

$$\int_{R^d} [u^m(t, x) - u_0^m(x)]h(x)dx + \int_0^t \int_{R^d} \langle \nabla[u^m[u^1(\theta, x) + u^2(\theta, x)]], \nabla h(x) \rangle dx d\theta$$
$$= \int_0^t \int_{R^d} u^m(\theta, x)[c_m - c_{m1}u_1(\theta, x) - c_{m2}u_2(\theta, x)]h(x)dx d\theta, \tag{10.2}$$

where $\langle y, g \rangle = \sum_{i=1}^{d} y_i g_i$ is the inner product in R^d.

To shed light to the structure of a stochastic process which should be associated with (10.1), we use an alternative though equivalent [12] definition of a generalized solution to this problem. To this end, we choose time-dependent test function $h \in C_0^\infty([0, \infty) \times R^d)$ and set $\nabla_k h(x) = \frac{\partial h(x)}{\partial x_k}$, $\Delta h(x) = \sum_{k=1}^{d} \frac{\partial^2 h(x)}{\partial x_k^2}$ and

$$\langle\langle u^m(t), h(t) \rangle\rangle = \int_{R^d} u^m(t, x)h(t, x)dx.$$

Definition 10.2 A pair of functions u^1, u^2 is called a generalized solution of (10.1) if it has the following properties:

(i) $u^1, u^2 \in L^\infty_{\text{loc}}([0, \infty); L^\infty(R^d))$ and $u^1, u^2 \ge 0$ a.e. in $(0, \infty) \times R^d$;

(ii) $\nabla u^m \in L^2_{\rm loc}((0,\infty)\times R^d)$;
(iii) for any test function $h \in C_0^\infty([0,\infty)\times R^d)$ with compact support

$$\int_0^\infty \langle\langle u^m(\theta), [\frac{\partial h(\theta)}{\partial\theta} + [u^1(\theta)+u^2(\theta)]\Delta h(\theta)]\rangle\rangle d\theta \tag{10.3}$$

$$+\int_0^\infty \langle\langle u^m(\theta), [c_m - c_{m1}u^1(\theta) - c_{m2}u^2(\theta)]h(\theta)\rangle\rangle d\theta = -\langle\langle u_0^m, h(0)\rangle\rangle,\ m=1,2.$$

Set

$$\frac{1}{2}M_u^2(x) = u^1(t,x)+u^2(t,x), \quad c_u^m(x) = c_m - c_{m1}u^1(t,x) - c_{m2}u^2(t,x)$$

and consider the Cauchy problem for a parabolic equation

$$\frac{\partial h^m(s,y)}{\partial s} + \frac{1}{2}M_u^2(y)\Delta h^m(s,y) + c_u^m h^m(s,y) = 0,\ h^m(t) = h^m \in C^2(R^d),\ 0\le s\le t. \tag{10.4}$$

Assume that $u^m(\theta, y)$ is a given bounded function twice differentiable in $y \in R^d$. Then, one can construct a probabilistic representation of the solution to the Cauchy problem (2). To this end, we consider a Wiener process $w(t) \in R^d$ defined on a given probability space $(\Omega, \mathcal{F}, P)$ and a couple of stochastic differential equations (SDEs)

$$d\xi(\theta) = M_u(\xi(\theta))dw(\theta), \quad \xi(s) = y, 0\le s\le\theta\le t, \tag{10.5}$$

$$d\eta^m(\theta) = c_u^m(\xi(\theta))\eta^m(\theta)d\theta, \quad \eta^m(s) = 1, \tag{10.6}$$

If we assume that there exists a solution $u = (u^1, u^2)$ to (10.1) such that u^m, $m = 1, 2$, are strictly positive, bounded, and twice differentiable in spatial argument, then we can deduce from the general theory [12] that the functions

$$h^m(s,y) = E[\eta^m(t)h(\xi_{s,y}(t))], \quad 0\le s\le\theta\le t, \tag{10.7}$$

are classical solutions of the Cauchy problem (2.5) for $m = 1, 2$; and hence, (10.7) defines a probabilistic representation of the classical solution to (2.5).

We construct a probabilistic representation of a regular generalized solution $u^m(t,x), m = 1, 2$ of (10.1) assuming that the solution $u^m(t,x)$ exists and unique. To derive the stochastic representation of $u^m(t,x)$, we have to modify (10.6) and apply some results from the Kunita stochastic flow theory.

10.2 Probabilistic Counterpart of a Parabolic System

To construct a probabilistic counterpart of the Cauchy problem (10.1) keeping in mind a priory assumptions of the previous section about existence and uniqueness of its regular generalized solution, we recall some notions and notations from the stochastic flow theory.

Assume as above that there exists a strictly positive twice differentiable generalized solution $u(t,x)$ of the problem (10.1) and consider a stochastic process $\xi(t)$ satisfying the SDE

$$d\xi(\theta) = M_u(\xi(\theta))dw(\theta), \quad \xi(0) = y \tag{10.8}$$

and its time reversal $\hat{\xi}(\theta)$ satisfying the SDE

$$d\hat{\xi}(\theta) = [M_u \nabla M_u](\hat{\xi}(\theta))d\theta + M_u(\hat{\xi}(\theta))d\tilde{w}(\theta), \quad \hat{\xi}(0) = x \tag{10.9}$$

with $M_u(x) = \sqrt{2[u^1(t,x) + u^2(t,x)]}$ and $\tilde{w}(\theta) = w(t-\theta) - w(t)$ for a fixed $t > \theta$.

Under the stated above a priori assumption, we can prove that there exists a unique solution $\xi(t)$ to (10.8) and its time reversal $\hat{\xi}(\theta)$ satisfies the stochastic integral equation

$$\hat{\xi}_{0,x}(\theta) = x - \int_\theta^t [M_u \nabla M_u](\hat{\xi}_{0,x}(\tau))d\tau - \int_\theta^t M_u(\hat{\xi}_{0,x}(\tau))d\tilde{w}(\tau), \tag{10.10}$$

where $0 \le \theta \le \tau \le t$. Set $\hat{\xi}_{t,x}(\theta) = \psi_{\theta,t}(x)$. Since the solution $\xi(\theta)$ of (10.8) is $\mathscr{F}_\theta$- measurable, then $\psi_{\theta,t} \in \mathscr{F}^{t-\theta}$, where $\mathscr{F}^t = \sigma\{\tilde{w}(s); 0 \le s \le t\} \vee \mathscr{N}$ and $\mathscr{N}$ are the null sets of $\mathscr{F}$. In addition under the above a priori assumptions, the mapping $\psi_{0,\theta} : x \mapsto \hat{\xi}_{0,\theta}(x)$ is differentiable.

Denote by $\mathbf{J}_t \equiv \mathbf{J}_{0,t} = \nabla\phi_{0,y}(t)$ the Jacobian matrix of the map $\phi_{0,t} : R^d \to R^d$. One can easily check that under the above a priori assumptions $\mathbf{J}_\theta$ exists and satisfies the linear stochastic equation

$$d\mathbf{J}_\theta = \mathbf{J}_{0,\theta}\langle \nabla M_u(\xi_{0,y}(\theta)), dw(\theta)\rangle, \quad \mathbf{J}_{0,0} = I. \tag{10.11}$$

Since $\mathbf{J}_{0,\theta}\hat{\mathbf{J}}_{0,\theta} = I$, we deduce by the Ito formula that $\hat{\mathbf{J}}_{0,\theta}$ satisfies the SDE

$$d\hat{\mathbf{J}}_{0,\theta} = \hat{\mathbf{J}}_{0,\theta}\|\nabla M_u(\xi_{0,x}(\theta))\|^2 d\theta - \hat{\mathbf{J}}_{0,\theta}\langle \nabla M_u(\xi_{0,x}(\theta)), dw(\theta)\rangle, \quad \hat{\mathbf{J}}_{0,0} = I. \tag{10.12}$$

Set $J_{0,t}(\omega) = \det \mathbf{J}_{0,t}(\omega)$ and note that

$$J_{0,t}(\omega) \equiv J(t) > 0 \quad \text{and} \quad J_{0,0}(\omega)) = 1.$$

Lemma 10.1 *Let $\mathbf{J}(t) = \mathbf{J}_{0,t}$ be a Jacobian matrix of the map $y \to \phi_{0,t}(y)$, where $\xi_{0,y}(t) = \phi_{0,t}(y)$ is a solution to (10.8). Then the Jacobian $J(\theta) = \det \mathbf{J}_{0,\theta}$ satisfies* *the equation*

$$dJ(\theta) = J(\theta)\langle \nabla M_u, dw(t)\rangle, \quad J(0) = 1. \tag{10.13}$$

Proof Recall that given a deterministic nondegenerate matrix $G(\theta)$ one can check that its determinant $\det G$ satisfies an ODE

$$d\det G(\theta) = \det G(\theta) Tr[G^{-1}(\theta) dG(\theta)].$$

Since the stochastic matrix $\mathbf{J}_{0,t}$ satisfying (10.11) is invertible and the determinant of a matrix is a multilinear function of matrix rows, we apply the Ito formula and observe that it satisfies the SDE

$$dJ(\theta) = J(\theta)\mathrm{Tr}(\hat{\mathbf{J}}(\theta) d\mathbf{J}(\theta)), \quad J(0) = 1.$$

which due to (10.12) yields (10.13). Recall that for a linear map Ito's formula for a stochastic differential coincides with the transformation law of a vector field since the correction term vanishes. □

Denote by

$$\mathscr{M}_u^m h = \frac{1}{2}[M_u]^2 \Delta h + c_u^m h \tag{10.14}$$

which is a dual operator to the operator $\mathscr{L}^m = \Delta[u^m[u^1 + u^2]] + c_u^m u^m$.

Consider a stochastic process $\gamma^m(\theta) = \eta^m(\theta) h(\xi(\theta)) J(\theta)$ where $\xi(\theta)$ and $J(\theta)$ satisfy (10.5) and (10.11), respectively, and the process $\eta^m(\theta)$ satisfies the following linear SDE

$$d\eta^m(\theta) = \tilde{c}_u^m(\xi(\theta))\eta^m(\theta) d\theta + C_u^m(\xi(\theta)\eta^m(\theta) dw(\theta), \quad \eta^m(0) = 1 \tag{10.15}$$

with coefficients $\tilde{c}_u^m$ and C_u^m to be specified in the lemma below.

Lemma 10.2 *Let coefficients $\tilde{c}_u^m$ and $\tilde{C}_u^m$ have the form*

$$\tilde{c}_u^m(\xi(\theta)) = c_u^m(\xi(\theta)) - \langle \nabla M_u(\xi(\theta)), \nabla M_u(\xi(\theta))\rangle, \quad C_u^m(\xi(\theta)) = -\nabla M_u(\xi(\theta)). \tag{10.16}$$

Then, the processes $\gamma^m(\theta) = \eta^m(\theta) h(\xi_{0,y}(\theta)) J(\theta), m = 1, 2,$ have stochastic differentials of the form

$$d\gamma^m(\theta) = \left[\frac{1}{2} M_u^2 \Delta h + c_u^m h\right](\xi_{0,y}(\theta))\eta^m(\theta) J(\theta) d\theta \tag{10.17}$$

$$+ M_u \nabla h(\xi_{0,y}(\theta))\eta^m(\theta) J(\theta) dw(\theta).$$

Proof We apply the Ito formula to evaluate $d\gamma^m(t)$

$$d\gamma^m(\theta) = d[\eta^m(\theta) h(\xi(\theta)) J^q(\theta)] = d[\eta^m(\theta)] h(\xi(\theta)) J(\theta) + \eta^m(\theta) d[h(\xi(\theta))] J(\theta)$$

$$+\eta^m(\theta)h(\xi(\theta))dJ(\theta)+d[\eta^m(\theta)]d[h(\xi(\theta))]J(\theta)$$

$$+\eta^m(\theta)d[h(\xi(\theta))]dJ(\theta)+d[\eta^q(\theta)]h(\xi(\theta))dJ(\theta).$$

Taking into account the expressions for $d\xi(t), dJ(t)$, and $d\eta^m(t)$ from (10.5), (10.13), and (10.15), we deduce

$$d\gamma^m(\theta)=\{\tilde{c}_u^m h+\frac{1}{2}M_u^2\Delta h+\langle C_u^m, M\nabla h\rangle+\langle\nabla M_u, M_u\nabla h\rangle\}(\xi(\theta))\eta^m(\theta)J(\theta)d\theta$$

$$+\langle C_u^m, h\nabla M_u\rangle](\xi(\theta))\eta^m(\theta)J(\theta)d\theta+\{C_u^m h+\nabla[M_u h]\}(\xi(\theta))\eta^m(\theta)J(\theta)dw(\theta).$$

Setting

$$C_u^m(\xi(\theta))=-\nabla M_u(\xi(\theta))$$

and

$$\tilde{c}_u^m(\xi(\theta))=c_u^m(\xi(\theta))+\langle\nabla M_u(\xi(\theta)), \nabla M_u(\xi(\theta))\rangle$$

we get

$$d\gamma^m(\theta)=\left[c_u^m(\xi(\theta))h(\xi(\theta))+\frac{1}{2}M_u^2(\xi(\theta))\Delta h(\xi(\theta))\right]\eta^m(\theta)J(\theta)d\theta$$

$$+M(\xi(\theta))\nabla h(\xi(\theta))\eta^m(\theta)J(\theta)dw(\theta).$$

□

Now, we can prove the following assertion.

Theorem 10.1 *Let a couple (u^1, u^2) be a generalized solution of (10.1). Then functions u^m admit probabilistic representations of the form*

$$u^m(t)=E[\zeta^m(t)\circ\psi_{0,t}],\quad m=1,2,$$

where $\psi_{0,t}(x)=\hat{\xi}_{0,x}(t)$ satisfies (10.9),

$$\zeta^m(t)=\exp\left\{\int_0^t n_u^m(\phi_{0,\theta})d\theta+\int_0^t\langle C_u^m(\phi_{0,\theta}), dw(\theta)\rangle\right\}u_0^m,$$

$n_u^m=\tilde{c}_u^m-\frac{1}{2}\|\nabla M_u\|^2$, $\tilde{c}_u^m=c_u^m+\|\nabla M_u\|^2\in R$,

$$\zeta^m(t)\circ\psi_{0,t}=\hat{\eta}^m(t)u_0^m\circ\psi_{0,t},$$

where $\hat{\eta}^m(t)=\exp\left\{\int_0^t n_u^m(\psi_{\theta,t})d\theta+\int_0^t\langle C_u^m(\psi_{\theta,t}), dw(\theta)\rangle\right\}$ *and coefficients c_u^m, C_u^m have the form (10.16).*

Proof Let $\phi_{0,t}(y) = \xi_{0,y}(t)$ be a solution to (10.5). Recall that under the assumption that $u^m(t)$ are bounded differentiable functions the existence of $\phi_{0,t}$ is justified by classical results of SDE theory as well as smooth dependence of $\xi_{0,y}(t)$ on the initial value y. Hence, $\psi_{0,t}$ does exist as well. This allows to define a random process $\zeta^m(t)$ by the following relation [4]

$$\int_{R^d} \zeta^m \circ \psi_{0,t}(x)h(x)dx = \int_{R^d} u_0^m(y)\eta^m(t)h \circ \phi_{0,t}(y)J(t)dy = \int_{R^d} u_0^m(y)\gamma^m(t,y)dy. \tag{10.18}$$

One can easily check that

$$\int_{R^d}\int_0^t u_0^m(y)d\gamma_y^m(\theta)dy = \int_{R^d} u_0^m(y)\gamma_y^m(t)dy - \int_{R^d} u_0^m(y)h(y)dy \tag{10.19}$$

$$= \int_{R^d} \hat{\eta}(t)u_0(\hat{\xi}(t))h(x)dx - \int_{R^d} u_0(x)h(x)dx.$$

On the other hand from (10.17), we deduce

$$E\left[\int_{R^d}\int_0^t u_0^m(y)d\gamma^m(\theta)dy\right] = E\left[\int_0^t\int_{R^d} u_0^m(y)d\left[\eta^m(\theta)h(\xi_{0,y}(\theta))J(\xi_{0,y}(\theta))\right]dy\right] \tag{10.20}$$

$$= E\left[\int_0^t\int_{R^d} u_0^m(y[\mathscr{M}_u^m]h(\xi_{0,y}(\theta))\eta^m(\theta)J(\theta))dyd\theta\right].$$

As a result, we get the equality

$$E\left[\int_{R^d} u_0^m(y)\gamma_y^q(t)dy\right] - \int_{R^d} u_0^m(y)h(y)dy \tag{10.21}$$

$$= E\left[\int_0^t\int_{R^d} u_0^m(y)[\mathscr{M}_u^m]h(\xi_{0,y}(\theta))\eta^m(\theta)J(\theta)dyd\theta\right].$$

By the change of variables $\xi_{0,y}(\theta) = x$ due to stochastic Fubini theorem, we deduce from (10.17)

$$E\left[\int_{R^d}\int_0^t u_0^m(y)d\gamma_y^m(\theta)dy\right] = E\left[\int_0^t\int_{R^d} [\hat{\eta}^m(\theta)u_0^m(\hat{\xi}_{0,x}(\theta))]\mathscr{M}_u^m h(x)dxd\theta\right] \tag{10.22}$$

$$= \int_0^t\int_{R^d} E[\hat{\eta}^m(\theta)u_0^m(\hat{\xi}_{0,x}(\theta))]\mathscr{M}_u^m h(x)dxd\theta$$

$$= \int_0^t\int_{R^d} \mathscr{L}_u^m E[\hat{\eta}^m(\theta)u_0^m(\hat{\xi}_{0,x}(\theta))]h(x)dxd\theta.$$

Hence from (10.18)–(10.22), we derive that $v^m(t,x) = E[\hat{\eta}^m(\theta)u_0^m(\hat{\xi}_{0,x}(\theta))]$ satisfy

$$\int_{R^d} v^m(t,x)h(x)dx - \int_{R^d} u_0^m(x)h(x)dx = \int_0^t \int_{R^d} \mathscr{L}_u^m v^m(\theta,x)h(x)dxd\theta$$

which results due to assumed above uniqueness of a solution to (10.1) that $v^m(t,x) = u^m(t,x)$ and hence

$$u^m(t,x) = E[\hat{\eta}^m(t)u_0^m(\hat{\xi}_{0,x}(t))].$$

10.3 Stochastic Counterpart of the Cauchy Problem for a System with Cross-Diffusion

In the previous section, we have derived a stochastic representation of a generalized solution of the Cauchy problem

$$\frac{\partial u^m}{\partial t} = \Delta[u^m[u^1+u^2]] + c_u^m u^m, \quad u^m(0,x) = u_{0m}(x), \quad m=1,2. \tag{10.23}$$

provided such solution exists.

In this section, our aim is to obtain a closed system of stochastic equations which can be treated as a stochastic counterpart of (10.23). To this end, it is not enough to have a stochastic representation of the solution u^m to (10.23) itself since coefficients of SDEs for $\hat{\xi}(\theta)$ and $\hat{\eta}^m(\theta)$ depend on ∇u^m. Hence, we need stochastic representations for spatial derivatives of $u^m(t,x)$.

Consider a system of SDEs

$$d\xi_{0,y}(\theta) = M_u(\xi_{0,y}(\theta))dw(\theta), \quad \xi_{0,y}(0) = y,$$

$$d\eta^m(\theta) = \tilde{c}_u^m(\xi_{0,y}(\theta))\eta^m(\theta)d\theta + C_u^m(\xi_{0,y}(\theta))\eta^m(\theta)dw(\theta), \quad \eta^m(0) = 1,$$

$$d\hat{\xi}_{0,x}(\theta) = [M_u\nabla M_u](\hat{\xi}_{0,x}(\theta))d\theta + M_u(\hat{\xi}_{0,x}(\theta))d\tilde{w}(\theta), \quad \hat{\xi}_{0,x}(0) = x, \tag{10.24}$$

$$d\hat{\eta}^m(\theta) = \tilde{c}_u^m(\hat{\xi}_{0,x}(\theta))\hat{\eta}^m(\theta)d\theta + C_u^m(\hat{\xi}_{0,x}(\theta))\hat{\eta}^m(\theta)dw(\theta), \tag{10.25}$$

$$\hat{\eta}^m(0) = 1, \quad m=1,2,$$

$$u^m(t,x) = E[\hat{\eta}^m(t)u_0^m(\hat{\xi}_{0,x}(t))]. \tag{10.26}$$

To make the system (10.24)–(10.26) closed, we need extra relations for functions $v_i^m(t,x) = \nabla_i u^m(t,x), i = 1,\ldots,d$, since coefficients of (10.24) and (10.25) depend on ∇u^m.

To derive these relations, we need some additional speculations based on results from [12]. By formal differentiation of the system

$$\frac{\partial u^m}{\partial t} = \Delta[u^m(u^1+u^2)] + c_u^m u^m, \quad u^m(0,x) = u_0^m(x), \; m=1,2. \tag{10.27}$$

we get a PDE for $v_i^m = \nabla_i u^m$

$$\frac{\partial v_i^m}{\partial t} = \Delta\{v_i^m(u^1+u^2)+u^m(v^1+v^2)\}+u^m\nabla_i c^m(u)+c^m(u)v_i^m, \quad v_i^m(0,x) = \nabla_i u_0^m(x). \tag{10.28}$$

In a similar way from

$$\frac{\partial h}{\partial \theta} + (u^1+u^2)\Delta h + c^m(u)h = 0, \quad h(t,y) = h(y), \tag{10.29}$$

we get a PDE for $g_i = \nabla_i h$

$$\frac{\partial g_i}{\partial \theta}+(u^1+u^2)\Delta g_i+(v_i^1+v_i^2)divg+\nabla_i c^m(u)h+c^m(u)g_i = 0, \quad g_i(0,y) = \nabla_i h(y). \tag{10.30}$$

In addition note that we can construct a stochastic representation of the solution to (10.30) in the form

$$G^m(\theta,y) = E[\beta^m(t)G_0(\xi_{\theta,y}(t))],$$

where $G(t,y) = \begin{pmatrix} h(t,y) \\ \nabla h(t,y) \end{pmatrix}$ and stochastic processes $\xi(\tau)$ and $\beta_{ik}^m(\tau)$ satisfy SDEs

$$d\xi(\tau) = \sqrt{2[u^1(\tau,\xi(\tau))+u^2(\tau,\xi(\tau))]}dw(\tau), \quad \xi(\theta) = y, 0 \le \theta \le \tau \le t,$$

$$d\beta^m(\tau) = n_u^m(\xi(t))\beta(\tau)d\tau + N_u^m(\xi(\tau))\beta^m(\tau)dw(\tau).$$

Here, $\beta^m(t) = (\beta_1^m(t), \beta_2(t)) \in R^2 \oplus (R^d \otimes R^2)$, $\beta_1^m = \nabla\eta^m(t)$, $\beta_2^m(t) = \mathbf{J}(t) \otimes \eta^m(t)$

$$\beta^m(\tau) = \begin{pmatrix} \nabla\eta^m(\tau) \\ \mathbf{J}(\tau)\otimes\eta^m(\tau) \end{pmatrix}, \quad n_u^m = \begin{pmatrix} c_u^m & \nabla c_u^m \\ 0 & 0\oplus c_u^m \end{pmatrix}, \quad N_u^m = \begin{pmatrix} 0 & 0 \\ 0 & \frac{[v^1+v^2]\delta}{\sqrt{2(u^1+u^2)}} \oplus 0 \end{pmatrix},$$

where δ is the Kronecker delta and $c \oplus a = a \otimes I + I \otimes c$ is an operator acting in $R^2 \otimes R^d$, $(c\oplus a)(\eta\otimes\mathbf{J}) = c\eta\otimes\mathbf{J}+\eta\otimes a\mathbf{J}$. Thus for $G_0(y) = G^m(0,y) = \begin{pmatrix} h(y) \\ \nabla h(y) \end{pmatrix}$, we obtain for a solution $G^m(\theta,y)$ of (10.29)–(10.30) an expression of the form

$$G^m(\theta,y) = E\left[\begin{pmatrix} \eta^m(t) & 0 \\ \nabla\eta^m(t) & \eta^m(t)\otimes\mathbf{J}^m(t) \end{pmatrix}\begin{pmatrix} h(\xi_{\theta,y}(t)) \\ \nabla h(\xi_{\theta,y}(t)) \end{pmatrix}\right]$$

$$= \begin{pmatrix} E[\eta^m(t)h(\xi_{\theta,y}(t))] \\ E[\nabla\eta^m(t)h(\xi_{\theta,y}(t)) + \eta^m(t)\nabla h(\xi_{\theta,y}(t))\mathbf{J}^m(t)] \end{pmatrix}.$$

To deduce the stochastic representation for the function $g_j = \nabla_j h$, we note that given the PDE system (10.29)–(10.30) we can derive its stochastic representation as follows. Let us rewrite the system (10.27), (10.28) in the form

$$\frac{\partial}{\partial t}\begin{pmatrix} u^m \\ v^m \end{pmatrix} = \mathscr{L}^m \left(u^m \; v^m\right), \quad m = 1, 2. \tag{10.31}$$

where

$$\mathscr{L}^m \begin{pmatrix} u^m \\ v^m \end{pmatrix} = \Delta\left[\begin{pmatrix} u^1 + u^2 & 0 \\ v^1 + v^2 & u^1 + u^2 \end{pmatrix}\begin{pmatrix} u^m \\ v^m \end{pmatrix}\right] + \begin{pmatrix} c_{11}^m & 0 \\ c_{21}^m & c_{22}^m \end{pmatrix}\begin{pmatrix} u^m \\ v^m \end{pmatrix}.$$

Consider as well a dual system derived from (10.31) as follows. Integrate over R^d a product of (10.31) and a vector test function $(h, g)^*$, where $g_j = \nabla_j h,\ j = 1, \dots, d$. As a result, we obtain a system of the form

$$\left\langle\!\!\left\langle \begin{pmatrix} u^m \\ v^m \end{pmatrix}\left[\frac{\partial}{\partial t}\begin{pmatrix} h \\ g \end{pmatrix} + \mathscr{Q}^m\begin{pmatrix} h \\ g \end{pmatrix}\right]\right\rangle\!\!\right\rangle = 0, \tag{10.32}$$

where

$$\mathscr{Q}^m\begin{pmatrix} h \\ g \end{pmatrix} = \begin{pmatrix} u^1 + u^2 & 0 \\ v^1 + v^2 & u^1 + u^2 \end{pmatrix}\Delta\begin{pmatrix} h \\ g \end{pmatrix} + \begin{pmatrix} c_{11}^m & 0 \\ c_{21}^m & c_{22}^m \end{pmatrix}\begin{pmatrix} h \\ g \end{pmatrix}.$$

Here and below, we denote by

$$\left\langle\!\!\left\langle \begin{pmatrix} u^m \\ v_i^m \end{pmatrix}\begin{pmatrix} h \\ g_i \end{pmatrix}\right\rangle\!\!\right\rangle = \begin{pmatrix} \int_{R^d} u^m(x)h(x)dx \\ \int_{R^d} v_i^m(x)g_i(x)dx \end{pmatrix}.$$

In the sequel, we take into account the relation $[v^1 + v^2]\Delta h = [v^1 + v^2]divg$ that allows to construct a proper stochastic representation of the backward Cauchy problem

$$\frac{\partial}{\partial \theta}\begin{pmatrix} h \\ g \end{pmatrix} + \mathscr{Q}^m\begin{pmatrix} h \\ g \end{pmatrix} = 0, \quad \begin{pmatrix} h(t) \\ g(t) \end{pmatrix} = \begin{pmatrix} h_0 \\ g_0 \end{pmatrix}, \quad 0 \le \theta \le t \tag{10.33}$$

based on results of [14]. To this end, we take into consideration the equality $[v^1 + v^2]\Delta h = [v^1 + v^2]divg$ that allows to construct a stochastic representation for a solution to (10.33). Along with (10.24), we consider a stochastic equation of the form

$$d\eta^m(\theta) = [\tilde{c}^m]^*(\xi(\theta))\eta^m(\theta)d\theta + [\tilde{C}^m]^*(\xi(\theta))(\eta^m(\theta), dw(\theta)), \quad \eta^m(s) = \gamma^m \tag{10.34}$$

with respect to the two component process $\eta^m(\theta) = \begin{pmatrix} \eta_1^m(\theta) \\ \eta_2^m(\theta) \end{pmatrix}$ with coefficients $\tilde{c}^m$ and C^m to be chosen below. Let $\zeta^m(t)$ maps γ^m to $\eta^m(\theta)$, that is

$$\zeta^m(\theta) = \begin{pmatrix} \zeta_{11}^m(\theta) & 0 \\ \zeta_{21}^m(\theta) & \zeta_{22}^m(\theta) \end{pmatrix}.$$

To simplify notation, we omit index m and define a stochastic test function

$$\kappa(\theta) = \begin{pmatrix} \kappa_1(\theta) \\ \kappa_2(\theta) \end{pmatrix} = \begin{pmatrix} \zeta_{11}(\theta) & 0 \\ \zeta_{21}(\theta) & \zeta_{22}(\theta) \end{pmatrix} \begin{pmatrix} h(\xi(\theta)) \\ g(\xi(\theta)) \end{pmatrix} J(\theta), \tag{10.35}$$

where $J(\theta)$ is a Jacobian of the stochastic transformation $y \to \xi_{s,y}(\theta)$. The stochastic differential of the process $\kappa(\theta)$ has the form $d\kappa(\theta) = \begin{pmatrix} d\kappa_1(\theta) \\ d\kappa_2(\theta) \end{pmatrix}$ with

$$d\kappa_1(\theta) = [\tilde{c}_{11}h + \frac{1}{2}M_u^2 \Delta h + \langle C_{11}, [M_u \nabla h + \nabla M_u h](\xi(\theta))\rangle \zeta_{11}(\theta) J(\theta)] d\theta$$

$$+\langle M_u \nabla h(\xi(\theta)), \nabla M_u\rangle \zeta_{11}(\theta) J(\theta) d\theta + \langle N_1(\xi(\theta)), dw(\theta)\rangle,$$

$$d\kappa_2^i(\theta) = \left[[\tilde{c}_{21}h + M_u \nabla M_u divg](\xi(\theta))\zeta_{21}^i(\theta) + \zeta_{22}(\theta)[\tilde{c}_{22}g_i + \frac{1}{2}M_u^2 \Delta g_i](\xi(\theta)) \right]$$

$$J(\theta)d\theta + \{C_{21}\zeta_{21}^i(\theta)[M_u \nabla h + \nabla M_u h](\xi(\theta)) + C_{22}\zeta_{22}(\theta)[M_u \nabla g_i + g_i \nabla M_u](\xi(\theta))$$

$$+\zeta_{21}^i(\theta) M_u \langle \nabla h, \nabla M_u\rangle(\xi(\theta)) + \zeta_{22}(\theta) M_u \langle \nabla g_i, \nabla M_u\rangle(\xi(\theta))\} J(\theta) d\theta$$

$$+\langle [N_{21}(\xi(\theta))\zeta_{21}^i(\theta) + N_{22}^i(\xi(\theta))\zeta_{22}(\theta)], dw(\theta)\rangle J(\theta).$$

Let us specify coefficients $\tilde{c}^m$ and C^m. As it was done in the previous section, we choose

$$C_{11}^m = -\nabla M_u, \quad \tilde{c}_{11}^m = c_u^m + \|\nabla M_u\|^2. \tag{10.36}$$

Next, we choose

$$C_{21}^m = -\nabla M_u, C_{22}^m = \frac{(v^1 + v^2)\delta}{M_u} - \nabla M_u, \tag{10.37}$$

$$[\tilde{c}_{21}^m]_i = \nabla_i c_u^m + \|\nabla M_u\|^2, \quad \tilde{c}_{22}^m = c_u^m + \|\nabla M_u\|^2. \tag{10.38}$$

We do not specify for the moment N_1^m and N_2^m since they do not take part in the probabilistic representation of u^m and v^m. Next, we proceed as in the previous section.

To get a closed counterpart of the system (10.1) in addition to Theorem 10.1, we state the following assertion.

Theorem 10.2 *Under assumptions of Theorem 10.1 both the functions $u^m(t,x)$ admit stochastic representations (10.30) and functions $(u^m, v_j^m = \nabla_j u^m)$ admit stochastic representations*

$$\begin{pmatrix} u^m(t,x) \\ \nabla_i u^m(t,x) \end{pmatrix} = E\left[\begin{pmatrix} \hat{\zeta}_{11}^m(t) & 0 \\ \hat{\zeta}_{21}^m(t) & \hat{\zeta}_{22}^m(\theta) \end{pmatrix} \begin{pmatrix} u_0^m(\hat{\xi}_{0,x}(t)) \\ v_i^m(\hat{\xi}_{0,x}(t)) \end{pmatrix}\right]. \tag{10.39}$$

Proof To verify the last assertion of the theorem, we note that we have the following matrix relations

$$\left\langle\!\left\langle \int_0^t \begin{pmatrix} u_0^m \\ v_{i0}^m \end{pmatrix} \begin{pmatrix} d\kappa_1^m(\theta) \\ d\kappa_2^m(\theta) \end{pmatrix} \right\rangle\!\right\rangle = \left\langle\!\left\langle \begin{pmatrix} u_0^m \\ v_{i0}^m \end{pmatrix} \begin{pmatrix} d\kappa_1^m(t) \\ d\kappa_2^m(t) \end{pmatrix} \right\rangle\!\right\rangle$$
$$- \left\langle\!\left\langle \begin{pmatrix} u_0^m \\ v_{i0}^m \end{pmatrix} \begin{pmatrix} d\kappa_1^m(0) \\ d\kappa_2^m(0) \end{pmatrix} \right\rangle\!\right\rangle.$$

On the other hand from (10.35), we deduce

$$E\left[\left\langle\!\left\langle \int_0^t \begin{pmatrix} u_0^m \\ v_{i0}^m \end{pmatrix} \begin{pmatrix} d\kappa^1(\theta) \\ d\kappa^2(\theta) \end{pmatrix} \right\rangle\!\right\rangle\right]$$
$$= E\left[\int_0^t \left\langle\!\left\langle \begin{pmatrix} u_0^m \\ v_{i0}^m \end{pmatrix} d\left[\begin{pmatrix} \zeta_{11}^m(\theta) & 0 \\ \zeta_{21}^m(\theta) & \zeta_{22}^m(\theta) \end{pmatrix} \begin{pmatrix} h(\xi_{0,\cdot}(\theta)) \\ g(\xi_{0,\cdot}(\theta)) \end{pmatrix} J(\theta)\right]\right\rangle\!\right\rangle\right]$$
$$= E\left[\int_0^t \left\langle\!\left\langle \begin{pmatrix} u_0^m \\ v_{i0}^m \end{pmatrix} \begin{pmatrix} \zeta_{11}^m(\theta) & 0 \\ \zeta_{21}^m(\theta) & \zeta_{22}^m(\theta) \end{pmatrix} \mathscr{Q}^m \begin{pmatrix} h(\xi_{0,\cdot}(\theta) \\ g(\xi_{0,\cdot}(\theta)) \end{pmatrix} J(\theta)\right\rangle\!\right\rangle d\theta\right].$$

By the change of variables $\xi_{0,y}(\theta) = x$ applying stochastic Fubini theorem, we get

$$E\left[\left\langle\!\left\langle \int_0^t \begin{pmatrix} u_0^m \\ v_{i0}^m \end{pmatrix}, \begin{pmatrix} d\kappa^1(\theta) \\ d\kappa^2(\theta) \end{pmatrix} \right\rangle\!\right\rangle\right]$$
$$= E\left[\int_0^t \left\langle\!\left\langle \begin{pmatrix} \hat{\zeta}_{11}^m(\theta) & 0 \\ \hat{\zeta}_{21}^m(\theta) & \hat{\zeta}_{22}^m(\theta) \end{pmatrix} \begin{pmatrix} u_0^m(\hat{\xi}_{0,\cdot}(\theta)) \\ v_{i0}^m(\hat{\xi}_{0,\cdot}(\theta)) \end{pmatrix} \mathscr{Q}^m \begin{pmatrix} h \\ g \end{pmatrix} \right\rangle\!\right\rangle d\theta\right]$$
$$= \int_0^t \left\langle\!\left\langle E\left[\begin{pmatrix} \hat{\zeta}_{11}^m(\theta) & 0 \\ \hat{\zeta}_{21}^m(\theta) & \hat{\zeta}_{22}^m(\theta) \end{pmatrix} \begin{pmatrix} u_0^m(\hat{\xi}_{0,\cdot}(\theta)) \\ v_{i0}^m(\hat{\xi}_{0,\cdot}(\theta)) \end{pmatrix}\right] \mathscr{Q}^m \begin{pmatrix} h \\ g \end{pmatrix} \right\rangle\!\right\rangle d\theta$$
$$= \int_0^t \left\langle\!\left\langle \mathscr{L}^m E\left[\begin{pmatrix} \hat{\zeta}_{11}^m(\theta) & 0 \\ \hat{\zeta}_{21}^m(\theta) & \hat{\zeta}_{22}^m(\theta) \end{pmatrix} \begin{pmatrix} u_0^m(\hat{\xi}_{0,\cdot}(\theta)) \\ v_{i0}^m(\hat{\xi}_{0,\cdot}(\theta)) \end{pmatrix}\right] \begin{pmatrix} h \\ g \end{pmatrix} \right\rangle\!\right\rangle d\theta.$$

Hence, we derive that the functions

$$\begin{pmatrix} \lambda^m(t,x) \\ \nabla\lambda^m(t,x) \end{pmatrix} = E\left[\begin{pmatrix} \hat{\zeta}_{11}^m(\theta) & 0 \\ \hat{\zeta}_{21}^m(\theta) & \hat{\zeta}_{22}^m(\theta) \end{pmatrix} \begin{pmatrix} u_0^m(\hat{\xi}_{0,x}(\theta)) \\ v_{i0}^m(\hat{\xi}_{0,x}(\theta)) \end{pmatrix}\right]$$

satisfy integral identities

$$\left\langle\!\!\left\langle \begin{pmatrix} \lambda^m(t) \\ \nabla\lambda^m(t) \end{pmatrix} \begin{pmatrix} h \\ g \end{pmatrix} \right\rangle\!\!\right\rangle - \left\langle\!\!\left\langle \begin{pmatrix} \lambda^m(0) \\ \nabla\lambda^m(0) \end{pmatrix} \begin{pmatrix} h \\ g \end{pmatrix} \right\rangle\!\!\right\rangle$$

$$= \left\langle\!\!\left\langle \mathcal{Q}^m \begin{pmatrix} \lambda^m(t) \\ \nabla\lambda^m(t) \end{pmatrix} \begin{pmatrix} h \\ g \end{pmatrix} \right\rangle\!\!\right\rangle$$

which yields due to the assumed uniqueness of a solution to (10.1) that

$$\begin{pmatrix} \lambda^m(t,x) \\ \nabla\lambda^m(t,x) \end{pmatrix} = \begin{pmatrix} u^m(t,x) \\ \nabla u^m(t,x) \end{pmatrix}$$

and hence

$$\begin{pmatrix} u^m(t,x) \\ \nabla u^m(t,x) \end{pmatrix} = E\left[\begin{pmatrix} \hat{\zeta}^m_{11}(t) & 0 \\ \hat{\zeta}^m_{21}(t) & \hat{\zeta}^m_{22}(t) \end{pmatrix} \begin{pmatrix} u^m_0(\hat{\xi}_{0,x}(t)) \\ v^m_{i0}(\hat{\xi}_{0,x}(t)) \end{pmatrix} \right].$$

As a result, we deduce from the last equalities that (10.31) holds and in addition

$$\nabla u^m_i(t,x) = E[\hat{\zeta}_{21}(t) u^m_0(\hat{\xi}_{0,x}(t)) + \hat{\zeta}^m_{22}(t) v^m_{i0}(\hat{\xi}_{0,x}(t))].$$

Remark 10.1 We have proved that under a priori assumption that there exists unique regular solution of the Cauchy problem (10.1) there exists a stochastic representation of this solution and moreover we derive a closed system of stochastic equations that can be considered without reference to this a priori assumption. Namely, we have shown that the system (10.24), (10.34) and (10.39) with coefficients given by (10.36)–(10.38) is a closed stochastic system which can be considered independently of (10.1).

At the next step starting with the system (10.24), (10.34) and (10.39) having the form

$$d\hat{\xi}_{0,x}(\theta) = [M_u \nabla M_u](\hat{\xi}_{0,x}(\theta))d\theta + M_u(\hat{\xi}_{0,x}(\theta))d\tilde{w}(\theta), \quad \hat{\xi}_{0,x}(0) = x,$$

$$d\hat{\zeta}^m(\theta) = \tilde{c}^m_u(\hat{\xi}(\theta))\hat{\zeta}^m(\theta)d\theta + C^m_u(\hat{\xi}(\theta)\hat{\zeta}^m(\theta)dw(\theta), \quad \hat{\zeta}^m(0) = I$$

with coefficients $\tilde{c}^m$, C^m given by (10.36)–(10.38) and

$$\begin{pmatrix} u^m(t,x) \\ \nabla u^m(t,x) \end{pmatrix} = E\left[\begin{pmatrix} \hat{\zeta}^m_{11}(\theta) & 0 \\ \hat{\zeta}^m_{21}(\theta) & \hat{\zeta}^m_{22}(\theta) \end{pmatrix} \begin{pmatrix} u^m_0(\hat{\xi}_{0,x}(\theta)) \\ v^m_0(\hat{\xi}_{0,x}(\theta)) \end{pmatrix} \right]$$

we will formulate conditions to ensure that the functions $u^m(t,x)$ defined by the last relation exist and give the required generalized solution of the problem (10.1). This will be done in the forthcoming chapter.

Acknowledgements The financial support of the RFBR Grant 15-01-01453 is gratefully acknowledged.

References

1. Belopolskaya, Ya.: Generalized solutions of nonlinear parabolic systems and vanishing viscosity method. J. Math. Sci. **133** 1207–1223 (2006)
2. Belopolskaya, Ya., Woyczynski, W.: Generalized solution of the Cauchy problem for systems of nonlinear parabolic equations and diffusion processes. Stoch. Dyn. **11**(1), 1–31 (2012)
3. Kunita H.: Stochastic Flows and Stochastic Differential Equations. Cambridge University Press, Cambridge (1990)
4. Kunita, H.: Stochastic flows acting on Schwartz distributions. J. Theor. Pobab. **7**(2), 247–278 (1994)
5. Kunita, H.: Generalized solutions of stochastic partial differential equations. J. Theor. Pobab. **7**(2), 279–308 (1994)
6. Shigesada, N., Kawasaki, K., Teramoto, E.: Spatial segregation of interacting species. J. Theor. Biol. **79**, 83–99 (1979)
7. Jüngel, A.: Diffusive and nondiffusive population models. In: Naldi, G., Pareschi, L., Toscani, G. (eds.) Mathematical Modeling of Collective Behavior in Socio-Economic and Life Sciences, pp. 397–425. Springer, Heidelberg (2010)
8. Desvilletes, L., Lepoutre, Th, Moussa, A.: Entropy, duality and cross diffusion. SIAM J. Math. Anal. **46**(1), 820–853 (2014)
9. Jüngel, A.: The boundedness-by-entropy method for cross-diffusion systems. Nonlinearity **28**, 1963–2001 (2015)
10. Galiano, G., Selgas, V.: On a cross-diffusion segregation problem arising from a model of interacting particles. Nonlinear Anal. Real World Appl. **18**, 34–49 (2014)
11. Fontbona, J., Meleard, S.: Non local Lotka-Volterra system with cross-diffusion in an heterogeneous medium. J. Math. Biol. **70**(4), 829–854 (2015)
12. Bogachev, V., Röckner, M., Shaposhnikov, S.: On uniqueness problems related to the Fokker-Planck-Kolmogorov equation for measures. J. Math. Sci. **179**(1), 7–47 (2011)
13. Protter, P.: Stochastic Integration and Differential Equations. Springer, Berlin (2010)
14. Belopolskaya, Ya., Dalecky, Yu.: Stochastic Equations and Differential Geometry. Kluwer Academic Publishers, Dordrecht (1990)

Chapter 11
Benefits and Application of Tree Structures in Gaussian Process Models to Optimize Magnetic Field Shaping Problems

Natalie Vollert, Michael Ortner and Jürgen Pilz

Abstract Recent years have witnessed the development of powerful numerical methods to emulate realistic physical systems and their integration into the industrial product development process. Today, finite element simulations have become a standard tool to help with the design of technical products. However, when it comes to multivariate optimization, the computation power requirements of such tools can often not be met when working with classical algorithms. As a result, a lot of attention is currently given to the design of computer experiments approach. One goal of this work is the development of a sophisticated optimization process for simulation based models. Within many possible choices, Gaussian process models are most widely used as modeling approach for the simulation data. However, these models are strongly based on stationary assumptions that are often not satisfied in the underlying system. In this work, treed Gaussian process models are investigated for dealing with non-stationarities and compared to the usual modeling approach. The method is developed for and applied to the specific physical problem of the optimization of 1D magnetic linear position detection.

Keywords Gaussian process surrogates · Non-stationarity · Simulation data
Tree models

11.1 Introduction

Gaussian process (GP) models have been widely used as emulators for time-consuming computer models, where the most common approach is adopted from spatial statistics and named Kriging [13]. This refers to a linear model with a

N. Vollert (✉) · M. Ortner
CTR Carinthian Tech Research AG, Europastraße 12, 9524 Villach, Austria
e-mail: natalie.vollert@ctr.at

M. Ortner
e-mail: michael.ortner@ctr.at

N. Vollert · J. Pilz
Department of Statistics, Alpen-Adria University of Klagenfurt,
Universitätsstraße 65-67, 9020 Klagenfurt, Austria
e-mail: juergen.pilz@aau.at

J. Pilz et al. (eds.), *Statistics and Simulation*, Springer Proceedings
in Mathematics & Statistics 231, https://doi.org/10.1007/978-3-319-76035-3_11

systematic departure realized as a stationary Gaussian random function. A major problem with this approach is the strong assumption of stationarity and homoscedasticity of the GPs, which is firstly difficult to verify and secondly often not valid. An efficient way to deal with this problem is to partition the input parameter space into regions and to fit individual, stationary GPs in each region. This method is referred to as treed Gaussian process modeling [6].

It is the ultimate goal of this work to develop an emulator based on GPs to model and optimize realistic physical systems using FEM data. This is done in the context of magnetic linear position detection where the magnetic field of a permanent magnet is emulated in the magneto-static limit. In such systems, a magnet moves relative to a magnetic sensor and the state of the magnet is determined from the field that is seen by the sensor. The advantages are wear-free measurements, high resolutions, low power requirements, and an excellent robustness against temperature and dirt with multiple applications in modern industries, e.g., in the detection of shifting shafts, flexible arm mechanisms, gearboxes or lift systems, [16]. To improve the signal stability while retaining cost-effectiveness, it is proposed in [9] to shape the magnetic field at the sensor by designing a compound magnet. However, even when dealing with a small number of constituents, the compound features multiple degrees of freedom which makes the modeling and optimization process difficult.

This work is intended to be a preliminary study for emphasizing advantages and also possible disadvantages of the treed GP models in comparison to the usual GPs. Thus, emulators of the magnetic field are constructed and investigated for both modeling approaches. To that end, the sample points for the construction of the models are generated from an analytical description for the magnetic field. Furthermore, at this early stage, the compound consists only of a single rectangular magnet, considerably reducing the number of parameters to better understand the potential and the difficulties of this method.

11.2 Magnetic Linear Position Detection

Magnetic position and orientation detection systems play an important role in modern industrial applications. Their features include contact-free measurement, low power requirements, and high resolutions combined with an excellent robustness against oil, grease, and dirt without the need for airtight seals or other environmental contamination control in harsh environments. Long life times up to decades and cost-effectiveness are especially interesting for the cost-driven automotive sector where magnetic sensors are increasingly used for gear shift detection, gas pedals, speed sensors, and many other applications.

State-of-the-art magnetic linear position detection systems feature a magnet that moves relative to a magnetic sensor which detects the magnetic field to determine the position of the magnet; see Fig. 11.1a. The magnetic field is generally not a linear function of the position of the magnet but typically features an even and an odd component; see Fig. 11.1b. It can be a sensitive task to find a bijective map that

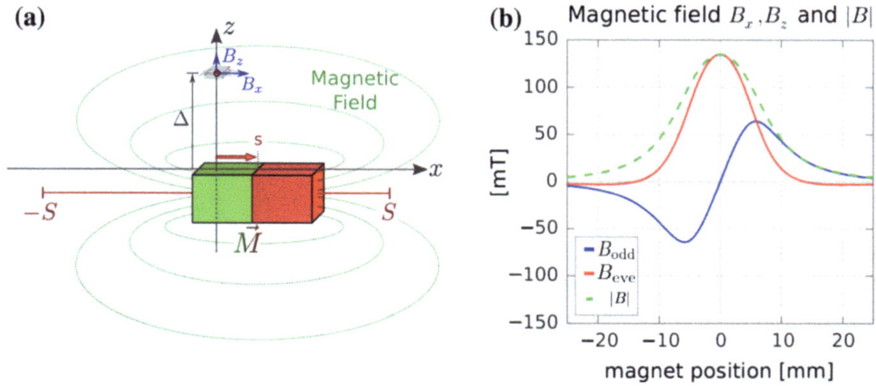

Fig. 11.1 **a** shows a sketch of a linear position detection system. A rectangular magnet with magnetization **M** oriented in the z-direction moves along the stroke $s \in [-S, S]$ in x-direction and generates a magnetic field with components B_x and B_z. The sensor is positioned on the positive z-axis at a distance Δ from the magnet called the airgap. **b** shows the magnetic field components detected by the sensor as a function of the position of the magnet for a typical setup with a cubical magnet with side length 10mm, a remanence field of one Tesla and an airgap of 5mm

relates the magnetic field to the position of the magnet. Distinction is essentially made between 1D and 2D magnetic position detection systems, where the former picks up both components of the magnetic field applying a 2D sensor, while the latter just detects the odd component with a simple 1D probe. For 1D position sensing, the linear range of the odd field component about the origin is used; see Fig. 11.1b. When compared to their 2D counterparts, 1D systems have a lot of shortcomings like small measurement ranges and an even smaller linear region as well as airgap instability. Despite these critical disadvantages, 1D systems are still used in modern industrial applications, solely due to their cost-effectiveness, as 1D sensors are much cheaper than 2D ones.

It is proposed in [9] to improve 1D magnetic position detection systems by designing a compound magnet which features a highly linear odd field component B_x along a given stroke while minimizing the magnet volume at the same time to reduce costs. The multiple shape parameters of the compound make the optimization a very time-consuming process when calculating the magnetic field by FEM means. In the following sections, a design of computer experiments approach is developed.

11.3 Gaussian Process Models

The statistical approach for computer experiments consists of two parts—experimental design and modeling. The designing refers to finding a set D_n of n points in the experimental domain T that optimally represents the entire domain; for further information, see [1, 5, 14, 15]. Then, data is collected based on the optimal design D_n and the relationship between the input variables $\mathbf{x_i} = (x_1, \ldots, x_s)^T$, $i = 1, \ldots, n$, and the output is modeled.

11.3.1 Kriging Setup

Among many different modeling approaches (see, e.g., [5]), especially Gaussian process models, also called Kriging models, are of main interest for computer experiments. Here, the response $Y(\mathbf{x})$ is treated as a realization of a stochastic process, i.e.,

$$Y(\mathbf{x}) = \mu(\mathbf{x}) + Z(\mathbf{x}), \tag{11.1}$$

where $\mu(\mathbf{x})$ is the trend function and $Z(\mathbf{x})$ is a primarily stationary Gaussian process with zero mean. There are different types of Kriging based on the definition of the trend function. The most general form is known as universal Kriging, where the trend function is specified by $\mu(\mathbf{x}) = \mathbf{f}(\mathbf{x})^T \beta$, i.e., as a regression model. Here, the function vector $\mathbf{f}$ is fixed, and the parameter vector β needs to be estimated. The ordinary Kriging approach defines a slightly simpler model, which has an unknown but constant trend, i.e., $\mu(\mathbf{x}) = \mu$. The covariance matrix of the Gaussian process $Z(\mathbf{x})$ is given by

$$Cov(Z(\mathbf{x_i}), Z(\mathbf{x_j})) = \sigma^2 R(\mathbf{x_i}, \mathbf{x_j}), \tag{11.2}$$

where $R(\mathbf{x_i}, \mathbf{x_j}) = Corr(Z(\mathbf{x_i}), Z(\mathbf{x_j}))$ is a given correlation function, scaled by the process variance σ^2 and $\mathbf{x_i}, \mathbf{x_j} \in D_n$. Most of the time, it is assumed that the stochastic process is stationary, i.e., $R(\mathbf{x_i}, \mathbf{x_j}) = R(\mathbf{x_i} - \mathbf{x_j}) = R(\mathbf{h})$. Among many possible correlation functions (see [11]), the Matérn class is of great importance and is given by

$$R(h) = \frac{2^{1-\nu}}{\Gamma(\nu)} \left(\frac{\sqrt{2\nu h}}{\theta} \right)^{\nu} K_{\nu} \left(\frac{\sqrt{2\nu h}}{\theta} \right), \tag{11.3}$$

where Γ is the gamma function, K_ν is a modified Bessel function, $h = |x_i - x_j|$, and ν, θ are positive parameters. The sample paths of a GP with the Matérn correlation function are $\lfloor \nu - 1 \rfloor$ times differentiable. Note, that, in general, the product correlation rule is used for multivariate input variables in computer experiments, i.e., $R(\mathbf{x_i}, \mathbf{x_j}) = \prod_{k=1}^{s} R_j(x_{ik} - x_{jk})$, see [3]. Usually, the parameters β, σ^2, ν, and θ are unknown and hence need to be estimated, e.g., by maximum likelihood estimation (MLE); see [5] for further details. When the parameters are specified, the model can be used to make predictions $Y(\mathbf{x_0})$ at untried points $\mathbf{x_0} \notin D_n$. Let $\mathbf{x_1}, \ldots, \mathbf{x_n} \in D_n$ be the set of design points and $\mathbf{y_D} = (y(\mathbf{x_1}), \ldots, y(\mathbf{x_n}))^T$ the corresponding data, then a linear predictor of $y(\mathbf{x_0})$ is given by

$$\hat{Y}(\mathbf{x_0}) = \lambda^T(\mathbf{x_0})\mathbf{y_D}. \tag{11.4}$$

Among all linear predictors, the best linear unbiased predictor (BLUP) is a common choice for prediction at untried points. This predictor minimizes the mean squared error (MSE)

$$\text{MSE}\left(\hat{Y}(\mathbf{x_0})\right) = \mathbb{E}\left(\lambda^T\mathbf{y_D} - \hat{Y}(\mathbf{x_0})\right)^2, \tag{11.5}$$

with respect to λ under the unbiased-constraint

$$\mathbb{E}\left(\lambda^T\mathbf{Y_D}\right) = \mathbb{E}\left(Y(\mathbf{x_0})\right). \tag{11.6}$$

Solving this optimization problem defines the BLUP as

$$\hat{Y}(\mathbf{x_0}) = \mathbf{f}^T\hat{\beta} + \mathbf{k}K_D^{-1}(\mathbf{y_D} - F\hat{\beta}), \tag{11.7}$$

where $\mathbf{f} = (f_1(\mathbf{x_0}), \ldots, f_k(\mathbf{x_0}))^T$, $K_D = \sigma^2 R_D$, $\mathbf{k} = (R(\mathbf{x_1}, \mathbf{x_0}), \ldots, R(\mathbf{x_n}, \mathbf{x_0}))$, $\hat{\beta}$ is the least squares estimator of β and F the design matrix, [13].

11.3.2 The Curse of Stationarity

A lot of research has been done concerning GPs and complex computer code modeling with a lot of examples and case studies where this approach was successfully demonstrated; see, e.g., [3]. Nevertheless, it has also been shown that especially the strong assumption of stationarity of the process can lead to problems, as many physical models exhibit a clear non-stationary behavior. To deal with this problem, non-stationary correlation functions can be used; see [10]; however, fitting fully non-stationary models quickly becomes difficult and computationally intractable. Another approach uses treed Gaussian process models (TGP); see, e.g., [6]. Here, the main idea is to divide the parameter space by making binary splits on single variables, i.e., a tree partition and fitting an independent GP model in each leaf; see Fig. 11.2.

This method has the advantage of a comparatively simple modeling of non-stationarity and an easier covariance matrix inversion as a result of data reduction in each leaf. It is also more likely that the trend functions in each leaf can be assumed to be simple functions or even just constants without losing information, making parameter estimation easier and reducing the risk of over-fitting. Furthermore, the partitioning yields perfect conditions for multi-core computing, which may further reduce computation time.

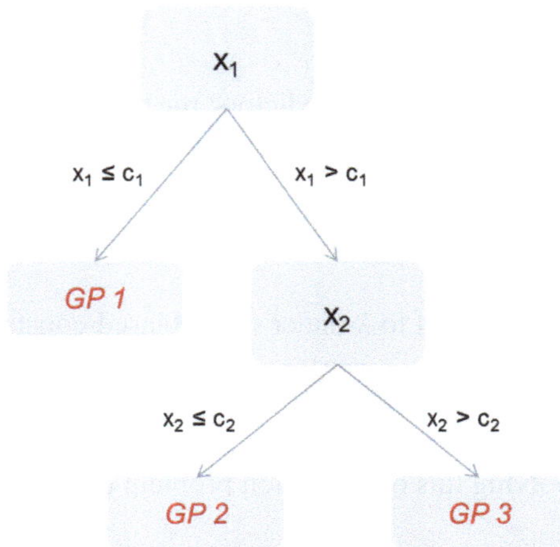

Fig. 11.2 Tree partitioning: division of the input space by binary splits. The two splits result in three leafs, i.e., three data sets—for *GP1*, all data points with $x_1 \leq c_1$ are used, *GP2* contains all data points with $x_1 > c_1$ and $x_2 \leq c_2$, and *GP3* includes the remaining data. An independent GP model is fitted in each of the three leafs

11.4 Case Study: Magnetic Field Shaping

In this section, different GP models are tested to describe the odd component B_x of the magnetic field along the stroke $s \in [-10, 10]$ mm of a rectangular magnet with sides 2a, 2b, and 2c aligned in x-,y-, and z-direction and a magnetization of $\mathbf{M} = (0, 0, x)$. In this first case study, the magnet volume V and side a are fixed to known, and realistic values and boundaries are given for the other parameters; see Table 11.1. The resulting GP model is then used to find the optimal values for c and x where the deviation of B_x along the stroke from a linear function with a slope of one millitesla per millimeter is minimal.

A CL_2-optimal latin hypercube design (see [5]) with $n = 50$ points for the parameters c and x with respective ten regularly spaced points along the stroke s is used to generate the data, a total of 500 points (c,x,s), of the final design. It is important to notice that the FEM simulation environment would always model the magnetic field along the entire stroke providing an arbitrary number of sample points for s and thus limiting the number of evaluations only for the parameters c and x. Without loss of generality, the data is generated using an analytical description of the magnetic

Table 11.1 Assumptions and constraints for the involved parameters

Parameter	Constraints
Δ	5 mm
V	500 mm^3
a	12 mm
b	$\frac{V}{8ac}$ mm
c	[0.1, 50] mm
x	[100, 1000] mT
s	[−10, 10] mm

field for ideal permanent magnets for testing the validity of the GP model, see [2]. A constant trend function and Matérn correlation function with $\nu = \frac{3}{2}$ are assumed for the GP models, and the DIviding RECTangles (DIRECT) algorithm is used for global optimization; see [7, 8]. The algorithms are implemented in R, making use of the packages `DiceKriging`, `DiceDesign`, `nloptr` ([4, 7, 12]).

It is known that for the parameter c, the stationarity assumption does not hold. For small values of c, the magnetic field varies strongly, while it is quite flat for larger values; see Fig. 11.3. Therefore, several GP models are investigated based on different splits for c and compared due to their ability to obtain the optimal values for c and x, which can be determined from the analytical model to be $c = 10.264815$ and $x = 997.9207$. The results are summarized in Table 11.2 and represented graphically in Fig. 11.4.

It can be seen from Table 11.2 and Fig. 11.4 that the TGP approach can really yield improvements and give an almost perfect fit despite the stationarity assumption, especially when using two splits on c. However, solutions can also get worse by bad splitting, where especially the last and extreme case in Table 11.2, i.e., when the border is drawn almost directly at the optimal value, emphasizes one of the major

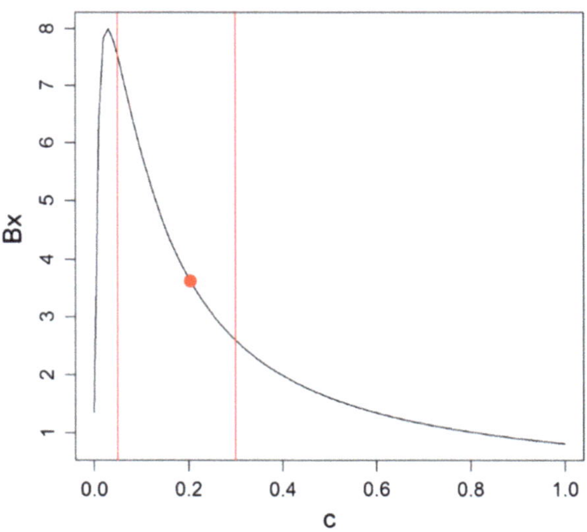

Fig. 11.3 Influence of the parameter c on the magnetic field B_x. The red point refers to the optimal value for c based on optimization of the analytical function, and the two red lines divide c into the parts used in the trees. The x-axis refers to the interval [0.1, 50] mapped onto [0, 1]

Table 11.2 Different GP models, based on the splits defined by *c border* and the related optimized parameter values

c border	c value	x value
none	9.443181	977.7832
15.07	9.614540	970.3704
$2.595 \wedge 15.07$	10.196923	996.9839
$10.264 \approx c_{opt}$	8.416667	845.2808

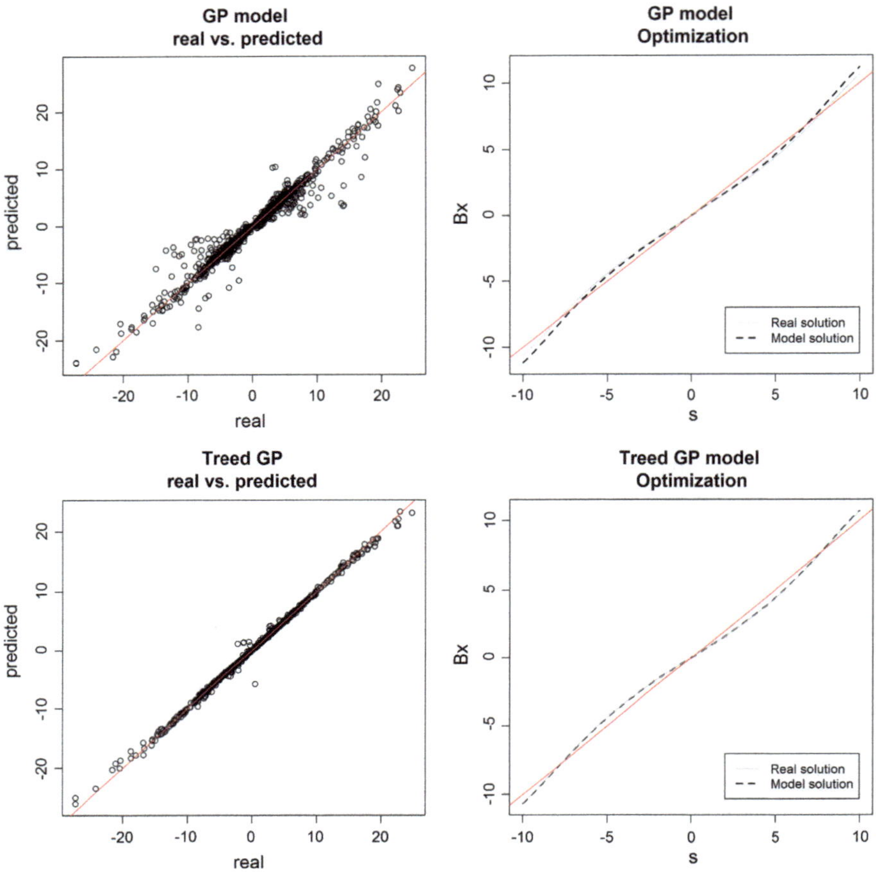

Fig. 11.4 The left-hand figures show real versus predicted outputs for 5000 arbitrary parameter combinations. The right-hand figures show the optimization solution based on the analytical equation and the models. The dashed line refers to the solution where the parameters obtained by the model with two splits are inserted into the analytical equation and the red line refers to a line with slope one in all pictures

drawbacks of treed structures. In this case, the estimated optimal values for c and x are far from being an acceptable solution. The reason for this lies in inaccuracies near the borders that occur due to the natural behavior of treed processes: at the border two processes, with probably completely different structures, melt together. This means that unless there is an sample point directly at the border, the two processes may not even meet at the same point leading to discontinuities. Assuming that there are enough border sample points, there remains the problem that differentiability of the process at the border will be never guaranteed, but rather very unlikely; see Fig. 11.5. However, the assumption of differentiability is crucial for many physical systems and hence should be also held in belonging models.

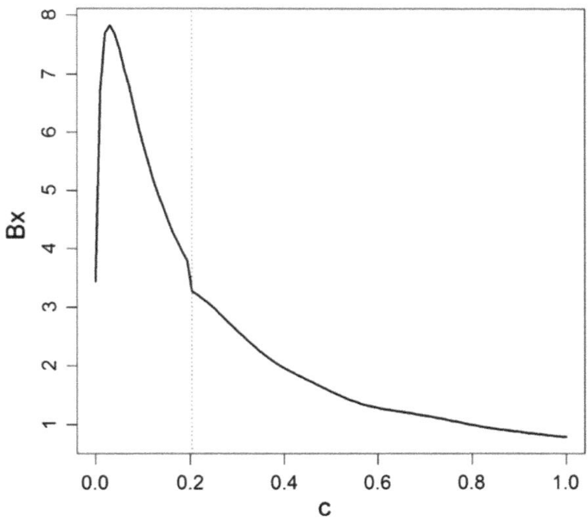

Fig. 11.5 It is shown how the magnetic field B_x changes along the parameter c. The red dotted line refers to the border which at the same time is the solution for the optimal c. The processes do melt together at the same point because there is a sample point directly at the border, however, the undesirable bend, and hence non-differentiability, is obvious

11.5 Conclusion and Outlook

It has been shown that treed Gaussian process models can be a powerful tool for the design of computer experiments, but great care must be taken with respect to the partitioning of the tree. Especially, predictions near borders can exhibit large errors and bad functional attributes. For optimization, it is crucial to grant good fitting of the GP model, especially near the optimum. However, it can never be guaranteed that the optimum is not located near or even directly at a border. Thus, actual research is strongly concerned with the construction of border processes that yield at least once continuously differentiable borders. Furthermore, also systematic and reasonable partitioning is currently under investigation, which should be achieved using an adapted genetic algorithm. From a physical point of view, more complex compound magnets with considerably more parameters will be implemented based on realistic, noisy FEM data to improve real-world magnetic linear position detection systems moving beyond the analytic description.

Acknowledgements This work is part of the Competence Centre ASSIC, which is funded within the R&D Program COMET - Competence Centers for Excellent Technologies by the Federal Ministries of Transport, Innovation and Technology (BMVIT), of Economics and Labor (BMWA). The funding program is managed on their behalf by the Austrian Research Promotion Agency (FFG), the Austrian provinces Carinthia and Styria provide additional funding.

References

1. Bursztyn, D., Steinberg, D.M.: Comparison of designs for computer experiments. J. Stat. Plan. Inference **136**, 1103–1119 (2006)
2. Camacho, J.M., Sosa, V.: Alternative method to calculate the magnetic field of permanent magnets with azimuthal symmetry. Revista Mexicana de Fisica E **59**, 8–17 (2013)
3. Currin, C., Mitchell, T.J., Morris, M.D., Ylvisaker, D.: Bayesian prediction of deterministic functions, with applications to the design and analysis of computer experments. J. Am. Stat. Assoc. **86**, 953–963 (1991)
4. Dupuy, D., Helbert, C., Franco, J.: Dicedesign and diceeval: two r packages for design and analysis of computer experiments. J. Stat. Softw. **65**(11), 1–38 (2015)
5. Fang, K.-T. Li, R. Sudjianto A.: *Design and Modeling for Computer Experiments*. Chapman & Hall/CRC (2006)
6. Gramacy, R.B., Lee, H.K.H.: Bayesian treed gaussian process models with an application to computer modeling. J. Am. Stat. Assoc. **103**, 1119–1130 (2008)
7. Johnson, S.G.: The nlopt nonlinear-optimization package. http://ab-initio.mit.edu/nlop (2008). Accessed 25 Nov 2015
8. Jones, D.R., Perttunen, C.D., Stuckman, B.E.: Lipschitzian optimization without the lipschitz constant. J. Optim. Theory Appl. **79**, 157–181 (1993)
9. Ortner, M.: Improving magnetic linear position measurement by field shaping. In: Conference proceedings - The 9th International Conference on Sensing Technology, Auckland, New Zealand, Dec. 8–Dec. 10 2015
10. Paciorek, C.J.: *Nonstationary Gaussian Processes for Regression and Spatial Modelling*. Ph.D thesis, Carnegie Mellon University (2003)
11. Rasmussen, C.E., Williams, C.K.I.: *Gaussian Processes for Machine Learning*. The MIT Press (2006)
12. Roustant, O., Ginsbourger, D., Deville, Y.: Dicekriging, diceoptim: two r packages for the analysis of computer experiments by kriging-based metamodeling and optimization. J. Stat. Softw. **51**(1), 1–55 (2012)
13. Sacks, J., Welch, W.J., Mitchell, T.J., Wynn, H.P.: Design and analysis of computer experiments. Stat. Sci. **4**, 409–435 (1989)
14. Santner, T.J., Williams, B.J., Notz, W.I.: Des. Anal. Comput. Exp. Springer, New York (2003)
15. Simpson, T.W., Lin, D.K.J., Chen, W.: Sampling strategies for computer experiments: design and analysis. Int. J. Reliab. Appl. **2**, 209–240 (2001)
16. Treutler, C.P.O.: Magnetic sensors for automotive applications. Sens. Actuators A **91**, 2–6 (2001)

Chapter 12
Insurance Models Under Incomplete Information

Ekaterina Bulinskaya and Julia Gusak

Abstract The aim of the chapter is optimization of insurance company performance under incomplete information. To this end, we consider the periodic-review model with capital injections and reinsurance studied by the authors in their previous paper for the case of known claim distribution. We investigate the stability of the one-step and multi-step model in terms of the Kantorovich metric. These results are used for obtaining almost optimal policies based on the empirical distributions of underlying processes.

Keywords Incomplete information · Periodic-review insurance model
Reinsurance · Capital injections · Optimization · Stability

12.1 Introduction

The primary goal of any insurer is redistribution of risks and indemnification of policyholders. This explains the popularity of reliability approach in actuarial sciences, that is, thorough analysis of ruin probability. Being a corporation insurance company has a secondary but very important goal, namely dividends payment to the shareholders. So, the alternative cost approach was started by De Finetti in 1957 (see [9]).

Thus, there arose the new research directions in actuarial sciences specific for modern period. They include, along with dividends payments (see, e.g., [1, 2, 11, 15]), reinsurance and investment problems (see, e.g., [4, 8, 13]). Hence, the treatment of complex models (see, e.g., [6]) and consideration of new classes of processes, such as martingales, diffusion, Lévy processes, or generalized renewal ones (see [7]), is needed. It turned out as well that discrete-time models sometimes are more realistic since reinsurance treaties have usually one-year duration, dividends are also paid at the end of financial year (see, e.g., [17]). Several types of objective functions and various methods are used to implement the stochastic models optimization (see, e.g., [19, 22]). It is also important to mention investigation of systems asymptotic

E. Bulinskaya (✉) · J. Gusak
Lomonosov Moscow State University, Moscow, Russia
e-mail: ebulinsk@yandex.ru

J. Pilz et al. (eds.), *Statistics and Simulation*, Springer Proceedings
in Mathematics & Statistics 231, https://doi.org/10.1007/978-3-319-76035-3_12

behavior and their stability with respect to parameters fluctuation and perturbation of underlying processes (see, e.g. [3, 5, 25]). Furthermore, in practice neither the exact values of parameters nor the processes distributions are known. Thus, it is important to study the systems behavior under incomplete information. If there is no a priori information at all it may be useful to employ the empirical processes.

The chapter is organized as follows. In Sect. 12.2, we gather some auxiliary results. The results concerning convergence in distribution in L_1 are transferred to Appendix. Section 12.3 contains a brief description of the model treated in the chapter (Sect. 12.3.1). Further parts of Sect. 12.3 are devoted to stability of the model under consideration. The case of unknown claim distribution is considered in Sect. 12.4. Finally, Sect. 12.5 presents conclusion and further research directions.

12.2 Preliminary Results

To investigate stability of the model, it is necessary to evaluate the difference between the objective functions calculated for two distributions close in some metric. For this purpose, we have chosen Kantorovich or Wasserstein L_1 metric.

12.2.1 Kantorovich or Wasserstein L_1 Metric

We begin by recalling the following definition given, e.g., in [23], see also [20].

Definition 12.1 For random variables (r.v.'s) X and Y defined on some probability space $(\Omega, \mathscr{F}, P)$ and possessing finite expectations, it is possible to define their distance on the base of Kantorovich metric in the following way

$$\kappa(X, Y) = \int_{-\infty}^{+\infty} |F(t) - G(t)|dt,$$

where F and G are the distribution functions (d.f.'s) of X and Y, respectively.

This metric coincides (see, e.g., [12] or [23]) with Wasserstein L_1 metric defined as $d_1(F, G) = \inf E|X - Y|$ where infimum is taken over all jointly distributed X and Y having marginal d.f.'s F and G. It is supposed that both d.f.'s belong to $\mathscr{C}_1$ consisting of all F such that $\int_{-\infty}^{+\infty} |x|\, dF(x) < \infty$.

Lemma 12.1 *The following statements are valid.*
1. Let $F^{-1}(t) = \inf\{x : F(x) \geq t\}$, *then* $d_1(F, G) = \int_0^1 |F^{-1}(t) - G^{-1}(t)|\, dt$.
2. $(\mathscr{C}_1, d_1)$ *is a complete metric space.*
3. For a sequence $\{F_n\}_{n\geq 1}$ *from* $\mathscr{C}_1$ *one has* $d_1(F_n, F) \to 0$ *if and only if* $F_n \xrightarrow{d} F$ *and* $\int_{-\infty}^{+\infty} |x|\, dF_n(x) \to \int_{-\infty}^{+\infty} |x|\, dF(x)$, *as* $n \to \infty$. *Here* $\xrightarrow{d}$ *denotes, as usual, convergence in distribution.*

The proof can be found in [12].

We are going to use also the notion of Lipschitz function.

Definition 12.2 A function f mapping a metric space (S_1, ρ_{S_1}) into a metric space (S_2, ρ_{S_2}) is called Lipschitz if there exists a constant $C \geq 0$ such that $\rho_{S_2}\left(f(s'), f(s'')\right) \leq C\rho_{S_1}(s', s'')$ for any $s', s'' \in S_1$, here ρ_{S_1}, ρ_{S_2} denote metrics in the corresponding spaces.

Now we can formulate

Lemma 12.2 *Let X, Y be nonnegative r.v.'s possessing finite expected values and $\kappa(X, Y) = \rho$. Assume also that $g : R^+ \to R^+$ is a non-decreasing Lipschitz function. Then $\kappa(g(X), g(Y)) \leq C\rho$ where C is the Lipschitz constant.*

Proof The distribution function of the random variable $g(X)$ can be calculated in a following way

$$F_{g(X)}(t) = P\{g(X) \leq t\} = P\{X \leq g^{-1}(t)\} = F_X\left(g^{-1}(t)\right),$$

where $g^{-1}(t)$ is defined as in Lemma 12.1. Similarly, one can write $F_{g(Y)}(t) = F_Y\left(g^{-1}(t)\right)$.

Since g is a non-decreasing Lipschitz function, we get the following sequence of equalities and inequalities

$$\begin{aligned}\kappa(g(X), g(Y)) &= \int_{R^+} |F_{g(X)}(t) - F_{g(Y)}(t)|dt = \int_{g^{-1}(R^+)} |F_X(s) - F_Y(s)|dg(s) \\ &= \int_{g^{-1}(R^+)} |F_X(s) - F_Y(s)|g'(s)ds \leq C\int_{g^{-1}(R^+)} |F_X(s) - F_Y(s)|ds \\ &\leq C\int_{R^+} |F_X(s) - F_Y(s)|ds = C\rho.\end{aligned}$$

In the first line, we have used the definition of Kantorovich metric and change of variables $t = g(s)$. As usually, $g^{-1}(R^+)$ is preimage of R^+. Then the properties of Lipschitz functions are employed. □

The next result enables us to estimate the difference between infimums of two functions.

Lemma 12.3 *Let functions $f_1(z)$, $f_2(z)$ be such that $|f_1(z) - f_2(z)| < \delta$ for some $\delta > 0$ and any $z > 0$. Then $|\inf_{z>0} f_1(z) - \inf_{z>0} f_2(z)| < \delta$.*

Proof Put $M_i = \inf_{z>0} f_i(z)$, $i = 1, 2$. According to definition of infimum, for any $\varepsilon > 0$, there exists $z_1(\varepsilon)$ such that $f_1(z_1(\varepsilon)) < M_1 + \varepsilon$. Therefore, $f_2(z_1(\varepsilon)) \leq f_1(z_1(\varepsilon)) + \delta < M_1 + \varepsilon + \delta$ implying $M_2 \leq f_2(z_1(\varepsilon)) < M_1 + \varepsilon + \delta$.

Letting $\varepsilon \to 0$ one gets immediately $M_2 \leq M_1 + \delta$. In a similar way, one establishes $M_1 \leq M_2 + \delta$, thus obtaining the desired result $|M_1 - M_2| < \delta$. □

12.2.2 Distance Between Empirical Functions

First of all we would like to establish that if the difference between two d.f.'s is small in the Kantorovich metric the same is true for the corresponding empirical functions. Thus, let $\{X_i = X_i(\omega)\}_{i=1}^n$ be a sample of size n from the population of r.v.'s with d.f. F. The empirical d.f. is given by $\mathsf{F}_n(\omega, t) = n^{-1}\sum_{i=1}^n I\{X_i \le t\}$, where $\omega \in \Omega$ and $I\{A\}$ is indicator of the set A. Suppose there exists another sample $Y_1, \dots, Y_n$ from the population of random variables with distribution function, say, G. The empirical distribution function for this sample is denoted by $\mathsf{G}_n(\omega, t)$. Note that we are going to assume further on the samples to consist of independent identically distributed (i.i.d.) r.v.'s.

Proposition 12.1 *Let $\kappa(F, G) = \rho$, then $P(\kappa(\mathsf{F}_n, \mathsf{G}_n) > \rho) \to 0$ as $n \to \infty$.*

Proof Obviously, $\int_{-\infty}^{+\infty} |\mathsf{F}_n(\omega, t) - \mathsf{G}_n(\omega, t)|dt$ does not exceed

$$\int_{-\infty}^{+\infty} |\mathsf{F}_n(\omega, t) - F(t)|dt + \int_{-\infty}^{+\infty} |\mathsf{G}_n(\omega, t) - G(t)|dt + \int_{-\infty}^{+\infty} |F(t) - G(t)|dt,$$

therefore we get $P\left(\kappa(\mathsf{F}_n, \mathsf{G}_n) > \varepsilon + \rho\right)$ is less than

$$P\left(\kappa(\mathsf{F}_n, F) > \frac{\varepsilon}{2}\right) + P\left(\kappa(\mathsf{G}_n, G)|dt > \frac{\varepsilon}{2}\right) + P\left(\kappa(F, G) > \rho\right). \tag{12.1}$$

The last term in (12.1) is equal to 0, since we assumed $\rho = \int_{-\infty}^{+\infty} |F(t) - G(t)|dt$. Two first terms tend to 0 as $n \to \infty$ for any $\varepsilon > 0$ due to convergence almost surely (a.s.) of empirical function to theoretical one in Kantorovich metric (see, e.g., [10]). Thus, we get the desired result. □

Remark 12.1 Since $\kappa(\mathsf{F}_n, F)$ and $\kappa(\mathsf{G}_n, G)$ tend to zero a.s., as $n \to \infty$, the statement of Proposition 12.1 can be rewritten as follows: $\limsup_{n\to\infty} \kappa(\mathsf{F}_n, \mathsf{G}_n) \le \rho$ if $\kappa(F,\ G) \le \rho$.

12.2.3 Convergence in Distribution for a Fixed t

Suppose for simplicity that two samples are independent. For each fixed $t \in R$ the difference $\mathsf{H}_n(\omega, t) =: \mathsf{F}_n(\omega, t) - \mathsf{G}_n(\omega, t)$ is a real-valued function of the random vector $(X_1, Y_1, \dots, X_n, Y_n)$ defined on a probability space $(\Omega, \mathscr{F}, P)$, namely

$$\mathsf{H}_n(\omega, t) = \frac{1}{n}\sum_{i=1}^n I\{X_i \le t\} - \frac{1}{n}\sum_{i=1}^n I\{Y_i \le t\} = \frac{1}{n}\sum_{i=1}^n \zeta_i(t), \tag{12.2}$$

where $\zeta_i(t) = I\{X_i \le t\} - I\{Y_i \le t\},\ i = \overline{1, n}$, are i.i.d. r.v.'s. Recall that

$$E\zeta_i(t) = EI\{X_i \le t\} - EI\{Y_i \le t\} = F(t) - G(t),$$
$$\mathrm{Var}\zeta_i(t) = \mathrm{Var}I\{X_i \le t\} + \mathrm{Var}I\{Y_i \le t\} = F(t) + G(t) - (F^2(t) + G^2(t)).$$

Since $\mathrm{Var}\zeta_i(t) < \infty$, the central limit theorem for i.i.d. r.v.'s gives

$$\frac{\sum_{i=1}^{n} \zeta_i(t) - n\,(F(t) - G(t))}{\sqrt{F(t) + G(t) - (F^2(t) + G^2(t))}\sqrt{n}} \xrightarrow{d} N(0,1),$$

where $N(0,1)$ is a standard normal variable. In other words,

$$\sqrt{n}\frac{\mathsf{H}_n(\omega,t) - (F(t) - G(t))}{\sqrt{F(t) + G(t) - (F^2(t) + G^2(t))}} \xrightarrow{d} N(0,1).$$

According to properties of convergence in distribution, we get immediately the following result.

Proposition 12.2 *For any $t \in R$*

$$\sqrt{n}\,|\mathsf{H}_n(\omega,t) - (F(t) - G(t))| \xrightarrow{d} \sqrt{F(t) + G(t) - (F^2(t) + G^2(t))}|N(0,1)|.$$

12.3 Stability of Insurance Model

We are going to study the stability of the periodic-review model of insurance company performance with capital injections and reinsurance introduced in [8].

12.3.1 Model Description

Let u be the initial surplus of insurance company. It is supposed that the surplus at the beginning of each period has to be maintained above some level $a > 0$. Denote by ξ_n the aggregate claim during the nth period. The sequence $\{\xi_n\}$ is assumed to consist of i.i.d. r.v.'s with a known d.f. F possessing a density and a finite mean γ. The company concludes at the end of each period the stop-loss reinsurance treaty. If the retention level is denoted by $z > 0$, then $c(z) = l\gamma - m\int_z^{+\infty} \overline{F}(t)\,dt$ is the insurer premium (net of reinsurance). Here we supposed that the insurer and reinsurer premiums are calculated on the base of expected value principle, and l and m are the corresponding safety coefficients. As usual $\overline{F}(t) = 1 - F(t)$.

It is necessary to choose the sequence of retention levels minimizing the total discounted injections during n periods.

One-period minimal capital injections are defined as follows

$$h_1(u) := \inf_{z>0} \mathsf{E}J(u,z), \quad \text{where} \quad J(u,z) = (\min(\xi, z) - (u-a) - c(z))^+ .$$

For the n-step model, $n \geq 1$, the company surplus $U(n)$ at time n is given by the relation

$$U(n) = \max(U(n-1) + c(z) - \min(\xi, z), a), \quad U(0) = u.$$

It was also proved in [8] that the minimal expected discounted costs $h_n(u)$ injected in company during n years satisfy the following Bellman equation

$$h_n(u) = \inf_{z>0}(\mathsf{E}J(u,z) + \alpha \mathsf{E}h_{n-1}(\max(u + c(z) - \min(\xi, z), a))), \quad h_0(u) = 0, \tag{12.3}$$

where $0 < \alpha < 1$ is the discount factor.

Put $h_n(u,z) := \mathsf{E}J(u,z) + \alpha \mathsf{E}h_{n-1}(\max(u + c(z) - \min(\xi, z), a))$ for $n \geq 1$. It was established that infimum of the function $h_n(u,z)$ is achieved for some $z > 0$ and function $h_n(u)$ determined by (12.3) is continuous in u.

12.3.2 One-Step Model

We are going to add the label X to all functions depending on ξ if $\xi \sim law(X)$. Putting $\Delta_1 := \sup_{u>a} |h_{1_X}(u) - h_{1_Y}(u)|$ we prove the following result.

Theorem 12.1 *Let X, Y be nonnegative r.v.'s possessing finite expectations, moreover, $\kappa(X,Y) = \rho$. Then*

$$\Delta_1 \leq (1 + l + m)\rho$$

where l and m are the safety loading coefficients of insurer and reinsurer premiums, respectively. Both premiums are calculated according to expected value principle and $1 < l < m$.

Proof Begin by estimating $|\mathsf{E}J_X(u,z) - \mathsf{E}J_Y(u,z)|$. Setting

$$C_X := -(u-a) - l\mathsf{E}X + m\mathsf{E}(X-z)^+, \quad C_Y := -(u-a) - l\mathsf{E}Y + m\mathsf{E}(Y-z)^+,$$

it is possible to write

$$\begin{aligned} |\mathsf{E}J_X(u,z) - \mathsf{E}J_Y(u,z)| &= |\mathsf{E}(\min(X,z) + C_X)^+ - \mathsf{E}(\min(Y,z) + C_Y)^+| \\ &\leq \underbrace{|\mathsf{E}(\min(X,z) + C_X)^+ - \mathsf{E}(\min(X,z) + C_Y)^+|}_{\delta_1(u,z)} \\ &+ \underbrace{|\mathsf{E}(\min(X,z) + C_Y)^+ - \mathsf{E}(\min(Y,z) + C_Y)^+|}_{\delta_2(u,z)}. \end{aligned}$$

Now we estimate separately $\delta_1(u,z)$ and $\delta_2(u,z)$.

$$\delta_1(u,z) \le \mathsf{E}|\,(\min(X,z)+C_X)^+ - (\min(X,z)+C_Y)^+\,| \le |C_X - C_Y| \le (l+m)\rho.$$

Applying Lemma 12.2 to r.v.'s X, Y and function $g(x) = (\min(x,z)+C_Y)^+$, we get

$$\delta_2(u,z) = |\mathsf{E}g(X) - \mathsf{E}g(Y)| = \left|\int_{R^+} \overline{F}_{g(X)}(t)dt - \int_{R^+} \overline{F}_{g(Y)}(t)dt\right|$$
$$\le \int_{R^+} |F_{g(X)}(t) - F_{g(Y)}(t)|dt = \kappa(g(X), g(Y)) \le \rho,$$

due to $g'(x) \le 1$. Hence using Lemma 12.3 and just obtained estimates for $\delta_1(u,z)$ and $\delta_2(u,z)$, it is easy to establish the desired result

$$\Delta_1 \le \sup_u |\mathsf{E}J_X(u,z) - \mathsf{E}J_Y(u,z)| \le (1+l+m)\rho.$$

□

12.3.3 Multi-step Model

Now we can prove the following result.

Lemma 12.4 *Function $h_n(u)$ defined by (12.3) is non-increasing in u.*

Proof Since $h_0(u) \equiv 0$ the statement of lemma is valid for $n = 0$. Due to the fact that $\max(u + c(z) - \min(\xi, z), a)$ is non-decreasing in u, we easily see that $h_{n-1}(\max(u + c(z) - \min(\xi, z), a))$ and its expectation are non-increasing in u if we assume $h_{n-1}(u)$ to be non-increasing. Furthermore, $J(u,z) = (\min(\xi, z) - (u - a) - c(z))^+$ does not increase in u; hence, the same is true for $\mathsf{E}J(u,z)$. Summing these results we conclude that $\mathsf{E}J(u,z) + \mathsf{E}h_{n-1}\,(\max(u + c(z) - \min(\xi, z), a))$ is non-increasing in u for any fixed z. It follows immediately that $h_n(u)$ is also non-increasing in u, as infimum in z of previous expression. So, we proved the desired result by means of mathematical induction. □

In the next lemma, we estimate the continuity modulus of function $h_n(u)$.

Lemma 12.5 *For each $n \ge 0$ and any $u \ge a$, $\Delta u \ge 0$ the following inequality is valid*

$$|h_n(u + \Delta u) - h_n(u)| \le C_n \Delta u,$$

where $C_n = (1 - \alpha^n)(1 - \alpha)^{-1}$.

Proof We use the mathematical induction and begin with $n = 0$. Since $h_0(u) \equiv 0$ it is clear that $|h_0(u + \Delta u) - h_0(u)| = 0$. Hence, one has $C_0 = 0 = (1 - \alpha^0)(1 - \alpha)^{-1}$.

Now assume that inequality $|h_{n-1}(u + \Delta u) - h_{n-1}(u)| \le C_{n-1}\Delta u$ is already established. Due to

$$|J(u+\Delta u, z) - J(u, z)|$$
$$= |\,(\min(\xi, z) - (u+\Delta u - a) - c(z))^+ - (\min(\xi, z) - (u - a) - c(z))^+\,| \le \Delta u$$

it follows immediately that $|\mathsf{E}J(u+\Delta u) - \mathsf{E}J(u, z)| \le \Delta u$.

Combining the induction assumption and obvious inequality

$$|\max(u+\Delta u + c(z) - \min(\xi, z), a) - \max(u + c(z) - \min(\xi, z), a)| \le \Delta u,$$

we get

$$|\mathsf{E}h_{n-1}(\max(u+\Delta u + c(z) - \min(\xi, z), a)) - \mathsf{E}h_{n-1}(\max(u + c(z) - \min(\xi, z), a))| \le C_{n-1}\Delta u.$$

Taking into account that $C_{n-1} = (1-\alpha^{n-1})(1-\alpha)^{-1}$ we can write

$$|h_n(u+\Delta u, z) - h_n(u, z)| \le (1+\alpha C_{n-1})\Delta u = C_n \Delta u.$$

Application of Lemma 12.3 with $f_1(z) = h_n(u+\Delta u, z)$ and $f_2(z) = h_n(u, z)$ leads us to the desired result ending the proof. □

Denote by $h_{n_X}(u)$ and $h_{n_Y}(u)$ the minimal injected capital during n years if the claim distribution coincides with $law(X)$ and $law(Y)$, respectively. Our aim is to investigate $|h_{n_X}(u) - h_{n_Y}(u)|$ under assumption $\kappa(X, Y) = \rho$. We put $\Delta_n = \sup_{u>a} |h_{n_X}(u) - h_{n_Y}(u)|$ to formulate the following result.

Theorem 12.2 *Let X, Y be nonnegative random variables having finite means and $\kappa(X, Y) = \rho$. Then*

$$\Delta_n \le \left(\sum_{i=0}^{n-1} \alpha^i C_{n-i}\right)(1+l+m)\rho,$$

here $0 < \alpha < 1$ is the discount factor, $1 < l < m$ are the safety loadings of insurer and reinsurer and C_k, $k \le n$, were defined in Lemma 12.5.

Proof We begin by estimation of $|h_{n_X}(u, z) - h_{n_Y}(u, z)|$. Since

$$(u-a) + l\mathsf{E}X - m\mathsf{E}(X-z)^+ = -C_X, \quad (u-a) + l\mathsf{E}Y - m\mathsf{E}(Y-z)^+ = -C_Y,$$

one can write

$$\max(u + c(z) - \min(X, z), a) = a - (C_X + \min(X, z))^-,$$

$$\max(u + c(z) - \min(Y, z), a) = a - (C_Y + \min(Y, z))^-,$$

where $(C_X + \min(X, z))^- = \min\{0, C_X + \min(X, z)\}$.

Hence, it is possible to get the following expression

$$|h_{n_X}(u,z) - h_{n_Y}(u,z)| \le \underbrace{|\mathsf{E}J_X(u,z) - \mathsf{E}J_Y(u,z)|}_{\delta_{1_n}(u,z)}$$
$$+\alpha \left|\mathsf{E}h_{n-1_X}\left(a-(C_X+\min(X,z))^-\right) - \mathsf{E}h_{n-1_Y}\left(a-(C_Y+\min(Y,z))^-\right)\right|.$$

The first summand in right-hand side of the last inequality is estimated in the one-step model as follows

$$\delta_{1_n}(u,z) \le (1+l+m)\rho.$$

The second summand can be bounded by the sum of three terms.

$$\begin{aligned}
&\left|\mathsf{E}h_{n-1_X}\left(a-(C_X+\min(X,z))^-\right) - \mathsf{E}h_{n-1_Y}\left(a-(C_Y+\min(Y,z))^-\right)\right| \\
&\le \underbrace{\left|\mathsf{E}h_{n-1_X}\left(a-(C_X+\min(X,z))^-\right) - \mathsf{E}h_{n-1_Y}\left(a-(C_X+\min(X,z))^-\right)\right|}_{\delta_{2_n}(u,z)} \\
&+ \underbrace{\left|\mathsf{E}h_{n-1_Y}\left(a-(C_X+\min(X,z))^-\right) - \mathsf{E}h_{n-1_Y}\left(a-(C_X+\min(Y,z))^-\right)\right|}_{\delta_{3_n}(u,z)} \\
&+ \underbrace{\left|\mathsf{E}h_{n-1_Y}\left(a-(C_X+\min(Y,z))^-\right) - \mathsf{E}h_{n-1_Y}\left(a-(C_Y+\min(Y,z))^-\right)\right|}_{\delta_{4_n}(u,z)}
\end{aligned}$$

According to definition of Δ_{n-1} for any $u \ge a$, we have $\left|h_{n-1_X}(u) - h_{n-1_Y}(u)\right| \le \Delta_{n-1}$, therefore

$$\delta_{2_n}(u,z) \le \Delta_{n-1}\int_R dF_X(t) = \Delta_{n-1}.$$

Using Lemma 12.2 for $g(x) = h_{n-1_Y}\left(a-(C_Y+\min(x,z))^-\right)$, one can write

$$\delta_{3_n}(u,z) \le C_{n-1}\rho.$$

To apply Lemma 12.2, it is necessary to verify that $g(x)$ is non-decreasing. This fact clearly follows from Lemma 12.4 due to the form of $g(x)$.

As follows from Lemma 12.5, for any $u \ge a$ one can use inequality $|h_{n-1_Y}(u+\Delta u) - h_{n-1_Y}(u)| \le C_{n-1}\Delta u$ to get

$$\delta_{4_n}(u,z) \le C_{n-1}|C_X - C_Y| \le C_{n-1}(l+m)\rho.$$

Combining the obtained results one gets

$$\begin{aligned}
|h_{n_X}(u,z) - h_{n_Y}(u,z)| &\le (1+l+m)\rho + \alpha\left(\Delta_{n-1} + C_{n-1}(1+l+m)\rho\right) \\
&= \Delta_1 + \alpha C_{n-1}\Delta_1 + \alpha\Delta_{n-1} = C_n\Delta_1 + \alpha\Delta_{n-1},
\end{aligned}$$

whence it follows

$$\Delta_n \le \sup_u |h_{n_X}(u,z) - h_{n_Y}(u,z)| \le C_n\Delta_1 + \alpha\Delta_{n-1}.$$

Since $C_1 = 1$ one gets immediately from the previous formula

$$\Delta_n \le C_n\Delta_1 + \alpha\Delta_{n-1} \le (C_n + \alpha C_{n-1})\Delta_1 + \alpha^2\Delta_{n-2}$$
$$\dots \le \sum_{i=0}^{n-2}\alpha^i C_{n-i}\Delta_1 + \alpha^{n-1}\Delta_1 = \left(\sum_{i=0}^{n-1}\alpha^i C_{n-i}\right)(1+l+m)\rho.$$

□

Remark 12.2 Letting n tend to infinity it is not difficult to establish that upper bound of Δ_n tends to $(1-\alpha)^{-2}(1+l+m)\rho$. In fact,

$$\sum_{i=0}^{n-1}\alpha^i C_{n-i} = \sum_{i=0}^{n-1}\frac{\alpha^i(1-\alpha^{n-i})}{1-\alpha} = \frac{1}{1-\alpha}\sum_{i=0}^{n-1}\alpha^i - \frac{1}{1-\alpha}n\alpha^n =$$
$$= \frac{1}{1-\alpha}\left(\frac{1-\alpha^{n-1}}{1-\alpha} - n\alpha^n\right) \to \frac{1}{(1-\alpha)^2},$$

as $n \to \infty$ and $0 < \alpha < 1$.

This result shows that the difference between the objective functions diminishes as the distance ρ between the claim distributions decreases. Thus, we have proved the stability of the model under consideration with respect to claim distribution perturbations.

The discount factor α describes the effect of reducing the value of money over time. Hence, it is natural that for α close to 1 the difference is larger than for small values of α.

12.4 Incomplete Information

Up to now, we assumed the claim distribution F per year to be known. In this case, it is possible to find the analytical solution of optimization problem. However in practice, the theoretical d.f. is usually unknown. It is understandable that for calculations the empirical d.f. F_n (n is the sample size) is taken instead of the theoretical one, since $\mathsf{F}_n(t) \to F(t)$ a.s. as $n \to \infty$.

For illustration, we formulate the result from [8] concerning one-step case and show what one can obtain if F is unknown. We need to introduce in addition to $c(z)$ defined in Sect. 12.3.1 the functions $r(z) = \int_z^{+\infty}\overline{F}(x)\,dx$, $k(z) = z + mr(z)$ and $g(z) = k(z) - l\gamma$, that is, $c(z) = l\gamma - mr(z)$ and $g(z) = z - c(z)$. Moreover, we put $z_* = F^{-1}(1 - m^{-1})$.

There exist three sets $D_1 = \{m > l > \gamma^{-1}k(z_*)\}$, $D_2 = \{\gamma^{-1}k(z_*) \geq l > \gamma^{-1}z_*\}$ and $D_3 = \{\gamma^{-1}z_* \geq l > 1\}$. It is obvious that $g(z_*) < 0$ in D_1, $g(z_*) \geq 0$ in $D_2 \cup D_3$ and $z_* - c(\infty) \geq 0$ in D_3. Put also $u_* = a + z_* - l\gamma$ and $u_1^* = a + k(z_*) - l\gamma = a + g(z_*)$. Moreover, it was established that inequalities $a > u_1^*$, $u_* < a \leq u_1^*$ and $a \leq u_*$ are equivalent to the relations $(l, m) \in D_1$, $(l, m) \in D_2$ and $(l, m) \in D_3$, respectively.

Recall that the optimal policy depends on system parameters l and m as follows.

Theorem 12.3 ([8]) 1. *If $(l, m) \in D_1$, then $h_1(u) = 0$ for all $u \geq a$. The optimal retention level $z_1(u) = z_*$.*
2. *If $(l, m) \in D_2$, then $h_1(u) = 0$ for $u \geq u_1^*$. The optimal retention level $z_1(u) = z_*$. For $u \in [a, u_1^*)$, the function $z_1(u)$ is the unique solution, for a fixed u, of the equation $u - a + c(z) = z_*$.*
3. *If $(l, m) \in D_3$, then for $u > u_*$ the results coincide with those of part 2, whereas for $u \in [a, u_*]$ it is optimal to use no reinsurance, that is, to take $z_1(u) = \infty$.*

We have reproduced only parts of Theorems 1, 2, and 3 proved in [8] pertaining to our investigation.

Denote by $z_*(n)$, $u_*(n)$, $u_1^*(n)$, and $\gamma(n)$ parameters z_*, u_*, u_1^*, and γ calculated using the empirical d.f. F_n instead of theoretical one.

Corollary 12.1 *For fixed a, l, and m the following relations take place a.s., as $n \to \infty$,*

$$z_*(n) \to z_*, \quad u_*(n) \to u_*, \quad u_1^*(n) \to u_1^*.$$

Proof It is well known that convergence in distribution is equivalent to convergence in quantile. That is, if $F_n \xrightarrow{d} F$, then $F_n^{-1} \xrightarrow{d} F^{-1}$ (quantiles converge in the continuity points of the limit function $F^{-1}(t)$, $0 < t < 1$), see [23]. Moreover, as follows from part 3 of Lemma 12.1, convergence in Kantorovich metric implies convergence in distribution, as well as convergence of expected values, and vice versa. If we take $F_n = \mathsf{F}_n$, then, according to [23], $d_1(\mathsf{F}_n, F) \to 0$ a.s., as $n \to \infty$. Hence, it is clear immediately that $z_*(n) = \mathsf{F}_n^{-1}(1 - m^{-1}) \to F^{-1}(1 - m^{-1}) = z_*$ a.s., as $n \to \infty$.

Since $u_*(n) = a + z_* - l\gamma(n)$, parameters a and l are fixed, whereas $|\gamma(n) - \gamma| \leq d_1(\mathsf{F}_n, F) \to 0$ a.s., as $n \to \infty$, the second statement of corollary is also valid.

Turning to the last statement of corollary, we can write $|r(z_*(n)) - r(z_*)| \leq d_1(\mathsf{F}_n, F) + |z_*(n) - z_*|$. Hence, one easily gets

$$|u_1^*(n) - u_1^*| \leq (m + l)d_1(\mathsf{F}_n, F) + (m + 1)|z_*(n) - z_*| \to 0, \quad \text{a.s.}$$

ending the proof. □

Remark 12.3 Since $z_1(u)$ is equal either to z_* or to $c^{-1}(z_* + a - u)$ for $(l, m) \in D_1 \cup D_2$ it follows immediately from Corollary 12.1 that optimal retention level calculated using empirical d.f. converges a.s. to theoretical one, as the sample size tends to infinity. For the set D_3, there exists also the possibility of no reinsurance.

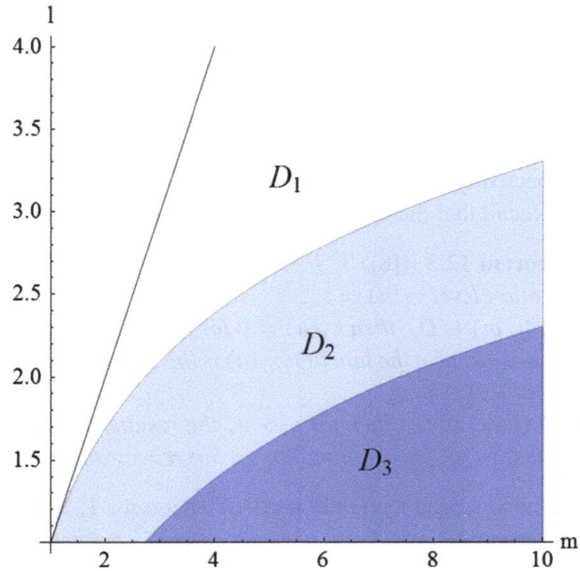

Fig. 12.1 Sets D_i for exponential distribution

The boundary between D_3 and D_2 is given by the curve $l = \varphi_1(m)$ where $\varphi_1(m) = \gamma^{-1}F^{-1}(1 - m^{-1})$, whereas the boundary between D_2 and D_1 is determined by $\varphi_2(m) = \varphi_1(m) + m\gamma^{-1}r(z_*)$. Thus, if we denote by $\varphi_i^{(n)}(m)$, $i = 1, 2$, the corresponding functions calculated on the base of empirical d.f., it is obvious that $\varphi_i^{(n)}(m) \to \varphi_i(m)$ a.s., as $n \to \infty$. So it is possible to specify entirely the "empirical" optimal policy for given parameters l, m, a, and u. Moreover, for a given initial capital u one can choose a providing zero additional costs entailed by capital injection.

The form of the sets $D_i, i = 1, 2, 3$, is depicted by Fig. 12.1 for exponential claim distribution.

It is also interesting to mention that for uniform, as well as, exponential distribution the boundaries $\varphi_i(m)$, $i = 1, 2$, do not depend on distribution parameters.

12.5 Conclusion and Further Research Directions

In this chapter, only the case of no a priori information about the claim distribution was treated for one-step model. The multi-step case is the next step. However to deal with it, we need to prove at first the existence of the so-called asymptotically optimal stationary policy. Then it will be possible to construct empirical asymptotically optimal policy, in other words, to propose a policy based on empirical distribution giving the same long-run injection cost per period as the above-mentioned stationary policy. These results will be published elsewhere. We plan also to carry out the sensitivity analysis as proposed in [18, 21, 24] for finding out the most important scalar parameters. Such analysis was already performed in [5] for two risk models.

12.6 Appendix

Here we prove some results concerning convergence in distribution in L_1 we plan to use in further investigation of two samples case.

Recall that $(X_1, Y_1), (X_2, Y_2), \ldots$ is a sequence of independent random vectors defined on a probability space $(\Omega, \mathscr{F}, P)$ taking values in R^2. Moreover, introduced in the previous Sect. 12.2.3 random variables $\zeta_i(t)$ for a fixed t can take values from the set $\{-1, 0, 1\}$. Hence, values of $\mathsf{H}_n(t, \omega)$ for a fixed n belong to the set $\{in^{-1} : i = \overline{-n, n}\}$ for any t, whereas mapping $\mathsf{H}_n(t, .) : \Omega \to R$ is measurable. Thus, the process $H_n(t, \omega)$ for a fixed n is jointly measurable in (t, ω), that is, it is $\mathscr{B}(R) \times \mathscr{F}$-measurable. As usually, $\mathscr{B}(R)$ is the Borel σ-algebra in R.

Theorem 12.4 *Let $X, X_i,\ i \in N$, be i.i.d. r.v.'s with d.f. F and let $Y, Y_i,\ i \in N$, be also i.i.d. r.v.'s but with d.f. G. Put*

$$\eta(t) := (I\{X > t\} - P(X > t)) - (I\{Y > t\} - P(Y > t)), \quad -\infty < t < \infty,$$

whereas $\eta_i,\ i \in N$, are the processes obtained by substitution of X_i instead of X and Y_i instead of Y in the last expression. Then

(a) The processes $\sum_{i=1}^n \eta_i/\sqrt{n} = \sqrt{n}(\mathsf{F}_n - \mathsf{G}_n - (F - G))$ converge in distribution in $L_1(R)$ to the process $B_1(F(t)) + B_2(G(t)),\ t \in R$, where B_1 and B_2 are two independent Brownian bridges, if and only if

$$\int_{-\infty}^{+\infty} \sqrt{F(t)(1 - F(t)) + G(t)(1 - G(t))}\, dt < \infty. \tag{12.4}$$

(b) (1) If the condition (12.4) is valid the sequence

$$\left\|\sum_{i=1}^{n} \eta_i/\sqrt{n}\right\|_{L_1} = \sqrt{n} \int_{-\infty}^{+\infty} |\mathsf{F}_n(\omega, t) - \mathsf{G}_n(\omega, t) - (F(t) - G(t))|\, dt, \quad n \in N,$$

is stochastically bounded.

(2) If the sequence $\left\|\sum_{i=1}^n \eta_i/\sqrt{n}\right\|_{L_1}$ is stochastically bounded, then

$$\sup_n E \left\|\sum_{i=1}^{n} (I\{\eta_i > t\} - P(\eta_i > t))/\sqrt{n}\right\|_{L_1} < \infty.$$

Proof According to [14] for any random element $\eta(t)$ from $L_1(R)$ such that $\int ||\eta||_{L_1} dP_\eta < \infty$ and $\int \eta dP_\eta = 0$ condition $\int_{-\infty}^{+\infty} \sqrt{E(\eta(t))^2} dt < \infty$ is equivalent to weak convergence of the measures generated by $\sum_{i=1}^{n} \eta_i(t)/\sqrt{n}$ to a Gaussian measure on $L_1(R)$. First, we show that this condition has the form (12.4) in our case.

Putting $\tilde{X}(t) = I\{X > t\} - P(X > t)$, $\tilde{Y}(t) = I\{Y > t\} - P(Y > t)$, for $s, t \in R$, we have, due to independence of X and Y combined with $E\tilde{X}(t) = E\tilde{Y}(t) = 0$,

$$\begin{aligned} cov(\eta(s), \eta(t)) &= E(\tilde{X}(s) - \tilde{Y}(s))(\tilde{X}(t) - \tilde{Y}(t)) = E\tilde{X}(s)\tilde{X}(t) + E\tilde{Y}(s)\tilde{Y}(t) \\ &= \min(F(t), F(s)) - F(t)F(s) + \min(G(t), G(s)) - G(t)G(s). \end{aligned}$$

Hence, according to the central limit theorem for R^k, $k \in N$, one has

$$(\eta(t_1), \ \ldots, \ \eta(t_k)) \xrightarrow{d} (B_1(F(t_1)) + B_2(G(t_1)), \ \ldots, \ B_1(F(t_k)) + B_2(G(t_k)))$$

for any sequence $t_1, \ldots, t_k$ with $t_i \in R$, $i = \overline{1, k}$. Using the result from [16], we see that processes $\sum_{i=1}^{n} \eta_i(t)/\sqrt{n}$ converge to the process $B_1(F(t)) + B_2(G(t))$ in $L_1(R)$ as $n \to \infty$. Thus paragraph (a) of the theorem and sufficiency of paragraph (b) are established.

Statement of paragraph (b2) is the immediate consequence of the proof of part (b) of Theorem 2.1 in [10]. □

References

1. Albrecher, H., Thonhauser, S.: Optimality results for dividend problems in insurance. Rev. R. Acad. Cien. Serie A. Mat. **103**(2), 295–320 (2009)
2. Avanzi, B.: Strategies for dividend distribution: a review. N. Am. Actuar. J. **13**(2), 217–251 (2009)
3. Bulinskaya, E.: Asymptotic analysis of insurance models with bank loans. In: Bozeman, J.R., Girardin, V., Skiadas, C.H. (eds.) New Perspectives on Stochastic Modeling and Data Analysis, pp. 255–270. ISAST, Athens, Greece (2014)
4. Bulinskaya, E., Gromov, A.: Asymptotic behavior of the processes describing some insurance models. Commun. Stat. Theory Methods **45**, 1778–1793 (2016)
5. Bulinskaya, E., Gusak, J.: Optimal control and sensitivity analysis for two risk models. Commun. Stat. Simul. Comput. **44**, 1–17 (2015)
6. Bulinskaya, E., Muromskaya, A.: Optimization of multi-component insurance system with dividend payments. In: Manca, R., McClean, S., Skiadas, Ch.H. (eds.) New Trends in Stochastic Modeling and Data Analysis. ISAST, Athens, Greece (2015)
7. Bulinskaya, E., Sokolova, A.: Asymptotic behaviour of stochastic storage systems. Mod. Probl. Math. Mech. **10**(3), 37–62 (2015) (in Russian)
8. Bulinskaya, E., Gusak, J., Muromskaya, A.: Discrete-time insurance model with capital injections and reinsurance. Methodol. Comput. Appl. Probab. **17**(4), 899–914 (2015)
9. De Finetti, B.: Su un'impostazione alternativa della teoria collettiva del rischio. Trans. XV-th Int. Congr. Actuar. **2**, 433–443 (1957)
10. Del Barrio, E., Giné, E., Matrán, C.: Central limit theorems for the Wasserstein distance between the empirical and the true distributions. Ann. Probab. **27**(2), 1009–1071 (1999)
11. Dickson, D.C.M., Waters, H.R.: Some optimal dividends problems. ASTIN Bulletin **34**, 49–74 (2004)

12. Dobrushin, R.L.: Prescribing a system of random variables by conditional distributions. Theory Probab. Appl. **15**(3), 458–486 (1970)
13. Eisenberg, J., Schmidli, H.: Optimal control of capital injections by reinsurance in a diffusion approximation. Blätter der DGVFM **30**, 1–13 (2009)
14. Jain, N.C.: Central limit theorems and related questions in Banah space. In: Proceedings of Symposia in Pure Mathematics, vol. 31, pp. 55–65. American Mathematical Society, Providence, RI (1977)
15. Kulenko, N., Schmidli, H.: Optimal dividend strategies in a Cramér-Lundberg model with capital injections. Insur. Math. Econ. **43**, 270–278 (2008)
16. Lawniczak, A.: The Levy-Lindeberg central limit theorem in Orlicz spaces. Proc. Amer. Math. Soc. **89**, 673–679 (1983)
17. Li, S., Lu, Y., Garrido, J.: A review of discrete-time risk models. Rev. R. Acad. Cien. Serie A. Mat. **103**(2), 321–337 (2009)
18. Oakley, J.E., O'Hagan, A.: Probabilistic sensitivity analysis of complex models: a Bayesian approach. J. R. Statist. Soc. B. **66**, Part 3, 751–769 (2004)
19. Peskir, G., Shiryaev, A.: Optimal Stopping and Free-Boundary Problems. Lectures in Mathematics ETH Zürich. Birkhäuser, Basel (2006)
20. Rachev, S.T., Klebanov, L., Stoyanov, S.V., Fabozzi, F.: The Methods of Distances in the Theory of Probability and Statistics. Springer, New York (2013)
21. Saltelli, A., Ratto, M., Andres, T., Campolongo, F., Cariboni, J., Gatelli, D., Saisana, M., Tarantola, S.: Global Sensitivity Analysis. The Primer. Wiley, New York (2008)
22. Schmidli, H.: Stochastic Control in Insurance. Springer, New York (2008)
23. Shorack, G.R., Wellner, J.A.: Empirical Processes with Application to Statistics. Wiley, New York (1986)
24. Sobol, I.M.: Sensitivity analysis for nonlinear mathematical models. Math. Model. Comput. Expt. **1**, 407–414 (1993)
25. Yang, H., Gao, W., Li, J.: Asymptotic ruin probabilities for a discrete-time risk model with dependent insurance and financial risks. Scand. Actuar. J. **1**, 1–17 (2016)

Chapter 13
Comparison and Modelling of Pension Systems

Christian Quast, Luboš Střelec, Rastislav Potocký, Jozef Kiseľák and Milan Stehlík

Abstract The purpose of this work is a comparison of pension systems of the selected countries—the pension systems and reforms of Austria, the Czech Republic, Slovakia, Sweden, Poland, and Chile will be our subjects of interest. Firstly, we focus on a short historical overview of the development and classification of pension systems in general. Consequently, the main part of this chapter deals with different scenarios, which should show whether the systems would be stable in the future. For these purposes, we developed utility in Mathematica. We tested normality of salary samples from Slovakia by robust tests for normality and computed pensions in several scenarios.

Keywords Pension systems and reforms · Modelling of pension systems
Lorenz curves · Gini coefficients · Robust testing for normality · Interest rates

C. Quast
Department of Applied Statistics, Johannes Kepler University, Linz, Austria
e-mail: qchristak@yahoo.de

L. Střelec
Department of Statistics and Operation Analysis, Mendel University in Brno,
Brno, Czech Republic
e-mail: lubos.strelec@mendelu.cz

R. Potocký
Department of Applied Mathematics and Statistics, Comenius University
in Bratislava, Bratislava, Slovak Republic
e-mail: potocky@fmph.uniba.sk

J. Kiseľák
Faculty of Science, Institute of Mathematics, P.J. Šafárik University
in Košice, Kosice, Slovakia
e-mail: jozef.kiselak@gmail.com

M. Stehlík (✉)
Linz Institute of Technology and Department of Applied Statistics,
Johannes Kepler University, Linz, Austria
e-mail: Milan.Stehlik@jku.at

J. Pilz et al. (eds.), *Statistics and Simulation*, Springer Proceedings
in Mathematics & Statistics 231, https://doi.org/10.1007/978-3-319-76035-3_13

13.1 Introduction

Pension systems are a rather new invention, in the history of humanity. In former tribal societies and high cultures (as ancient Egypt, ancient Rome, and ancient China), there was also no real need for such systems. First, the populations were rather young, not many old people in comparison with the whole population and secondly one can doubt that such systems could be established and maintained by such ancient cultures. The first care system for elderly people besides the own family was the so-called Knappschaften, which was kind of social miners insurances. The next big step toward a widespread social security and pension system was initiated by the Bismarck's social reform. As a starting point, one can refer to the so-called Kaiserliche Botschaft (of November the 17th 1881). In the following years, the German Reichstag enacted several different social laws. The law for the pension insurance, the so-called Invaliditts- und Alterssicherung 1889 (Gesetzliche Rentenversicherung = GRV), became effective on January 1, 1891.

Generally, there are three so-called pillars or tiers, which define pension systems. These pillars or tiers are used by OECD. For more you can see classification of the pension system of the analyzed countries (see Table 13.1). One must say that these two terms sometimes are used synonymously. The first tier is mandatory and redistributive. The goal of this tier is to prevent people from old-age poverty. This first tier is divided into three main types. Basic schemes pay kind of flat-rate benefits where an additional retirement income does not change the entitlement.

The aim of this chapter is to simulate the stability of pension system. For this purpose, we focus on three pension systems—Austrian, Slovakian, and Swedish pension systems. We illustrate this problem at a pay-as-you-go pillar studied by [5] and [6]. Therein, the probability of oversizing the limiting value of pillar is studied under normality (see [6] p. 241) and for the light-tailed claims (therein pp. 241–243). Reference [6] considered the Cramer–Lundberg model in the case of a homogeneous portfolio with the attention focused on ruin probability for it under both light or heavy tails. They illustrated such situation in the setup of oversizing of the limiting value

Table 13.1 Classification of the pension systems of the analyzed countries

Taxonomy of selected pension systems					
	First tier			Second tier	
	Public			Public	Private
	Resource-tested	Basic	Minimum	Type	Type
Austria				DB	
Czech Republic		Yes	Yes	DB	
Chile	Yes		Yes		DC
Poland			Yes	NDC	DC
Slovak Republic			Yes	Points	DC
Sweden			Yes	NDC	DC

of the fund for the pay-as-yo-go pillar in Slovakia (see also [5]). Reference [4] gives further consequences for insurance. We continue in research of sequence of papers [1, 7].

13.2 Comparison of Pension Systems in Analyzed Countries

13.2.1 Austrian Pension System

The Austrian pension system consists of three different pillars. The main pillar is a public pay-as-you-go system. The former “Abfertigung,” the Austrian form of the severance pay, was expanded to the “Abfertigung Neu.” It is entirely funded by the employers. In a major pension reform in the early 2000s, a voluntary pension tier was established. The so-called Geförderte Staatliche Zukunftsvorsorge systematically is a state-aided funding principle.

According to the OECD taxonomy, the Austrian pay-as-you-go system is a defined-benefit public schema. There is also a so-called income-tested top-up for low-income pensions (Ausgleichszulage). The normal pension age is 65 for men and 60 for women. However, one must say that Austria has one of the lowest real retirement age of all OECD countries. On average, the Austrians retire at 58.1 (old age and disability pension combined). A factor that will stress the Austrian pension system for many years to come is the long transition period of the harmonization of women’s pension age. Not until 2033, the retirement age of women will reach equality. The conditions to receive pension payments are the following. One has to pay 180 months of contributions within the last 30 years, or 300 months during the complete working career. There is an exception to this rule. Since 2005, it is possible to receive pension payments with only 7 years of contribution, if the remaining insurance period of 8 years can be reached, by child-raising periods.

13.2.2 Chilean Pension System

In 1980, Chile replaced its pay-as-you-go public pension system with a system of individual accounts, the Chilean model. It is based on three tiers. The first tier is a poverty prevention tier, the second is an individual accounts tier, and the third is a voluntary saving tier. Next, I will describe the tiers in more detail.

First Tier

For all people who are older than 65 years and pass means test and lived in Chile for at least 20 years, and who did not contribute to individual accounts the state pays a basic pension of 75000 pesos, about 154$ per month (wage indexed started from

2008). There is also a second form of state-paid pension, the Pension Solidarity Complement (PSC). It is paid for people who contributed to individual accounts and pass means test. The amount and the calculation of the PSC depend on the height of the pension of the individual accounts tier.

Second Tier

The second tier is the major pension tier in Chile. It is a mandatory individual accounts system. Each employee contributes 10% of his/her wage or salary earnings into individual accounts. The contribution into the system is capped up to 67.4 UF (unidades de formento, a Chilean term which is used in many purposes, including pension contributions. In 2012, one UF equals about $22.46). The employers directly forward the contribution to a so-called AFP (Administradora de Fondos de Pensiones, these are private managed pension funds). Each employee chooses his/her desired AFP. An important point in the Chilean Pension System is that the employers generally do not contribute to the individual accounts, they only have to contribute to a survivor and disability insurance for their employees, and therefore they have to pay about 1.49% of the employees wage. Concerning the AFPs, one can say that during the time the employee can switch them at any time. But have to pay a certain fee for that. There are 5 AFPs, Funds A to E, which have different levels of risk and potential return. All AFPs must adhere to the rules drawn up by the government. The pension is calculated based on the accumulated assets. Age and gender are taken into account. There is the possibility of early retirement, if the pension equals at least 80% of the Pension Solidarity Complement. The assets accumulated can be withdrawn in four different ways. Also for funeral expenses, 15 UFs are reserved from the account balance.

Third Tier

This is a voluntary system. Workers can contribute to saving products which are authorized by the Chilean government, such as voluntary savings accounts managed by AFPs, mutual funds, and other savings products. Contributors may pay up to 50 UF per month to this pension tier. There is also the possibility to transfer savings accounts to the individual accounts, to increase future monthly pension annuity. Contributors receive certain tax preferences for this kind of payments. The government also tried to encourage employers with tax incentives, to contribute to voluntary savings accounts for their employees.

13.2.3 Slovakian Pension System

Due to the fact that Slovakia was not an independent state until January 1, 1993, apart from a short period between 1939 and 1945, a historical summary makes no real sense. Since the pension reform of 2005, the Slovakian pension system consists of a reformed PAYG (Pay-as-you-go) state pension system and a funded pension system, which is divided into a mandatory personal pension tier and a voluntary pension tier.

Since the pension reform of 2005, people entering the labor market and all self-employed have to participate in the new reformed system. It consists of a social insurance public pension pillar and a funded pension pillar. People younger than 52 who already paid into the former pension system can choose if they also want to enter the mandatory private saving tier. The legal retirement age is 62 years for men and as of 2015 also for women. People gain eligibility after at least 10 years of contribution. The height of the pension benefits is calculated according to a point formula. Each contributor earns annual pension points (ratio of individual earnings to economy-wide average earnings). The sum of the pension points over the career multiplied by the pension point value is the pension entitlement. A point is worth 8.9955 Euro (2009) and indexed to average earnings. Pension payments are indexed to the arithmetic average of earnings growth and inflation.

There is no minimum pension, however a minimum pension base that is equal to the minimum wage of 295.5 Euro. In the new system, an incentive mechanism is established. The pension payments are increased by 0.5 percent for each 30-day period worked beyond retirement age. On the other hand, the pension is reduced the same percentage for each 30-day period worked less the retirement age. Nevertheless, there are three conditions necessary for receiving early retirement payments. Not before the age of 60, the fifteen-year contribution and the minimum pension have to be higher than 223.2 Euro.

13.2.4 Swedish Pension System

Sweden had one of the most generous pension systems in the world. Due to financial difficulties during the eighties, Sweden decided to overcome the former pension system, which was a combination of a flat-rate basic pension and an earnings-related, contribution-financed, defined-benefit pension system. Within only a few years, Sweden changed its pension system considerable. It is now a multi-pillar system, which in its present design is considered as one of the most stable and reliable in the world. In the following, we will describe this new system. The Swedish pension system can be divided into three different pillars. The most important part is the national pension system. It accounts for about 3/4 of the pension payments and consists of three tiers. Further, there exists an occupational pillar, which accounts for about a fifth of the payments. Finally, there is also a voluntary fund-based pillar and it accounts only for 5% of the payments.

The Swedish national pension system is based on three tiers. In the following classification, labeling starts with 0. The tier zero is a guaranteed pension. The first tier is the so-called income pension, a pension system meanly based on a pay-as-you-go scheme. The last tier of the national pension system is a fund-based premium pension (bonus-pension). For people who were born before 1938, there applies the old ATP system. For persons born between 1938 and 1953, there applies a mixture of the old and the new reformed system.

Table 13.2 Income values converted in EUR, 2000–2010

Year	Austria	Sweden	Slovakia	Czech Republic
2000	1.987,42	2.076,96	379,41	480,73
2001	2.002,92	2.177,46	410,44	522,87
2002	2.034,92	2.266,79	448,48	564,55
2003	2.064,33	2.344,95	476,83	597,50
2004	2.091,67	2.411,95	525,29	635,17
2005	2.142,00	2.467,78	573,39	667,10
2006	2.208,33	2.523,62	622,75	710,82
2007	2.288,17	2.557,12	668,72	762,13
2008	2.354,58	2.713,45	723,03	821,59
2009	2.378,08	2.802,78	744,50	848,93
2010	2.392,92	2.847,44	769,00	867,84
N	11	11	11	11
μ	2.176,85	2.471,85	576,53	679,93
σ	154,78	249,65	138,84	133,52

13.3 Dissimilarity of Income Levels

Due to the fact that incomes and wages are the basis of future pensions, we give a short overview of the different income levels of the above countries and check them according to their statistical similarity. In the following table, the income values are converted in EUR (Table 13.2).

13.4 Modeling of Pension Systems

Here, we continue in research based on [5]. This approach originally deals with the Slovakian pension system. Their fear is based on assumption that the 1st pension pillar, so-called a pay-as-you-go system, is not sufficient to cover the liabilities of the future pensioners, because the number of contributors in relation to the pensioners worsens, so this fear is comprehensible. Therein is considered a closed group of Slovakian people, all aged 50 in the year 1998, and interest is in the estimation of the total claim amount for this group in the year 2010 when the members are supposed to retire. For this purpose, they also assume a linear relationship between the salary S_t and pension P_t at time t.

Therefore, [5] is interested in estimation of the probabilities $P\left(\sum_{k=1}^{N} X_k > C\right)$, where X_i are individual monthly claims of the members of the above-mentioned group and C is a critical (limiting) value of the fund representing the amount the fund has gathered from the contributions of the active members or from other sources. It is possible to consider N as a constant or a random variable as it was treated in [5, 8]. In [6], the case that N is a random variable was considered. Then following [5], it is quite natural to choose a binomial model for N, namely $N \sim bi(n, p)$ with $n = 130000$ and p representing the probability of surviving a 50-year person from the group to the age 62 years. Note that such probabilities are regularly published by Slovak Statistical Office (see [9]). Then, one is looking for the largest C such that $P(\sum_{k=1}^{N} X_k > C) = p$ with p given in advance, e.g., 0.1 or 0.05.

Typically, it is possible to model salaries as normal variables in short terms and lognormal at long terms. In [5] is used the normal distribution which led to the following upper bound

$$\bar{p} = 1 - \Phi\left(\frac{C/(kN_t) - \mu}{\sigma}\right). \tag{13.1}$$

Here, Φ is cdf of standardized normal distribution, C is a critical level as given above, μ and σ^2 are parameters of normal distribution of salaries, $k = \frac{P_t}{S_t}$, and N_t is the number of claims.

Consequently, we will simulate the example given in the mentioned paper [5] and we will also show other settings based on estimated Austrian and Swedish numbers. For the implementation of the model, in the following designated as simply tool, we used the mathematical programming language Mathematica Version 8.0.

At the beginning, we will reconstruct the example of the paper [5]. Therefore, we need the average maximum Slovakian salaries from 1998 to 2002, which are shown in the following table (note that this data was used for testing for normality in the paper [10]):

As it is mentioned above, typically it is possible to model salaries as normal variables in short terms and lognormal at long terms. In [5] is used the normal distribution which led to the upper bound in Eq. (13.1). In the case of Table 13.3, we have $\hat{\mu} = 29396.4$ and $\hat{\sigma} = 3903.35$. Therefore, the first screenshot of the tool is shown in Figs. 13.1 and 13.2, which show the development of (13.1), given $N_t = 130000$ and $k \in (0.5, 0.67)$ and $C \in (15 * 10^6, 29 * 10^8)$.

Table 13.3 Slovakian Salaries (Slovakian Koruna), 1998–2002

Year	1998	1999	2000	2001	2002
Salary	24233	26862	30021	31825	34041

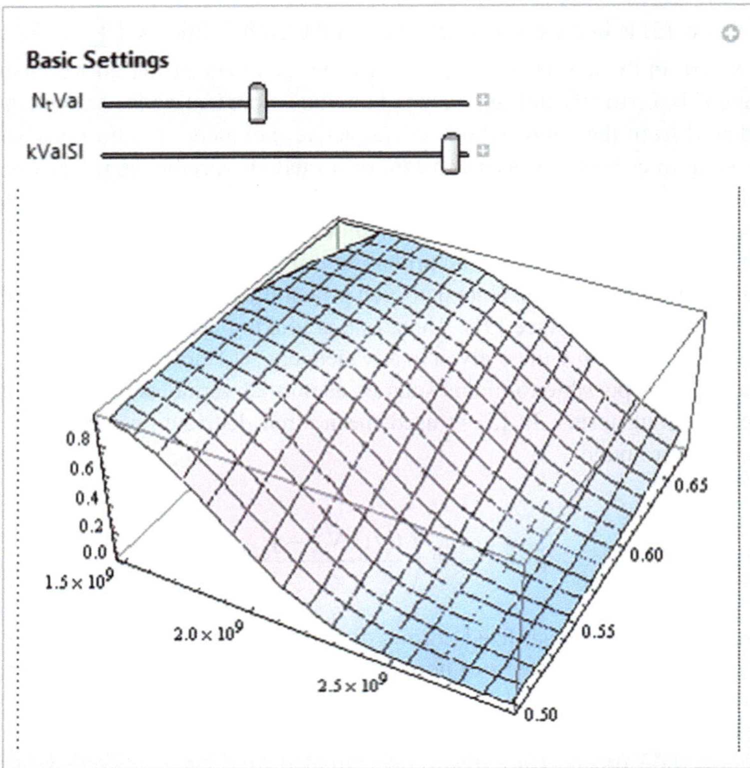

Fig. 13.1 Slovakian wages

We also implement the same model for the minimum wages (for reasons of simplification we assume $N_t = 130000$). Next, Table 13.4 presents average Slovakian minimum and maximum wages and Figs. 13.3 and 13.4 show the different development of the ruin probability when we use average Slovakian minimum and maximum wages.

From Fig. 13.4, we can see that if all Slovaks only would receive minimum average wage, there would not be any problems with future pension payments at all. The ruin probability is practically zero. On the other hand, if ever Slovak would earn the maximum average wage the ruin probabilities are very high (pink surface) many different settings.

Alternatively, we want to show the situation of Austrian incomes. In addition, the Austrian incomes we got from Statistik Austria source—see Table 13.5. As we can see from this table, the Austrian wages moved slower than the Slovakian ones. Therefore,

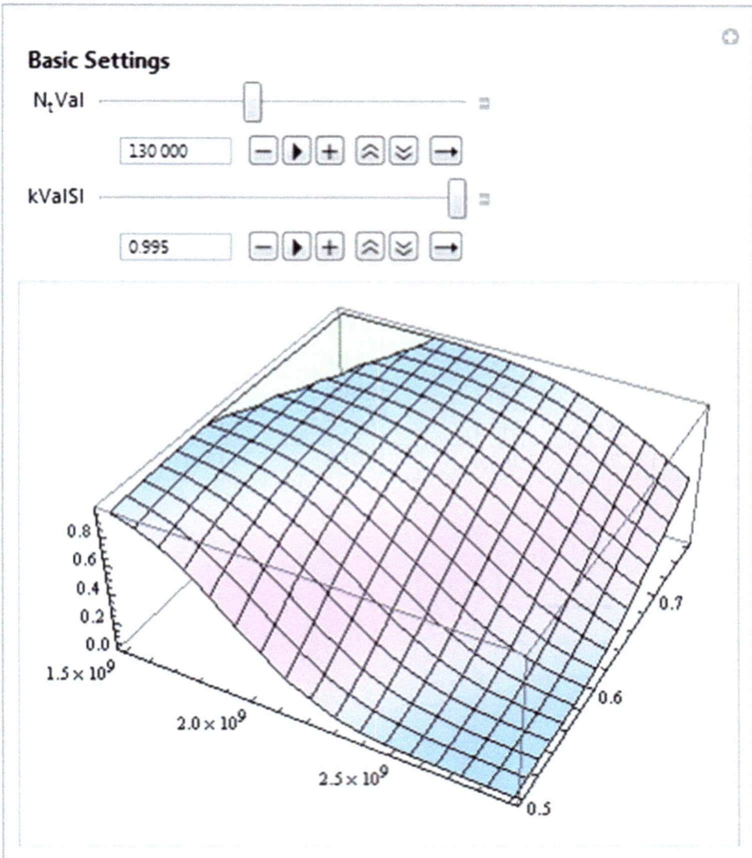

Fig. 13.2 Slovakian wages with active sliders

Fig. 13.5 shows the basic model with the Austrian situation, given the wages from Table 13.5 and the following starting settings: $N_t = 75500$ and $k \in (0.5, 0.67)$ and $C \in (10 * 10^8, 20 * 10^8)$.

Finally, we also show the development of p (ruin probability) for the Swedish incomes—data are also presented in Table 13.5. Consequently, Fig. 13.6 shows the basic model with the Swedish situation, given the wages from Table 13.5 and the following starting settings: $N_t = 124000$ and $k \in (0.5, 0.67)$ and $C \in (6 * 10^9, 3 * 10^{10})$.

Table 13.4 Monthly mean brutto salary in Slovakia (EUR), 1992–2013 [9]

Year	Max. salary group	Min. salary group	Year	Max. salary group	Min. salary group
1992	255.6	138.3	2003	1148.1	294.7
1993	329.4	152.6	2004	1315.6	314.8
1994	386.4	172.6	2005	1418.1	339.9
1995	451.2	199.2	2006	1511.6	364.9
1996	645.9	210.8	2007	1609.4	398.2
1997	827.4	187.9	2008	1705.1	431.5
1998	807.7	206.9	2009	1728.9	474.9
1999	895.4	214	2010	1790	491
2000	1000.7	226.1	2011	1835	503
2001	1060.8	242.1	2012	1923	521
2002	1134.7	284.4	2013	1934	532

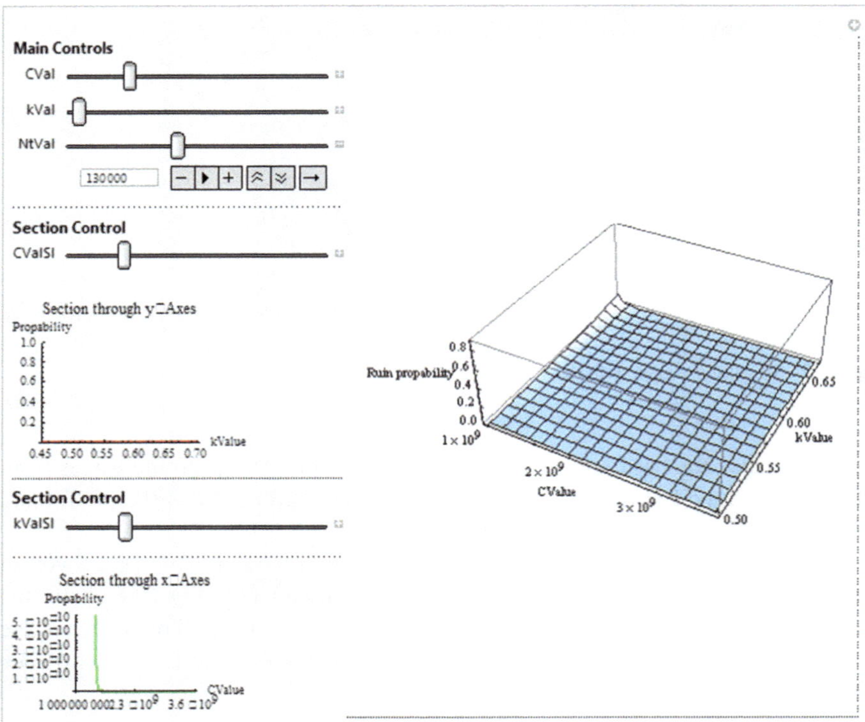

Fig. 13.3 Slovakian wages—minimum average wages 1998–2007

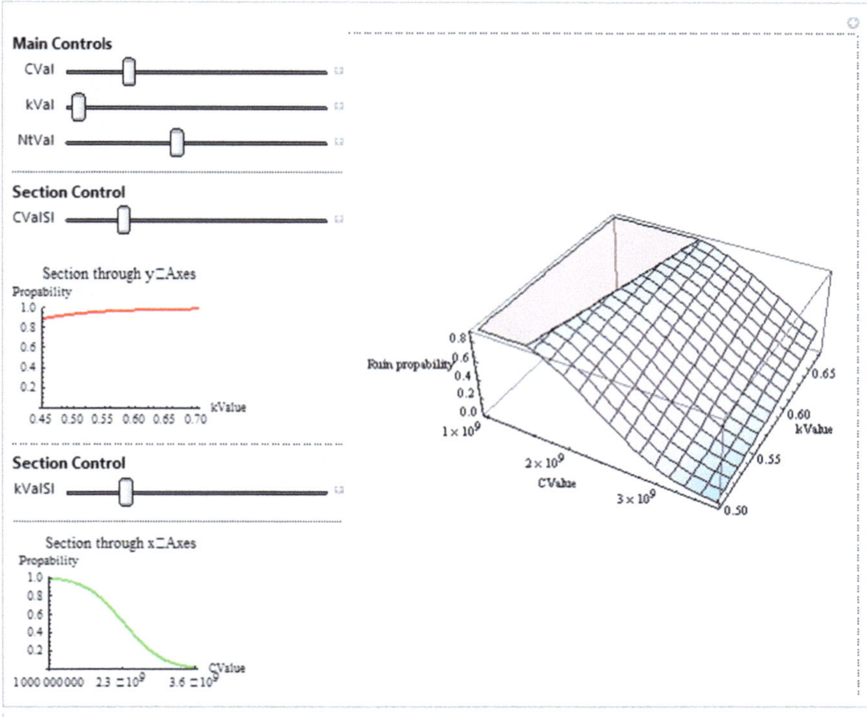

Fig. 13.4 Slovakian wages – maximum average wages 1997–2007

Table 13.5 Austrian average salaries (Euro) and Swedish average salaries (1000 Swedish krona), 1998–2007

Year	Austria	Sweden	Year	Austria	Sweden
1998	22857	182.0	2003	24772	222.7
1999	23311	190.7	2004	25100	227.9
2000	23849	200.9	2005	26500	234.7
2001	24035	210.5	2006	27458	242.0
2002	24419	217.4	2007	28262	251.9

13.5 Calculated Gini Coefficients and Lorenz Curves

This chapter concentrates on the wage distribution. Therefore, the earnings distributions of the different countries are shown. Concrete the deciles, out of this a measure for evenly distribution is calculated, namely the Gini coefficient. The Lorenz curve is linked with the Gini coefficient. These measures are calculated with the R-Package `ineq`.

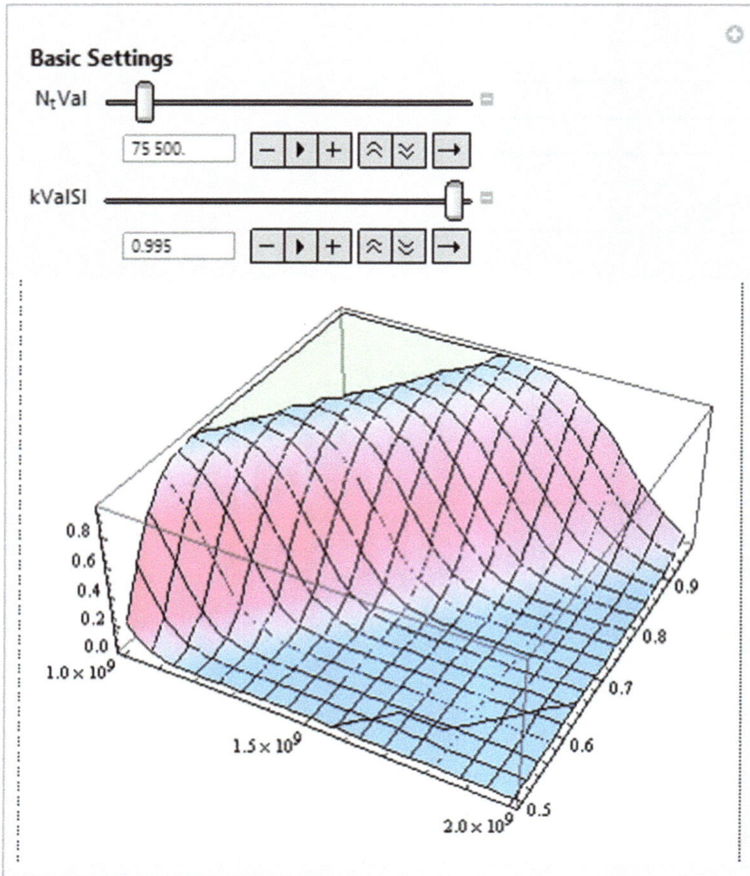

Fig. 13.5 Austrian wages

13.5.1 Calculation of Gini Coefficient

The below-mentioned table consists of the available income distribution. The data are mainly from ILO, the International Labor Organization. This leads to a more or less unified data set. Only for Sweden, there is no suitable data, so the Gini coefficient is calculated based on data from Eurostat. We considered another income distribution for Austria and form data of Statistik Austria. The reason for that is that the first decile of the Austrian income data of ILO looks unreasonably low. Also, the ratio of last and first decile (83.3) is unreasonably high. This is typically a characteristic of low-income and developing countries. In contrast to the ILO data, the data provided by Statistics Austria are based on annual wages (Table 13.6).

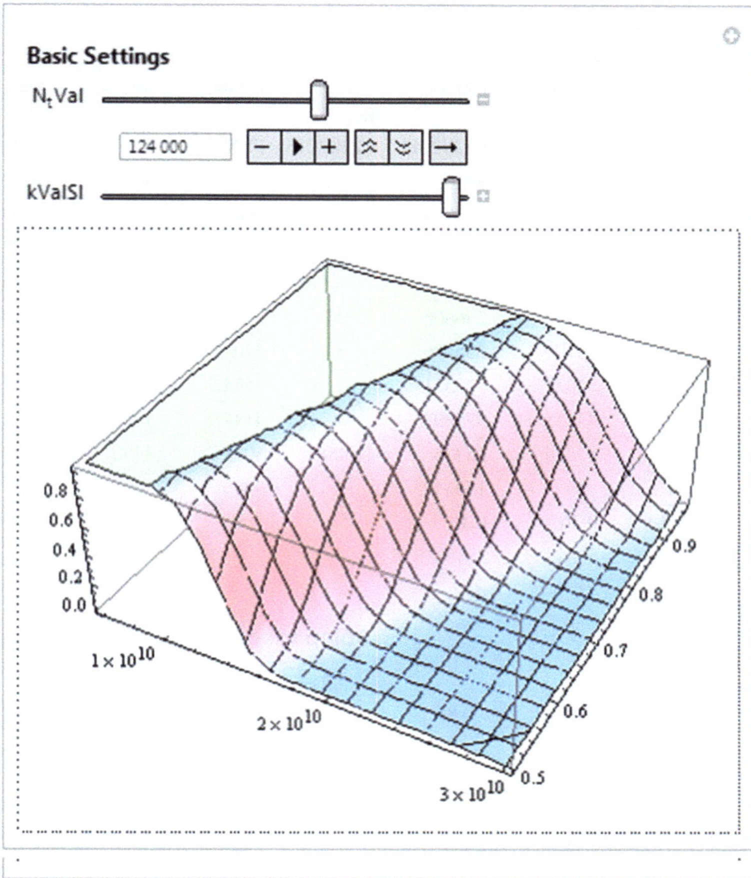

Fig. 13.6 Sweden wages

13.5.2 Lorenz Curves

In this section, Lorenz curves for all countries are shown. Therefore, Fig. 13.7 shows the Lorenz curves of all considered countries, i.e., for Austria, Chile, the Czech Republic, Poland, Slovakia, and Sweden.

13.6 Impact of Interest Rates on Pensions

Here, we study the influence of interest rates on pensions (see [13]). Generally, there are three main points that lead to low fund returns.

- High fund management fees.

Table 13.6 Countries and their mean monthly earnings of employees by decile (local currency/most recently of data) and the Gini coefficient

Decile	Austria	Austria	Chile	Czech Rep.	Poland	Slovakia	Sweden
	EUR/2011	EUR/2012	CLP/2011	CZK/2013	PLN/2010	EUR/2013	SEK/2013
Decile1	87	2400	89805	11972	1350	386	122709
Decile2	407	7309	167754		1660.5	469	155295
Decile3	920	13232	191513		2010.9	554	182202
Decile4	1412	19031	217659		2360.7	637	206667
Decile5	1854	24540	256606	22557	2719.6	718	229912
Decile6	2269	29700	305286		3104.2	815	253738
Decile7	2688	35327	375511		3564.2	934	280526
Decile8	3218	43215	475303		4144.4	1106	316268
Decile9	4079	57736	657366	41600	5073.2	1452	373978
Decile10	7247		1534495		9440.2		
Gini coefficient	0.438	0.367	0.43	0.259	0.314	0.224	0.181

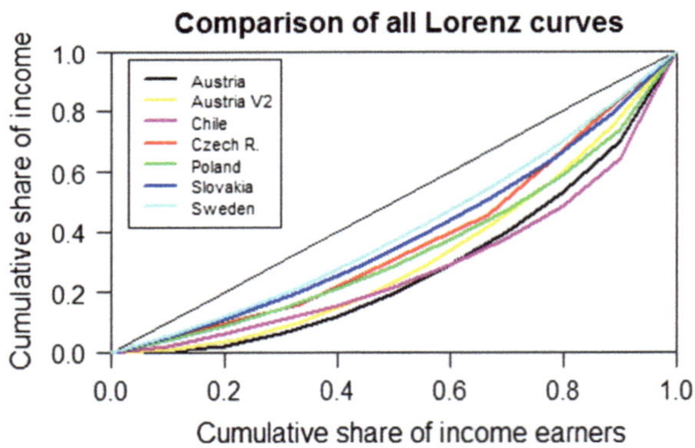

Fig. 13.7 Comparison of Lorenz curves

- Fund mismanagement.
- Lower than expected interest rates.

In [13] the following scenario based on the Slovakian data from Table 13.4 was considered. In this table the monthly mean gross salary is shown for both rich and poor males who were 45 years old in 1993 (max. and min. salary) and who invested in a fund with a certain interest rate until 2009. The authors assumed a contribution rate $u = 0.09$, and fix interest rates of $r \in \{0.005, 0.01, 0.02\}$, and additionally a non-fix interest function $r(t) = 0.05exp(-t/10)$, whereas t is the calendar year 1993.

With this parameters and the following equation of equivalence, they calculated the pension height and the replacement rate:

Table 13.7 Estimation of pension at age 62 for 45 year old male, $r(t) = 0.05exp(-t/10)$

Distribution	r	v	Pmax	Pmin
Weibull	0.005	0.27154	3056.08	842.3
$\hat{\gamma} = 0.033$	0.01	0.30135	3298.08	913.12
$\hat{\beta} = 1.548$	0.02	0.36914	3827.27	1069.53
	r(t)	0.24407	2292.01	620.108
Gamma	0.005	0.21724	3056.07	842.3
$\hat{\gamma} = 0.084$	0.01	0.2437	3298.09	913.12
$\hat{\beta} = 2.297$	0.02	0.3039	3827.27	1069.54
	r(t)	0.19283	2179.2	589.59
Logistic	0.005	0.41675	3056.08	842.3
$\hat{\mu} = 27.35$	0.01	0.46088	3298.08	913.13
$\hat{\sigma} = 9.948$	0.02	0.56116	3827.27	1069.53
	r(t)	0.37605	2331	630.657
Makeham	0.005	0.158	3855.45	1021.24
	0.01	0.1344	3310.29	872.22
	0.02	0.1193	3062.15	804.8
	r(t)	0.1085	2400.89	649.566

$$\sum_{t=1}^{17} 0.95 \times 0.09 \times X_{t+1992} \times (1 + r_t)^{17-t} {}_t p_{45} =$$

$$= \sum_{t=0}^{\infty} 0.95 \times v \times P \times (1 + r_t)^{-t} {}_t p_{62}.$$

Here, the left-hand side (LHS) and right-hand side (RHS) mean the following. LHS: Left side sums up contributions during working life (45–62). Parameter of the LHS: 0.95 is a constant which discounts the contribution by 5% (normally the fund fee). The constant $0.09 = u$ is the contribution rate, X_{t+1992} is the salary in year $t + 1992$ (see table), r_t is the interest rate in year t, and ${}_t p_{45}$ stands for the probability a person aged $x = 45$ survive the next t years. These probabilities were modeled with different distributions that generally fit mortality rates quite well.

RHS: Right side is life annuity of the surviving pensioner, v stands for replacement rate, and P is the pension.

The equation was then solved and resulted in the following results for different mortality distributions and interest rates (Table 13.7).

Out of this concrete numbers of the replacement rate and the pension height, the chapter also concluded the following. The more realistic non-fix interest rates lead to the lowest pension and replacement rate. And maybe the most important conclusion is that for the poorer males the expected pensions are too low in comparison with

Table 13.8 Expected value of pension at age 62 for 45 years old male with fixed v for two groups salary

	σ	$\mathbb{E}[P_{max}]$	Std. err.	$\mathbb{E}[P_{min}]$	Std. err.
$f(t) = 0.05\exp\left(-\frac{t}{10}\right)$	0.001	3704.093	1.303	998.555	0.353
	0.01	3786.651	13.267	1016.706	3.657
	0.05	6982.14	119.479	1966.152	35.305

Table 13.9 Expected value of pension at age 62 for 45 years old male with fixed v for two groups salary

	σ	$\mathbb{E}[P_{max}]$	Std. err.	$\mathbb{E}[P_{min}]$	Std. err.
$f(t) = 0.02 + 0.05\exp\left(-\frac{t}{10}\right)\cos t$	0.001	3287.102	1.100	851.710	0.284
	0.01	3357.465	11.183	871.762	2.929
	0.05	6087.512	106.88	1570.891	27.392

minimal pension of 250 Euros guaranteed in the first pension pillar. So consequently they should rather stay in the 1st pension pillar (see [13]).

13.6.1 Computation of Pension Under Stochastic Interest Rates: An Example

Now consider that paths of interest rate are given by the process

$$r_t = f(t) + \sigma\, W_t,$$

where $f \in C[t_0, \infty)$ (Figs. 13.8 and 13.9).

Obviously, r_t is normally distributed with $\mathbb{E}[r_t] = f(t)$ and $\mathrm{Var}[r_t] = \sigma^2 t$. The number of replications was 10^4 (Tables 13.8 and 13.9).

13.7 Testing for Normality – RT Class Tests

The general RT class is based on robustification of the classical Jarque-Bera test. The general RT class test statistic is defined by [11] for the purpose of robust testing for normality against Pareto tails and more analyzed in [12].

For the example purposes, we consider some classical non-robust tests of normality with higher power against the broad scale of alternative distributions—the

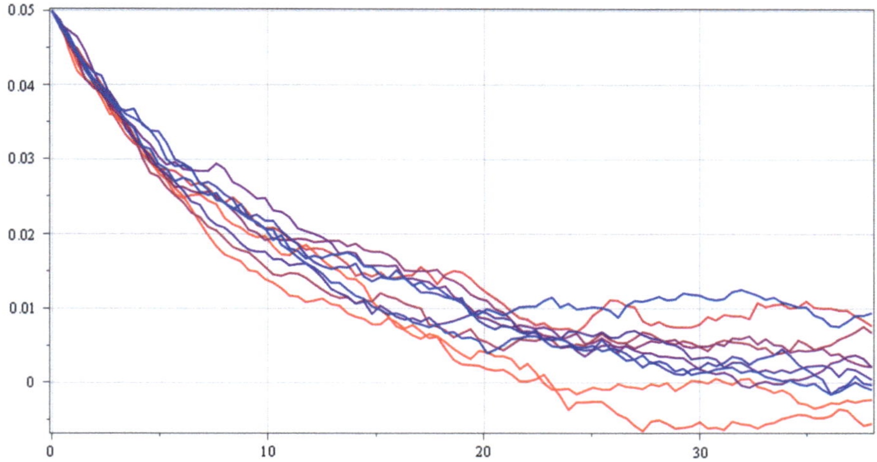

Fig. 13.8 Ten paths of r_t with monotonic expectation

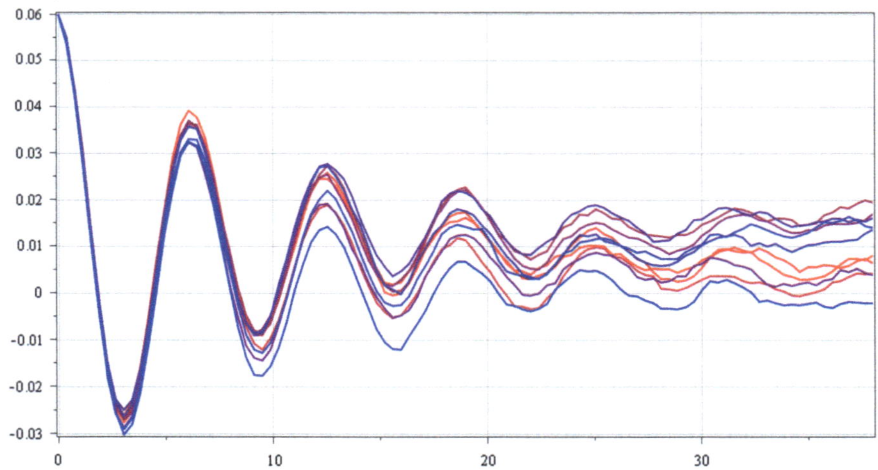

Fig. 13.9 Ten paths of r_t with oscillatory expectation

Shapiro–Wilk test (SW) as the most popular omnibus test of normality for a general use, the Jarque-Bera test (JB) as the most widely adopted omnibus test of normality in finance and related fields, and the Anderson-Darling test (AD) and the Lilliefors test (LT) as the most famous tests of normality based on the empirical distribution function – accompanied with several new tests for normality based on robust characteristics, in particular, the medcouple test (MC-LR) introduced by [2], the robust Jarque-Bera test (RJB) introduced by [3], and the selected robust tests from the RT class, namely MMRT1, MMRT2, TTRT1 and TTRT2 – for more details of these RT class tests see [12]. We also suppose the data set of max. and min. salary group for Slovakia presented in Table 13.4.

Table 13.10 Test statistics and p values of analyzed normality tests for Slovakian data of max. and min. salary group

	Max. salary		Min. salary	
	Statistic	p-value	Statistic	p-value
AD	0.333	0.487	0.708	0.055
JB	1.248	0.303	1.955	0.135
LT	0.119	0.630	0.160	0.191
RJB	1.024	0.354	1.320	0.256
SW	0.945	0.305	0.897	0.038
MC_{LR}	1.198	0.591	5.525	0.039
$MMRT1$	1.118	0.417	2.642	0.119
$MMRT2$	1.137	0.421	2.836	0.092
$TTRT1$	2.367	0.427	4.874	0.200
$TTRT2$	1.013	0.504	2.014	0.258

Based on results presented in Table 13.10, we can conclude that the hypothesis of normality of analyzed data sets is not rejected by the majority of tests for normality, at 5% significance level. Only Shapiro–Wilk test rejects the hypothesis of normality in the case of minimum salary data, at 5% significance level. We can also see higher robustness of the TTRT1, TTRT2, MC-LR, and RJB tests in comparison with the classical normality tests such as the classical Jarque-Bera test, Shapiro-Wilk test, etc.

13.8 Summary

As conclusion, we can say that there are a few basic pension system concepts, which are combined in different ways. Consequently, each pension system of the three countries is unique. From our simulation study, we can see that in the future each country would face difficulties financing their pension system, because of the rising of the old dependency rate.

For proper pension system management, one should at least use two different approaches. Namely, ruin probability and a kind of income distribution measure, and their suitable data representation (curves, indices) ROC-shaped curves have similarities to probability distribution of the ruin, so we can use the indices of the ROC curve on it. For the income distribution point of view, we used the Lorenz curves and Gini coefficients.

In a society, a certain level of financial balancing is wishful. Therefore and because of the 80:20 rule ($\sim$20% of fund owners, hold $\sim$80% of the fund assets), the wealthy should invest in private pension fund. The so generated taxes could be redistributed to the poorer in the pension system.

Acknowledgements Luboš Střelec was supported by the grant No. GA16-07089S of the Czech Science Foundation. Milan Stehlík acknowledges Fondecyt Proyecto Regular N 1151441 and the LIT-2016-1-SEE-023 project modec. Rastislav Potocký was supported by Vega grant 2/0047/15.

References

1. Adams, J.H.: A nonlinear regression model of incurred but not reported losses. In: CASE Forum Summer, pp. 1–14 (2007)
2. Brys, G., Hubert, M., Struyf, A.: Goodness-of-fit tests based on a robust measure of skewness. Comput. Stat. **23**, 429–442 (2008)
3. Gel, Y.R., Gastwirth, J.L.: A robust modification of the Jarque Bera test of normality. Econ. Lett. **99**, 30–32 (2008)
4. Potocký, R.: Modelling of the claims for non-life insurance. Forum Statisticum Slovacum **3**(4), 122–126 (2007)
5. Potocký, R., Stehlík, M.: Analysis of pensions in the 1st pilar under the expected demographic development. In: Proceedings of 10th Slovak Conference on Demography, Smolenice (2005)
6. Potocký, R., Stehlík, M.: Stochastic models in insurance and finance with respect to basel II. JAMSI, **3**(2), 237–245 (2007)
7. Potocký, R., Stehlík, M.: Improved nonlinear regression modeling of parameters of IBNR reserves. Commun. Dependability Qual. Manag. **11**(4), 54–60 (2008)
8. Potocký, R., Waldl, H., Stehlík, M.: On sums of claims and their applications in analysis of pension funds and insurance products. Prague Econ. Pap. **3**, 349–370 (2014)
9. Statistical database of indicators of economic and social-economic development in the Slovak Republic, Statistical Yearbook of Slovakia, 1998–2013
10. Stehlík, M., Střelec, L.: On normality assumptions for claims in insurance. Acta Universitatis Agriculturae et Silviculturae Mendelianae Brunensis **57**(3), 141–146 (2009)
11. Stehlík, M., Fabián, Z., Střelec, L.: Small sample robust testing for normality against Pareto tails. Commun. Stat. - Simul. Comput. **41**(7), 1167–1194 (2012)
12. Stehlík, M., Střelec, L., Thulin, M.: On robust testing for normality in chemometrics. Chemom. Intell. Lab. Syst. **130**, 98–108 (2014)
13. Stehlík, M., Potocký, R., Kiselak, J., Jordanova, P.: On generalized interest rate dynamics. Appl. Math. Inf. Sci. **9**(2L), 325–338 (2015)

Chapter 14
Markowitz Problem for a Case of Random Environment Existence

Alexander Andronov and Tatjana Jurkina

Abstract Classical Markowitz model considers n assets with $R_1, R_2, \ldots, R_n$ random profitability and $r_1, r_2, \ldots, r_n$ relevant average, $\sigma_1^2, \sigma_2^2, \ldots, \sigma_n^2$ variances, and $\sigma_{\mu,\nu}$, $\mu, \nu = 1, \ldots, n$ covariance. The portfolio is built of these assets, by using weighting coefficients $\omega_1, \omega_2, \ldots, \omega_n$, where ω_μ is the share of asset cost μ in the whole portfolio value. The profitability of such portfolio is a random value $F(\omega) = \omega_1 R_1 + \omega_2 R_2 + \ldots + \omega_n R_n$. The cumulative hazard of the portfolio at preassigned value of average profitability $r*$ can be measured by dispersion $DF(\omega)$. It is necessary to determine weighting coefficients by such a way, that minimizes dispersion $DF(\omega)$ given assigned value of $r*$. A more general supposition considered in this chapter: It is supposed that a random environment exists. The last is described by a continuous-time irreducible Markov chain with k states and known matrix of transition intensities $\lambda = (\lambda_{i,j})_{k\times k}$. The reward rate depends on a state of the random environment. For this case, the parameters of Markowitz model are derived.

Keywords Markov chain · Continuous time · Markovic problem

14.1 Introduction

One of the classical problems of the portfolio theory is the portfolio determination problem with the minimal variance and given average risk $r*$, which is formulated by Markowitz in 1952 [6–8]. There are n assets with $R_1, R_2, \ldots, R_n$ random profitability and $r_1, r_2, \ldots, r_n$ corresponding averages, $\sigma_1^2, \sigma_2^2, \ldots, \sigma_n^2$ variances, and $\sigma_{\mu,\nu}$, $\mu, \nu = 1, \ldots, n$ covariance. Note, that $\sigma_{\mu,\mu} = \sigma_\mu^2$.

The portfolio is built of these assets, by using $\omega_1, \omega_2, \ldots, \omega_n$ weighting coefficients, where ω_μ is the share of the μ asset cost in the whole portfolio cost. Let $\omega = (\omega_1, \omega_2, \ldots, \omega_n)$ is the corresponding vector. The profitability of such portfolio

A. Andronov (✉) · T. Jurkina
Transport and Telecommunication Institute, Lomonosova 1, Riga 1019, Latvia
e-mail: lora@mailbox.riga.lv

T. Jurkina
e-mail: ju_ta@mits.lv

J. Pilz et al. (eds.), *Statistics and Simulation*, Springer Proceedings
in Mathematics & Statistics 231, https://doi.org/10.1007/978-3-319-76035-3_14

is a random variable

$$F(\omega) = \omega_1 R_1 + \omega_2 R_2 + \ldots + \omega_n R_n.$$

The average and the variance of the portfolio are:

$$EF(\omega) = \omega_1 r_1 + \omega_2 r_2 + \ldots + \omega_n r_n,$$

$$DF(\omega) = \sum_{\mu=1}^{n} \sum_{\nu=1}^{n} \omega_\mu \omega_\nu \sigma_{\mu,\nu} = \sum_{\mu=1}^{n} \sum_{\nu \neq \mu}^{n} \omega_\mu \omega_\nu \sigma_{\mu,\nu} + \sum_{\mu=1}^{n} \omega_\mu^2 \sigma_\mu^2.$$

The cumulative risk of the portfolio with pre-assigned value of average profitability $r*$ can be measured by variance $DF(\omega)$, which positive value of square root is the standard deviation of the profitability.

Markowitz problem is formulated like this:

To minimize dispersion

$$DF(\omega) = \sum_{\mu=1}^{n} \sum_{\nu \neq \mu}^{n} \omega_\mu \omega_\nu \sigma_{\mu,\nu} + \sum_{\mu=1}^{n} \omega_\mu^2 \sigma_{\mu,\mu} \tag{14.1}$$

under constraints

$$EF(\omega) = \omega_1 r_1 + \omega_2 r_2 + \ldots + \omega_n r_n = r*,$$

$$\omega_1 + \omega_2 + \ldots + \omega_n = 1, \quad \omega_\mu \geq 0, \quad \mu = 1, 2, \ldots, n. \tag{14.2}$$

Classical solution of Markowitz problem is the following. The Lagrange multipliers are introduced and Lagrangian is compiled:

$$L(\omega) = \sum_{\mu=1}^{n} \sum_{\nu \neq \mu}^{n} \omega_\mu \omega_\nu \sigma_{\mu,\nu} + \sum_{\mu=1}^{n} \omega_\mu^2 \sigma_\mu^2 -$$
$$- (\omega_1 r_1 + \omega_2 r_2 + \ldots + \omega_n r_n - r*)\lambda - (\omega_1 + \omega_2 + \ldots + \omega_n - 1)\gamma.$$

With the purpose of Lagrangian minimization should be take partial derivatives on $\omega_1, \omega_2, \ldots, \omega_n$, λ and γ, and equate ones to zero. As a result, we have a system of $n + 2$ equations relatively unknowns $\omega_1, \omega_2, \ldots, \omega_n$, λ, and γ:

$$\frac{\partial}{\partial \omega_\mu} L(\omega) = \sum_{\nu \neq \mu}^{n} \omega_\nu \sigma_{\mu,\nu} + 2\omega_\mu \sigma_\mu^2 - \lambda r_\mu - \gamma = 0, \quad \mu = 1, 2, \ldots, n,$$

$$\frac{\partial}{\partial \lambda} L(\omega) = r * -(\omega_1 r_1 + \omega_2 r_2 + \ldots + \omega_n r_n) = 0, \tag{14.3}$$
$$\frac{\partial}{\partial \gamma} L(\omega) = 1 - (\omega_1 + \omega_2 + \ldots + \omega_n) = 0.$$

This system is a linear one and has a simple solution. Let us rewrite one in a matrix form. We denote $(n+2)$-dimensional vector of the unknowns as $x = (\omega_1, \omega_2, \ldots, \omega_n, \lambda, \gamma)^T$, $(n+2)$-dimensional vector of free terms as $\beta = (0, 0, \ldots, 0, r*, 1)^T$, and the elements of the matrix A of conditions

$$A_{\mu,\mu} = 2\sigma_\mu^2, \quad \mu = 1, 2, \ldots, n;$$
$$A_{\mu,v} = \sigma_{\mu,v}, \quad \mu, v = 1, 2, \ldots, n, \quad v \neq \mu; \quad A_{\mu,n+1} = -r_\mu; \quad A_{\mu,n+2} = -1; \tag{14.4}$$
$$A_{n+1,v} = r_v, \quad v = 1, 2, \ldots, n; \quad A_{n+1,n+1} = A_{n+1,n+2} = 0;$$
$$A_{n+2,v} = 1, \quad v = 1, 2, \ldots, n; \quad A_{n+2,n+1} = A_{n+2,n+2} = 0.$$

Now, we can rewrite the system equations as

$$Ax = \beta. \tag{14.5}$$

The solution is the following:

$$x = A^{-1}\beta, \tag{14.6}$$

where A^{-1} means the inverse matrix for A.

Now, the question arises: How variances $\sigma_1^2, \sigma_2^2, \ldots, \sigma_n^2$ and covariances $\sigma_{\mu,v}$, $\mu, v = 1, \ldots, n$, can be determined? These values can be obtained naturally if to consider a random environment initially. Namely, a rewards increment is a constant for each state of the random environment, but different for various states. A randomness of resulting reward arises because a sojourn time in each state is a random variable.

Further, a more general supposition will be accepted: For each state of the random environment, reward increasing is a random vector with normal distribution. For this case, formulas for the parameters of Markowitz model are derived.

The chapter is organized as follows. Sects. 14.2 and 14.3 contain a description and needed results about the random environment. The last is gotten as finite irreducible continuous-time Markov chain. The main results are presented in Sect. 14.4. The numerical example is considered in Sect. 14.5. The Conclusion ends the exposition.

14.2 Random Environment

Random environment is described by a continuous-time Markov chain $X(t)$, $t > 0$, with k states $1, 2, \ldots, k$, and matrix of transition intensities $\lambda = (\lambda_{i,j})_{k\times k}$ [4, 9]. Let Λ_i denote total transition intensity for the state i: $\Lambda_i = \sum_{j=1}^{k} \lambda_{i,j}$, and $\Lambda = (\Lambda_1, \Lambda_2, \ldots, \Lambda_k)^T$.

Let $P_{i,j}(t) = P\{X(t) = j|X(0) = i\}$ be transition probability of Markov chain $X(t)$, and $P(t) = (P_{i,j}(t))_{k\times k}$ be the corresponding matrix. If all eigenvalues of matrix $A = \lambda - \Lambda$ are different, then probabilities $P(t) = (P_{i,j}(t))_{k\times k}$ can be represented simply. Let χ_i and ν_i, $i = 1, \ldots, k$, be the eigenvalue and the corresponding eigenvector of A, $\chi = (\chi_1, \ldots, \chi_k)^T$, $\nu = (\nu_1, \ldots, \nu_k)$ be the matrix of the eigenvectors and $\bar{\nu} = \nu^{-1} = (\bar{\nu}_1^T, \ldots, \bar{\nu}_k^T)^T$ be the corresponding inverse matrix (here, $\bar{\nu}_\eta$ is the ηth row of $\bar{\nu}$). Then [1–3]

$$P(t) = exp(tA) = \nu diag(exp(\chi\ t))\nu^{-1} = \sum_{i=1}^{k} \nu_i exp(t\chi_i)\bar{\nu}_i. \tag{14.7}$$

Now, we suppose that reward $R_\mu(t)$ of the μth asset during time t depends on a state of the random environment and is accumulated. At beginning, we suppose that an increasing of R_μ during time $u < t$ in the state i is constant $\rho_\mu^{(i)}u$. Now, the gotten rewards during time t are dependent random variables $R_1(t), R_2(t), \ldots, R_n(t)$, because all assets operate in the same random environment. Further, we suppose that the rewards increasing are random variables. For both cases, we must calculate constant parameters $r_1, r_2, \ldots, r_n, \sigma_1^2, \sigma_2^2, \ldots, \sigma_n^2, \sigma_{\mu,\nu}, \mu, \nu = 1, \ldots, n$ of Markovitz problem. It can be made if there are known means, variances, and covariances of sojourn times of the random environment in the various states during time t.

14.3 Analysis of Sojourn Time for the Random Environment

This analysis can be performed by standard methods of continuous-time Markov chain theory. Let $T_j(t)$ be sojourn time of the random environment in the states j during time t, $T(t) = (T_1(t), T_2(t), \ldots, T_k(t))$. We begin with average sojourn times during time t in various states of the random environment, if initial state is i: $\tau_{i,j}(t) = E(T_j|X(0) = i)$, $j = 1, \ldots, k$. The corresponding vector $\tau_i(t) = (\tau_{i,1}(t), \tau_{i,2}(t), \ldots, \tau_{i,k}(t))$ can be calculated by the known formula: If $P_i(t)$ is the ith row of matrix (14.7), then

$$\tau_i(t) = \int_0^t P_i(u)du = \int_0^t \sum_{\zeta=1}^{k} \nu_{i,\zeta} exp(\chi_\zeta u)\bar{\nu}_\zeta du = \sum_{\zeta=1}^{k} \nu_{i,\zeta}\bar{\nu}_\zeta \int_0^t exp(\chi_\zeta u)du.$$

There exists unique zero eigenvector among all eigenvalues, let it has number one: $\chi_1 = 0$. Then

$$\tau_i(t) = \nu_{i,1}\bar{\nu}_1 t - \sum_{\zeta=2}^{k} \nu_{i,\zeta} \frac{1}{\chi_\zeta}(1 - exp(t\chi_\zeta))\bar{\nu}_\zeta. \tag{14.8}$$

For the mixed second moment of the sojourn time in the states $j, j* = 1, \ldots, k$ on the interval $(0, t)$ we have

$$E(T_j(t)T_{j*}(t)|X(0) = i) =$$

$$= \int_0^t P_{i,j}(u)E(T_{j*}(t-u)|X(0) = j)du + \int_0^t P_{i,j*}(u)E(T_j(t-u)|X(0) = j*)du. \tag{14.9}$$

Now, we can calculate the covariance $C^{(i)}_{j,j*}(t)$ of sojourn times in the jth and $j*$th states during time t for the initial state i:

$$C^{(i)}_{j,j*}(t) = E(T_j(t)T_{j*}(t)|X(0) = i) - \tau_{i,j}(t)\tau_{i,j^*}(t). \tag{14.10}$$

Let $C^{(i)}(t) = (C^{(i)}_{j,j*}(t))$ be the covariance matrix for initial state i.

14.4 Calculation of Parameters of Markowitz Problem

Such parameters are $r_1, r_2, \ldots, r_n, \sigma_1^2, \sigma_2^2, \ldots, \sigma_n^2, \sigma_{\mu,\nu}, \mu, \nu = 1, \ldots, n$. We suppose that operation time t and the initial state i of the random environment are known and are the same for all assets. If rewards increment for fixed time and the same state of the random environment X are constant, then for initial state i

$$r_\mu = \sum_{j=1}^{k} \rho_\mu^{(j)} \tau_{i,j}(t),$$

$$\sigma_{\mu,\nu} = \sum_{j=1}^{k} \sum_{j*=1}^{k} \rho_\mu^{(j)} C^{(i)}_{j,j*}(t) \rho_\nu^{(j*)}.$$

Now, we are able to realize Markovic model.

Further, the more general problem will be considered. We suppose that increasing $R(t+u) - R(t)$ of reward $R(t) = (R_1(t), \ldots, R_n(t))^T$ during time u in the state i is a normal distributed random multivariate variable $Z^{(i)}u = (Z_1^{(i)}, \ldots, Z_n^{(i)})^T u$ with a mean $u\rho^{(i)} = u(\rho_1^{(i)}, \ldots, \rho_n^{(i)})^T$ and covariance matrix $uC^{(i)} = u(c^{(i)}_{\mu,\nu})_{n\times n}$. These increasing values for various states of the random environment are independent and are additive. Let $Z_\mu = (Z_\mu^{(1)}, \ldots, Z_\mu^{(k)})$, $Z = (Z_1^T, \ldots, Z_n^T)^T = (Z_\mu^{(i)})_{n\times k}$.

Let $T(t) = (T^{(1)}(t), \ldots, T^{(k)}(t))$ be a vector of the sojourn time for different states of random environment during time t. Then

$$R(t) = \begin{pmatrix} R_1(t) \\ \ldots \\ R_n(t) \end{pmatrix} = ZT(t)^T = (Z_1^T, \ldots, Z_n^T)^T \begin{pmatrix} T_1(t) \\ \ldots \\ T_k(t) \end{pmatrix}.$$

Because vectors $T = (T_1, \ldots, T_k)$ and $Z_\mu = (Z_\mu^{(1)}, \ldots, Z_\mu^{(k)})$, $\mu = 1, \ldots, n$ are independent, then

$$E(R(t)) = E\left(\begin{pmatrix} R_1(t) \\ \ldots \\ R_n(t) \end{pmatrix}\right) = E(Z)E(T(t)^T) = E((Z_1^T, \ldots, Z_n^T)^T)E\left(\begin{pmatrix} T_1(t) \\ \ldots \\ T_k(t) \end{pmatrix}\right).$$

Let us calculate the corresponding covariance matrix:

$$\begin{aligned} Cov(R(t)) = E[(R(t) - E(R(t)))(R(t) - E(R(t)))^T] = \\ = E\big[(ZT(t)^T - E(Z)E(T(t)^T))(ZT(t)^T - E(Z)E(T(t)^T))^T\big] = \\ = E\big[ZT(t)^T T(t)Z^T\big] - E(Z)E(T(t))^T E(T(t))E(Z)^T = \\ = E\big[ZE(T(t)^T T(t))Z^T\big] - E(Z)E(T(t))^T E(T(t))E(Z)^T. \end{aligned}$$

But

$$\begin{aligned} E\big[(Z - E(Z))E(T(t)^T T(t))(Z - E(Z))^T\big] = \\ = E\big[ZE(T(t)^T T(t))Z^T\big] - E(Z)E(T(t))^T T(t))E(Z)^T, \end{aligned}$$

therefore,

$$Cov(R(t)) = E\big[(Z - E(Z))E(T(t)^T T(t))(Z - E(Z))^T\big] + E(Z)Cov(T(t))E(Z)^T.$$

Let $W(t) = E(T(t)^T T(t))$. We must calculate the square matrix

$$M = (M_{\mu,\nu}) = E\big[(Z - E(Z))W(t)(Z - E(Z))^T\big].$$

We have:

$$\begin{aligned} M_{\mu,\nu} = E\big((Z_\mu - E(Z_\mu))W(t)(Z_\nu - E(Z_\nu))^T\big) = \\ = E\Big(\sum_{i=1}^{k}\sum_{j=1}^{k}(Z_\mu^{(i)} - E(Z_\mu^{(i)}))W_{i,j}(t)(Z_\nu^{(j)} - E(Z_\nu^{(j)}))\Big) = \end{aligned}$$

$$
= \sum_{i=1}^{k}\sum_{j=1}^{k} W_{i,j}(t)E((Z_{\mu}^{(i)} - E(Z_{\mu}^{(i)}))(Z_{v}^{(j)} - E(Z_{v}^{(j)}))) =
$$

$$
= \sum_{i=1}^{k}\sum_{j=1, j\neq i}^{k} W_{i,j}(t)E((Z_{\mu}^{(i)} - E(Z_{\mu}^{(i)}))(Z_{v}^{(j)} - E(Z_{v}^{(j)}))) +
$$

$$
+ \sum_{i=1}^{k} W_{i,i}(t)E((Z_{\mu}^{(i)} - E(Z_{\mu}^{(i)}))(Z_{v}^{(i)} - E(Z_{v}^{(i)}))) =
$$

$$
= \sum_{i=1}^{k} W_{i,i}(t)E((Z_{\mu}^{(i)} - E(Z_{\mu}^{(i)}))(Z_{v}^{(i)} - E(Z_{v}^{(i)}))) = \sum_{i=1}^{k} W_{i,i}(t)c_{\mu,v}^{(i)}.
$$

Finally, we get

$$
Cov(R(t)) = \sum_{i=1}^{k} E(T(t)^{T}T(t))_{i,i}C^{(i)} + E(Z)Cov(T(t))E(Z)^{T}.
$$

If $Z = z$ is constant matrix, then $C^{(i)} = 0$, $E(Z) = z$ and the usual expression arises:

$$
Cov(R(t)) = Cov(ZT(t)^{T}) = zCov(T(t))z^{T} = E(Z)Cov(T(t))E(Z)^{T}.
$$

14.5 Numerical Example

Our example supposes the following initial data. The random environment has three states: $k = 3$. Transition intensities between states of the random environment are the following:

$$
\lambda = \begin{pmatrix} 0 & 0.2 & 0.3 \\ 0.4 & 0 & 0.1 \\ 0.2 & 0 & 0 \end{pmatrix}.
$$

The number of considered assets $n = 5$ with the following values per unit sojourn time in the ith states: the mean reward $\rho^{(i)} = (\rho_1^{(i)}, \ldots, \rho_n^{(i)})$ and the covariance matrix $C^{(i)} = (c_{\mu,v}^{(i)})_{n\times n}$. Corresponding matrices are the following:

$$
\rho = (\rho^{(1)}\ \ \rho^{(2)}\ \ \rho^{(3)}) = \begin{pmatrix} \rho_1^{(1)} & \rho_1^{(2)} & \rho_1^{(3)} \\ \rho_2^{(1)} & \rho_2^{(2)} & \rho_2^{(3)} \\ \rho_3^{(1)} & \rho_3^{(2)} & \rho_3^{(3)} \\ \rho_4^{(1)} & \rho_4^{(2)} & \rho_4^{(3)} \\ \rho_5^{(1)} & \rho_5^{(2)} & \rho_5^{(3)} \end{pmatrix} = \begin{pmatrix} 1 & 2 & 3 \\ 1 & 1 & 1 \\ 1 & 0 & 3 \\ 2 & 1 & 0 \\ 3 & 2 & 1 \end{pmatrix}.
$$

$$C^{(1)} = C^{(3)} = \begin{pmatrix} 1 & -0.3 & 0 & 0 & 0.3 \\ -0.3 & 1 & 0 & 0 & -0.5 \\ 0 & 0 & 1 & 0 & 0 \\ 0 & 0 & 0 & 1 & 0 \\ 0.3 & -0.5 & 0 & 0 & 1 \end{pmatrix}, \quad C^{(2)} = \begin{pmatrix} 1&0&0&0&0 \\ 0&1&0&0&0 \\ 0&0&1&0&0 \\ 0&0&0&1&0 \\ 0&0&0&0&1 \end{pmatrix}.$$

Now, we present gotten results for time $t = 15$ and given average risk $r* = 20$. The vectors $(r_1, \ldots, r_n)^T$ of mean rewards for different assets and initial states $X(0)$ are the following:

$$E(R(15)|X(0) = 1) = \begin{pmatrix} 31.23 \\ 15 \\ 27.07 \\ 13.77 \\ 28.77 \end{pmatrix}, \quad E(R(15)|X(0) = 2) = \begin{pmatrix} 31.56 \\ 15 \\ 24.18 \\ 13.45 \\ 28.45 \end{pmatrix},$$

$$E(R(15)|X(0) = 3) = \begin{pmatrix} 35.09 \\ 15 \\ 32.21 \\ 9.91 \\ 24.91 \end{pmatrix}.$$

The covariance matrices $(\sigma_{\mu,\nu})$ of rewards for different activities and initial states $X(0)$ are the following:

$$Cov(R(15)|X(0) = 1) = \begin{pmatrix} 156.70 & -32.08 & 50.59 & -39.44 & -7.36 \\ -32.08 & 117.26 & 0 & 0 & -53.47 \\ 50.59 & 0 & 202.99 & -50.59 & -50.59 \\ -39.44 & 0 & -50.59 & 156.70 & 39.44 \\ -7.36 & -53.47 & -50.59 & 39.44 & 156.70 \end{pmatrix},$$

$$Cov(R(15)|X(0) = 2) = \begin{pmatrix} 143.37 & -26.01 & 46.40 & -35.27 & -9.26 \\ -26.01 & 108.09 & 0 & 0 & -45.35 \\ 46.40 & 0 & 196.75 & -46.40 & -46.40 \\ -35.27 & 0 & -46.40 & 143.37 & 35.27 \\ -9.26 & -43.35 & -46.40 & 35.27 & 143.37 \end{pmatrix},$$

$$Cov(R(15)|X(0) = 3) = \begin{pmatrix} 170.39 & -37.818 & 48.72 & -38.08 & -0.268 \\ -37.81 & 132.12 & 0 & 0 & -63.02 \\ 48.72 & 0 & 208.46 & -48.72 & -48.72 \\ -38.08 & 0 & -48.72 & 170.39 & 38.08 \\ -0.268 & -63.02 & -48.72 & 38.08 & 170.39 \end{pmatrix}.$$

Table 14.1 Convergence of the simulated rewards to the true expectation

N	5	50	100	500	1000	10000	50000
1	21.290	19.815	19.653	20.065	20.142	19.996	19.990
2	18.839	19.740	19.507	20.065	20.137	19.986	20.019
3	22.470	19.652	19.800	20.133	20.116	19.976	19.985

About system of linear equations (14.5), the vector of coefficients $\beta = (0\ \ 0\ \ 0\ \ 0\ \ 0\ \ 20\ \ 1)^T$ and the matrix of restrictions (for X(0) = 1 only):

$$A(X(0)=2) = \begin{pmatrix} 286.73 & -26.01 & 46.40 & -35.27 & -9.26 & -31.56 & -1 \\ -26.01 & 216.19 & 0 & 0 & -43.35 & -15 & -1 \\ 46.40 & 0 & 393.49 & -46.40 & -46.40 & -24.18 & -1 \\ -35.27 & 0 & -46.40 & 286.73 & 35.27 & -13.45 & -1 \\ -9.26 & -43.35 & -46.402 & 35.27 & 286.73 & -28.45 & -1 \\ 31.56 & 15 & 24.18 & 13.45 & 28.45 & 0 & 0 \\ 1 & 1 & 1 & 1 & 1 & 0 & 0 \end{pmatrix}.$$

Optimal solutions for different initial states are the following:

$$x(X(0)=1) = (0.119\ \ 0.359\ \ 0.119\ \ 0.262\ \ 0.141\ \ -3.216\ \ 121.036)^T,$$

$$x(X(0)=2) = (0.125\ \ 0.335\ \ 0.136\ \ 0.250\ \ 0.153\ \ -2.369\ \ 98.067)^T,$$

$$x(X(0)=3) = (0.122\ \ 0.328\ \ 0.113\ \ 0.248\ \ 0.190\ \ -2.248\ \ 103.936)^T.$$

The five first elements of the vector x correspond to optimal solution $\omega^* = (\omega_1^*, \omega_2^*, \omega_3^*, \omega_4^*, \omega_5^*)$.

The simulation study has been performed to verify these formulas. Let us present gotten results for initial state of the random environment $X(0) = 0$. Table 14.1 contains simulated average rewards for different numbers N of the runs. The second, the third, and the fourth rows of the table present three various realizations of the considered process. We see how the average rewards converge to the true expectation $r^* = 20$.

It allows us to conclude that the gotten solution satisfies given constraint with respect to r^*.

Minimal values of the variances of the profitable (14.1) are the following:

$$D(F(\omega^*)|X(0)=1) = \omega^*(X(0)=1)^T Cov(R(t)|X(0)=1)\omega^*(X(0)=1) = 22.713,$$

$$D(F(\omega^*)|X(0)=2) = \omega^*(X(0)=2)^T Cov(R(t)|X(0)=2)\omega^*(X(0)=2) = 20.336,$$

$$D(F(\omega^*)|X(0)=3) = \omega^*(X(0)=3)^T Cov(R(t)|X(0)=3)\omega^*(X(0)=3) = 22.974.$$

It is interesting to compare these results with results when we consider mistakenly that rewards per unit time for all states of random environment are not random variables: Ones are constants $\rho^{(i)} = (\rho_1^{(i)}, \ldots, \rho_n^{(i)})^T$ and all covariances $C^{(i)} = (c_{\mu,\nu}^{(i)})_{n\times n}$ equal zero. In this case, optimal solutions for different initial states are the following:

$$x(X(0) = 1) = (0.145\ \ 0.649\ \ 0.036\ \ 8.328 \times 10^{-3}\ \ 0.162\ \ 0.403\ \ -6.046)^T,$$

$$x(X(0) = 2) = (0.157\ \ 0.654\ \ 0.022\ \ 3.049 \times 10^{-3}\ \ 0.163\ \ 0.377\ \ -5.659)^T,$$

$$x(X(0) = 3) = (0.142\ \ 0.670\ \ 0.042\ \ 1.438 \times 10^{-3}\ \ 0.144\ \ 0.363\ \ -5.448)^T.$$

In this case, the following values of the variances have place:

$$D(F(\omega^*)|X(0) = 1) = \omega^*(X(0) = 1)^T Cov(R(t)|X(0) = 1)\omega^*(X(0) = 1) = 39.364,$$

$$D(F(\omega^*)|X(0) = 2) = \omega^*(X(0) = 2)^T Cov(R(t)|X(0) = 2)\omega^*(X(0) = 2) = 38.599,$$

$$D(F(\omega^*)|X(0) = 3) = \omega^*(X(0) = 3)^T Cov(R(t)|X(0) = 3)\omega^*(X(0) = 3) = 47.351.$$

We see that a difference is essential.

14.6 Conclusion

Classical portfolio model of Markowitz has been considered for a case when the random environment exists. It is shown that it changes optimal portfolio essentially.

References

1. Andronov, A., Gertsbakh, I.B.: Signatures in Markov-modulated processes. Stoch. Models **30**, 1–15 (2014)
2. Andronov, A.M.: Parameter statistical estimates of Markov-modulated linear regression. In: Statistical Methods of Parameter Estimation and Hypothesis Testing, vol. 24, pp. 163–180. Perm State University, Perm, Russia (1992) (in Russian)
3. Bellman, R.: Introduction to Matrix Analysis. McGraw-Hill book company, Inc., New York (1969)
4. Kijima, M.: Markov Processes for Stochastic Modeling. Chapman & Hall, London (1997)
5. Lyuu, Y.-D.: Financial Engineering and Computation: Principles. Mathematics, Algorithms. Cambridge University Press, Cambridge (2002)
6. Markowitz, H.M.: Portfolio selection. J. Financ. **7**(1), 77–91 (1952)
7. Markowitz, H.M.: Mean-Variance Analysis in Portfolio Choice and Capital Markets. Blackwell, Oxford (1987)
8. Markowitz, H.M.: The general mean-variance portfolio selection problem. Philos. Trans. R. Soc. A **347**(1684), 543–549 (1994)
9. Pacheco, A., Tang, L.C., Prabhu, N.U.: Markov-Modulated Processes and Semiregenerative Phenomena. World Scientific, New Jersey, London (2009)

Part IV
Testing and Classification Problems in Statistics

Chapter 15
Signs of Residuals for Testing Coefficients in Quantile Regression

Sergey Tarima, Peter Tarassenko, Bonifride Tuyishimire, Rodney Sparapani, Lisa Rein and John Meurer

Abstract We introduce a family of tests for regression coefficients based on signs of quantile regression residuals. In our approach, we first fit a quantile regression for the model where an independent variable of interest is not included in the set of model predictors (the null model). Then signs of residuals of this null model are tested for association with the predictor of interest. This conditionally exact testing procedure is applicable for randomized studies. Further, we extend this testing procedure to observational data when co-linearity between the variable of interest and other model predictors is possible. In the presence of possible co-linearity, tests for conditional association controlling for other model predictors are used. Monte Carlo simulation studies show superior performance of the introduced tests over several other widely available testing procedures. These simulations explore situations when normality of regression coefficients is not met. An illustrative example shows the use of the proposed tests for investigating associations of hypertension with quantiles of hemoglobin A1C change.

Keywords Conditionally exact test · Quantile regression · Hypothesis testing Diabetes

---

S. Tarima (✉) · B. Tuyishimire · R. Sparapani · L. Rein · J. Meurer
Institute for Health and Society, Medical College of Wisconsin, Milwaukee, WI, USA
e-mail: starima@mcw.edu

B. Tuyishimire
e-mail: btuyishimire@mcw.edu

R. Sparapani
e-mail: rsparapani@mcw.edu

L. Rein
e-mail: lrein@mcw.edu

J. Meurer
e-mail: jmeurer@mcw.edu

P. Tarassenko
International Department of Management, Tomsk State University, Tomsk, Russia
e-mail: ptara@mail.tsu.ru

J. Pilz et al. (eds.), *Statistics and Simulation*, Springer Proceedings
in Mathematics & Statistics 231, https://doi.org/10.1007/978-3-319-76035-3_15

15.1 Introduction

Quantile regression has been widely used in various applied disciplines since 1978 [1] and generally testing hypotheses about regression coefficients plays the key role in answering subject area research questions. Statistical inference for quantile regression is thoroughly covered in [2].

Hypothesis testing in quantile regression traditionally relies on asymptotic normality of the estimates of regression coefficients, or on computationally intensive resampling procedures.

In this manuscript, we show via simulation examples that there are situations where the large sample properties are not yet applicable to testing regression coefficients. To resolve these testing difficulties, we suggest to test conditional independence between the variable of interest and signs of model residuals.

Section 15.2 reviews hypothesis testing procedures available for quantile regression. A new approach to hypothesis testing is introduced in Sect. 15.3. This approach is compared with the methods implemented in the R package *quantreg* in Sect. 15.4. An illustrative example on associations with upper and lower quantiles of hemoglobin A1C change is presented in Sect. 15.5. A brief summary concludes the chapter.

15.2 Quantile Regression and Hypothesis Testing

The quantile regression model can be expressed in terms of random variables as

$$\mathbf{Y} = \mathbf{X}\beta + \epsilon, \tag{15.1}$$

where $\mathbf{Y} = (Y_1, \ldots, Y_n)^T$ is a column of continuous responses, $\mathbf{X}$ is a fixed $n \times (p+1)$ design matrix with elements X_{ij} where the first column identically equal to 1 ($\mathbf{X}_0 \equiv 1$), $\beta = \left(\beta_0, \ldots, \beta_p\right)^T$ is a column of regression coefficients, and $\epsilon = (\epsilon_1, \ldots, \epsilon_n)$ is a vector of independent continuous random variables. The index i is used to enumerate independent experimental units (subjects), $i = 1, \ldots, n$, and j enumerates regression coefficients, $j = 0, \ldots, p$. The columns of $\mathbf{X}$ are denoted by $\mathbf{X}_j$ and $\mathbf{X}_{i\cdot}$ are its rows. The distributions of ϵ_i, $F_i(u) = Pr\left(\epsilon_i < u\right)$, are not known but ϵ_i share the same quantile, $F_i\left(0\right) = \tau, \forall i$.

Following [2] quantile regression coefficients can be estimated by minimizing $\sum_{i=1}^{n} \rho_\tau(y_i)$, where ρ_τ is a weighted loss function.

The first and most common estimating procedure for quantile regression is based on the LAD loss function

$$\rho_\tau^{(LAD)}(y) = y(\tau - I(y < 0)) = |y| \cdot |\tau - I(y < 0)|,$$

which is implemented in the R package "*quantreg*". The sign based loss function

$$\rho_\tau^{(SB)}(y) = \text{sgn}(y)(\tau - I(y < 0)) = |\tau - I(y < 0)|,$$

where $\text{sgn}(u) = \{-1, u<0;\ \ 1, u>0\}$ was suggested for quantile regression in [3].

The loss functions, $\rho_\tau^{(LAD)}(y)$ and $\rho_\tau^{(SB)}(y)$, rely on the same weights, $|\tau - I(y < 0)|$, but the LAD uses the actual values of residuals, y, whereas the SB uses only $\text{sgn}(y)$.

Alternative approaches modify $\rho_\tau^{(LAD)}(y)$ with kernel or nearest neighbor smoothing, or add a penalty term [4].

For a chosen $\rho_\tau(\cdot)$, the minimum of $\sum_{i=1}^n \rho_\tau(y_i)$ is reached at $\hat{\beta} = \left(\hat{\beta}_0, \ldots, \hat{\beta}_p\right)$, and under certain regularity conditions $\sqrt{n}\left(\hat{\beta} - \beta\right)$ convergences to a zero-mean normal variate. For an i.i.d. case, $F_i(\cdot) \equiv F(\cdot)$,

$$\sqrt{n}\left(\hat{\beta} - \beta\right) \rightarrow N_{p+1}\left(\mathbf{0}, \frac{\tau(1-\tau)}{f^2(0)}\mathbf{D}^{-1}\right)$$

in distribution, where $f(u) = F'(u)$ and $\mathbf{D} = \lim_{n\to\infty} \frac{1}{n} \sum_{i=1}^n \mathbf{X}_{i.}^T \mathbf{X}_{i.}$. More generally,

$$\sqrt{n}\left(\hat{\beta} - \beta\right) \rightarrow N_{p+1}\left(\mathbf{0}, \tau(1-\tau)\mathbf{U}^{-1}\mathbf{D}\mathbf{U}^{-1}\right)$$

in distribution, where $\mathbf{U} = \lim_{n\to\infty} \frac{1}{n} \sum_{i=1}^n f_i(0)\mathbf{X}_{i.}^T \mathbf{X}_{i.}$.

The asymptotic normality of $\hat{\beta}$ is the most popular approach to make statistical inference. In the *quantreg* package, there are multiple methods for estimating standard errors (SE) of the components $\hat{\beta}$. The group of asymptotic methods in Table 15.1 summarizes estimating procedures for SEs available in the R package "quantreg".

In addition, Table 15.1 lists a rank-based approach, where the confidence interval is produced by inverting a rank test, see [13], the sign based method, where the SB criterion is resampled under the null [3], and a nonparametric bootstrap method [7].

We modify the originally proposed SB criterion [3] and resample the test statistic

$$T_{SB} = \text{sgn}\left(\hat{\epsilon}\right)^T \mathbf{Z}_1 \left(\mathbf{Z}_1^T \mathbf{Z}_1\right)^{-1} \mathbf{Z}_1^T \text{sgn}\left(\hat{\epsilon}\right),$$

where

$$\mathbf{Z_1} = \left(\mathbf{I} - \mathbf{R}\left(\mathbf{R}^T\mathbf{R}\right)^{-1}\mathbf{R}^T\right)\mathbf{X_1}$$

is a column of model residuals after fitting the ordinary least squares regression, $\mathbf{X_1}$ on $\mathbf{X_2}, \ldots, \mathbf{X_p}$, $\mathbf{R} = \left(\mathbf{X_0}, \mathbf{X_2}, \ldots, \mathbf{X_p}\right)$, and $\hat{\epsilon}$ is a column of quantile regression residuals fitted under $H_0 : \beta_1 = 0$. The test statistic T_{SB} has a similar structure to the sign-based criterion [3] with the design matrix $\mathbf{X}$ substituted by $\mathbf{Z_1}$ and all weights set to one.

Resampling under H_0 produces the P-value for testing H_0. Under H_0, the distribution of $\text{sgn}\left(\hat{\epsilon}\right)$ is Bernoulli with $P\left(\text{sgn}\left(\hat{\epsilon}\right) = -1\right) = \tau$ and $P\left(\text{sgn}\left(\hat{\epsilon}\right) = 1\right) = 1 - \tau$. The $\mathbf{Z}_1$ can be resampled from an assumed and estimated parametric

Table 15.1 Inference methods for hypothesis testing

Group	Short description	Citation
Asymptotic	The asymptotic covariance matrix under the i.i.d. assumption	[1]
Asymptotic	A Huber sandwich estimate of the covariance matrix	[5]
Asymptotic	Kernel estimates of $f(0)$, $f(\cdot)$ is the density of ϵ_i	[6]
Asymptotic (bootstrap SE)	Nonparametric bootstrap	[7]
Asymptotic (bootstrap SE)	A bootstrap procedure	[8]
Asymptotic (bootstrap SE)	Monte Carlo marginal bootstrap (MCMB)	[9], [10]
Asymptotic (bootstrap SE)	A generalized bootstrap	[11]
Asymptotic (bootstrap SE)	A Wild bootstrap	[12]
Rank-based	Rank based confidence intervals	[13]
Sign-based	Resampling of the SB criterion under H_0	[3]
Bootstrap	Nonparametric bootstrap (NPboot)	[7]

distribution, or from an empirical distribution. For a fixed design matrix $\mathbf{X}$, $\mathbf{Z}_1$ stays constant.

In Sect. 15.3, a new approach to testing H_0 is considered. The conditional independence testing

$$\text{sgn}(\epsilon) \perp \mathbf{X}_1 \Big| \mathbf{X}_2, \ldots, \mathbf{X}_p$$

is considered instead. The SB test is a conditional independence test under the assumption that $(\mathbf{X}_1, \mathbf{X}_2, \ldots, \mathbf{X}_p)$ came from a p-dimensional normal distribution.

15.3 Methods

Without loss of generality, we consider testing $H_0 : \beta_1 = 0$, a scalar or a vector of possibly multidimensional $\mathbf{X}_1$. From the conditional independence $\text{sgn}(\hat{\epsilon}) \perp \mathbf{X}_1 \big| \mathbf{X}_2, \ldots, \mathbf{X}_p$ the null on β_1 immediately follows.

If a researcher investigates the effect of covariate $\mathbf{X}_1$ on τ^{th}-level quantile controlling for other variables, we first fit a quantile regression model under H_0:

$$Y_i = \beta_0 + \beta_2 X_{i2} + \cdots + \beta_p X_{ip} + \epsilon_i.$$

Then we estimate $\hat{\epsilon}_i = Y_i - \hat{Y}_i$, where $\hat{Y}_i = \hat{\beta}_0 + \hat{\beta}_2 X_{i2} + \cdots + \hat{\beta}_p X_{ip}$. Here $\hat{Y}_i$ is an estimate of τ-level quantile conditional on X_{ij} $(j = 2, \ldots, p)$. To differentiate model residuals calculated by different estimating procedures a superscript is added. The residuals obtained by the LAD criterion are denoted as $\hat{\epsilon}^{(LAD)}$ and $\hat{\epsilon}^{(SB)}$ are used with the SB criterion. Since asymptotic properties of the SB and LAD quantile regressions are the same and SB is very computationally intensive, the simulation studies reported in Tables 15.2 and 15.3 rely on LAD residuals only.

The conditional independence $\text{sgn}(\hat{\epsilon}) \perp \mathbf{X}_1 \big| \mathbf{X}_2, \ldots, \mathbf{X}_p$ can be tested in multiple ways but in this manuscript we focus only on two.

The first method is LADLR, which refers to testing conditional independence via the logistic regression model when the residuals are modeled by

$$Pr\left(\text{sgn}\left(\hat{\epsilon}^{(LAD)}\right) = 1\right) = \frac{\exp\left(\alpha_0 + \alpha_1 \mathbf{X}_1 + \cdots + \alpha_p \mathbf{X}_p\right)}{1 + \exp\left(\alpha_0 + \alpha_1 \mathbf{X}_1 + \cdots + \alpha_p \mathbf{X}_p\right)}.$$

The conditional independence in this case leads to $H_0 : \alpha_1 = 0$. The model parameters are estimated by the vector $\hat{\alpha} = \left(\hat{\alpha}_0, \ldots, \hat{\alpha}_p\right)$, the maximum likelihood estimators of the vector of unknown logistic regression parameter $\alpha = \left(\alpha_0, \ldots, \alpha_p\right)$ and the asymptotic normality of the regression coefficients is used for testing H_0.

The second method (SB) is the SB test based on resampling T_{SB} where $\hat{\epsilon}$ are LAD residuals.

15.4 Simulations

To compare the conditional independence testing versus previously available methods, we performed several simulation experiments with 10, 000 repetitions under the null and 2, 000 under each alternative.

15.4.1 *Conditional Independence Tests Versus Tests Relying on Asymptotic Normality, n = 100*

We performed 144 Monte-Carlo simulation experiments and summarized the results in 36 tables (supplementary data, available from the corresponding author on a separate request). Each table aggregated results of four simulation experiments (one under H_0 and three under alternatives). For every experiment, the outcome Y was either normal, $N(\mu, \sigma^2)$, or log-normal, $LN(\mu, \sigma^2)$, with $\mu = \beta_0 + \beta_1 X_1 + \beta_2 X_2$, $\beta_0 = 0$, $\beta_2 = 1$, $\sigma = 2$, and β_1 takes values 0 (the null), and 0.5, 1, 1.5 (three alternatives).

For the experiments where X_1 was considered to be a continuous variable, (X_1, X_2) were generated from a bivariate normal with zero mean $(EX_1 = EX_2 = 0)$, unit variances ($Var(X_1) = Var(X_2) = 1$), and the correlation $Corr(X_1, X_2) = \rho$ taking values 0, 0.4, and 0.8. To consider a dichotomous version the variable of interest X_1, a new variable X_1^d (=1, if $X_1 > 0$; =0 otherwise) was considered instead. This categorization makes the correlation between X_2 and X_1^d not equal to ρ; rather, the parameter ρ becomes the point biserial correlation between X_1^d and X_2. In addition, the use of X_1^d leads to $\mu = \beta_0 + \beta_1 X_1^d + \beta_2 X_2$. Simulations considered three quantiles: $0.1, 0.5, 0.9$ at $n = 100$.

Thus, two distributions (normal and lognormal), two types of the variable of interest X_1 (continuous) or X_1^d (categorical), three different correlation structures, $\rho \in \{0, 0.4, 0.8\}$, three quantiles, $\tau \in \{0.1, 0.5, 0.9\}$, and four values for β_1 $(0, 0.5, 1, 1.5)$ generated 144 simulation experiments.

The general conclusion after reviewing these 36 Tables is two-fold: (1) in Gaussian scenarios, asymptotic methods show similar power properties when compared with methods based on testing for conditional independence, but (2) if the assumption of normality is violated and the central limit theorem is not yet applicable, the asymptotic methods fail whereas methods based on conditional independence continue to show reasonable control of type 1 error as well as demonstrating adequate power.

Among the fifteen hypothesis testing approaches investigated through 144 experiments, we left only four promising tests for further simulations: LADLR, SB, MCMB, and NPboot.

The experiments at $n = 100$ allowed us to exclude from further consideration the testing procedures with inferior operational characteristics. We excluded as inferior the procedures relying on asymptotic properties (see Table 15.1) with the exception of MCMB. These procedures showed unacceptable control for type I error and power for lognormal simulation studies. The rank based procedure also showed inadequate type I error control and was excluded from further consideration.

The MCMB procedure was not suitable for small sample sizes and it often results in errors when $n = 100$. Similarly, nonparametric bootstrap was also known to have issues with small samples. This is why we decided to investigate these two using larger than $n = 100$ samples.

15.4.2 Conditional Independence Tests Versus Bootstrap Tests, n = 200

Then, in the competitive group, we left LADLR, SB, MCMB, and NPboot.

In simulations reported in Table 15.2, we investigated at $n = 200$ more "difficult" scenarios for most testing procedures: loglinear model (an example of a non-Gaussian case), highly correlated predictors (co-linearity) and both binary and continuous form of a predictor of interest.

Table 15.2 shows that LADLR and SB have similar performance, but LADLR shows a slightly better type I error control. The LADLR is easy to implement, since

Table 15.2 Statistical Power. Data were generated from a lognormal distribution with $\mu = \beta_1 X_1^d + X_2$ and $\sigma = 2$, $X_1^d = I(X_1 > 0)$, X_1 and X_2 are correlated standard normals with $\rho = 0.8$. Under the null ($\beta_1 = 0$) 10, 000 simulations were performed and 2000 under each alternative

LADLR	SB	MCMB	NPboot	β_1	τ
0.0637	0.0703	0.0408	0.0301	0.00	0.1
0.1795	0.1935	0.1290	0.1125	0.50	0.1
0.4595	0.4755	0.3355	0.3600	1.00	0.1
0.7485	0.7680	0.6050	0.6690	1.50	0.1
0.0584	0.0620	0.0550	0.0390	0.00	0.5
0.3150	0.3185	0.2695	0.2635	0.50	0.5
0.6820	0.6795	0.6345	0.6400	1.00	0.5
0.9315	0.9350	0.9070	0.9180	1.50	0.5
0.0538	0.0564	0.0752	0.0567	0.00	0.9
0.1550	0.1570	0.2260	0.2090	0.50	0.9
0.3300	0.3390	0.4690	0.4555	1.00	0.9
0.5230	0.5245	0.7325	0.7145	1.50	0.9

all we need is to run a logistic regression model on quantile regression residuals fitted under H_0, whereas SB needs resamples from the distribution of residuals under the null. The MCMB procedure showed less stable type I error control, but this MCMB bootstrap is also used by "*quantreg*" for estimating standard errors and thus relies on asymptotic normality. The NPboot showed the best performance for upper quantile modeling but was overly conservative which comes with lower power for modeling lower quantiles.

15.4.3 Conditional Independence Tests Versus Bootstrap Tests, n = 300, Five Predictor Case

Table 15.3 reports 72 simulation experiments defined by the continuous and categorical predictor of interest (X_1^d or X_1), $\tau \in \{0.2, 0.5, 0.8\}$, $\rho \in \{0, 0.4, 0.8\}$, and $\theta \in \{0, 0.5, 1.0, 1.5\}$.

In these simulation experiments $(X_1, X_2, \ldots, X_5)$ were generated from a five dimensional normal distribution with zero mean and an exchangeable covariance matrix. The exchangeable covariance matrix was defined by unit variances and the correlation ρ. The categorical predictor of interest was defined by $X_1^d = I(X_1 > 0)$.

The Y for continuous predictor of interest were generated from a lognormal distribution with $\mu = \theta X_1 + X_2 + .. + X_5$ and $\sigma = 2$, and for the categorical case $\mu = \theta X_1^d + X_2 + .. + X_5$.

A careful inspection of the results clearly shows that the LADLR was the preferred choice. LADLR outperformed SB for the categorical predictor of interest and

Table 15.3 Statistical power

Categorical (X_1^d)				Continuous (X_1)						
LADLR	MCMB	SB	NPboot	LADLR	MCMB	SB	NPboot	θ	τ	ρ
0.0490	0.0361	0.0860	0.0187	0.0490	0.0338	0.0517	0.0217	0.0	0.2	0.0
0.2350	0.1835	0.2765	0.1470	0.7155	0.5850	0.7205	0.5640	0.5	0.2	0.0
0.7325	0.5900	0.6920	0.5575	0.9990	0.9820	0.9990	0.9855	1.0	0.2	0.0
0.9690	0.9090	0.9375	0.9130	1.0000	0.9985	1.0000	0.9990	1.5	0.2	0.0
0.0558	0.0390	0.0525	0.0257	0.0509	0.0398	0.0521	0.0236	0.0	0.5	0.0
0.2605	0.1840	0.2440	0.1600	0.7390	0.6555	0.7420	0.6325	0.5	0.5	0.0
0.7430	0.6505	0.7020	0.6235	0.9995	0.9935	0.9995	0.9935	1.0	0.5	0.0
0.9755	0.9395	0.9655	0.9440	1.0000	1.0000	1.0000	1.0000	1.5	0.5	0.0
0.0462	0.0326	0.0321	0.0229	0.0458	0.0366	0.0478	0.0213	0.0	0.8	0.0
0.1505	0.0895	0.1115	0.0860	0.4560	0.3825	0.4595	0.3440	0.5	0.8	0.0
0.4740	0.2935	0.3875	0.3325	0.9425	0.8835	0.9430	0.8830	1.0	0.8	0.0
0.7830	0.5825	0.6960	0.6615	0.9990	0.9910	0.9990	0.9875	1.5	0.8	0.0
0.0659	0.0323	0.0879	0.0190	0.0503	0.0350	0.0529	0.0186	0.0	0.2	0.4
0.2395	0.1380	0.2545	0.1085	0.4520	0.3135	0.4550	0.2745	0.5	0.2	0.4
0.6420	0.4740	0.6130	0.4295	0.9420	0.8410	0.9430	0.8110	1.0	0.2	0.4
0.9245	0.8120	0.8985	0.7835	0.9965	0.9665	0.9960	0.9385	1.5	0.2	0.4
0.0515	0.0312	0.0486	0.0226	0.0522	0.0365	0.0541	0.0206	0.0	0.5	0.4
0.1910	0.1085	0.1635	0.1105	0.3775	0.2785	0.3785	0.2345	0.5	0.5	0.4
0.5420	0.3615	0.5025	0.3840	0.8760	0.7555	0.8765	0.7490	1.0	0.5	0.4
0.8395	0.6480	0.8015	0.6845	0.9820	0.9420	0.9825	0.9300	1.5	0.5	0.4
0.0253	0.0172	0.0159	0.0158	0.0463	0.0302	0.0478	0.0171	0.0	0.8	0.4
0.0580	0.0405	0.0325	0.0520	0.1580	0.1015	0.1610	0.0700	0.5	0.8	0.4
0.1605	0.1220	0.0925	0.1450	0.4755	0.3000	0.4810	0.2690	1.0	0.8	0.4
0.2625	0.2645	0.1730	0.2830	0.7430	0.5305	0.7420	0.4570	1.5	0.8	0.4
0.1083	0.0313	0.1116	0.0171	0.0475	0.0271	0.0496	0.0139	0.0	0.2	0.8
0.2910	0.1130	0.2825	0.0835	0.1735	0.1030	0.1730	0.0740	0.5	0.2	0.8
0.6250	0.3405	0.6150	0.2730	0.4800	0.3165	0.4895	0.2485	1.0	0.2	0.8
0.8695	0.6040	0.8570	0.5490	0.7550	0.5445	0.7585	0.4540	1.5	0.2	0.8
0.1055	0.1262	0.0334	0.0716	0.0481	0.0328	0.0493	0.0191	0.0	0.5	0.8
0.2465	0.2935	0.1155	0.1875	0.1175	0.0700	0.1190	0.0495	0.5	0.5	0.8
0.4265	0.4600	0.2730	0.3380	0.2995	0.1890	0.3020	0.1505	1.0	0.5	0.8
0.6065	0.6285	0.4880	0.4885	0.4920	0.3085	0.4920	0.2365	1.5	0.5	0.8
0.0490	0.3740	0.0002	0.1211	0.0474	0.0260	0.0475	0.0147	0.0	0.8	0.8
0.0600	0.4905	0.0000	0.1635	0.0705	0.0350	0.0725	0.0185	0.5	0.8	0.8
0.0875	0.5805	0.0010	0.2010	0.1325	0.0580	0.1340	0.0380	1.0	0.8	0.8
0.1090	0.6580	0.0005	0.2435	0.2070	0.0780	0.2085	0.0435	1.5	0.8	0.8

was better than the nonparametric bootstrap. The most problematic scenario for all four considered methods was highly collinear predictors and the categorized version of X_1.

15.5 Illustrative Example

To illustrate the practical use of testing for conditional independence we extracted a deidentified sample of 10, 000 primarily type 2 Diabetes Mellitus (DM) patients from a large databank of medical records of mainly Milwaukee metro area residents. Following our inclusion criteria these 10, 000 DM patients had at least one year of follow up as defined by their billing data. Further we limited our attention to subjects with two sequential Hemoglobin A1C (A1C) assessments 3 to 12 months apart and the initial A1C at 7 or higher. Thus, the sample size decreased to 2460.

A1C measures severity of Diabetes and is the key measure physicians and their patients focus on [14]. A1C below 7 is often the goal of diabetes management [15], but a goal which is difficult to achieve [16]. Thus, instead of focusing on this goal we investigate the change in A1C.

The mean and median A1C changes in our data are -0.4 and -0.3, but these two characteristics only describe central tendency and do not capture all spectrum of ΔA1C responses. To expand our scope, we also look at 0.2-level quantile = -1.1 (the best 20%) and 0.8-level quantile = 0.5 (the worst 20%).

To target our research interest, we will investigate associations between ΔA1C and hypertension (a prevalent and costly comorbidity) controlling for effects of other factors. Since age is often associated with hypertension as well as with A1C dynamics, we investigate the effect of hypertension separately for two age groups (< 65 and 65+). To be able to compare our models in a side by side manner we included predictors significant in one quantile regression model in the sets of predictors for the other two models. Table 15.4 reports the three quantile regression models. The MCMB bootstrap was used to calculate standard errors.

P-values for significance of hypertension for each age group were calculated by three different methods (LADLR, MCMB, and NPboot). Table 15.5 shows that the conclusion may be different. Nonparametric bootstrap never showed significance which is consistent with our simulations where NPboot was overly conservative. MCMB on the other hand was somewhat closer to LADLR and found the same significance with the exception of $\tau = 0.8$. Since colinearity for large samples is not an issue and the simulation studies ensured us that LADLR has better operational characteristics we rely on LADLR.

Table 15.4 Three quantile regression models. Regression coefficients (EST) reported along with standard errors (SE) estimated by MCMB method

VARIABLE	$\tau = 0.2$ EST(SE)	$\tau = 0.5$ EST(SE)	$\tau = 0.8$ EST(SE)
Intercept	−1.139(0.186)	−0.256(0.215)	0.791(0.351)
Age >= 65, Hypertension = Y	−0.671(0.427)	−0.802(0.315)	−0.507(0.341)
Age < 65, Hypertension = Y	−0.345(0.153)	−0.215(0.122)	−0.15(0.227)
Age > = 65	0.403(0.41)	0.344(0.316)	−0.174(0.356)
Time b/w A1C tests (per 1 year)	0.68(0.367)	0.524(0.303)	0.98(0.46)
Baseline A1C	−0.965(0.05)	−0.582(0.07)	−0.277(0.084)
Current insulin = Yes	0.196(0.15)	0.556(0.128)	0.293(0.197)
Ordered insulin = Yes	0.676(0.163)	0.36(0.145)	0.588(0.268)
Annual charges (up to $380)	0.152(0.172)	0.282(0.139)	0.338(0.213)
Annual charges ($381–$1294)	0.293(0.165)	−0.1(0.185)	−0.281(0.271)
Annual charges ($1295–$4584)	−0.042(0.188)	−0.209(0.183)	−0.187(0.266)

Table 15.5 Table of p-values for variables of interest

	LADLR	MCMB	NPboot	τ
Age <65, Hypertension = Yes	0.0052	0.0112	0.1382	0.2
	0.1026	0.0745	0.1360	0.5
	0.3237	0.4852	0.1446	0.8
Age ≥65, Hypertension = Yes	0.2698	0.0595	0.1380	0.2
	0.0179	0.0112	0.1368	0.5
	0.0285	0.2599	0.1364	0.8

15.5.1 Implementation

The implementation of the proposed approach is easy, and below, we show an artificial example for regression coefficient testing in 0.8 quantile modeling. Suppose in the dataset "d", the variable "y" is the study outcome and "x1" is the variable of interest. The control variables in this dataset are "x2", "x3", "x4". The R code for this artificial example starts with fitting the quantile regression model under the null. Then, signs of residuals are calculated and saved into "a". Finally, the conditional association between "a" and "x1" is tested via the logistic regression model.

```
library(quantreg)
attach(d)
fit <- rq(y ~ x2 + x3 + x4, tau=0.8)
a<- 1*(o > predict(fit))
f0 <- glm(a ~ x2 + x3 + x4, family=binomial)
f1 <- glm(a ~ x1 + x2 + x3 + x4, family=binomial)
anova(f1,f0)$table$pvalue
```

15.6 Summary

In this manuscript, we suggest an alternative way of hypothesis testing for quantile regression. Our approach relies on testing for conditional association between the signs of residuals of quantile regression and the variable of interest. Testing for conditional independence is conceptually different from the array of widely available asymptotic methods and bootstrap. Asymptotic properties are often not applicable, especially if the underlying distribution is skewed, or when the sample sizes are not large enough. As shown in our simulation experiments, conditional independence based hypothesis testing has substantially better control for type I error and power.

Simulation experiments also show that the performance of these new methods is similar to nonparametric bootstrap. The bootstrap however is very computationally intensive and reliable estimation of P-values, especially reaching significance at lower cutoffs (say, 0.01), require large number of resamples. Bootstrap does not always work well for smaller sample sizes showing discreteness and multimodality of the bootstrap distribution. Conditional independence testing has no such issues.

We considered a few methods for conditional independence testing, some are applicable only for randomized studies, others work well for observational studies. One of the easiest to implement was the logistic regression model fitted on signs of residuals of quantile regression under the null hypothesis, where the signs were the binary outcome. These models do not require any resampling. Some resampling was required for calculating P-values of the sign-based test statistic suggested in [3], which resampled from the Bernoulli distribution and was substantially faster than the nonparametric bootstrap.

The illustrative example showed that association between hypertension and the 0.8 level quantile of A1C change would be missed for older adults if we rely on asymptotic properties of regression coefficients or on nonparametric bootstrap.

Overall, we conclude that conditional independence testing is superior to others considered in this chapter and is applicable for a wide range of scenarios.

Acknowledgements Funding for this project was provided by the Advancing Healthier Wisconsin Research and Education Program under award 9520277. This publication was also supported by the National Center for Advancing Translational Sciences, National Institutes of Health, through

Grant Number UL1TR001436. Its contents are solely the responsibility of the authors and do not necessarily represent the official views of the NIH.

References

1. Bassett, G., Koenker, R.: Asymptotic theory of least absolute error regression. J. Am. Stat. Assoc. **78**, 618–622 (1978)
2. Koenker R.W.: Quantile Regression, Cambridge University Press (2005)
3. Tarassenko, P.F., Tarima, S.S., Zhuravlev, A.V., Singh, S.: On sign-based regression quantiles. J. Stat. Comput. Simul. **85**, 1420–1441 (2015)
4. Koenker, R.W.: Additive models for quantile regression: model selection and confidence bandaids. Braz. J. Probab. Stat. **25**, 239–262 (2011)
5. Huber, P.J.: The behavior of maximum likelihood estimates under nonstandard conditions. Proc. Fifth Berkeley Symp. Math. Stat. Probability **I**, 221–33 (1967)
6. Powell, J.L.: Estimation of monotonic regression models under quantile restrictions. In: Barnett, W.A., Powell, J.L., Tauchen, G. (eds.), Nonparametric and Semiparametric Methods in Econometrics and Statistics. Cambridge, Cambridge University Press
7. Efron, B., Tibshirani, R.: An Introduction to the Bootstrap. Chapman & Hall/CRC, Boca Raton (1993)
8. Parzen, M.I., Wei, L., Ying, Z.: A resampling method based on pivotal estimating functions. Biometrika **81**, 341–350 (1994)
9. He, X., Hu, F.: Markov chain marginal bootstrap. J. Am. Stat. Assoc. **97**, 783–795 (2002)
10. Kocherginsky, M., He, X., Mu, Y.: Practical confidence intervals for regression quantiles. J. Comput. Graph. Stat. **14**, 41–55 (2005)
11. Bose, A., Chatterjee, S.: Generalized bootstrap for estimators of minimizers of convex functions. J. Stat. Plan. Inf **117**, 225–239 (1997)
12. Feng, X., He, X., Hu, J.: Wild bootstrap for quantile regression. Biometrika **98**, 995–999 (2011)
13. Koenker, R.W.: Confidence Intervals for regression quantiles. In: Mandl, P., Huskova, M. (eds.) Asymptot. Stat., pp. 349–359. Springer, New York (1994)
14. Koenig, R.J., Cerami, A.: Hemoglobin A1C and diabetes mellitus. Ann. Rev. Med. **31**, 29–34 (1980)
15. Diabetes Care Standards of medical care in diabetes-2014. **37**(S1), S14–S80 (2014)
16. Teoh, H., Home, P., Leiter, L.A.: Should A1C targests be individualized for all people with diabetes? Arguments Against Diabetes Care **34**(S2), S191–S196 (2011)

Chapter 16
Classification of Multivariate Time Series of Arbitrary Nature Based on the ϵ-Complexity Theory

Boris Darkhovsky and Alexandra Piryatinska

Abstract The problem of classification of relatively short multivariate time series generated by different mechanisms (stochastic, deterministic or mixed) is considered. We generalize our theory of the ϵ-complexity, which was developed for scalar continuous functions, to the case of vector-valued functions from Hölder class. The methodology for classification of multivariate time series based on the ϵ-complexity parameters is proposed. The results on classification of simulated data and real data (EEG records of alcoholic and control groups) are provided.

Keywords Multivariate time series · Classification · Epsilon-complexity

16.1 Introduction

Classification of multivariate time series is an important problem in numerous applications (e.g. applications in medicine, biology, finance). At the present time, a large number of different classifiers (see e.g. [4]) are available in the literature, which allow to separate multi-dimensional data into classes with a good accuracy, if the characteristic features of the data are well selected. However, success in solving of this problem strongly depends on how well the features were selected. In our opinion, the features selection problem is the essential step in classification procedure. Currently, the creation of the feature space in case of time series is based on a priori information about data generation mechanisms. If such information is available to researchers (e.g. it is known that the time series is a stationary random process), then

B. Darkhovsky
Institute for Systems Analysis, FRC CSC RAS, Higher School of Economics,
9 pr.60-letiya Oktyabrya, Moscow 117312, Russia
e-mail: darbor2004@mail.ru

A. Piryatinska (✉)
San Francisco State University, 1600 Holloway Ave, San Francisco,
CA 94132, USA
e-mail: alpiryat@sfsu.edu

J. Pilz et al. (eds.), *Statistics and Simulation*, Springer Proceedings
in Mathematics & Statistics 231, https://doi.org/10.1007/978-3-319-76035-3_16

the characteristics of the observed processes (such as spectral characteristics) can be chosen as features for the classification problem.

However, prior information on data generating mechanism is not always available. A typical example is the EEG signal which according to most experts is among the most complex physical signals. Currently, there are no generally accepted models of its generation. Modern EEGs record brain signals for several dozens of channels simultaneously; i.e. we are dealing with a multivariate time series. It is clear that all of the components of a series are interconnected. However, it is not clear in advance how to select features which are useful in classification of different states of the brain. Usage of standard statistical procedures (e.g. spectrum estimation, the correlation dimension) is not fully justified in that case, since, as we know (see e.g. [9]) the EEG signal is a non-stationary process.

For financial time series some biological problems and etc. the situation is similar, there are no established models of the observed processes. This circumstance significantly complicates the selection of features for solving classification problems.

The question arises whether it is possible to find such characteristics of a multivariate time series, which on the one hand would not depend on the mechanism of its generating, and on the other hand would enable us to select features for further classification.

We believe that the ϵ-complexity of a continuous function which was proposed in our paper [2] is such a characteristic. This concept is in line with the general idea of Kolmogorov on "complexity of an object". His idea can be expressed as follows: *A "complex" object requires a lot of information for its reconstruction and, for a "simple" object, little information is needed*, and "complexity" of an object should be measured by the length of its shortest description [6, 7].

In our paper ([2]), the theory of the ϵ-complexity of continuous functions defined on a compact set in finite-dimensional space was developed. It was shown that the ϵ-complexity of "almost all" functions satisfying Hölder conditions are effectively characterized by pairs of real numbers, which we call the *ϵ-complexity parameters (or coefficients)*.

For analysis of multivariate time series, we need to extend our theory into the case of continuous vector-functions from Hölder class. Therefore, in this chapter, we generalize the concept of the ϵ-complexity to that case and obtain an effective characterization of the ϵ-complexity for continuous vector-functions. This fact enables us to propose new features for classification of multivariate time series which does not use *any prior information* on data generating mechanisms.

The chapter is organized as follows. In Sect. 16.2, we provide a definition of the ϵ-complexity of continuous vector-functions and give the theoretical results which are the consequence of the general theory. In Sect. 16.3, we present our classification methodology. In Sect. 16.4, we provide the results of simulations and application of our methodology for classification of EEG signals into two groups: alcoholic and control.

16.2 Theoretical Results

In this section, we provide necessary results from the general theory of the ϵ-complexity and generalize them to the case of vector-functions from Hölder class.

16.2.1 The ϵ-Complexity of Continuous Vector-Functions

Let us consider a continuous vector-function $x(t) = (x_1(t), \dots, x_d(t))$, $t \in [0, 1]$. Let $R_i \stackrel{\text{def}}{=} \max_{t\in[0,1]} |x_i(t)|$, $i \in I \stackrel{\text{def}}{=} \{1, \dots, d\}$. We will assume that $\min_{i\in I} R_i > 0$. Suppose that the values of the ith component $x_i(\cdot)$, $i \in I$ of the function $x(\cdot)$ are known only at points of a uniform grid with spacing h, and let $\mathscr{F}$ be a family of approximation methods.

Let $\hat{x}_i(\cdot)$ be an estimate of the ith component of vector-function $x(\cdot)$ based on its values at the grid points by one of the methods from family $\mathscr{F}$.

Definition 16.1 The function $x_i(\cdot)$ is called *$\mathscr{F}$-nontrivial (correspondingly, totally nontrivial)*, if it can not be recovered with arbitrary small error by methods $\mathscr{F}$ (respectively, by any enumerable collection of methods) for any $h > 0$. The vector-function $x(\cdot)$ is called *$\mathscr{F}$-nontrivial (correspondingly, totally nontrivial)* if all its components are *$\mathscr{F}$-nontrivial (respectively, totally nontrivial).*

Denote by $\tilde{I} \stackrel{\text{def}}{=} \{i \in I : x_i(\cdot) \text{ is } \mathscr{F} - \text{nontrivial function}\}$. Put

$$\delta_i^{\mathscr{F}}(h) = \inf_{\hat{x}_i(\cdot)\in\mathscr{F}} \sup_{t\in[0,1]} |x_i(t) - \hat{x}_i(t)|,\ i \in I.$$

The function $\delta_i^{\mathscr{F}}(h)$ is called *absolute recovery error of component $x_i(\cdot)$ by methods $\mathscr{F}$*. Put ($\forall\epsilon \geq 0$)

$$h_x^*(\epsilon, \mathscr{F}) = \begin{cases} \inf\{h \leq 1 : \sum_{i\in\tilde{I}} \frac{\delta_i^{\mathscr{F}}(h)}{R_i} > \epsilon\}, \text{ if } \tilde{I} \neq \emptyset \\ 1, \qquad\qquad\qquad\qquad \text{in opposite case} \end{cases} \tag{1}$$

We call $\frac{\delta_i^{\mathscr{F}}(h)}{R_i}$ *the related recovery error of component $x_i(\cdot)$ by methods $\mathscr{F}$.*

Definition 16.2 *The number*

$$\mathbb{S}_x(\epsilon, \mathscr{F}) = -\log h_x^*(\epsilon, \mathscr{F})$$

is called the $(\epsilon, \mathscr{F})$-complexity of an individual continuous vector-function $x(\cdot)$.

This definition is a generalization of the main definition from [2] where it was given for scalar functions. Thus, the $(\epsilon, \mathscr{F})$-complexity of a vector-function is the logarithm of the minimum number of function values required for its recovery by methods from family $\mathscr{F}$ with a relative error no more than epsilon. In other words, it is "the shortest" description of the vector-function. Therefore, our definition is in line with Kolmogorov's idea mentioned in the introduction.

Let $\mathscr{T}$ be a set of totally nontrivial vector-functions satisfying the Hölder condition, which means that for any $(t, s) \in [0, 1] \times [0, 1]$

$$\sum_{i \in I} |x_i(t) - x_i(s)| \leq L|t - s|^p, \; L > 0, \; p > 0.$$

Due to the fact that the considered vector-functions have finite number of components, it is possible (as in the scalar case) to show that $\mathscr{T}$ is everywhere dense in the set of vector-functions satisfying Hölder conditions. In other words, "almost any" Hölder vector-function is totally nontrivial, i.e. has totally nontrivial components.

The theorem below immediately follows from the general theory (see, [2]) in case the vector-function $x(\cdot)$ has a finite number of components and all components satisfy Hölder conditions.

Theorem 16.1 *For any vector-function $x(\cdot)$ from a dense subset of $\mathscr{T}$, and any (sufficiently small) $r > 0$, $\gamma > 0$, there exist $\alpha > 0$, $\Delta > 0$, $\mathbb{A}$, $\mathbb{B}$, $|\mathbb{B}| \geq b(x(\cdot)) > 0$, family of approximation methods $\mathscr{F}^*$, functions $\theta(\epsilon)$, $\xi(\epsilon)$ and set $M \subset [\alpha, \alpha + \Delta]$, with the Lebegue measure $\mu(M) > \Delta - r$, such that on the set M for all $\mathscr{F} \supseteq \mathscr{F}^*$ the following relations hold*

$$\mathbb{S}_x(\epsilon, \mathscr{F}) = \mathbb{A} + \mathbb{B} \log \epsilon + \theta(\epsilon) \log \epsilon + \xi(\epsilon), \; \sup_{\epsilon \in M} \max \left(|\theta(\epsilon)|, \; |\xi(\epsilon)|\right) \leq \gamma \tag{16.1}$$

Let us now consider functions from Hölder class and start with a scalar function. It is known that a scalar function $x(t)$, $t \in [0, 1]$ belongs to $C^{k,p}$ class, if it can be represented as follows:

$$x(t + h) = x(t) + x'(t)h + \cdots + \frac{1}{k!} x^{(k)}(t)h^k + r(t, h)h^k$$

where $\max_{t \in [0,1]} |r(t, h)| \leq Lh^p$, $0 < p \leq 1$, $L > 0$.

It is clear that a function of a $C^{0,p}$ class is just a continuous function satisfying Hölder condition, and all derivatives of functions from $C^{k,p}$ class up to kth order satisfy Hölder conditions (which for derivatives up to $(k - 1)$th order become Lipschitz conditions).

Let $x(t)$, $t \in [0, 1]$ be a function from $C^{k,p}$. We will say that the vector-function $z(t) \stackrel{\text{def}}{=} \left(x(t), x'(t), \ldots, x^{(k)}(t)\right)$ *is conjugated* to $x(t)$, and we state a problem of estimation of vector-functions $z(t)$ based on its values at a uniform grid by methods from the family $\mathscr{F}$ (i.e. described above problem).

By definition of $C^{k,p}$ class, $z(t)$ is a continuous vector-function such that all its components satisfying Hölder conditions. Therefore, for vector-function $z(t)$, one can use the Definition 16.2 and Theorem 16.1 to obtain the analogy of the Theorem 16.1 for scalar function of $C^{k,p}$ class using its conjugate vector-function.

Now we consider the vector-function $x(t) = (x_1(t), \ldots, x_d(t))$, $t \in [0, 1]$ and assume that each $x_i(t)$ $(i = 1, \ldots, d)$ belongs to C^{k_i,p_i} class. Then, taking into account the above statement for the scalar function of $C^{k,p}$ class, we can reduce the problem of function reconstruction $x(t)$ based on its values on a uniform grid to the problem of reconstruction of "expanded" vector-function $\tilde{x}(t)$, where to each component $x_i(t)$ we assign its k_i derivatives. It is easy to see that dimension of that vector-function is equal $(d + \sum\limits_i k_i)$. Therefore, the problem of reconstruction of the vector-function $x(t)$ based on its values at uniform grid is reduced to the problem of reconstruction of an expended vector-function $\left(x_1(t), x_1'(t), \ldots, x_1^{(k_1)}(t), x_2(t), x_2'(t), \ldots, x^{(k_2)}(t), \ldots, x_d(t), x_d'(t), \ldots, x_d^{(k_d)}(t)\right)$, and we can use given earlier in this section arguments to obtain an analogue of Theorem 16.1.

16.2.2 *The ϵ-Complexity of a Continuous Function Given on a Uniform Grid*

In modern applications, we mostly deal with vector-functions known only on the discrete set of values (i.e. with a finite set of samples). We assume that these sets of values are restrictions of continuous vector-functions (respectively, the vector-functions whose components are functions from C^{k_i,p_i} classes $(i = 1, \ldots, d)$) at some uniform grid on the unit interval. Let us show how the definition of $(\epsilon, \mathcal{F})$-complexity should be extended to this case. We will start from the continuous vector-function.

Let an $\mathcal{F}$ nontrivial continuous vector-function $x(t)$ is given by its n values (i.e. by n vectors in $\mathbb{R}^d$). Consider the following procedure. Chose $0 < S < 1$ and discard $[(1 - S)n]$ values of the sample (here $[a]$ denotes an integer part of a). Then, we reconstruct the values of the vector-function in the discarded points using the retained points and family of approximation methods $\mathcal{F}$ and find the best approximation (i.e. approximation with the smallest relative error).

Let us consider the value $h_x^*(\epsilon, \mathcal{F})$ which was introduced in (1) and assume that $[h_x^*(\epsilon, \mathcal{F})n] \gg 1$. If the unit interval has n values of continuous vector-function, then the interval of length $h_x^*(\epsilon, \mathcal{F})$ contains $[h_x^*(\epsilon, \mathcal{F})n]$ values, and therefore, the number of vector-function values sufficient to reconstruct it with the absolute error not larger then ϵ is equal $n^* = \left[n/[h_x^*(\epsilon, \mathcal{F})n]\right]$.

Similarly, to the case of continuous argument, we give the following definition:

Definition 16.3 The value

$$\mathcal{S}_n(x(\cdot), \epsilon, \mathcal{F}) = \log \frac{n}{[h_x^*(\epsilon, \mathcal{F})n]} \tag{16.2}$$

is called the $(\epsilon, \mathscr{F})$-complexity of an individual continuous vector-function $x(\cdot)$, which is given by a discrete set of values on the uniform grid.

It follows from the Definition 16.3 that the $(\epsilon, \mathscr{F})$-complexity of an individual continuous vector-function $x(\cdot)$, which is given by a discrete set of values can be measured as a *logarithm of the fraction of function values* needed to recover the components of the vector-function with a sum (by components) of relative errors not larger than ϵ.

The theorem below follows from Theorem 16.1, Definition 16.3 and obvious relationship of $(\epsilon, \mathscr{F})$-complexity of continuous vector-functions and vector-functions given by the discrete set of values (as in [2]).

Theorem 16.2 *For any vector-function $x(\cdot)$ from some dense subset of $\mathscr{T}$, given by its n values on a uniform grid, and for any (sufficiently small) $\kappa > 0, \delta > 0$, and $n \geq n_0(x(\cdot))$ there exist a family of approximation methods $\mathscr{F}^*$, numbers $0 < \alpha(n, x(\cdot)) < \beta(n, x(\cdot)) < 1$, $A(n, x(\cdot))$, $B(n, x(\cdot))$ with $|B(\cdot)| \geq c(n, x(\cdot))$ for some constant $c(n, x(\cdot)) > 0$, functions $\rho(S)$, $\zeta(S)$, and a set $M \subset Q = [\alpha(\cdot), \beta(\cdot)]$, $\mu(M) > \mu(Q) - \delta$ such that, under the family of approximation $\mathscr{F} \supseteq \mathscr{F}^*$ for $S \in M$ the following relationships hold*

$$\log \epsilon = A + B \log S + \rho(S) \log S + \zeta(S), \quad \sup_{S \in M} \max(|\rho(S)|, |\zeta(S)|) \leq \kappa. \tag{16.3}$$

It follows from the above theorem that in case of sufficiently rich family of approximation methods $\mathscr{F}$ and sufficiently large sample size n, for vector-functions satisfying the Hölder condition and defined by their n values on a uniform grid the $(\epsilon, \mathscr{F})$-complexity is characterized by a pair of real numbers (A, B). Namely,

$$\log \epsilon \approx A + B \log S \tag{16.4}$$

where the meaning of $\approx$ is clear from the Theorem 16.2.

Let us consider the case of vector-functions which for each ith component is given by their values on a uniform grid and belongs to C^{k_i, p_i} class $(i = 1, \ldots, d)$. The definition of the $(\epsilon, \mathscr{F})$-complexity for such vector-function can be obtained by application of the Definition 16.3 to the conjugate (or "extended") vector-function (see previous section). Thus, instead of the derivatives, we use appropriate differences; for example, instead of the first derivative, the difference $x(t + 1) - x(t)$, $t = 1, \ldots, n - 1$ is used. For sufficiently high-sampling rate, the differences are approximately equal to the corresponding derivatives multiplied by the length of the sampling interval. Since $(\epsilon, \mathscr{F})$ -complexity of the function remains unchanged when it is multiplied by a constant, we assume that the $(\epsilon, \mathscr{F})$-complexity of "extended" vector-function will be close to the corresponding value of continuous vector-function. This suggests that for vector-functions, ith component of which belongs to the C^{k_i, p_i} class, and given by its values on a uniform grid, using "extension" with the inclusion of the relevant differences the relationship (16.4) holds.

Parameters A, B in relationship (16.4) are new *features of the time series* that are proposed to be used for the classification of the "short" time series, e.g. "short" EEG-recordings. These features are independent from the data generating mechanism and are *model-free*.

16.3 Classification Methodology

In this section, we will describe our methodology for the classification of multivariate time series. This methodology contains two steps, the first step is an estimation of the ϵ-complexity parameters for the time series and transformed time series. These parameters will be used as features for classification algorithms. The second step is the utilization of well-known classifiers such as random forest [1] and support vector machine (see e.g. [4]).

Let us assume that our multivariate time series is a restriction of a continuous vector-function $x(t) = (x_1(t), \ldots, x_d(t))$, $t \in [a, b]$ at the uniform grid.

Step 1. Algorithm for estimation of the ϵ-complexity parameters.

1. Normalize each component of the multivariate time series $x_i(t)$, i.e. replace our original components of the multivariate time series by $x_i(t)/\max_t(|x_i(t)|)$.
2. Select S, the fraction of the remaining points as follows: $S_1 = 50\%$, $S_2 = 33\%$, $S_3 = 29\%$, $S_4 = 25\%$, $S_5 = 22.5\%$, $S_6 = 20\%$.
3. For each fixed S and for each component of the multivariate time series, discard the values of the functions at points which are placed uniformly, or almost uniformly, according to the following scheme: Let $x_i^1, x_i^2, x_i^3, \ldots, x_i^n$ be the values of a function on a grid.

    a. $S_1 = 50\%$: Values of $x_i^2, x_i^4, \ldots, x_i^{2j}, \ldots$; or $x_i^1, x_i^3, \ldots, x_i^{2j+1}, \ldots$; are discarded. Notice we have two different ways to discard function values;
    b. $S_2 = 33\%$:Values of $x_i^1, x_i^4, x_i^7, x_i^{10}, \ldots$; or $x_i^2, x_i^5, x_i^8, x_i^{11}, \ldots$; or $x_i^3, x_i^6, x_i^9, x_i^{12}, \ldots$; are discarded. We have three different placements of discarded values;
    c. The procedures are similar in the case $S_3 = 29\%$, $S_4 = 25\%$, $S_5 = 22.5\%$ and $S_6 = 20\%$.

4. For each S_k and for each of those placements, we consider all possible reconstructions of the function by piece-wise polynomials up to fourth degree and select the one which provides the minimal error of reconstruction. Record this value of the minimal error.
5. For the same S_k, we consider other placements of the retained points and repeat the procedure. Record the obtained minimal errors.
6. Then, we take a mean of the recorded errors calculated over all placements for each component of multivariate time series.
7. Take the sum of the mean errors over all component. It is our estimate of ϵ_k in the case of S_k.

8. Repeat the procedure for $k = 1, \ldots, 6$.
9. Consider points $(\log(S_k), \log(\epsilon_k))$ and find the best linear fit

$$\log \epsilon \approx A + B \log S \tag{16.5}$$

using the least squares method.

Step 2. Classification. In the next step, we use the calculated ϵ-complexity coefficients as well as ϵ-complexity coefficients of first, second, third and fourth differences as an input to the supervised classifiers such as random forest and support vector machine. The employment of differences corresponds to the analysis of derivatives of the multivariate time series. Since, a priori, we did not know the features of the time series which are useful for classification, we propose to test the different combinations of the ϵ-complexity coefficients of the original series and the series of finite differences to find the best set of features for classification process.

The results will be evaluated using the Out-Of-Bag (OOB) [1] error in case of the random forest and k-fold cross-validation procedure (see, e.g. [3, 5]) in both cases to be able to compare the performance of two classifiers.

16.4 Results of Classification Methodology for Simulated and EEG data

16.4.1 Simulation Results

Let us first illustrate the performance of the algorithm for estimation of ϵ-complexity coefficients and dependence (16.4) on the simulated data.

Example 1. We simulated a multivariate time series with the following components:

- ARMA(3,2): $\left(1 - \sum_{i=1}^{2} \phi^i L^i\right) X_t = \left(1 - \sum_{i=1}^{2} \theta^i L^i\right) \epsilon_t, \ r = 1, \ldots, 4, \ L^k X_t = X_{t-k}$. where $\phi = (-0.1, -0.3, 0.1)$, $\theta = (-0.2, 0.1)$; Here and below, $L^k X_t = X_{t-k}$ is the shift operator, ϵ_t standard gaussian white noise.
- ARMA(3,2) where $\phi = (0.4, 0.3, 0.4)$, $\theta = (0.5, 0.4)$;
- FARIMA: $(1 + \phi_1 L - \phi_2 L^2)(1 - L)^{0.35} X_t = (1 + \theta_1 L + \theta_2 L^2)\epsilon_t$. where $\phi = (0.2, -0.40)$, $\theta = (0.4, 0.2)$;
- Logistic map: $x(t) = ax(t-1)\,(1 - x(t-1))$, where $a = 3.98$;
- Quadratic map: $x(t) = x^2(t-1) - 2$;
- Mackey-Glass equation: $\frac{dx}{dt} = a\dfrac{x(t-13)}{1 + x(t-13)^c} - bx$, where $a = 0.1$, $b = 0.2$, $c = 9.7$.

Notice that the first three components are stochastic processes and the last three components are trajectories of the chaotic deterministic processes.

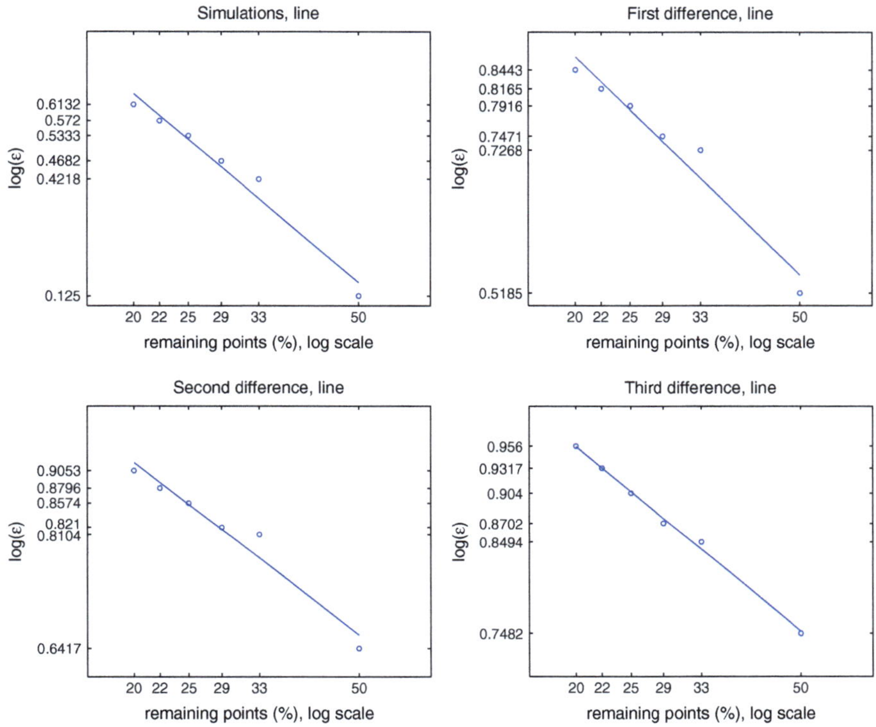

Fig. 16.1 Example of affine dependance of multivariate time series (top left) and its first (top right), second (bottom left) and third (bottom right) differences

We apply the above algorithm to this multivariate time series as well as to multivariate time series which are formed from the first, second and third differences of each component of original time series. In our simulations, we choose $n = 200$ points. The typical examples of such simulation are presented in Fig. 1. The circles correspond to the values $(\log(S_i), \log(\epsilon_i))$, and the straight line is the fitted regression line whose coefficients are ϵ-complexity coefficients of the original time series, first difference, second difference and third differences (top left, top right, bottom left, bottom right correspondingly). One can observed the dependence (16.4) holds well for these cases (Fig. 16.1).

Example 2 Now we will demonstrate the efficiency of our methodology to the simulated data. For it, we simulate two groups of multivariate time series. Both groups of time series have the same types of underline processes as in Example 1 but two different sets of coefficients. The components of vector-processes and their coefficients are listed below.

- ARMA(3,2) coefficients. Group 1: $\phi = (-0.1, 0.3, 0.1)$, $\theta = (0.2, 0.1)$; Group 2: $\phi = (0.5, -0.7, 0.9)$, $\theta = (0.5, 0.6)$;

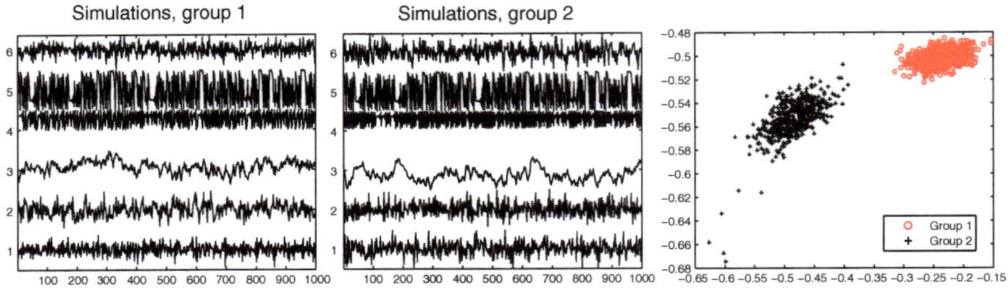

Fig. 16.2 Simulation results. Examples of the multivariate time series from Group 1 (left), from group 2 (middle). Plot of ϵ-complexity coefficients (A, B) for two groups, red circles correspond to group 1 and black crosses correspond to group 2 (right)

- ARMA(3,2) process coefficients. Group 1: $\phi = (0.4, 0.3, 0.4)$, $\theta = (0.1, -0.5)$; Group 2: $\phi = (-0.2, -0.3, -0.8)$, $\theta = (0.2, 0.1)$
- FARIMA process with coefficients Group 1: $\phi = (0.1, -0.5)$; $\theta = (0.6, 0.01)$; $d = 0.35$; Group 2: $\phi = (0.2, -0.4)$; $\theta = (0.4, 0.02)$; $d = 0.35$;
- Logistic map: with coefficients Group 1: $\alpha = 3.98$, Group 2: $\alpha = 3.87$.
- Quadratic map. The same components for both groups.
- Mackey Glass equation: with coefficients Group 1: $a = 0.1$, $b = 0.2$, $c = 9.7$ Group 2: $a = 0.14$, $b = 0.19$, $c = 9.6$

We simulate 500 replications for each group of the above multivariate time series with six components. To get some variability in the processes, the Gaussian noise with zero mean and s.d.=0.005 is added to each coefficient. Then their ϵ-complexity coefficients (A, B) are estimated. Figure 16.2 gives examples of multivariate time series generated by above processes for group one (left plot) and group two (middle plot). The right plot of Fig. 16.2 shows the ϵ-complexity coefficients (A, B) for all simulated time series. The red circles correspond to group one and black crosses correspond to group two. One can see that we got a perfect separation in this example. In this case, both classification algorithms give 100% accuracy on the cross-validation (Fig. 16.2).

16.4.2 Application to the Classification of the EEG-data

Now we will demonstrate our methodology on the EEG-data with two groups of subjects. The data came from a large study which was performed at the Neurodynamics Laboratory, State University of New York Health Center. The purpose of that study was to examine EEG correlates of genetic predisposition to alcoholism. Data contains measurements from 64 electrodes placed on subject's scalps which were sampled at 256 Hz (3.9-msec epoch) for 1 s. The data are publicly available at https://archive.ics.uci.edu/ml/datasets/EEG+Database.

Table 16.1 (Results for the Random Forest (RF) and Support Vector Machine (SVM) classifiers)

		Accuracy (in %)	FP (in %)	FN (in %)
RF	OOB	87.18	12.0	13.6
RF	95% CI	(86.0,88.0)	(10.4, 13.0)	(12.6,15.7)
RF	test set	86.3%	9.2	16.8
SVM	10 f	87.2	8.9%	16.7.0%
SVM	95% CI	(86.7,87.9)	(8.0, 9.7)	(15.6,17.4)
SVM	test	84.3%	9.7%	18.8%

There were two groups of subjects: alcoholic and control. Each subject was exposed to either a single stimulus (S1 or S2) or to two stimuli (S1 and S2) which were pictures of objects chosen from the 1980 Snodgrass and Vanderwart picture set ([8]).

In this chapter, we provide only an example of our approach. Two data sets were analysed (in database they are called: training data and validation data sets). Each of them contains data from 20 subjects, 10 alcoholics and 10 controls. For each of the subject, 10 runs are given for each type of stimuli (in total, we got 600 EEG records for each data set, 300 records for each group). [1]

At first, we consider a training data set. We estimated the ϵ-complexity coefficients (A_i, B_i) for the original time series and ϵ-complexity coefficients of first, second, third and fourth differences (ADk_i, BDk_i) $(k = 1, 2, 3, 4,\ i = 1, \ldots, 600)$. Each combination of the set of the ϵ-complexity coefficients we feed into supervised classifiers such random forest (RF) and support vector machine (SVM). Then, we performed 10-fold cross-validation to select the best combination of the features. This step is performed using R project software and package "RandomForest" for the random forest classifier and package "e1071" for the SVM. We also perform 10-fold cross-validation using the "cart" package. We found that $(A_i, B_i, AD2_i, BD2_i)$ (complexity coefficients of original time series and their second differences) give the best result on 10-fold cross-validation, and we decided to use this set of the features.

The results for the OOB and the 10-fold cross-validation for random forest and SVM classifiers are presented in Table 16.1. In this table, we provide the accuracy of these classifiers and the percentage of false negative and false positive cases. False positive cases are the cases in which we classify the subjects from control groups as subject from alcoholic group, and false negative cases are the cases in which we classify a subject from alcoholic group as a subject from control group. To get 95% bootstrap confidence intervals (CI), we performed 10,000 replications of our experiments using random re-sampling of the data. We also trained our classifiers on training set and validate results on the test set. These results are also presented in the table below.

[1] We thank Henri Begleiter of the Neurodynamics Laboratory at the State University of New York Health Center in Brooklyn for this data set.

16.5 Conclusions

In this chapter, we proposed the methodology for separation of multivariate time series into two groups without any information on data generating mechanism. This methodology is based on the concept of ϵ-complexity of a continuous vector-function. Here, we extended our definition of ϵ-complexity of a continuous function to the case of vector-function. This definition is consistent with the idea of the Kolmogorov complexity of objects.

Our numerical experiments and results on EEG data analysis suggest that the proposed methodology can be widely used.

References

1. Breiman, L.: Random forests. Mach. Learn. **45**(1), 5–32 (2001)
2. Darkhovsky, B., Piryatinska, A.: New approach to the segmentation problem for time series of arbitrary nature. Proc. Steklov Inst. Math. **287**(1), 54–67 (2014)
3. Efron, B., Tibshirani, R.: Improvements on cross-validation: the 632+ bootstrap method. J. Am. Stat. Assoc. **92**(438), 548–560 (1997)
4. Hastie, T., Tibshirani, R., Friedman, J., Franklin, J.: The elements of statistical learning: data mining, inference and prediction. Math. Intell. **27**(2), 83–85 (2005)
5. Kohavi, R., et al.: A study of cross-validation and bootstrap for accuracy estimation and model selection. In: Ijcai, vol. 14, pp. 1137–1145 (1995)
6. Kolmogorov, A.: Combinatorial foundations of information theory and the calculus of probabilities. Russ. Math. Surv. **38**(4), 29–40 (1983)
7. Li, M., Vitányi, P.: An introduction to Kolmogorov complexity and its applications. Springer Science & Business Media, New York (2013)
8. Snodgrass, J.G., Vanderwart, M.: A standardized set of 260 pictures: norms for name agreement, image agreement, familiarity, and visual complexity. J. Exp. psychol. Hum. Learn. Mem. **6**(2), 174 (1980)
9. Subha, D.P., Joseph, P.K., Acharya, R., Lim, C.M.: Eeg signal analysis: a survey. J. Med. Syst. **34**(2), 195–212 (2010)

Chapter 17
EEG, Nonparametric Multivariate Statistics, and Dementia Classification

Patrick Langthaler, Yvonne Höller, Zuzana Hübnerová, Vítězslav Veselý and Arne C. Bathke

Abstract We are considering the problem of performing statistical inference with functions as independent or dependent variables. Specifically, we will work with the spectral density curves of electroencephalographic (EEG) measurements. These represent the distribution of the energy in the brain on different frequencies and therefore provide important information on the electric activity of the brain. We have data of 315 patients with various forms of dementia. For each individual patient, we have one measurement on each of 17 EEG channels. We will look at three different methods to reduce the high dimensionality of the observed functions: 1. Modeling the functions as linear combinations of parametric functions, 2. The method of relative power (i.e., integration over prespecified intervals, e.g., the classical frequency bands), and 3. A method using random projections. The quantities that these methods return can then be analyzed using multivariate inference, for example, using the R package npmv (Ellis et al., J Stat Softw 76(1): 1–18, 2017, [4]). We include a simulation study comparing the first two methods with each other and consider the advantages and shortcomings of each method. We conclude with a short summary of when which method may be used.

P. Langthaler (✉) · A. C. Bathke
Paris-Lodron-University Salzburg, Hellbrunner Str. 34, Salzburg, Austria
e-mail: langthalerpa@stud.sbg.ac.at

A. C. Bathke
e-mail: arne.bathke@sbg.ac.at

P. Langthaler · Y. Höller
Paracelsus Medical University Salzburg, Strubergasse 21, Salzburg, Austria
e-mail: yvonne.hoeller@sbg.ac.at

Y. Höller
Department of Neurology, Christian Doppler Medical Centre and Centre of Cognitive Neuroscience, Paracelsus Medical University Salzburg, Ignaz Harrer Str. 79, Salzburg, Austria

Z. Hübnerová · V. Veselý
Brno University of Technology, Technická 2896/2, Brno, Czech Republic
e-mail: hubnerova@fme.vutbr.cz

V. Veselý
e-mail: vesely.v@fme.vutbr.cz

J. Pilz et al. (eds.), *Statistics and Simulation*, Springer Proceedings in Mathematics & Statistics 231, https://doi.org/10.1007/978-3-319-76035-3_17

Keywords Dimension reduction · Functional data · Multivariate inference
Random projections · Rank statistics

17.1 Introduction

Drawing statistical inference from data where the variables of interest are functions instead of vectors or scalars can be problematic. In this contribution, we chose the strategy of reducing the functions' dimensionality to a fixed finite number of variables, which are then amenable to more traditional statistical analysis. For most of the chapter, we will treat the quantities derived from the functions as the dependent variables and the diagnostic group as the independent variable. We will give one example of the functions as the independent variables in Sects. 17.2.4 and 17.2.5.

For multivariate testing, we will use the R package npmv [4], which provides a well-validated approach to nonparametric multivariate data analysis.

We present three methods for reducing the functional responses to a vector of variables:

1. Modeling the functions as a linear combination of simple functions which can be completely determined by six parameters.
2. Using so-called relative power on certain intervals, which is calculated by integrating the functions over the intervals and dividing by the total integral.
3. Using random projections into a lower-dimensional subspace. This is done using the R package RPEnsemble [2].

The first method can be seen as an additive regression model in which each patient yields a single functional observation, and the estimated parameters are then compared between different diagnostic groups. To our knowledge, this kind of modeling of spectral density curves has never been used before.

The second method has in some variation been used in quantitative EEG research for a long time (e.g., [11]) and has established itself as a standard method. Among clinicians and neuroscientists, it is known as analysis of the power in the classical frequency bands, which are commonly termed *delta, theta, alpha, beta, and gamma*.

The mathematical basis for the third method is the Johnson–Lindenstrauss Lemma [7]. We are using the R package RPEnsemble [1, 2] for implementation. As far as we are aware, random projections are not commonly used in neurological research of this kind.

17.1.1 Notation

Our data consists of observations (functions) from 315 patients. We had the two factors:

- *Diagnostic Group*, consisting of the levels *Alzheimer's, Mild Cognitive Impairment (MCI), Subjective Cognitive Complaint (SCC), Depression with Cognitive Impairment (DCI)*, and *No Diagnosis*.
- *EEG Channel* consisting of the levels *C3, C4, Cz, F3, F4, F7, F8, Fz, O1, O2, P3, P4, Pz, T3, T4, T5*, and *T6*. The letters represent different areas of the brain (*C* = *Central*, *F* = *Frontal*, *O* = *Occipital*, *P* = *Parietal*, and *T* = *Temporal*). The digits (and the *z*) specify the location in more detail. Even numbers refer to the *right* hemisphere of the brain, odd numbers to the *left* hemisphere. A *z* means *central*, that is, in the lateral center of the head. The positions do conform with the 10–20 system for standardized acquisition.

Each patient belongs to exactly one diagnostic group, and each patient is measured exactly once on each of the 17 channels. We excluded patients belonging to the *No Diagnosis* group. This way we obtained 243 patients with complete records. Each observation is given as a series of points (x_i, y_i), where the x_i, $i \in \{1, \ldots, N\}$ are the same for every observation and the x_i are equidistant. In our dataset, the x_i represented 211 different, equidistant frequencies between 0 and 41 Hz on which the *power* (i.e., the square of the signal strength at that frequency) was measured. The y_i correspond to these measured values. So the point (x_i, y_i) for a specific patient means that at frequency x_i, the power of y_i was measured. Technically, more indices could be used for the patient number and level of the between and within-subject factor. For notational convenience, we omit those indices here.

17.2 Method: Modeling the Data as Realizations of Parameterized Functions

This method interprets each observation as a function of a small number of parameters. Reasonable estimates for the parameters can be found, for example, with a least squares procedure. Multivariate analysis can then be performed on these coefficients.

17.2.1 Normalizing

In order to make our parameters only correspond to the shape of the functions and not to the total integral, we will standardize them. This also has the advantage of needing one less parameter as we will see later on. Let $y_1^*, \ldots, y_N^*$ be the observed values. We then approximate the integral of a function by

$$I := \frac{x_N - x_1}{N} \sum_{i=1}^{N} y_i^* . \tag{17.1}$$

Note that this is just the closed Newton–Cotes formula of degree 1. We then set $y_i := \frac{y_i^*}{I}$ for $i \in \{1, \ldots, N\}$. Then the pairs (x_i, y_i) define the standardized curve.

17.2.2 Estimation of Parameters

In order to estimate the parameters from a given standardized curve, we model it as the sum of integrable functions. Let $f_1(\theta_1; x), \ldots, f_p(\theta_p; x)$ be integrable functions, such that for all $i = 1, \ldots, p$: $\theta_i \in \mathbb{R}^{k_i}$ for some $k_i \in \mathbb{N}$. Then we define $\theta := (\theta_1, \ldots, \theta_p) \in \mathbb{R}^{\sum_{i=1}^{p} k_i}$ and

$$f(\theta; x) := \sum_{i=1}^{p-1} a_i \cdot f_i(\theta_i; x) + (1 - \sum_{i=1}^{p-1} a_i) \cdot f_p(\theta_p; x) \tag{17.2}$$

We further request that $\int_{x_1}^{x_N} f_i(\theta_i;\ x)dx = 1 \quad \forall \theta_i \in \mathbb{R}^{k_i}$ and $\int_{x_1}^{x_N} f(\theta;\ x)dx = 1$ $\forall \theta \in \mathbb{R}^{\sum_{i=1}^{p} k_i}$. This, in combination with the standardization, allows us to write $1 - \sum_{i=1}^{p-1} a_i$ instead of a_p. In order to estimate the parameters $a_1, \ldots, a_{p-1}$ as well as $\theta_{1,1}, \ldots \theta_{1,k_1}, \ldots, \theta_{p,1}, \ldots \theta_{p,k_p}$, we minimize the following sum of squares:

$$SSQ = \sum_{i=1}^{N} (f(\theta; x_i) - y_i)^2 \tag{17.3}$$

with respect to those parameters. Only in special cases can we find a closed analytical expression for the values of the parameters that minimize *SSQ*. Usually we have to resort to numerical methods.

17.2.2.1 Using Weight Functions

Sometimes, certain regions of the domain of the function to be estimated might be more important than others. For example, if they correspond with a hypothesis that we want to test. In this case, we can use a weight function

$$w : \mathbb{R} \longrightarrow [0, \infty)$$

and minimize

$$SSQ^* = \sum_{i=1}^{N} (f(\theta; x_i) - y_i)^2 \cdot w(x_i) \tag{17.4}$$

instead. When choosing $w(x_i) = 1 \quad \forall i$ we get Eq. (17.3). In order to make the models comparable, one has to make sure that $\sum_{i=1}^{N} w(x_i) = c$ for some constant c.

Restricting the Range of Parameters

If we have a theoretically motivated desire for a number of our parameters to be within a certain subset of $\mathbb{R}$, we can modify SSQ in such a way that estimated parameters falling out of their respective ranges are penalized. If, for example, we want the parameters to satisfy $\theta_{j,k} \in A_{j,k}$, we can minimize

$$SSQ^* = \sum_{i=1}^{N} (f(\theta; x_i) - y_i)^2 + \sum_{j=1}^{p} \sum_{k=1}^{k_j} c_j g(d(\theta_{j,k}, A_{j,k})) \qquad (17.5)$$

Here g is the loss function, for example, $g(x) = |x|$ or $g(x) = x^2$. Furthermore, $d(x, A) := \inf_{y \in A} d(x, y)$ where d is some metric, usually the euclidean metric. The c_j are smoothing parameters that scale the loss function.

17.2.3 Applying This Method

When looking at the power spectral density curves of our dataset, we can see two major features that all of them have in common:

- A general decline of power with increasing frequency.
- A peak somewhere between approximately 5 and 15 Hz (the so-called dominant rhythm, or peak frequency, linked to individual alpha frequency or brain rate).

The first feature can be modeled well by a function of the form

$$f_1(\lambda; x) = \frac{x^{-\lambda}}{\int_{x_6}^{x_{211}} x^{-\lambda} dx} \qquad (17.6)$$

where λ determines the rate of decline. The peak we decided to model with

$$f_2(\mu, \sigma; x) = \frac{\frac{1}{\sqrt{2\pi\sigma^2}} e^{-\frac{(x-\mu)^2}{2\sigma^2}}}{\int_{x_6}^{x_{211}} \frac{1}{\sqrt{2\pi\sigma^2}} e^{-\frac{(x-\mu)^2}{2\sigma^2}} dx} \qquad (17.7)$$

which is the scaled probability density function of a normal distribution. μ tells us the position of the peak on the x-axis, whereas σ describes the breadth of the peak. It was important to us to model the peak in such a way as to identify its position, since we conjectured that it changed with age and even more with pathological aging [6].

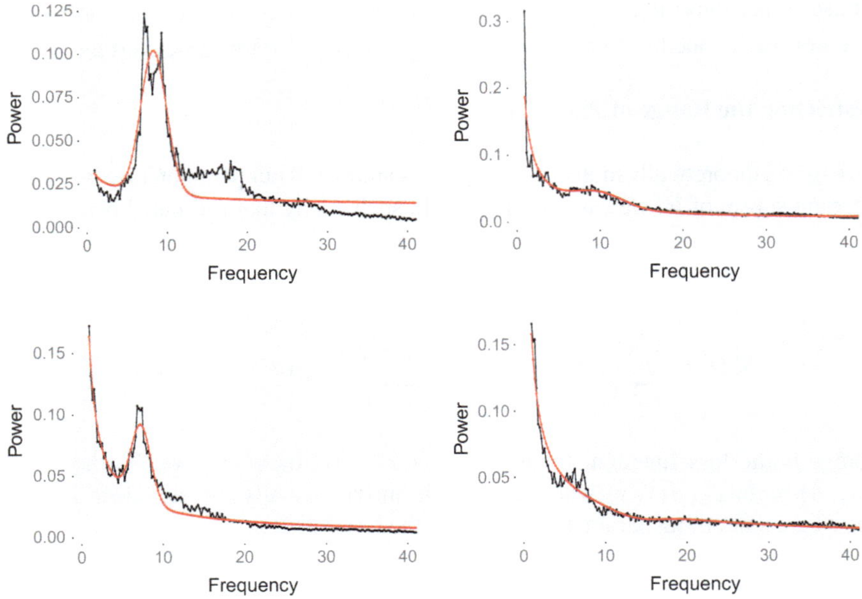

Fig. 17.1 Examples of the two function model

When applying this model we can see that it is often not satisfactory as can be seen in Fig. 17.1.

Therefore, we added a third function:

$$f_3(ncp;\ x) = \frac{\frac{e^{-\frac{1}{2}(x+ncp)}}{2^{\frac{3}{2}}} \sum_{j=0}^{\infty} \frac{x^{\frac{3}{2}+j-1} ncp^j}{2^{2j}\Gamma(\frac{3}{2}+j)j!}}{\int_{x_6}^{x_{211}} \frac{e^{-\frac{1}{2}(x+ncp)}}{2^{\frac{3}{2}}} \sum_{j=0}^{\infty} \frac{x^{\frac{3}{2}+j-1} \lambda^j}{2^{2j}\Gamma(\frac{3}{2}+j)j!} dx} \quad (17.8)$$

which is the scaled probability density function of a noncentral chi-squared distribution with 3 degrees of freedom.

The final model looks like this:

$$f(a,\ b,\ \lambda,\ \mu,\ \sigma,\ ncp;\ x) = af_1(\lambda;\ x) + (1-a-b)f_2(\mu,\ \sigma;\ x) + bf_3(ncp;\ x) \quad (17.9)$$

Examples can be seen in Fig. 17.2.

Overall, we have the parameters $a,\ b,\ \lambda,\ \mu,\ \sigma$, and ncp. In order to test for differences between groups, we used the package npmv with the parameters as dependent variables and diagnostic group as independent variable.

Note: We removed the first 5 observation points for each observation. This was done because the very first observation point at 0 Hz is meaningless, while for very low frequencies (we chose ≈1 Hz as cutoff) the measurements are unreliable. We did this for every method.

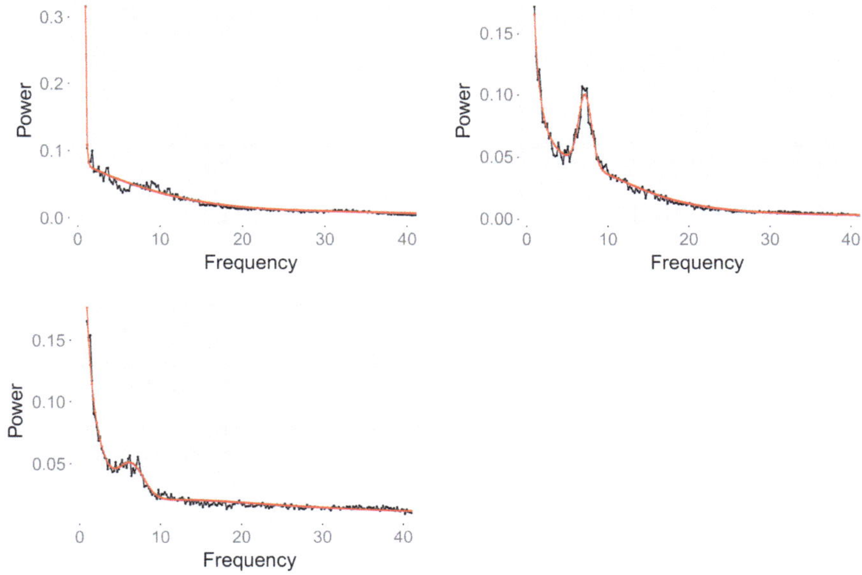

Fig. 17.2 Examples of the three function model

17.2.4 *Hierarchical Clustering of the Channels Within Each Diagnostic Group*

We also performed an agglomerative hierarchical clustering of the different EEG channels within each diagnostic group. Each EEG channel was represented by the six-dimensional vector $(a, b, \lambda, \mu, \sigma, ncp)$. Parameter σ was log transformed to obtain less skewed sample. Obtained dendrograms based on the Mahalanobis distance of the clusters can be seen in Fig. 17.3. The clusters suggest that one may use one of the two symmetrical measurements (left/right hemisphere of the brain) which are typically highly correlated. This is advantageous because it reduces the numerical dimension of responses without loss of information.

17.2.5 *Multicategorical Response Model of Diagnostic Groups*

A multicategorical response model [5] with diagnostic groups as dependent variable and all channels parameters as independent variables can be also applied. In our case, the model had full column rank design matrix of size 729×309. It should be noted that the usual Newton–Rhapson method leading to iterative weighted least squares method did not converge and trust region algorithm [3] must have been used to find the

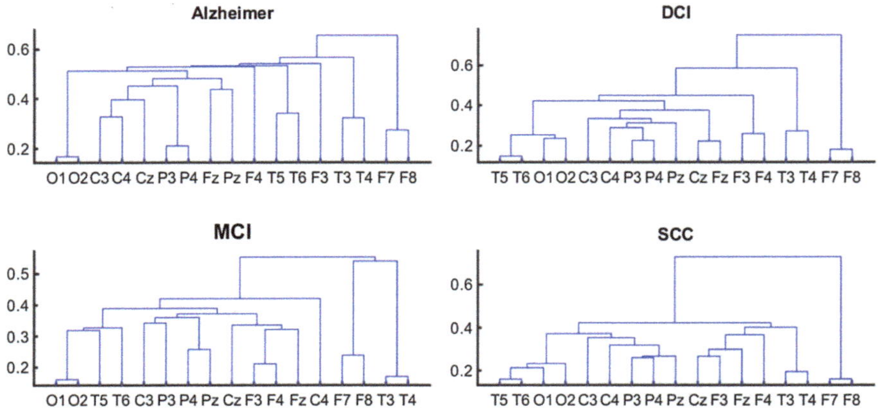

Fig. 17.3 Hierarchical clustering dendrograms of the EEG channels. The vertical distances represent the Mahalanobis distances between the six-dimensional means of the two corresponding clusters

maximum likelihood estimates of the unknown parameters of the multicategorical response model. Using a stepwise procedure, significant parameters and channels with respect to prediction of the probability of having considered types of dementia could have been identified. Note that the choice of neglected channels differed from the approach in Sect. 17.2.4 since they reflect the dependence of the probabilities of the diagnostic groups on the channel parameters.

When the channels' interactions are taken into account in the multicategorical response model, a strong rank deficiency in the design matrix is encountered. Similarly to [12], we considered a sparse parameter estimation technique based on BPA4—a four-step modification of the Basis Pursuit Algorithm [10]. We were searching for the sparse parameter estimates in model for the whole sample as well as a limited sample of patients with either Alzheimer's disease or Mild Cognitive Impairment (as in Sect. 17.4.1).

17.3 Method: Simplification by Integration

Another often used method for analyzing power spectral density curves (e.g., [11]) is to compare the relative power of certain intervals. By relative power over the interval $[a, b]$ for some integrable function h, we mean

$$\frac{\int_a^b h(x)dx}{\int_{x_1}^{x_n} h(x)dx}. \tag{17.10}$$

Some studies also use the absolute power, which is just the numerator in expression (17.10), or ratios of different relative/absolute powers. Since we have no analytical expression for the power spectral density curves (this is what we want to estimate), we can approximate this expression via numerical integration, similar to Eq. (17.1). The following intervals are often used in EEG research:

- delta (0–4 Hz)
- theta (4–8 Hz)
- alpha (8–13 Hz)
- beta (13–30 Hz)
- gamma (more than 30 Hz).

17.3.1 Applying This Method

Since we needed 6 parameters for the previous method, we decided to use 6 intervals for this method in order to get a fair comparison. Since the frequencies we measured were only 0.195 Hz apart, we decided to simply use the neighboring frequencies of an interval for numeric integration, instead of interpolating the exact frequencies. We, therefore, used the following frequencies:

- delta (0–3.91 Hz)
- theta (3.91–8.01 Hz)
- lower alpha (8.01–10.16 Hz)
- higher alpha (10.16–13.09 Hz)
- beta (13.09–30.08 Hz)
- gamma (30.08–41.03 Hz).

The two subdivisions of the alpha range are motivated by the finding that these ranges react differently to specific cognitive tasks [8]. In order to test for differences between groups, we used the package npmv [4], using the six relative power values as dependent variables and diagnostic groups as independent variable.

17.4 Method: Projecting into a Subspace

This method is built around the R package RPEnsemble [2]. Details on the mathematical theory can be read in [1]. The basic idea behind the package is the so-called Johnson–Lindenstrauss Lemma [1]. This lemma states that for $x_1, \cdots, x_n \in \mathbb{R}^p$, $\varepsilon \in (0, 1)$ and $d > \frac{8\log(n)}{\varepsilon^2}$, there exists a linear map $f : \mathbb{R}^p \to \mathbb{R}^d$ such that

$$(1-\varepsilon)||x_i - x_j||^2 \leq ||f(x_i) - f(x_j)||^2 \leq (1+\varepsilon)||x_i - x_j||^2, \tag{17.11}$$

for all $i, j = 1, \cdots, n$. Since this map nearly preserves pairwise distances, classification problems can be solved equivalently in $\mathbb{R}^d$ instead of $\mathbb{R}^p$ and multivariate inference can be done on the coordinates of $f(x_i)$, $i = 1, \cdots, n$ instead of

x_i, $i = 1, \cdots, n$. The package attempts to find this map via randomly generating projections and then choosing the projection which works best for classifying (i.e., has the most correct classifications) a test set using Linear Discriminant Analysis, Quadratic Discriminant Analysis, a K-Nearest Neighbors method, or other classification methods.

A limitation of this method is that the package only provides methods for data in which the factor variable (in our case diagnostic group) has exactly two levels. Another potential limitation is the fact that the values provided by the package (i.e., the coordinates of the observed values in the low-dimensional space) are linear combinations of some of the original coordinates. Therefore, they may not be easy to interpret and the results may not be replicable when choosing different x-values on which the functions are measured.

17.4.1 Applying This Method

Usually one splits the data into a training and test set for this method. When using it to test for differences between the groups, however, we used the whole dataset as training set. We modified the function RPChoose from the package RPEnsemble in order to return the projection matrix used. We then applied the matrix onto the observations and tested for differences in the resulting coordinates using the package npmv [4].

Since RPEnsemble only works for group factors with a factor level of two, we decided to limit our sample to patients with either Alzheimer's disease or Mild Cognitive Impairment, since we expected to see the most interesting differences between these two groups, out of all two-group combinations.

17.5 Simulation Study

We decided to do a simulation study to compare the two methods, *modeling the data as parametric functions* and *simplification by integration*, that is, the first and second method described in this chapter. We chose to restrict the simulation study to these two methods since they both can be implemented such that they have the same number of parameters, namely six. The number of parameters that the data can be reduced to via the method *projecting into a subspace* depends on the sample size via the formula in the Johnson–Lindenstrauss Lemma. The larger the sample size, the larger the number of parameters required. Even if we chose a very small sample size of 5 per group, resulting in 10 overall observations, and set the maximum value for ε to 1, we still had $d > 18.42$. Thus, we would have to project into a 19-dimensional subspace at the very least, which makes this method incomparable with the other two.

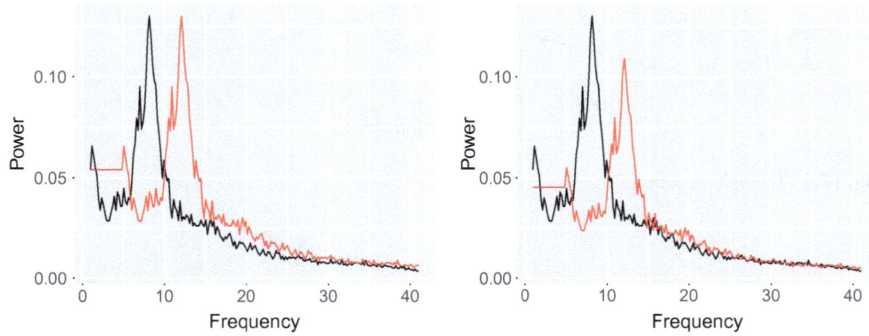

(a) Shift without normalization afterwards (b) Shift with normalization afterwards

Fig. 17.4 Example of a shift effect. Original normalized curve is black and shifted curve is red

We generated our data for simulation as follows: We limited our whole data to observations of the biggest diagnostic group (Depression with Cognitive Impairment) and one channel (F4) in order to acquire a homogeneous sample. These 69 observations were the pool from which we drew. For each constellation of a sample size, a certain effect, and one of the two methods, we then drew two random samples with the given sample size out of the pool. We always left the first sample unchanged, applied an effect to the second sample and then extracted the parameter estimates. The actual testing was done with the ANOVA-type test provided by the R package npmv [4].

There were two kinds of effects that we applied to the second sample: A *Shift Effect* and an *Additive Triangle Effect*. For a shift effect, we shifted each observation by a certain number of grid points to the right and the new values that would appear on the left would be held constant at the leftmost value of the original observation. So shifting the observation $\{(x_1, y_1), (x_2, y_2), (x_3, y_3), \ldots, (x_N, y_N)\}$ to the right by 3 grid points will result in the observation $\{(x_1, y_1), (x_1, y_1), (x_1.y_1), (x_1, y_1), (x_2, y_2), (x_3, y_3), \ldots, (x_{N-4}, y_{N-4}), (x_{N-3}, y_{N-3})\}$. This can be seen graphically in Fig. 17.4a. Since the first method (modeling the data as parametric functions) requires the integral to be 1, we normalized the shifted observations again after shifting. An example of this can be seen in Fig. 17.4b. This of course did not only introduce a *horizontal* effect but also a *vertical* one.

An *Additive Triangle Effect* was created by adding a triangle function to all observations in the second sample. Such a function can be seen in Fig. 17.5. The base of the triangle was always the whole domain of the functional observations (i.e., the interval $[0, 41.0156]$), and the x-coordinate of the peak was always exactly the grid point in the middle, i.e., 20.5078. So the strength of the effect was solely determined by the height of the peak. In order for effect sizes to be comparable between methods, we normalized the observations for both methods before adding the triangle function and then normalized again for the method of modeling the data by parametric functions. An example of a normalized curve with an added triangle function can be

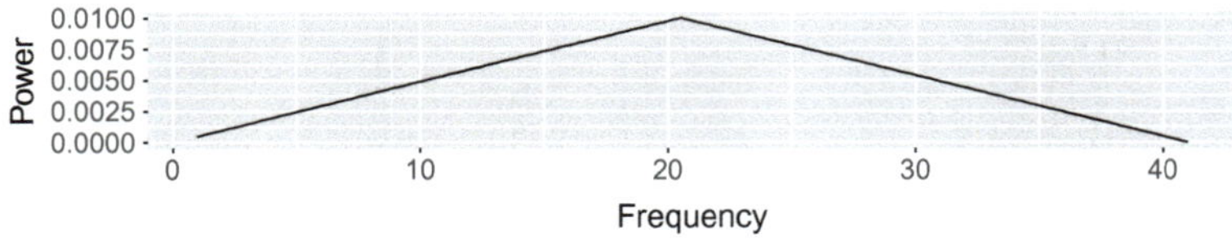

Fig. 17.5 Triangle function

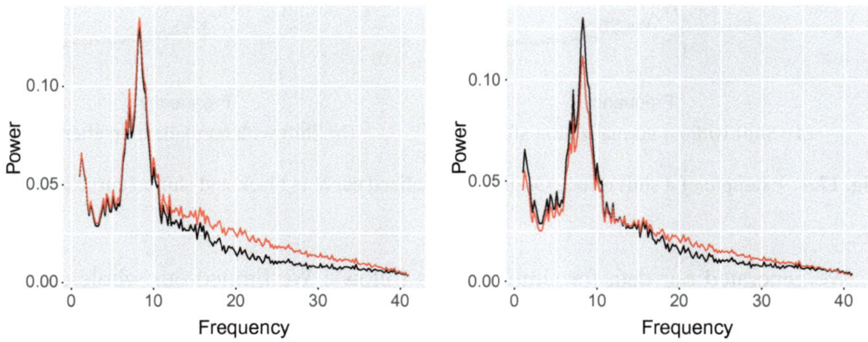

(a)Added Triangle without normalization afterwards

(b) Added Triangle with normalization afterwards

Fig. 17.6 Example of an Additive Triangle Effect. Original normalized curve is black and curve with triangle effect is red

seen in Fig. 17.6a, and the same curve after being normalized again can be seen in Fig. 17.6b.

We looked at three different shifting effects: 10, 15 and 20, which corresponded to 1.9531 Hz, 2.93 Hz, and 3.9063 Hz, respectively.

For the additive triangle effect, we chose the three heights: 0.01, 0.02, and 0.03.

For each combination of sample size, effect, and method, we ran 1000 simulation runs. We originally planned for 10000 but decided that this would take up too much computational time. For example, the simulation for sample size 20, shift effect of 10 and the method of modeling the observations as parametric curves took about 142 mins. The relative frequencies of p-values smaller than 0.05 out of all 1000 p-values can be seen in Table 17.1.

Generally speaking, we observed an increase in power both with increasing sample size and effect size. For sample sizes smaller than 20, both methods were conservative. Most of the time, the integration (relative power) method actually outperformed the parameterized function modeling approach.

Table 17.1 Results of the simulation study

			Effect						
			No Effect	Shift			Triangle		
				10	15	20	0.01	0.02	0.03
Sample size	5	Parameterized functions	0.031	0.05	0.285	0.592	0.057	0.156	0.275
		Integration	0.027	0.117	0.144	0.196	0.102	0.354	0.661
	10	Parameterized functions	0.038	0.15	0.714	0.986	0.146	0.524	0.791
		Integration	0.044	0.442	0.688	0.838	0.291	0.847	0.991
	20	Parameterized functions	0.048	0.386	0.992	1	0.356	0.935	1
		Integration	0.052	0.949	0.999	1	0.636	0.999	1

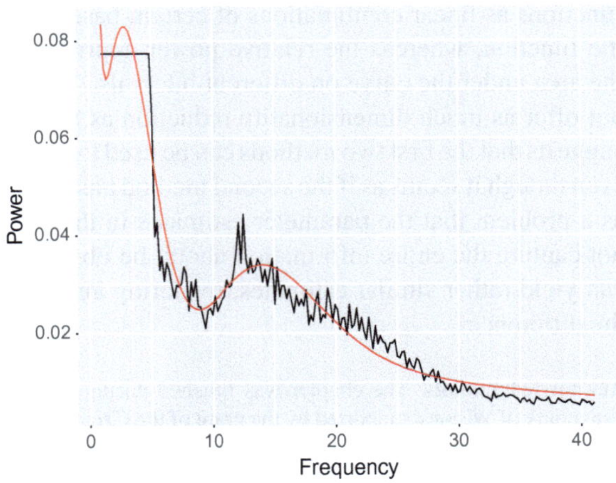

Fig. 17.7 Example of fit achieved by the first method for a shifted observation

There is an important caveat regarding both methods: Differences in the extracted parameters might not increase as differences in the curves themselves increase. For example, it is entirely possible that a shift by a certain amount does not change the relative value of the integral at all, giving the relative power method no additional power above the type 1 error rate for that particular scenario. This was also a problem for the function modeling method. In the shift scenario, for example, it was often not the peak that was modeled by the mean of the normal density component, but the constant part that had been shifted in. An example can be seen in Fig. 17.7. While in this scenario the parameters do differ as a result of the effect, the parameters cannot be interpreted as before. Indeed, the mean of the normal distribution might not correspond to the peak in the alpha range. It is, therefore, also possible for the first method to imagine a scenario where a certain possibly large effect might not lead to any significant change in the extracted parameter estimates.

17.6 Conclusion

We considered three methods for reducing functional EEG responses to a finite-dimensional response vector, in order to use multivariate statistical inference methods. While the integration (relative power) approach is commonly used in EEG research concerning pathological aging, the other two methods to our knowledge are not used. Our interest in analyzing alternatives to the relative power approach comes from the fact that it is not known whether the traditional frequency bands provide an optimal partition of the whole frequency domain. For example, it is often assumed that pathological aging is associated with a shift of the peak frequency from the alpha range to the theta range [9]. However, the shift might also take place within the alpha range, not changing the relative power of the alpha interval significantly. Moreover, the normal aging process is also associated with a slight shift of the peak, further complicating the matter [9].

Which method to use depends on the specific problem. Modeling the response functions as linear combinations of certain base functions emphasizes the shape of the function, whereas the relative power approach emphasizes the distribution of the area under the curve on different intervals. The random projection method does not offer as much dimensionality reduction as the other two. Our simulation study suggests that the first two methods can be used to pick up differences between groups, even though it seems as if the second method has an edge over the first. It still remains as a problem that the parameter estimates in the functional modeling approach do not capture the entire information about the observed curves. Very different curves can yield rather similar estimates, rendering any statistical test powerless to reveal the differences.

Acknowledgements The chapter was finished during a research stay of the third author at the University of Warsaw supported by the grant of the Czech Ministry of Education, Youth and Sports.

References

1. Cannings, T.I., Samworth, R.J.: Random projection ensemble classification. arXiv:1504.04595 (2015)
2. Cannings, T.I., Samworth, R.J.: RPEnsemble: Random projection ensemble classification (2016). R package version 0.3
3. Coleman, T.F., Li, Y.: An interior trust region approach for nonlinear minimization subject to bounds. SIAM J. Optim. **6**(2), 418–445 (1996)
4. Ellis, A.R., Burchett, W.W., Harrar, S.W., Bathke, A.C.: Nonparametric inference for multivariate data: the R package npmv. J. Stat. Softw. **76**(1), 1–18 (2017)
5. Fahrmeir, L., Tutz, G.: Multivariate statistical modelling based on generalized linear models. Springer, New York (1994)
6. Ihl, R., Dierks, T., Martin, E.M., Frölich, L., Maurer, K.: Importance of the EEG in early and differential diagnosis of dementia of the Alzheimer type. Fortschritte der Neurologie-Psychiatrie **60**(12), 451–459 (1992)
7. Johnson, W.B., Lindenstrauss, J.: Extensions of Lipschitz mappings into a Hilbert space. Contemp. math. **26**(189–206), 1 (1984)

8. Klimesch, W., Doppelmayr, M., Russegger, H., Pachinger, T., Schwaiger, J.: Induced alpha band power changes in the human EEG and attention. Neurosci. Lett. **244**(2), 73–76 (1998)
9. Rossini, P.M., Rossi, S., Babiloni, C., Polich, J.: Clinical neurophysiology of aging brain: from normal aging to neurodegeneration. Prog. Neurobiol. **83**(6):375–400 (2007)
10. Shaobing, S.S., Donoho, D.L., Saunders, M.A.: Atomic decomposition by basis pursuit. SIAM J. Sci. Comput. **20**(1), 33–61 (1998)
11. Vecchio, F., Babiloni, C., Lizio, R., Fallani, F.V. Blinowska, K., Verrienti, G., Frisoni, G., Rossini, P.M.: Resting state cortical EEG rhythms in Alzheimer's disease: toward eeg markers for clinical applications: a review. Suppl. Clin. Neurophysiol. **62**, 223–236 (2012)
12. Veselý, V., Tonner, J., Hrdličková, Z., Michálek, J., Kolář, M.: Analysis of PM10 air pollution in Brno based on generalized linear model with strongly rank-deficient design matrix. Environmetrics **20**(6), 676–698 (2009)

Chapter 18
Change Point in Panel Data with Small Fixed Panel Size: Ratio and Non-ratio Test Statistics

Barbora Peštová and Michal Pešta

Abstract The main goal is to develop and, consequently, compare stochastic methods for detecting whether a structural change in panel data occurred at some unknown time or not. Panel data of our interest consist of a moderate or relatively large number of panels, while the panels contain a small number of observations. Testing procedures to detect a possible common change in means of the panels are established. Ratio and non-ratio type test statistics are considered. Their asymptotic distributions under the no change null hypothesis are derived. Moreover, we prove the consistency of the tests under the alternative. The advantage of the ratio statistics compared to the non-ratio ones is that the variance of the observations neither has to be known nor estimated. A simulation study reveals that the proposed ratio statistic outperforms the non-ratio one by keeping the significance level under the null, mainly when stronger dependence within the panel is present. However, the non-ratio statistic incorrectly rejects the null in the simulations more often than it should, which yields higher power compared to the ratio statistic.

Keywords Change point · Panel data · Change in mean · Hypothesis testing
Structural change · Ratio type statistics

18.1 Introduction

The problem of an unknown common change in means of the panels is studied here, where the panel data consist of N panels and each panel contains T observations

B. Peštová
Department of Medical Informatics and Biostatistics, Institute of Computer Science, The Czech Academy of Sciences, Pod Vodárenskou věží 271/2, 18207 Prague, Czech Republic
e-mail: pestova@cs.cas.cz

M. Pešta (✉)
Faculty of Mathematics and Physics, Department of Probability and Mathematical Statistics, Charles University, Sokolovská 49/83, 18675 Prague, Czech Republic
e-mail: michal.pesta@mff.cuni.cz

J. Pilz et al. (eds.), *Statistics and Simulation*, Springer Proceedings in Mathematics & Statistics 231, https://doi.org/10.1007/978-3-319-76035-3_18

over time. Various values of the change are possible for each panel at some unknown common time $\tau = 1, \ldots, N$. The panels are considered to be independent, but this restriction can be weakened. In spite of that, observations within the panel are usually not independent. It is supposed that a common unknown dependence structure is present over the panels.

Tests for change point detection in the panel data have been proposed only in case when the panel size T is sufficiently large; i.e., T increases overall limits from an asymptotic point of view, cf. [4] or [7]. However, the change point estimation has already been studied for finite T not depending on the number of panels N; see [2] or [12]. The remaining task is to develop testing procedures to decide whether a common change point is present or not in the panels, while taking into account that the length T of each observation regime is fixed and can be relatively small.

The chapter is structured as follows: Sect. 18.2 introduces a change point model for panel data together with stochastic assumptions. Ratio and non-ratio type test statistics for the change point detection are proposed in Sect. 18.3. The asymptotic behavior of the considered test statistics is derived in Sect. 18.4, which covers the main theoretical contribution. Section 18.5 contains a simulation study that compares the test based on the ratio statistic against the non-ratio type test. It numerically emphasizes the advantages and disadvantages of the proposed procedure. Proofs are given in the Appendix.

18.2 Panel Change Point Model

Let us consider the panel change point model

$$Y_{i,t} = \mu_i + \delta_i I\{t > \tau\} + \sigma\varepsilon_{i,t}, \quad 1 \le i \le N, \ 1 \le t \le T; \tag{18.1}$$

where $I\{\cdot\}$ is an indicator function, $\sigma > 0$ is an unknown variance-scaling parameter, and T is fixed, not depending on N. The possible *common change point time* is denoted by $\tau \in \{1, \ldots, T\}$. A situation where $\tau = T$ corresponds to *no change* in means of the panels. The means μ_i are panel-individual. The amount of the break in mean, which can also differ for every panel and may depend on N, is denoted by δ_i. Furthermore, it is assumed that the sequences of panel disturbances $\{\varepsilon_{i,t}\}_t$ are independent and within each panel the errors form a weakly stationary sequence with a common correlation structure. This can be formalized in the following assumption.

Assumption A1 The vectors $[\varepsilon_{i,1}, \ldots, \varepsilon_{i,T}]^\top$ from a probability space

$$\rho_t = \mathsf{Corr}\left(\varepsilon_{i,s}, \varepsilon_{i,s+t}\right) = \mathsf{Cov}\left(\varepsilon_{i,s}, \varepsilon_{i,s+t}\right), \quad \forall s \in \{1, \ldots, T-t\},$$

which is independent of the lag s, the cumulative autocorrelation function

$$r(t) = \mathsf{Var} \sum_{s=1}^{t} \varepsilon_{i,s} = \sum_{|s|<t} (t - |s|)\rho_s,$$

and the shifted cumulative correlation function

$$R(t, v) = \mathsf{Cov} \left(\sum_{s=1}^{t} \varepsilon_{i,s}, \sum_{u=t+1}^{v} \varepsilon_{i,u} \right) = \sum_{s=1}^{t} \sum_{u=t+1}^{v} \rho_{u-s}, \quad t < v$$

for all $i = 1, \ldots, N$ and $t, v = 1, \ldots, T$.

The sequence $\{\varepsilon_{i,t}\}_{t=1}^{T}$ can be viewed as a part of a *weakly stationary* process. Note that the dependent errors within each panel do not necessarily need to be linear processes. For example, GARCH processes as error sequences are allowed as well. The assumption of independent panels can indeed be relaxed, but it would make the setup much more complex. Consequently, probabilistic tools for dependent data need to be used (e.g., suitable versions of the central limit theorem). Nevertheless, assuming that the claim amounts for different insurance companies are independent is reasonable. Moreover, the assumption of a common homoscedastic variance parameter σ can be generalized by introducing weights $w_{i,t}$, which are supposed to be known. Being particular in actuarial practice, it would mean to normalize the total claim amount by the premium received, since bigger insurance companies are expected to have higher variability in total claim amounts paid.

The aim is to test the *null hypothesis* of no change in the means

$$H_0 : \tau = T$$

against the *alternative* that at least one panel has a change in mean

$$H_1 : \tau < T \quad \text{and} \quad \exists i \in \{1, \ldots, N\} : \delta_i \neq 0.$$

18.3 Ratio Versus Non-ratio Test Statistic

Detection of change point in panel data can be considered as a structural stability issue in high-dimensional time series. References [3, 8] discuss the analysis of panel data with possible change points in case of stationary and non-stationary (random walk) errors. We propose a *ratio type statistic* to test H_0 against H_1, because this type of statistic does not require estimation of the nuisance parameter for the variance. Generally, this is due to the fact that the variance parameter simply cancels out from the nominator and denominator of the statistic. A competitive and traditional way for testing the change in panel means could be a usage of *non-ratio* (CUSUM) type statistics, for example a maximum or minimum of properly standardized or modified sums. For surveys on ratio type test statistics, we refer to [5, 6, 10].

Our particular panel change point non-ratio test statistic is

$$\mathscr{C}_N(T) = \frac{1}{\sqrt{N}} \max_{t=1,\ldots,T-1} \left| \sum_{i=1}^{N} \sum_{s=1}^{t} \left(Y_{i,s} - \overline{Y}_{i,T}\right) \right|,$$

which is going to be compared with the ratio test statistics

$$\mathscr{R}_N(T) = \max_{t=2,\ldots,T-2} \frac{\max_{s=1,\ldots,t} \left|\sum_{i=1}^{N} \sum_{r=1}^{s} \left(Y_{i,r} - \overline{Y}_{i,t}\right)\right|}{\max_{s=t,\ldots,T-1} \left|\sum_{i=1}^{N} \sum_{r=s+1}^{T} \left(Y_{i,r} - \widetilde{Y}_{i,t}\right)\right|},$$

where $\overline{Y}_{i,t}$ is the average of the first t observations in panel i and $\widetilde{Y}_{i,t}$ is the average of the last $T-t$ observations in panel i, i.e.,

$$\overline{Y}_{i,t} = \frac{1}{t} \sum_{s=1}^{t} Y_{i,s} \quad \text{and} \quad \widetilde{Y}_{i,t} = \frac{1}{T-t} \sum_{s=t+1}^{T} Y_{i,s}.$$

The latter ratio statistic has already been elaborated in [11]. It will be demonstrated by simulations that $\mathscr{R}_N(T)$ keeps the theoretical significance level, while $\mathscr{C}_N(T)$ does not.

18.4 Asymptotic Results

Firstly, we derive the behavior of the test statistics under the null hypothesis of no change.

Theorem 1 (Under Null) *Under hypothesis H_0 and Assumption A1*

$$\mathscr{C}_N(T) \xrightarrow[N\to\infty]{\mathscr{D}} \sigma \max_{t=1,\ldots,T-1} \left| X_t - \frac{t}{T} X_T \right|$$

and

$$\mathscr{R}_N(T) \xrightarrow[N\to\infty]{\mathscr{D}} \max_{t=2,\ldots,T-2} \frac{\max_{s=1,\ldots,t} \left|X_s - \frac{s}{t} X_t\right|}{\max_{s=t,\ldots,T-1} \left|Z_s - \frac{T-s}{T-t} Z_t\right|},$$

where $Z_t := X_T - X_t$ and $[X_1, \ldots, X_T]^\top$ is a multivariate normal random vector with zero mean and covariance matrix $\boldsymbol{\Lambda} = \{\lambda_{t,v}\}_{t,v=1}^{T,T}$ such that

$$\lambda_{t,t} = r(t) \quad \textit{and} \quad \lambda_{t,v} = r(t) + R(t,v), \; t < v.$$

For testing purposes, it is necessary to estimate variance nuisance parameter σ as well as covariance matrix $\boldsymbol{\Lambda}$ in case of the test based on $\mathscr{C}_N(T)$. Although in case of

$\mathscr{R}_N(T)$, its limiting distribution does not depend on the variance parameter σ, but it depends on the unknown correlation structure of the panel change point model. The way of the variance parameter and covariance structure estimation is shown in Sect. 18.4.1. Note that in case of independent observations within the panel, the covariance matrix $\boldsymbol{\Lambda}$ is simplified such that $r(t) = t$ and $R(t, v) = 0$.

Next, we show how the test statistics behave under the alternative.

Assumption A2 $\lim_{N\to\infty} \frac{1}{\sqrt{N}} \left|\sum_{i=1}^{N} \delta_i\right| = \infty$.

Theorem 2 (Under Alternative) *If $\tau \leq T - 3$, then under Assumptions A1, A2 and alternative H_1*

$$\mathscr{C}_N(T) \xrightarrow[N\to\infty]{\mathsf{P}} \infty \quad \textit{and} \quad \mathscr{R}_N(T) \xrightarrow[N\to\infty]{\mathsf{P}} \infty. \tag{18.2}$$

Note that $\delta_i \equiv \delta_i(N)$ may depend on N. Assumption A2 is satisfied, for instance, if $0 < \delta \leq \delta_i \; \forall i$ (a common lower change point threshold) and $\delta\sqrt{N} \to \infty$, $N \to \infty$. Another suitable example of δ_is for the condition in Assumption A2 can be $0 < \delta_i = KN^{-1/2+\eta}$ for some $K > 0$ and $\eta > 0$. Or $\delta_i = Ci^{\alpha-1}\sqrt{N}$ may be used as well, where $\alpha \geq 0$ and $C > 0$. The assumption $\tau \leq T - 3$ means that there are at least three observations in the panel after the change point. It is also possible to redefine the test statistic by interchanging the nominator and the denominator of $\mathscr{R}_N(T)$. Afterward, Theorem 2 for the modified test statistic would require three observations before the change point, i.e., $\tau \geq 3$. Note that the assertion of Theorem 2 for non-ratio statistic $\mathscr{C}_N(T)$ can be weakened by omitting $\tau \leq T - 3$.

Theorem 2 says that in presence of a structural change in the panel means, the test statistics explode above all bounds. Hence, the procedures are consistent and the asymptotic distributions from Theorem 1 can be used to construct the tests.

18.4.1 Estimation of the Covariance Structure

The estimation of the covariance matrix $\boldsymbol{\Lambda}$ from Theorem 1 requires panels as vectors with elements having common mean (i.e., without a jump). Therefore, it is necessary to construct an estimate for a possible change point. A *consistent estimate* of the change point τ in the panel data is proposed in [12] as

$$\widehat{\tau}_N := \arg\min_{t=2,\ldots,T} \frac{1}{w(t)} \sum_{i=1}^{N} \sum_{s=1}^{t} (Y_{i,s} - \overline{Y}_{i,t})^2, \tag{18.3}$$

where $\{w(t)\}_{t=2}^{T}$ is a sequence of weights specified in [12]. However, any other estimate of τ that is consistent, i.e., $\lim_{N\to\infty} \P[\widehat{\tau}_N = \tau] = 1$, can be used instead of $\widehat{\tau}_N$ from (18.3).

Since the panels are considered to be independent and the number of panels may be sufficiently large, one can estimate the correlation structure of the errors

$[\varepsilon_{1,1}, \ldots, \varepsilon_{1,T}]^\top$ empirically. We base the errors' estimates on *residuals*

$$\widehat{e}_{i,t} := \begin{cases} Y_{i,t} - \overline{Y}_{i,\widehat{\tau}_N}, & t \leq \widehat{\tau}_N, \\ Y_{i,t} - \widetilde{Y}_{i,\widehat{\tau}_N}, & t > \widehat{\tau}_N. \end{cases} \tag{18.4}$$

Then, the empirical version of the autocorrelation function is

$$\widehat{\rho}_t := \frac{1}{\widehat{\sigma}^2 NT} \sum_{i=1}^{N} \sum_{s=1}^{T-t} \widehat{e}_{i,s} \widehat{e}_{i,s+t}.$$

Consequently, the kernel estimation of the cumulative autocorrelation function and shifted cumulative correlation function is adopted in lines with [1]:

$$\widehat{r}(t) = \sum_{|s|<t} (t - |s|) \kappa \left(\frac{s}{h} \right) \widehat{\rho}_s,$$

$$\widehat{R}(t, v) = \sum_{s=1}^{t} \sum_{u=t+1}^{v} \kappa \left(\frac{u-s}{h} \right) \widehat{\rho}_{u-s}, \quad t < v;$$

where $h > 0$ stands for the window size and κ belongs to a class of kernels

$$\Big\{ \kappa(\cdot) : \mathbb{R} \to [-1, 1] \,\Big|\, \kappa(0) = 1,\ \kappa(x) = \kappa(-x),\ \forall x,\ \int_{-\infty}^{+\infty} \kappa^2(x) \mathrm{d}x < \infty,$$
$$\kappa(\cdot) \text{ is continuous at 0 and at all but a finite number of other points} \Big\}.$$

Finally, the variance parameter σ for the limiting distribution of $\mathscr{C}_N(T)$ from Theorem 1 can also be estimated by $\widehat{\sigma}^2 := \frac{1}{NT} \sum_{i=1}^{N} \sum_{s=1}^{T} \widehat{e}_{i,s}^2$.

18.5 Simulations

A simulation experiment was performed to study the *finite sample* properties of the test statistics for a common change in panel means. In particular, the interest lies in the empirical *sizes* of the proposed tests, i.e., tests based on ratio test statistic $\mathscr{R}_N(T)$ and non-ratio test statistic $\mathscr{C}_N(T)$, under the null hypothesis and in the empirical *rejection* rate (power) under the alternative. Random samples of panel data (5000 each time) are generated from the panel change point model (18.1). The panel size is set to $T = 10$ and $T = 25$ in order to demonstrate the performance of the testing approaches in case of small and intermediate panel length. The number of panels considered is $N = 50$ and $N = 200$.

The correlation structure within each panel is modeled via random vectors generated from iid, AR(1), and GARCH(1,1) sequences. The considered AR(1) process

Table 18.1 Empirical size (1−specificity) of the test under H_0 for test statistics $\mathscr{R}_N(T)$ and $\mathscr{C}_N(T)$ using the asymptotic critical values, considering a significance level of 5%, weight function $w(t) = t^2$, and smoothing window width $h = 2$

T	N	Innovations	IID		AR(1)		GARCH(1,1)	
10	50	N(0, 1)	0.052	0.066	0.067	0.176	0.054	0.065
		t_5	0.049	0.075	0.068	0.178	0.054	0.071
		Centered χ_3^2	0.051	0.076	0.063	0.179	0.055	0.072
	200	N(0, 1)	0.050	0.067	0.061	0.175	0.050	0.062
		t_5	0.052	0.073	0.065	0.179	0.052	0.063
		Centered χ_3^2	0.055	0.075	0.069	0.177	0.052	0.061
25	50	N(0, 1)	0.054	0.060	0.068	0.220	0.053	0.055
		t_5	0.052	0.055	0.068	0.210	0.054	0.057
		Centered χ_3^2	0.054	0.057	0.059	0.212	0.053	0.059
	200	N(0, 1)	0.051	0.061	0.070	0.199	0.049	0.061
		t_5	0.047	0.059	0.069	0.187	0.048	0.054
		Centered χ_3^2	0.045	0.060	0.060	0.191	0.047	0.059

has coefficient $\phi = 0.3$. In case of GARCH(1,1) process, we use coefficients $\alpha_0 = 1$, $\alpha_1 = 0.1$, and $\beta_1 = 0.2$, which according to [9, Example 1] gives a strictly stationary process. In all three sequences, the innovations are obtained as iid random variables from a standard normal $\mathsf{N}(0, 1)$, student t_5, or centered χ_3^2 distribution. Let us remark that a random variable X from the centered χ_3^2 distribution means that $X + 3$ has a χ^2 distribution with three degrees of freedom. Simulation scenarios are produced as all possible combinations of the above-mentioned settings.

When using the asymptotic distributions from Theorem 1, the variance parameter and the covariance matrix are estimated as proposed in Sect. 18.4.1 using the Parzen kernel

$$\kappa_P(x) = \begin{cases} 1 - 6x^2 + 6|x|^3, & 0 \le |x| \le 1/2; \\ 2(1 - |x|)^3, & 1/2 \le |x| \le 1; \\ 0, & \text{otherwise.} \end{cases}$$

The Bartlett (triangular) window was tried as well yielding similar results than the Parzen one.

Several values of the smoothing window width h are tried from the interval [2, 5], and all of them work fine providing comparable results. To simulate the asymptotic distributions of the test statistics, 2000 multivariate random vectors are generated using the pre-estimated variance parameter and covariance matrix. To access the theoretical results under H_0 numerically, Table 18.1 provides the empirical size (one minus specificity) of the asymptotic tests based on $\mathscr{R}_N(T)$ and $\mathscr{C}_N(T)$, where the significance level is $\alpha = 5\%$.

On one hand, it may be seen that the approach based on ratio type statistic $\mathscr{R}_N(T)$ gives the test size close to theoretical value 0.05. As expected, the best results are achieved in case of independence within the panel, because there is no information overlap between two consecutive observations. The precision of not rejecting the null is increasing as the number of panels is getting higher and the panel is getting longer as well. On the other hand, the test sizes from non-ratio type statistic $\mathscr{C}_N(T)$ are higher than the theoretical value of 0.05, especially when stronger dependence within the panel is considered. This means that the non-ratio test rejects the null hypothesis more frequently and, hence, incorrectly.

The performance of both testing procedures under H_1 in terms of the empirical rejection rates is shown in Table 18.2, where the change point is set to $\tau = \lfloor T/2 \rfloor$ and the change sizes δ_i are independently uniform on $[1, 3]$ in 33, 66% or in all panels.

One can conclude that the power of both tests increases as the panel size and the number of panels increase, which is straightforward and expected. Moreover, higher power is obtained when a larger portion of panels is subject to have a change in mean. The test power drops when switching from independent observations within the panel to dependent ones. Innovations with heavier tails (i.e., t_5) yield smaller power than innovations with lighter tails. Asymmetric error distribution (i.e., centered χ_3^2) gives smaller power than the standard normal distribution of errors. The other considered symmetric error distribution (i.e., t_5) yields only slightly higher power in most of the cases than the asymmetric centered χ_3^2 distribution. Generally, ratio type statistic $\mathscr{R}_N(T)$ provides lower power than non-ratio type statistic $\mathscr{C}_N(T)$ in all scenarios. However, this is among other things due to the fact that the $\mathscr{C}_N(T)$-based test rejects the null more often than it should.

Finally, an early change point is discussed very briefly. We stay with standard normal innovations, iid observations within the panel, the size of changes δ_i being independently uniform on $[1, 3]$ in all panels, and the change point is $\tau = 3$ in case of $T = 10$ and $\tau = 5$ for $T = 25$. The empirical sensitivities of both tests for small values of τ are shown in Table 18.3.

When the change point is not in the middle of the panel, the power of the test generally falls down. The source of such decrease is that the left or right part of the panel possesses less observations with constant mean, which leads to a decrease of precision in the correlation estimation.

18.6 Conclusions

In this chapter, we consider the change point problem in *panel data with fixed panel size*. Occurrence of common breaks in panel means is tested. We compare the *ratio and the non-ratio type test statistic* from a theoretical point of view and by simulations as well. The asymptotic properties of both test statistics are derived. Under the null hypothesis of no change, the test statistics weakly converges to functionals of the multivariate normal random vector with zero mean and covariance structure depending on the intra-panel covariances. The asymptotic distribution of the non-

Table 18.2 Empirical sensitivity (power) of the test under H_1 for test statistics $\mathscr{R}_N(T)$ and $\mathscr{C}_N(T)$ using the asymptotic critical values, considering a significance level of 5%, weight function $w(t) = t^2$, and smoothing window width $h = 2$

$H_1(\%)$	T	N	Innovations	IID		AR(1)		GARCH(1, 1)	
33	10	50	N(0, 1)	0.235	1.000	0.256	0.999	0.193	1.000
			t_5	0.174	0.999	0.202	0.996	0.201	0.999
			Centered χ^2_3	0.175	0.999	0.210	0.995	0.204	0.999
		200	N(0, 1)	0.453	1.000	0.486	1.000	0.387	1.000
			t_5	0.360	1.000	0.393	1.000	0.389	1.000
			Centered χ^2_3	0.349	1.000	0.360	1.000	0.362	1.000
	25	50	N(0, 1)	0.376	1.000	0.394	0.992	0.312	1.000
			t_5	0.294	1.000	0.301	0.993	0.312	1.000
			Centered χ^2_3	0.291	1.000	0.295	0.991	0.310	1.000
		200	N(0, 1)	0.685	1.000	0.699	0.995	0.584	1.000
			t_5	0.561	1.000	0.565	1.000	0.590	1.000
			Centered χ^2_3	0.526	1.000	0.555	1.000	0.579	1.000
66	10	50	N(0, 1)	0.450	1.000	0.491	1.000	0.386	1.000
			t_5	0.360	1.000	0.377	1.000	0.390	1.000
			Centered χ^2_3	0.366	1.000	0.403	1.000	0.388	1.000
		200	N(0, 1)	0.774	1.000	0.807	1.000	0.677	1.000
			t_5	0.642	1.000	0.692	1.000	0.688	1.000
			Centered χ^2_3	0.639	1.000	0.682	1.000	0.675	1.000
	25	50	N(0, 1)	0.688	1.000	0.694	1.000	0.581	1.000
			t_5	0.558	1.000	0.570	1.000	0.594	1.000
			Centered χ^2_3	0.534	1.000	0.530	1.000	0.569	1.000
		200	N(0, 1)	0.951	1.000	0.959	1.000	0.905	1.000
			t_5	0.874	1.000	0.888	1.000	0.906	1.000
			Centered χ^2_3	0.835	1.000	0.860	1.000	0.901	1.000
100	10	50	N(0, 1)	0.641	1.000	0.667	1.000	0.563	1.000
			t_5	0.519	1.000	0.547	1.000	0.546	1.000
			Centered χ^2_3	0.529	1.000	0.568	1.000	0.548	1.000
		200	N(0, 1)	0.928	1.000	0.945	1.000	0.868	1.000
			t_5	0.844	1.000	0.869	1.000	0.872	1.000
			Centered χ^2_3	0.843	1.000	0.881	1.000	0.873	1.000
	25	50	N(0, 1)	0.873	1.000	0.884	1.000	0.792	1.000
			t_5	0.760	1.000	0.771	1.000	0.789	1.000
			Centered χ^2_3	0.737	1.000	0.749	1.000	0.758	1.000
		200	N(0, 1)	0.997	1.000	0.997	1.000	0.985	1.000
			t_5	0.977	1.000	0.982	1.000	0.986	1.000
			Centered χ^2_3	0.964	1.000	0.967	1.000	0.965	1.000

Table 18.3 Empirical sensitivity of the test for small values of τ under H_1 for test statistics $\mathscr{R}_N(T)$ and $\mathscr{C}_N(T)$ using the asymptotic critical values, considering a significance level of 5%, weight function $w(t) = t^2$, and smoothing window width $h = 2$

T	τ	N	H_1, iid, N(0, 1)		T	τ	N	H_1, iid, N(0, 1)	
10	3	50	0.551	1.000	25	5	50	0.629	1.000
		200	0.867	1.000			200	0.927	1.000

ratio statistic depends also on the unknown variance parameter. In spite of that, the asymptotic distribution of the ratio statistic is free of this nuisance parameter. As shown in the chapter, the variance parameter and the covariances can be estimated and, consequently, used for testing whether a change in means occurred or not. This is indeed feasible, because both test statistics under the alternative converge to infinity in probability. Furthermore, the whole stochastic theory behind requires relatively simple assumptions, which are not too restrictive.

A simulation study illustrates that even for small panel size, the investigated approach based on ratio statistic $\mathscr{R}_N(T)$ works fine. It *keeps the significance level* under the null, while various simulation scenarios are considered. Besides that, the power of this test is reasonably high. The procedure based on non-ratio (CUSUM) statistic $\mathscr{C}_N(T)$ does not firmly keep the theoretical significance level. Even though the power for test based on the non-ratio statistic is higher than in case for the ratio statistic, the *non-ratio type test should not be used for small fixed panel lengths*, because of the demonstrated imperfection of not keeping the significance level under the null.

18.7 Appendix: Proofs

Proof (*of Theorem* 1) Let us define

$$U_N(t) := \frac{1}{\sigma\sqrt{N}} \sum_{i=1}^{N} \sum_{s=1}^{t} (Y_{i,s} - \mu_i).$$

Using the multivariate Lindeberg–Lévy CLT for a sequence of T-dimensional iid random vectors $\{[\sum_{s=1}^{1} \varepsilon_{i,s}, \ldots, \sum_{s=1}^{T} \varepsilon_{i,s}]^\top\}_{i\in\mathbb{N}}$, we have under H_0

$$[U_N(1), \ldots, U_N(T)]^\top \xrightarrow[N\to\infty]{\mathscr{D}} [X_1, \ldots, X_T]^\top,$$

since $\mathsf{Var}\,[\sum_{s=1}^{1} \varepsilon_{1,s}, \ldots, \sum_{s=1}^{T} \varepsilon_{1,s}]^\top = \boldsymbol{\Lambda}$. Indeed, the tth diagonal element of the covariance matrix $\boldsymbol{\Lambda}$ is $\mathsf{Var} \sum_{s=1}^{t} \varepsilon_{1,s} = r(t)$ and the upper off-diagonal element on position (t, v) is

$$\mathsf{Cov}\left(\sum_{s=1}^{t}\varepsilon_{1,s}, \sum_{u=1}^{v}\varepsilon_{1,u}\right) = \mathsf{Var}\sum_{s=1}^{t}\varepsilon_{1,s} + \mathsf{Cov}\left(\sum_{s=1}^{t}\varepsilon_{1,s}, \sum_{u=t+1}^{v}\varepsilon_{1,u}\right)$$
$$= r(t) + R(t, v), \quad t < v.$$

Moreover, let us define the reverse analogue to $U_N(t)$, i.e.,

$$V_N(t) := \frac{1}{\sigma\sqrt{N}}\sum_{i=1}^{N}\sum_{s=t+1}^{T}(Y_{i,s} - \mu_i) = U_N(T) - U_N(t).$$

Hence,

$$U_N(s) - \frac{s}{t}U_N(t) = \frac{1}{\sigma\sqrt{N}}\sum_{i=1}^{N}\left\{\sum_{r=1}^{s}\left[(Y_{i,r} - \mu_i) - \frac{1}{t}\sum_{v=1}^{t}(Y_{i,v} - \mu_i)\right]\right\}$$
$$= \frac{1}{\sigma\sqrt{N}}\sum_{i=1}^{N}\sum_{r=1}^{s}\left(Y_{i,r} - \overline{Y}_{i,t}\right)$$

and, consequently,

$$V_N(s) - \frac{T-s}{T-t}V_N(t) = \frac{1}{\sigma\sqrt{N}}\sum_{i=1}^{N}\left\{\sum_{r=s+1}^{T}\left[(Y_{i,r} - \mu_i) - \frac{1}{T-t}\sum_{v=t+1}^{T}(Y_{i,v} - \mu_i)\right]\right\}$$
$$= \frac{1}{\sigma\sqrt{N}}\sum_{i=1}^{N}\sum_{r=s+1}^{T}\left(Y_{i,r} - \widetilde{Y}_{i,t}\right).$$

Using the Cramér–Wold device, we end up with

$$\max_{t=1,\dots,T-1}\left|U_N(t) - \frac{t}{T}U_N(T)\right| \xrightarrow[N\to\infty]{\mathscr{D}} \max_{t=1,\dots,T-1}\left|X_t - \frac{t}{T}X_T\right|$$

and

$$\max_{t=2,\dots,T-2}\frac{\max_{s=1,\dots,t}\left|U_N(s) - \frac{s}{t}U_N(t)\right|}{\max_{s=t,\dots,T-1}\left|V_N(s) - \frac{T-s}{T-t}V_N(t)\right|}$$
$$\xrightarrow[N\to\infty]{\mathscr{D}} \max_{t=2,\dots,T-2}\frac{\max_{s=1,\dots,t}\left|X_s - \frac{s}{t}X_t\right|}{\max_{s=t,\dots,T-1}\left|(X_T - X_s) - \frac{T-s}{T-t}(X_T - X_t)\right|}.$$

□

Proof (*of Theorem* 2) Considering $\mathscr{C}_N(T)$, we have under alternative H_1 that

$$
\begin{aligned}
&\frac{1}{\sigma\sqrt{N}}\left|\sum_{i=1}^{N}\sum_{s=1}^{\tau}\left(Y_{i,s}-\overline{Y}_{i,T}\right)\right|\\
&=\frac{1}{\sigma\sqrt{N}}\left|\sum_{i=1}^{N}\sum_{s=1}^{\tau}\left(\mu_i+\sigma\varepsilon_{i,s}-\frac{1}{T}\sum_{v=1}^{T}(\mu_i+\sigma\varepsilon_{i,v})-\frac{1}{T}\delta_i\right)\right|\\
&=\frac{1}{\sqrt{N}}\left|\sum_{i=1}^{N}\sum_{s=1}^{\tau}\left(\varepsilon_{i,s}-\overline{\varepsilon}_{i,T}\right)-\frac{\tau}{\sigma T}\sum_{i=1}^{N}\delta_i\right|=\mathscr{O}_{\mathsf{P}}(1)+\frac{\tau}{\sigma T\sqrt{N}}\left|\sum_{i=1}^{N}\delta_i\right|\xrightarrow{\mathsf{P}}\infty,\quad N\to\infty,
\end{aligned}
$$

where $\overline{\varepsilon}_{i,T}=\frac{1}{\tau}\sum_{v=1}^{T}\varepsilon_{i,v}$.

In case of $\mathscr{R}_N(T)$, let $t=\tau+1$. Then under alternative H_1, it holds that

$$
\begin{aligned}
&\frac{1}{\sigma\sqrt{N}}\max_{s=1,\ldots,\tau+1}\left|\sum_{i=1}^{N}\sum_{r=1}^{s}\left(Y_{i,r}-\overline{Y}_{i,\tau+1}\right)\right|\geq\frac{1}{\sigma\sqrt{N}}\left|\sum_{i=1}^{N}\sum_{r=1}^{\tau}\left(Y_{i,r}-\overline{Y}_{i,\tau+1}\right)\right|\\
&=\frac{1}{\sigma\sqrt{N}}\left|\sum_{i=1}^{N}\sum_{r=1}^{\tau}\left(\mu_i+\sigma\varepsilon_{i,r}-\frac{1}{\tau+1}\sum_{v=1}^{\tau+1}(\mu_i+\sigma\varepsilon_{i,v})-\frac{1}{\tau+1}\delta_i\right)\right|\\
&=\frac{1}{\sqrt{N}}\left|\sum_{i=1}^{N}\sum_{r=1}^{\tau}\left(\varepsilon_{i,r}-\overline{\varepsilon}_{i,\tau+1}\right)-\frac{\tau}{\sigma(\tau+1)}\sum_{i=1}^{N}\delta_i\right|\\
&=\mathscr{O}_{\mathsf{P}}(1)+\frac{\tau}{\sigma(\tau+1)\sqrt{N}}\left|\sum_{i=1}^{N}\delta_i\right|\xrightarrow{\mathsf{P}}\infty,\quad N\to\infty,
\end{aligned}
$$

where $\overline{\varepsilon}_{i,\tau+1}=\frac{1}{\tau+1}\sum_{v=1}^{\tau+1}\varepsilon_{i,v}$.

Since there is no change after $\tau+1$ and $\tau\leq T-3$, then by Theorem 1 we obtain

$$
\frac{1}{\sigma\sqrt{N}}\max_{s=\tau+1,\ldots,T-1}\left|\sum_{i=1}^{N}\sum_{r=s+1}^{T}\left(Y_{i,r}-\widetilde{Y}_{i,\tau+1}\right)\right|\xrightarrow[N\to\infty]{\mathscr{D}}\max_{s=\tau+1,\ldots,T-1}\left|Z_s-\frac{T-s}{T-\tau}Z_{\tau+1}\right|.
$$

□

Acknowledgements The authors would like to thank an anonymous referee for the suggestions that improved this chapter. Institutional support to Barbora Peštová was provided by RVO:67985807. The research of Michal Pešta was supported by the Czech Science Foundation project "DYME—Dynamic Models in Economics" No. P402/12/G097.

References

1. Andrews, D.W.K.: Heteroskedasticity and autocorrelation consistent covariance matrix estimation. Econometrica **59**(3), 817–858 (1991)
2. Bai, J.: Common breaks in means and variances for panel data. J. Econom. **157**(1), 78–92 (2010)

3. Bai, J., Carrion-I-Silvestre, J.L.: Structural changes, common stochastic trends, and unit roots in panel data. Rev. Econ. Stud. **76**(2), 471–501 (2009)
4. Chan, J., Horváth, L., Hušková, M.: Change-point detection in panel data. J. Stat. Plan. Infer. **143**(5), 955–970 (2013)
5. Csörgő, M., Horváth, L.: Limit Theorems in Change-Point Analysis. Wiley, Chichester (1997)
6. Horváth, L., Horváth, Z., Hušková, M.: Ratio tests for change point detection. In: Balakrishnan, N., Peña, E.A., Silvapulle, M.J. (eds.) Beyond Parametrics in Interdisciplinary Research: Festschrift in Honor of Professor Pranab K. Sen, vol. 1, pp. 293–304. IMS Collections, Beachwood, Ohio (2009)
7. Horváth, L., Hušková, M.: Change-point detection in panel data. J. Time Ser. Anal. **33**(4), 631–648 (2012)
8. Im, K.S., Lee, J., Tieslau, M.: Panel LM unit-root tests with level shifts. Oxford B. Econ. Stat. **67**(3), 393–419 (2005)
9. Lindner, A.M.: Stationarity, mixing, distributional properties and moments of GARCH(p, q)-processes. In: Andersen, T.G., Davis, R.A., Kreiss, J.P., Mikosch, T. (eds.) Handbook of Financial Time Series, pp. 481–496. Springer, Berlin (2009)
10. Madurkayová, B.: Ratio type statistics for detection of changes in mean. Acta Universitatis Carolinae: Mathematica et Physica **52**(1), 47–58 (2011)
11. Peštová, B., Pešta, M.: Testing structural changes in panel data with small fixed panel size and bootstrap. Metrika **78**(6), 665–689 (2015)
12. Peštová, B., Pešta, M.: Erratum to: Testing structural changes in panel data with small fixed panel size and bootstrap. Metrika **79**(2), 237–238 (2016)

Chapter 19
How Robust Is the Two-Sample Triangular Sequential T-Test Against Variance Heterogeneity?

Dieter Rasch and Takuya Yanagida

Abstract Reference (Rasch, Kubinger and Moder (2011b). Stat. Pap. 52, 219–231.) [4] showed that in case that nothing is known about the two variances it is better to use the approximate Welch test instead of the two-sample t-test for comparing means of two continuous distributions with existing first two moments. An analogue approach for the triangular sequential t test is not possible because it is based on the first two derivatives of the underlying likelihood functions. Extensive simulations have been done and are reported in this chapter. It is shown that the two-sample triangular sequential t test in most interesting cases holds the type I and type II risks when variances are unequal.

Keywords Comparing expectations · t test · Welch test · Triangular sequential t-test · Unequal variances

19.1 Comparing Two Means of Continuous Distributions

More details about the tests below and their robustness against non-normality can be found in Rasch and Schott [6] or [5].

We restrict ourselves to location parameters of two independent samples from two continuous distributions with existing first two moments. For testing the equality of means of those distributions [2] showed by simulation experiments that tests based on normal assumptions can be applied even if the distribution are skewed or have considerable kurtosis. Scale parameters however are sensitive against deviations from normality. The authors defined robustness as follows:

D. Rasch (✉)
University of Natural Resources and Life Sciences, Vienna, Austria
e-mail: d_rasch@t-online.de

T. Yanagida
University of Applied Sciences Upper Austria, Vienna, Austria
e-mail: takuya.yanagida@fh-linz.at

J. Pilz et al. (eds.), *Statistics and Simulation*, Springer Proceedings in Mathematics & Statistics 231, https://doi.org/10.1007/978-3-319-76035-3_19

Definition 1 Let $\mathbf{d}_\alpha$[1] be a confidence estimation based on an experimental design V_n of size n concerning a parameter θ of a class G of distributions with (nominal) confidence coefficient $1-\alpha_{act}(0<\alpha_{nom}<1)$ in G. For an element $h \in H \supset G$ of a class H of distributions which contains G, we denote by $1-\alpha_{act}$ the actual confidence coefficient of $\mathbf{d}_\alpha$. Then, we call $\mathbf{d}_\alpha(1-\varepsilon)$ robust in H if $\max_{h \in H} |\alpha_{nom}-\alpha_{act}| \leq \varepsilon$.

Due to the fact that a test for testing a null hypothesis $H_0 : \theta = \theta_0$ can be performed by accepting H_0 if θ_0 is inside the confidence interval and reject it otherwise; Definition 1 includes the robustness of a test concerning the significance level α_{nom}.

Reference [2] used for G the family of univariate normal $(N(\mu, \sigma^2)-)$ distributions and for H the Fleishman system of distributions.

Definition 2 A distribution belongs to the Fleishman system [1] if its first four moments exist and if it is the distribution of the transform

$\mathbf{y} = a + b\mathbf{x} + c\mathbf{x}^2 + d\mathbf{x}^3$

where $\mathbf{x}$ is a standard normal random variable (with mean 0 and variance 1).

By a proper choice of the coefficient a, b, c and d the random variable y will have any quadruple of first four moments $(\mu, \sigma^2, \gamma_1), \gamma_2)$. By γ_1 and γ_2, we denote the skewness (standardized third moment) and the kurtosis (standardized fourth moment) of any distribution respectively. For instance, any normal distribution (i.e. any element of G) with mean μ and variance σ^2 can be represented as a member of the Fleishman system by choosing $a = \mu$, $b = \sigma$ and $c = d = 0$. This shows that we really have $H \supset G$ as demanded in Definition 1.

It is known that all probability and empirical distributions (with existing fourth-order moment) fulfil the inequality

$$\gamma_2 \geq -2\,(g_2 \geq g_1^2 - 2)$$

Here g_1 and g_2 are estimates of γ_1 and γ_2, respectively.

The equality sign defines a parabola in the (γ_1, γ_2)-plane $\{(g_1, g_2)$-plane$\}$.

In Fig. 19.1, the position of the (g_1, g_2)-values calculated for the 144 characters from agricultural data in that parabola are shown (weakly printed). The six (γ_1, γ_2)-values used by [2] are shown as bold. As it can be seen these values cover the range of empirical values quite good (due to symmetry negative skewness was not regarded). [2] used in Definition 1 the value $\in = 0.1$ so that a test with a nominal risk $\alpha_{nom} = 0.05$ is considered as 90%-robust as long as $0.04 \leq \alpha_{act} \leq 0.06$.

All tests below have been found to be at least 90%-robust.

Therefore in the following, we exemplify everything for expectations of normal distributions.

We independently sample n_1 and n_2 observations, respectively, from each of two continuous distributions (population 1 and 2) with existing fourth moment having potentially different expectations μ_1 and μ_2. That is, the null hypothesis is $H_0 : \mu_1 = \mu_2$.

---

[1]Random variables are boldt print.

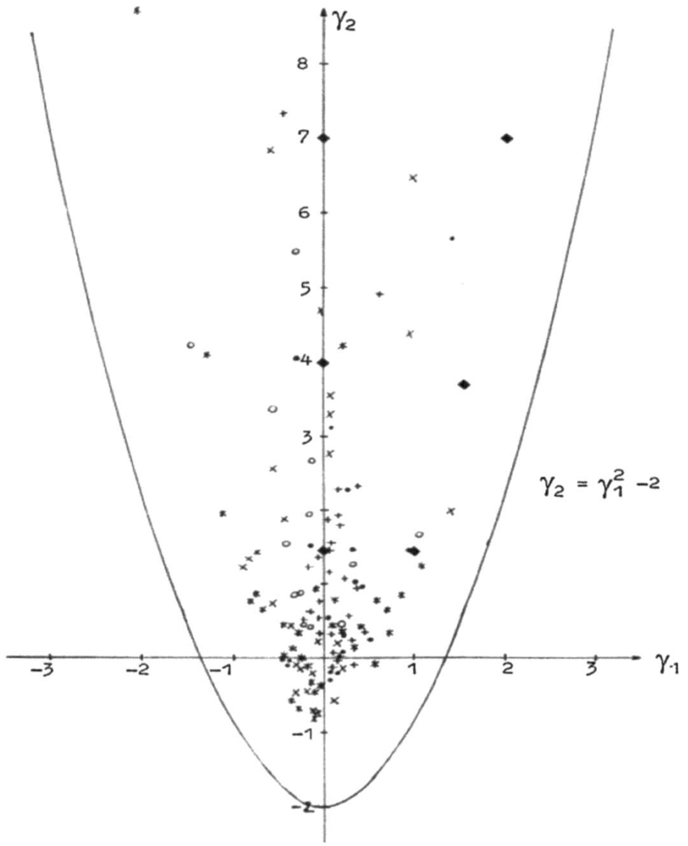

Fig. 19.1 Values of empirical skewness g_1 and kurtosis g_2 of 144 characters in a (γ_1, γ_2)-plane, by the parameters (γ_1, γ_2) of the six distributions of the Fleishman system used by [2]

The one-sided alternative hypothesis is then $H_A : \mu_1 > \mu_2$, or that is to say $H_A : \delta = \mu_1 - \mu_2 > 0$.

The two-sided alternative hypothesis is then $H_A : \mu_1 \neq \mu_2$, or that is to say $H_A : \delta = \mu_1 - \mu_2 \neq 0$.

Given that the null hypothesis is true, for any α-test, the value of the power function is equal to α for all sample sizes n_1 and n_2. Given that the alternative hypothesis is true, the value of the power function depends on the actual value of δ and the sample sizes n_1 and n_2. Thus, when we try for a certain type II risk of, for instance $\beta = 0.10$, we must fix the δ as well. In the following, we restrict ourselves to normal distributions because there is a wide range of distributions with considerable values of skewness and kurtosis parameters where the tests based on normality assumptions work well [2].

19.1.1 The Two-Sample T Test

Assuming that

- both distributions are normal and
- they have common variances $\sigma^2 = \sigma_2^2 = \sigma^2$

the two-sample t-test based on the test statistic

$$t = \frac{\overline{y}_1 - \overline{y}_2}{s}\sqrt{\frac{n_1 n_2}{n_1 + n_2}} \tag{19.1}$$

with

$$\mathbf{s} = \frac{\sum_{i=1}^{n_1}(\mathbf{y}_{1i} - \overline{y}_1)^2 + \sum_{i=1}^{n_2}(\mathbf{y}_{2i} - \overline{y}_2)}{n_1 + n_2 - 2} \tag{19.2}$$

is the most powerful unbiased test for all α. The test statistic (19.1) is non-centrally t-distributed with $n_1 + n_2 - 2$ degrees of freedom. Under the null hypothesis, (19.1) is (centrally) t-distributed.

19.1.2 The Welch Test

If the assumption of equal variances is either not fulfilled or it is not known if it is fulfilled an approximate t-test is used. The distribution of

$$\mathbf{t}^* = \frac{\overline{y}_1 - \overline{y}_2 - (\mu_1 - \mu_2)}{\sqrt{\frac{s_1^2}{n_1} + \frac{s_2^2}{n_2}}}, \mathbf{s}_k^2 = \frac{1}{n_k - 1}\sum\nolimits_{i=1}^{n_k}(\mathbf{y}_{ik} - \overline{\mathbf{y}}_k)^2, k = 1, 2$$

was derived by [11] from this stems the name Welch-test.

To test
$H_0 : \mu_1 = \mu_2, \sigma_1^2, \sigma_2^2$ arbitrary
against
a)
$H_A : \mu_1 > \mu_2, \sigma_1^2, \sigma_2^2$ arbitrary
or b)
$H_A : \mu_1 \neq \mu_2, \sigma_1^2, \sigma_2^2$ arbitrary,
we use the statistic

$$t^* = \frac{\overline{y}_1 - \overline{y}_2}{\sqrt{\frac{s_1^2}{n_1} + \frac{s_2^2}{n_2}}}, \tag{19.3}$$

and reject H_0 if

(a) t^* exceeds the $(1-\alpha)$-quantile or
(b) $|t^*|$ exceeds the $(1-\frac{\alpha}{2})$-quantile of the central t-distribution with
(c) $f^* = \frac{\left(\frac{s_1^2}{n_1}+\frac{s_2^2}{n_2}\right)^2}{\frac{s_1^4}{n_1^2(n_1-1)}+\frac{s_2^4}{n_1^2(n_1-1)}}$ degrees of freedom, respectively.

Reference [4] showed that in case that nothing is known about the two variances it is better to use always the approximate Welch test instead of the two-sample t test. Also, pretesting the hypothesis of equality of variances and to continue with the t test in case of acceptation and with the Welch-test in case of rejection is not preferable.

To determine the sizes of the two samples the approximate formulae

$$n_1 \approx \left\lceil \frac{\sigma_1(\sigma_1+\sigma_2)}{\delta^2}[\{t(f^*;P)+t(f^*;1-\beta)\}]^2 \right\rceil \text{ and } n_2 \left\lceil \frac{\sigma_2\sigma_1}{n \quad _1} \right\rceil \tag{19.4}$$

can be used by putting $P = 1-\alpha$ in the one-sided and $P = 1-\alpha/2$ in the two-sided case. A rough estimation of the unknown variances can be obtained using the anticipated range of the character in question (the difference of maximal and minimal outcome) in the two distribution, respectively, divided by six, and the result may be used as an estimate for σ_1 and σ_2 respectively.

19.1.3 The Sequential Triangular T-Test

The first paper on sequential analysis (or design) was written during World War II by Abraham Wald. Namely Wald, A. [8] Sequential Analysis of Statistical Data; Theory Statist. Res. Group Rep. 75, Columbia University. The first easy accessible publication was [9] and the first book [10]. Wald developed the so-called probability ratio test what is now called the likelihood ratio test, a term we will use in future. In triangular designs, the continuation region is closed and in triangular form. It is based on an asymptotic test described in Rasch and schott [6] and in Sect. 5.4 in [3] where also some of the theory of sequential tests can be found. Triangular tests have been developed by Whitehead (1992) [12] and [7].

By the triangular sequential test, we test in the one-sided case
$H_0: \mu_1 = \mu_2, \sigma_1^2 = \sigma_2^2 = \sigma^2$ arbitrary
against
$H_A: \mu_1 > \mu_2, \sigma_1^2 = \sigma_2^2 = \sigma^2$ arbitrary

Putting $\theta = \frac{\mu_1-\mu_2}{\sigma} = \frac{\delta}{\sigma}$, we calculate from the n_1 and n_2 observations the maximum-likelihood-estimate (non-random) s^2 obtained from (19.2).

Then, we calculate

$$z_n = \frac{n_1 n_2}{n_1+n_2}\frac{\overline{y}_1-\overline{y}_2}{s}, \; v_n = \frac{n_1 n_2}{n_1+n_2}\frac{z_n^2}{2(n_1+n_2)}. \tag{19.5}$$

and accept H_0 , if $z_n \leq a + bv_n$. The triangle is defined by the two lines $a + bv_n$ and $-a + 3bv_n$ If z_n leaves this triangle for $z_n \leq -a + 3bv_n$ or meets the boundaries, H_A is accepted. The two constants a and b have to be chosen as follows:

$$a = \frac{1}{\theta}\left(1 + \frac{z_{1-\beta}}{z_{1-\alpha}}\right) \ln\left(1 + \frac{1}{2\alpha}\right) \tag{19.6}$$

$$b = \frac{\theta_1}{2\left(1 + \frac{z_{1-\beta}}{z_{1-\alpha}}\right)} \tag{19.7}$$

with the P-quantiles z_P of the standard normal distribution.

The two boundary lines meet in the point $(v_{\max}; z_{\max}) = \left(\frac{a}{b}; 2a\right)$.

If just this point is met, then accept H_A. This point defines the maximum sample size. It is larger than the size needed for the fixed sample size problem with the same precision, but the latter is larger than the average sample size of the triangular test.

Unfortunately, there exists no Welch-type approach for the sequential triangular test. It is the aim of this chapter to investigate the behaviour of the test above if variances are unequal.

19.2 The Robustness of the Two-Sample Triangular Sequential Test Against Variance Heterogeneity a Simulation Study

Because the two variances are unknown, we at first assume that sample 1 stems from the distribution with the larger variance. Then, we can proceed as follows: the anticipated range of the character in question (the difference of maximal and minimal outcome) has to be divided by six, and the result may be used as an estimate for σ_1. Now we use in the simulation experiment $\theta = \frac{\mu_1 - \mu_2}{\sigma_1}$ with $\theta = 0, 2, 0.4, 0.6, 0.8$, and 1.0. All simulation conditions were investigated with the nominal risks $\alpha_{nom} = 0.05$; $\beta_{nom} = 0.1$ and 0.2. Data were simulated in R version 3.2.3 (R Core Team, 2015) based on a normal distribution with $\sigma_1 = 10$ and σ_2 ranging 1 to 10 with an increment of 1.

In sum, 100,000 runs were conducted using the R packages seqtest [13] for each simulation condition. By N_{fix} we denote the sum of the two sample sizes and from (19.4). Some of our results are shown below: In the Tables 19.1, 19.2, 19.3, 19.4, 19.5, 19.6, 19.7, 19.8, 19.9, and 19.10 α_{act} and β_{act} are the relative frequencies of wrongly rejecting or accepting the null hypothesis in the 100,000 runs, respectively. ASN is the average sample number (in both samples) over all runs and N_{fix} is the size of both samples needed when using the fixed sample Welch test; thus, $N_{fix} = n_1 + n_2$ with values on the r.h.s from (19.4). In Tables 19.1, 19.2, 19.3, 19.4, 19.5, 19.6, 19.7, 19.8, 19.9, and 19.10 the simulation results are given.

Table 19.1 Simulation results for $\beta_{nom} = 0.1$ and $\theta = 0.2$

$H_0: \mu_1 \geq \mu_2$ *versus* $H_A: \mu_1 < \mu_2$

σ_1	10	10	10	10	10	10	10	10	10	10
σ_2	1	2	3	4	5	6	7	8	9	10
α_{act}	0.050	0.050	0.050	0.048	0.049	0.049	0.050	0.049	0.049	0.050
β_{act}	0.007	0.008	0.010	0.015	0.019	0.028	0.039	0.054	0.074	0.097
$ASN\|\|\nu_1$	466.492	465.976	466.870	465.106	466.145	465.311	464.990	464.544	465.676	465.525
$ASN\|\nu_2$	368.015	373.852	383.785	397.452	413.209	433.397	452.942	474.224	495.472	516.542
N_{fix}	260	310	364	421	484	550	620	696	775	860

Table 19.2 Simulation results for $\beta_{nom} = 0.1$ and $\theta = 0.4$

$H_0: \mu_1 \geq \mu_2$ *versus* $H_A: \mu_1 < \mu_2$

σ_1	10	10	10	10	10	10	10	10	10	10
σ_2	1	2	3	4	5	6	7	8	9	10
α_{act}	0.052	0.051	0.051	0.049	0.051	0.049	0.048	0.048	0.049	0.049
β_{act}	0.007	0.008	0.010	0.013	0.019	0.026	0.037	0.052	0.069	0.092
$ASN\|\nu_1$	118.470	118.608	118.338	118.156	118.687	118.242	118.344	118.178	118.416	118.824
$ASN\|\nu_2$	94.185	95.975	98.642	102.348	106.394	111.171	116.718	121.891	127.249	132.071
N_{fix}	67	79	92	107	123	139	156	176	195	216

Table 19.3 Simulation results for $\beta_{nom} = 0.1$ and $\theta = 0.6$

$H_0: \mu_1 \geq \mu_2$ *versus* $H_A: \mu_1 < \mu_2$

σ_1	10	10	10	10	10	10	10	10	10	10
σ_2	1	2	3	4	5	6	7	8	9	10
α_{act}	0.055	0.054	0.054	0.051	0.050	0.050	0.048	0.050	0.049	0.048
β_{act}	0.007	0.008	0.010	0.012	0.018	0.025	0.036	0.049	0.069	0.091
$ASN\|\nu_1$	53.183	53.395	53.418	53.426	53.359	53.514	53.532	53.438	53.752	53.762
$ASN\|\nu_2$	43.512	44.398	45.564	47.219	49.253	51.345	53.731	55.989	58.435	60.884
N_{fix}	30	36	42	49	55	64	71	79	89	98

Table 19.4 Simulation results for $\beta_{nom} = 0.1$ and $\theta = 0.8$

$H_0: \mu_1 \geq \mu_2$ *versus* $H_A: \mu_1 < \mu_2$

σ_1	10	10	10	10	10	10	10	10	10	10
σ_2	1	2	3	4	5	6	7	8	9	10
α_{act}	0.061	0.061	0.059	0.055	0.054	0.052	0.052	0.050	0.051	0.050
β_{act}	0.006	0.007	0.009	0.012	0.016	0.024	0.033	0.048	0.066	0.086
$ASN\|\nu_1$	30.340	30.482	30.590	30.558	30.737	30.790	30.816	30.845	30.792	30.832
$ASN\|\nu_2$	25.754	26.156	26.900	27.865	28.994	30.242	31.463	32.930	34.219	35.361
N_{fix}	18	21	24	28	33	36	40	46	51	56

Table 19.5 Simulation results for $\beta_{nom} = 0.1$ and $\theta = 1.0$

$H_0 : \mu_1 \geq \mu_2$ *versus* $H_A : \mu_1 < \mu_2$

σ_1	10	10	10	10	10	10	10	10	10	10
σ_2	1	2	3	4	5	6	7	8	9	10
α_{act}	t 0.071	0.068	0.065	0.060	0.057	0.054	0.053	0.052	0.052	0.052
β_{act}	0.006	0.007	0.008	0.012	0.015	0.020	0.030	0.046	0.058	0.081
$ASN\|\mu_1$	19.725	19.834	19.856	20.007	20.079	20.191	20.201	20.150	20.197	20.211
$ASN\|\mu_2$	17.578	17.929	18.295	18.905	19.456	20.492	21.238	21.984	22.745	23.807
N_{fix}	9	14	16	19	22	24	27	30	34	36

Table 19.6 Simulation results for $\beta_{nom} = 0.2$ and $\theta = 0.2$

$H_0 : \mu_1 \geq \mu_2$ *versus* $H_A : \mu_1 < \mu_2$

σ_1	10	10	10	10	10	10	10	10	10	10
σ_2	1	2	3	4	5	6	7	8	9	10
α_{act}	0.049	0.050	0.049	0.050	0.049	0.049	0.050	0.048	0.049	0.049
β_{act}	0.031	0.034	0.040	0.050	0.063	0.081	0.104	0.130	0.159	0.194
$ASN\|\mu_1$	337.641	337.645	336.633	337.074	337.077	336.947	337.236	337.682	336.342	337.323
$ASN\|\mu_2$	318.856	323.103	330.800	340.625	352.361	365.580	379.303	392.092	403.067	414.979
N_{fix}	189	224	263	305	349	398	448	504	560	620

Table 19.7 Simulation results for $\beta_{nom} = 0.2$ and $\theta = 0.4$

$H_0 : \mu_1 \geq \mu_2$ *versus* $H_A : \mu_1 < \mu_2$

σ_1	10	10	10	10	10	10	10	10	10	10
σ_2	1	2	3	4	5	6	7	8	9	10
α_{act}	0.054	0.052	0.051	0.052	0.050	0.050	0.048	0.049	0.049	0.049
β_{act}	0.028	0.033	0.038	0.048	0.060	0.077	0.099	0.126	0.154	0.189
$ASN\|\mu_1$	85.923	85.786	85.891	85.615	85.922	85.982	86.089	86.221	86.068	85.927
$ASN\|\mu_2$	81.530	82.890	85.169	87.907	91.047	93.957	97.617	100.947	104.048	107.083
N_{fix}	48	57	67	78	88	100	115	127	142	158

Table 19.8 Simulation results for $\beta_{nom} = 0.2$ and $\theta = 0.6$

$H_0 : \mu_1 \geq \mu_2$ *versus* $H_A : \mu_1 < \mu_2$

σ_1	10	10	10	10	10	10	10	10	10	10
σ_2	1	2	3	4	5	6	7	8	9	10
α_{act}	0.059	0.058	0.055	0.055	0.052	0.050	0.049	0.049	0.049	0.049
β_{act}	0.027	0.031	0.035	0.044	0.057	0.073	0.095	0.120	0.150	0.182
$ASN\|\mu_1$	38.599	38.655	38.833	38.926	39.071	39.079	39.062	39.060	39.128	39.212
$ASN\|\mu_2$	37.663	38.286	39.262	40.589	41.988	43.528	45.100	46.643	47.986	49.283
N_{fix}	23	26	31	36	40	46	52	57	64	72

Table 19.9 Simulation results for $\beta_{nom} = 0.2$ and $\theta = 0.8$

$H_0: \mu_1 \geq \mu_2$ versus $H_A: \mu_1 < \mu_2$										
σ_1	10	10	10	10	10	10	10	10	10	10
σ_2	1	2	3	4	5	6	7	8	9	10
α_{act}	0.068	0.065	0.063	0.058	0.056	0.054	0.053	0.052	0.051	0.051
β_{act}	0.025	0.030	0.035	0.043	0.054	0.072	0.090	0.115	0.142	0.174
$ASN\|\mu_1$	22.174	22.189	22.351	22.336	22.527	22.521	22.614	22.619	22.607	22.565
$ASN\|\mu_2$	22.299	22.631	23.272	23.988	24.792	25.675	26.513	27.43	28.226	28.860
N_{fix}	14	16	18	21	24	27	30	34	38	42

Table 19.10 Simulation results for $\beta_{nom} = 0.2$ and $\theta = 1.0$

$H_0: \mu_1 \geq \mu_2$ versus $H_A: \mu_1 < \mu_2$										
σ_1	10	10	10	10	10	10	10	10	10	10
σ_2	1	2	3	4	5	6	7	8	9	10
α_{act}	0.078	0.072	0.068	0.063	0.061	0.057	0.056	0.054	0.053	0.054
β_{act}	0.022	0.025	0.031	0.039	0.049	0.065	0.084	0.111	0.133	0.168
$ASN\|\mu_1$	14.472	14.623	14.658	14.768	14.832	14.877	14.879	14.923	14.911	14.892
$ASN\|\mu_2$	15.287	15.429	15.863	16.226	16.623	17.388	17.979	18.478	18.927	19.318
N_{fix}	14	16	18	21	24	27	30	34	38	42

19.3 Discussion

As it can be seen from the tables, the empirical first-kind risk α_{act} is approximately equal to the nominal one or the test at least 90%-robust if $\theta \leq 0.7$. If $\theta > 0.7$, the test is only applicable if $\frac{\sigma_2}{\sigma_1} > 0.5$. The empirical second-kind risk β_{act} is small if the variances are unequal and monotonically increasing with increasing variance in the second sample reaching approximately the nominal second-kind risk if both variances are equal. The average sample numbers $ASN|\mu_1$ and $ASN|\mu_2$ at μ_1 and μ_2, respectively, are for $\sigma_2 < 4$ larger than the size of the Welch test, for $\sigma_2 = 4$ approximately equal to the size of the Welch test and for larger σ_2 smaller than the size of the Welch test (Table 19.9).

Summarizing we may say that the use of the two-sample triangular sequential test holds both nominal risks as long as $\frac{\sigma_1^2}{\sigma_2^2} > 10$ The empirical second-kind risk β_{act} is very small for small values of σ_2 on cost of a high average sample size. But if nothing is known about the actual value of σ_2, there is no improvement possible by using a larger nominal second-kind risk. We finally can recommend the use of the two-sample triangular sequential test even if variances possibly are unequal but $\frac{\sigma_1^2}{\sigma_2^2}$ is expected to be smaller than 10.

References

1. Fleishman, A.J.: A method for simulating non-normal distributions. Psychometrika **43**, 521–532 (1978)
2. Rasch, D., Guiard, V.: The robustness of parametric statistical methods. Psychol. Sci. **46**, 175–208 (2004)
3. Rasch, D., Pilz, J., Gebhardt, A., Verdooren, R.L.: Optimal Experimental Design with R. Chapman and Hall, Boca Raton (2011a)
4. Rasch, D., Kubinger, K.D., Moder, K.: The two-sample t test: pre-testing its assumptions does not pay off. Stat. Pap. **52**, 219–231 (2011b)
5. Rasch, D., Kubinger, K.D., Yanagida, T.: Statistics in Psychology using R and SPSS. Wiley, New York (2011c)
6. Rasch, D., Schott, D.: Mathematical Statistics, Wiley, Oxford (2018)
7. Schneider, B.: An interactive computer program for design and monitoring of sequential clinical trials. In: Proceedings of the XVIth international biometric conference, pp. 237–250. Hamilton, New Zealand (1992)
8. Wald, A.: Sequential analysis of statistical data. Theory Statistical Research Group Report 75, Columbia University (1943)
9. Wald, A.: On cumulative sums of random variables. Ann. Math. Stat. **15**, 283–296 (1944)
10. Wald, A.: Sequential Analysis. Wiley, New York (1947), Whitehead, J.: The Design and Analysis of Sequential Clinical Trial, 2nd edn. Chichester, Ellis Horwood (1997), Whitehead, J.: The Design and Analysis of Sequential Clinical Trials, 2. rev. edn. Wiley, New York (1997)
11. Welch, B.L.: The generalization of Students problem when several different population variances are involved. Biometrika **34**, 2835 (1947)
12. Whitehead, J.: The Design and Analysis of Sequential Clinical Trials, Ellis Horwood, Chichester (1992)
13. Yanagida, T.: Seqtest: sequential triangular test. R package version 0.1-0 (2016). http://CRAN.R-project.org/package=seqtest

Part V
Clinical Trials and Design of Experiments

Chapter 20
Performances of Poisson–Gamma Model for Patients' Recruitment in Clinical Trials When There Are Pauses in Recruitment or When the Number of Centres is Small

Nathan Minois, Guillaume Mijoule, Stéphanie Savy, Valérie Lauwers-Cances, Sandrine Andrieu and Nicolas Savy

Abstract To predict the duration of a clinical trial is a question of paramount interest. To date, the more elaborated model is the so-called Poisson–gamma model introduced by Anisimov and Fedorov in 2007. Theoretical performances of this model are asymptotic and have been established under assumptions especially on the recruitment rates by centre which are assumed to be constant in time. In order to evaluate the practical use of this model, ranges of validity have to be assessed. By means of simulation studies, authors investigate, on the one hand, the impact of the number of centres involved, of the average recruitment rate, of the duration of recruitment and of the interim time of analysis on the expected duration of the trial and, on the other hand, two strategies of estimation of the trial duration accounting for breaks

N. Minois · S. Savy · S. Andrieu
INSERM UMR 1027, University of Toulouse III, 31073 Toulouse, France
e-mail: nathan.minois@inserm.fr

S. Savy
e-mail: sm.savy@gmail.fr

G. Mijoule
University of Paris XI, 91405 Orsay, France
e-mail: guillaume.mijoule@gmail.com

V. Lauwers-Cances
Epidemiology Unit, CHU Purpan, 31062 Toulouse, France
e-mail: lauwers-cances.v@chu-toulouse.fr

S. Andrieu
Epidemiology Unit of Toulouse CHU, 31073 Toulouse, France
e-mail: sandrine.andrieu@univ-tlse.fr

N. Savy (✉)
Toulouse Institute of Mathematics, University of Toulouse III,
31062 Toulouse, France
e-mail: nicolas.savy@math.univ-toulouse.fr

J. Pilz et al. (eds.), *Statistics and Simulation*, Springer Proceedings
in Mathematics & Statistics 231, https://doi.org/10.1007/978-3-319-76035-3_20

in recruitment (period during which centres do not recruit) which are compared and discussed. These investigations yield to guidelines on the use of Poisson–gamma processes to model recruitment dynamics regarding these issues.

Keywords Clinical trials · Recruitment time · Bayesian statistics · Cox processes

20.1 Introduction

In order to get marketing authorization, a new product has to succeed in clinical trials. A clinical trial is based on statistical considerations in order to show the product efficiency, taking into account the variability of the environment. It is a well-known fact that the power of the statistical test involved is linked to the number of patients one deals with. If an inadequate number of enrolled patients is used, the study may fail to reject the null hypothesis due to lack of power. The number of patients to include, usually called necessary sample size, is thus a fixed parameter of the trial. Its computation is now standard in trial protocols and mandatory for most of the publications. It is a surprising fact that, on the one side, much effort has been devoted in computing the necessary sample size for clinical trials, while on the other side, relatively little attention is focused on improving the prediction of the recruitment process. Indeed, till now, most of techniques used by pharmaceutical companies are based on deterministic models and various ad hoc techniques. "Patient recruitment and retention remains until now more of an art rather than a science" [15].

The problem of predicting patients' recruitment and evaluating the recruitment duration in clinical trials is of paramount interest for planning trials because of scientific, economic and ethical reasons. Ethical concern because it is not satisfactory to continue a study in vain. Economical concern because a clinical trial is an expensive study in itself and, as the duration of the trial is included in the duration of the exclusive right to exploit the drug, a delay generates an enormous loss of incomes. And scientific concern because new drugs are increasingly developed and approved by regulatory agencies, and when accrual rates are too low, there may be new information available during the enrolment period such as the results of other trials or a change in the understanding of the underlying biology. For these reasons, stopping or continuing a trial is a decision with huge consequences and to develop some objective tools, based on scientific criteria, would be useful to decide.

Few authors have considered the problem of patients' recruitment modelling. The reader can refer to [9] for a systematic review of the existing models. As far as we know, the pioneer work is one of [14] where an estimation of the study duration is proposed as a function of inclusion duration and based on data from previous clinical trials. Let us cite [11] for a model of recruitment by Poisson processes. In [16], a model for multicentric trial based on Poisson process is introduced. However, Poisson processes depend on only one parameter, the enrolment rate, and [10] have noticed that the use of the historic mean is too simple. It is thus necessary to take into consideration variability in the rate.

Poisson–gamma model introduced in [7] assumes that the patients arrive at different centres according to Poisson processes with the rates viewed as independent gamma-distributed random variables. The procedure of parameters estimation at interim stage using empirical Bayesian techniques has been suggested in [7]. The model has been validated using data from a large number of real trials [3]. The Poisson–gamma model was developed further for predicting recruitment process at initial and interim stages [1], to account for the situations when the centres opening dates may not be known and assumed to be uniformly distributed in some intervals [2, 12], some centres can be closed or open in the future [6]. Finally, sensitivity analyses to errors in parameters' estimation can be found in [12]. Poisson-gamma model can be used as a basis for developing techniques for the analysis of the effect of centre stratification on randomization [4], for predictive event modelling [5], for predicting randomization process [6] and for management of dropout.

The Poisson–gamma approach on patients recruitment modelling is now popular, but two questions of paramount interest emerge. First, for which values of the recruitment parameters (number of centres, average recruitment rate for each centre, duration of the trial, interim time of analysis), the model is relevant? Second, is the assumption on the rate, which is assumed constant in time, realistic. These questions are investigated in this chapter by means of simulation studies. The first question is easy to investigate by varying the parameters of the model. The second is much more difficult. A particular setting, of practical interest is to consider breaks in recruitment. A break is defined as a period during which a centre does not recruit any patient (holidays, weekend,..). These information are observed and can be collected, but, in practice, it is a huge and complicated work. Two strategies of estimation of recruitment duration are proposed in this chapter accounting or not breaks. These strategies are compared in terms of bias in estimation and in terms of predictive performances. These investigations allow us to deal with the question: Is it really useful to enrich the model in order to take into account breaks in recruitments? These results are deepened in [13] where a third strategy of analysis is considered along with a comparison of the strategies.

The chapter is organized as follows. Section 20.2 describes the Poisson–gamma model, the estimation procedure is given, and the computation of the expected duration of the trial is discussed. Section 20.3 explains the strategy used to take into account breaks in the recruitment model. The data generation procedures of the two simulation studies which are the keystone of our results are explained in Sect. 20.4. The results are presented and discussed in Sect. 20.5. Finally, the chapter ends with a concluding Sect. 20.6 where a few recommendations are proposed.

20.2 The Poisson–Gamma Model Without Breaks in Recruitment

This section presents the standard Poisson–gamma model as formulated in [8]. Consider a multicentric clinical trial where C centres are involved to recruit n patients. Denote u_i the opening date of the ith centre which is assumed to be observed. The recruitment process of centre i is denoted $\{N_i(t),\ t \geq u_i\}$ and is modelled by a Poisson process of rate λ_i. The global inclusion process is $N = \sum_{i=1}^{C} N_i$. The parameter of interest is the stopping time:

$$T = \left\{ \inf_{t \geq 0} \ : \ N(t) = n \right\}.$$

In the sequel, we consider, for any i, λ_i as a random variable which is gamma distributed with parameters (α, β) whose probability density function is as follows:

$$p_{\alpha,\beta}(x) = \kappa e^{-\beta x} x^{\alpha-1} \mathbf{1}_{\{x>0\}},$$

where κ is a normalizing constant.

20.2.1 *Estimation*

In most setting, parameters (α, β) are unknown. To estimate these parameters, an empirical Bayesian strategy may be used. Fix an interim time of analysis t_1. Data collected on $[0, t_1]$ are used to calibrate the model. For any centre i, denote $\tau_{1,i} = (t_1 - u_i) \vee 0$ the duration of activity up to t_1 of centre i and $k_{1,i} = N_i(t_1)$ the number of patients recruited by centre i up to t_1. Notice that $\{(\tau_{1,i}, k_{1,i})\ , i = 1, \ldots, C\}$ are observed data.

Theorem 20.1 ([8]) *Maximum likelihood estimation $(\hat{\alpha}, \hat{\beta})$ of the parameters (α, β) is obtained by maximization of the function:*

$$M_C^{\Gamma}(\alpha, \beta) = \alpha \ln(\beta) - \ln \Gamma(\alpha) + \frac{1}{C} \sum_{i=1}^{C} \left[\ln \Gamma(\alpha + k_{1,i}) - (\alpha + k_{1,i}) \ln(\beta + \tau_{1,i}) \right].$$

20.2.2 *Prediction*

Theorem 20.2 ([8]) *Consider $\hat{\lambda}_{1,i}$ a random variable of distribution $\Gamma(\hat{\alpha} + k_{1,i}, \hat{\beta} + \tau_{1,i})$. The so-called forward rate knowing $\{N_i(t_1) = k_{1,i}\}$ in centre i is the function defined as*

$$t \to \hat{\lambda}_{1,i}.\mathbf{1}_{\{\max(t_1,u_i)\leq t)\}}. \tag{20.1}$$

Given, $n_1 = \sum_{i=1}^{C} k_{1,i}$*, the predictive recruitment process N expresses, for any* $t > t_1$ *as:*

$$N(t) = n_1 + \bar{N}_1(t), \qquad where \quad \bar{N}_1(t) = \sum_{i=1}^{C} \bar{N}_{1,i}(t),$$

and $\bar{N}_{1,i}$ *is a Cox process whose rate is given by* (20.1) *and starting at time* t_1*.*

20.2.3 Expected Duration

Consider $\bar{n}_1 = n - n_1$, the number of patients remaining to recruit after t_1 and the remaining inclusion time $\bar{T} = \left\{\inf_{t\geq 0} : \bar{N}_1(t) = \bar{n}_1\right\}$.

Theorem 20.3 ([6, 8]) *Denote* $\hat{\Lambda}_1 = \sum_{i=1}^{C} \hat{\lambda}_{1,i}$.

- *Assume that all the centres are initiated at time* 0 *(*$u_i = 0$*, for any* i*). Then* $\bar{T}$ *is* $\gamma(\bar{n}_1, \hat{\Lambda}_1)$*-distributed.*
- *Assume that all the centres are initiated at the same time (*$u_i = u > 0$*, for any* i*). Denote* $\tau_1 = (t_1 - u) \vee 0$*. Then,* $\bar{T}$ *is* $P_{VI}\left(\bar{n}_1, \hat{\alpha}C + n_1, \hat{\beta} + \tau_1\right)$ *distributed where* $P_{VI}(n, a, b)$ *denotes the Pearson VI distribution whose probability density function is:*

$$p_{n,a,b}(x) = \frac{1}{\mathscr{B}(n,a)} \frac{x^{n-1}b^a}{(x+b)^{n+a}},$$

  where $\mathscr{B}(a,b) = \int_0^1 x^{a-1}(1-x)^{b-1}dx$ *is the beta function.*
- *In practice, the* $\tau_{1,i}$*'s may be different. The distribution of* $\bar{T}$ *can be approximated for large n by a* $P_{VI}\left(\bar{n}_1, \hat{A}_1, \hat{B}_1\right)$ *distribution with*

$$\hat{A}_1 = \frac{\left(\sum_{i=1}^{C} \hat{m}_{1,i}\right)^2}{\sum_{i=1}^{C} \hat{v}_{1,i}}, \quad \hat{B}_1 = \frac{\sum_{i=1}^{C} \hat{m}_{1,i}}{\sum_{i=1}^{C} \hat{v}_{1,i}} \quad where \ \hat{m}_{1,i} = \frac{\hat{\alpha} + k_{1,i}}{\hat{\beta} + \tau_{1,i}}, \quad \hat{v}_{1,i} = \frac{\hat{\alpha} + k_{1,i}}{(\hat{\beta} + \tau_{1,i})^2}.$$

As a consequence of Theorem 20.2, the expression of the expected duration of the trial is as follows:

$$\mathbf{E}[T] = \begin{cases} t_1 + \bar{n}_1 \frac{\hat{B}_1}{\hat{A}_1 - 1} & \text{if } \hat{A}_1 > 1 \\ +\infty & \text{if } 0 < \hat{A}_1 \leq 1. \end{cases}$$

20.3 The Poisson–Gamma Model with Breaks in Recruitment

Assume that the recruitment process of centre i stops at sometimes denoted $b_{i,j}$ for a period denoted $d_{i,j}$. As in previous section, fix an interim time of analysis t_1. Data collected on $[0, t_1]$ will be used to calibrate the model. For centre i, the data collected are, the number of patients recruited by centre i up to t_1 denoted $k_{1,i}$, the number of breaks up to t_1: $j_{1,i} = \inf\left\{j \ : \ b_{i,j} < t_1, \quad \text{and} \quad b_{i,j} + d_{i,j} \geq t_1\right\}$, $(b_{1,i,j}, \ j = 1, \ldots, , j_{1,i})$ and $(d_{1,i,j}, \ j = 1, \ldots, , j_{1,i})$ the breaks times and durations up to t_1. The duration of activity up to t_1 is thus given by

$$\tau_{1,i} = \left(t_1 - u_i - \sum_{j=1}^{j_{1,i}} d_{1,i,j}\right) \vee 0.$$

The recruitment process for centre i, still denoted N_i, is a non-homogeneous Cox process of intensity governed by λ_i which is $\gamma(\alpha, \beta)$ distributed. Indeed, the rate for centre i is time dependent and expresses by:

$$t \to A(\lambda_i, t) = \lambda_i \, \mathbf{1}_{\{t \notin \mathscr{D}_{1,i}\}} \, \mathbf{1}_{\{t > u_i\}} \,, \tag{20.2}$$

with $\mathscr{D}_{1,i}$ is the set of time t such that there exists $j \in \{1, 2, \ldots, j_{1,i}\}$ verifying $t \geq b_{1,i,j}$ and $t \leq b_{1,i,j} + d_{1,i,j}$.

20.3.1 Estimation

The following theorem ensures that (α, β) are estimated following the same strategy as in Sect. 20.2. Only the definition of $\tau_{1,i}$ differs.

Theorem 20.4 ([13]) *Maximum likelihood estimation* $(\hat{\alpha}, \hat{\beta})$ *of the parameters* (α, β) *are obtained by maximization of the function:*

$$M_C^{\Gamma}(\alpha, \beta) = \alpha \ln(\beta) - \ln \Gamma(\alpha) + \frac{1}{C} \sum_{i=1}^{C} \left[\ln \Gamma(\alpha + k_{1,i}) - (\alpha + k_{1,i}) \ln(\beta + \tau_{1,i})\right].$$

20.3.2 Prediction

When considering breaks, the difficulty comes from the Cox process N modelling the recruitment which is non-homogeneous because of potential breaks in the dynamic. To overpass this difficulty, consider $\tilde{N}$ a homogeneous Cox process, starting at t_1, of

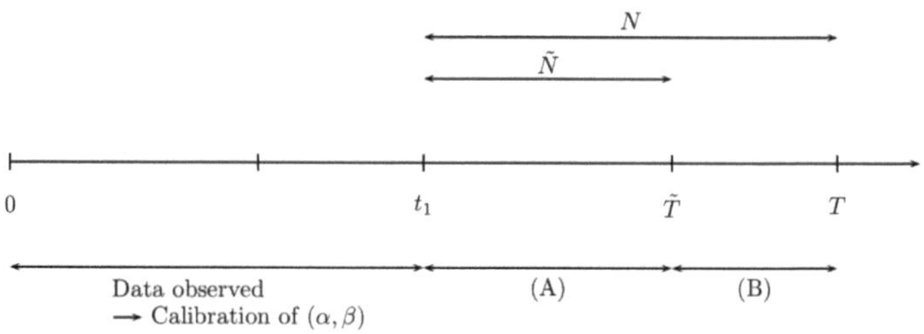

Fig. 20.1 Processes involved in the prediction of T

intensity given by

$$t \to \sum_{i=1}^{C} \hat{\lambda}_{1,i} \, \mathbf{1}_{\{t \geq t_1\}}.$$

Processes N and $\tilde{N}$ have the same intensities, but the first one allows breaks, while the second one does not (see Fig. 20.1).

Consider $T = \left\{\inf_{t\geq 0} \; : \; N(t) = n\right\}$ the "true" duration of the clinical trial and $\tilde{T} = \left\{\inf_{t\geq 0} \; : \; \tilde{N}(t) = n\right\}$. Obviously $\tilde{T} \leq T$. In Fig. 20.1, the duration (A) is the remaining time of the study if there were no breaks after t_1 while the duration (B) explains as the estimated cumulated breaks duration.

20.3.3 Expected Duration

The expected duration cannot be estimated directly but, noticing that $\mathbb{E}[T] = \mathbb{E}[\tilde{T}] + \mathbb{E}[T - \tilde{T}]$, an estimation can be proposed, since $\mathbb{E}[\tilde{T}]$ is related to a homogeneous Cox process thus Theorem 20.3 gives us an estimation of $\mathbb{E}[\tilde{T}]$ and, assuming that the cumulated breaks duration is proportional to the duration of the follow up, $\mathbb{E}[T - \tilde{T}]$ can be estimated by:

$$BC_1 = \frac{\mathbb{E}[\tilde{T}]}{\sum_{i=1}^{C}(t_1 - u_i)} \sum_{i=1}^{C} \sum_{j=1}^{j_{1,i}} d_{1,i,j}. \tag{20.3}$$

The simulation study of Sect. 20.4.2 aims to quantify the bias when $\mathbb{E}[T - \tilde{T}]$ is estimated by BC_1.

20.4 Data Generation Procedures for Simulation Studies

20.4.1 Sensitivity of the Model to Its Parameters

Poisson–gamma model depends on parameter $\theta = (C, \alpha, T, t_1)$, C the number of centres, (α, β) the parameters of the gamma distribution, T the duration of the trial and t_1 the interim time of analysis. Sensitivity of the model to the parameter is assessed by means of a simulation study. Simulation run r consists in choosing a configuration θ_r with $C \in \{1, 2, ..., 30\}$, $\alpha \in \{1, 1.025, 1.050, \ldots, 3.5\}$, $T \in \{50, 100, 150\}$ and $t_1 \in \{T/2, 2T/3\}$. For such a range of parameters, β is usually observed in practice to be fixed to 2. These values have been chosen in coherence with literacy [7] and in such a way that the error of prediction is large enough to be observed. This yields to $R = 18000$ simulation runs. The data generation procedure splits in two steps:

Step 1: Consider a Poisson–gamma process involving C centres and (α, β) the parameters of the gamma distribution.

1. Generate a global recruitment process $\{N^r(t),\ \ 0 \leq t \leq 2T\}$. The value $2T$ is sufficiently large for having a solution at next step.
2. Identify T_0^r the first time verifying $N^r(T_0^r) = N^r$ where $N^r = \alpha TC/\beta$ is the average number of patients to be recruited.

Step 2: Given the interim time t_1.

1. The parameters (α, β) of the Poisson–gamma model are estimated applying Theorem 20.1 from data collected on $[0, t_1]$.
2. The expected duration for the recruitment to reach N^r patients (T_1^r) is computed through the application of Theorem 20.2 at interim time t_1.

The performance of the model at interim time t_1 is measured by means of the absolute error defined by:

$$E_{\theta_r} = |T_1^r - T_0^r|. \tag{20.4}$$

20.4.2 Impact of Breaks on Recruitment Modelling

In order to evaluate the performance of the model when breaks in the recruitment occur, a simulation study is performed. Consider a multicentric trial involving $C = 60$ centres. We aim to recruit $n = 720$ patients in 365 days. In order to investigate different approaches of the breaks dynamic, different scenarios are proposed. Scenarios differ by the breaks generation procedure (times of breaks and durations of breaks). The scenarios are as follows:

- **Scenario 1: Exponential generation**. The instants and durations of breaks are generated according to exponential distributions. The breaks times are exponentially distributed of intensity $\frac{1}{60}$, and this means a break appears on average every

60 days. The breaks durations are exponentially distributed of intensity $\frac{1}{14}$, and this means the average breaks duration is 14 days.
- **Scenario 2: Multinomial generation**. The instants of breaks are generated according to an exponential distribution of parameter $\frac{1}{60}$, meanwhile the durations are generated according to a multinomial distribution. Five levels of duration (2, 4, 8, 16 and 32 days) are involved. The corresponding probability vector is built in such a way that it ensures that the total durations for each level are the same, (the breaks of 2 days happen twice more than the one of 4 days for instance).
- **Scenario 3: Deterministic generation**. The instants and durations of the breaks are generated by hand: two days by week for weekends, and one week every two months for holidays.

Recruitment dynamics are generated involving breaks, themselves generated according to the scenarios defined above. Whole the dynamic is known thus the true duration denoted T_0 of the trial is known. The study consists in considering the data collected on $[0, t_1]$ and to make use of the results of Sects. 20.2 and 20.3 to estimate the duration of the trial. In order to answer to the question "Is it useful to collect the information about breaks?", two strategies of analysis of the dataset are considered:

- **Strategy 1: not taking into account the breaks**. The breaks times and durations are not collected. The parameters of the Poisson–gamma model for recruitment are estimated following results of Sect. 20.2. The expected duration is denoted T_1 and is computed by means of Theorem 20.3.
- **Strategy 2: taking into account all the breaks**. The breaks times and durations are collected. This allow us to make use of the estimation of the trial duration as explained in Sect. 20.3.3. The expected duration is denoted T_2.

For a sake of simplicity, all centres are initiated at $t = 0$ ($u_i = 0$ for all i). The data generation procedure splits in two steps:

Step 1: The generation of $R = 1000$ recruitment processes $\{N^r(t),\ 0 \leq t \leq T_0^r\}$, $1 \leq r \leq R$, where T_0^r denotes the first time verifying $N^r(t) = 720$.

1. Generate the breaks according to the scenario 1, 2 and 3 considered for a period of 730 days. The duration of 730 days is arbitrary and chosen in order to be sure to catch the true duration of the trial.
2. Generate the rates according to a $\Gamma(2, 60.8)$ distribution. The parameters (2, 60.8) of the gamma distribution are the one chosen by [7] to ensure a realistic recruitment dynamic.
3. Consider the modified rate function as defined in Eq. (20.2).
4. Generate the recruitment process up to 730 days.
5. Identify T_0^r and shrink the recruitment process to $[0, T_0^r]$.

Step 2: Given an interim time $t_1 = 182$ days. For each simulation run $r = 1, \ldots, R$ and each strategy $s = 1, 2$,

1. Estimate parameters (α_s^r, β_s^r) of the gamma distribution applying Theorem 20.1 for $s = 1$ or Theorem 20.4 for $s = 2$ from data collected on $[0, t_1]$.

2. Compute the expected duration of the trial T_s^r through the application of Theorem 20.2 for $s = 1$ or following strategies explained in Sect. 20.3.3 for $s = 2$.

The performances of the model at interim time t_1 are measured by means of the absolute error defined by:

$$E_{s,s'} = \frac{1}{R}\sum_{r=1}^{R} |T_s^r - T_{s'}^r|, \qquad \text{for } s = 0, 1, 2,\ s' = 0, 1, 2 \text{ and } s \neq s'. \tag{20.5}$$

20.5 Results and Discussion

20.5.1 Sensitivity of the Model to Its Parameters

The results of the simulation study performed as detailed in Sect. 20.4.1 are illustrated by Fig. 20.2. Each sub-figure corresponds to fixed values of T and t_1 and is the plot of the 3000 simulation runs varying with the value of C in abscissa and $\alpha/2$, the average rate, in ordinate. For each value of (C, α) correspond a black dot, if the absolute error E_{θ_r} defined by (20.4) is greater than $0.05 \times T$ which corresponds to a relative error in prediction greater than a threshold of 5%. Notice that an error of 5% corresponds to a few days and is very small in practice. This value has been chosen because for larger values, the Poisson–gamma is so powerful that there are a too small number of black dots. Each row of Fig. 20.2 corresponds to a value of T (50 weeks on top, 100 weeks in the middle and 150 weeks on the bottom), while each column corresponds to a value of t_1 ($T/2$ on the left and $2T/3$ on the right).

Comparing the two columns of graphs, Fig. 20.2 illustrates that the model in more relevant when the interim time is late and quantifies the benefit. Comparing the rows, the same phenomenon is observable. Larger the duration of recruitment is, lesser the error of prediction is. Both these results are consistent with the model since the volume of information collected up to the interim time t_1 increases with the duration of the trial and with the interim time.

The role of C and α can be identified on each graph. The error decreases with C whatever the value of α and decreases with α whatever the value of C. It is important to notice that this effect is more pronounced for the number of centres which appears to be the most important parameter. If C is large, the model is relevant even for small value of α, but for small value of α, the model is less relevant whatever the value of C. For ending, notice that the minimal value $C = 20$ stated in [7] can be diminished if the average rate is large enough or if the interim time is late.

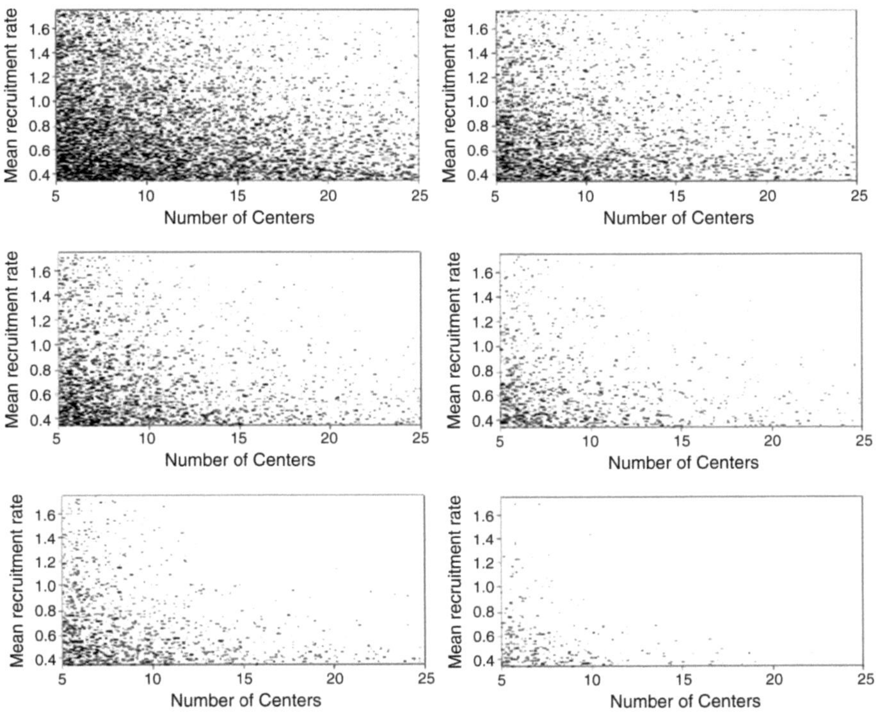

Fig. 20.2 Performance of Poisson–gamma model, black dot corresponds to a configuration for which the absolute error is larger than $0.05 \times T$ (in abscissa, the number of centres and in ordinate the average rate). First (respectively, second and third) row corresponds to a trial duration of 50 (respectively, 100 and 150) weeks. First (respectively, second) column corresponds to a interim analysis at time $T/2$ (respectively, $2T/3$)

20.5.2 Impact of Breaks on Recruitment Modelling

For each scenario, the mean duration (over the simulation runs) of the simulated recruitment dynamic together with its 95% confidence interval (the 25th and 975th values of the sorted sample) is identified. For strategy p ($p = 1, 2$), the expected trial duration and its 95% confidence interval are computed. For strategy p, the bias is assessed by the average (over r) of the absolute errors between the expected durations (T_p^r) and the true value (T_0^r) of the trial duration, $E_{0,p}$ defined by (20.5). The value of $E_{0,p}$, its 95% confidence interval and the parameter is denoted $S_{0,p}$, the proportion of overestimation is defined as the number of runs for which the expected duration computed by means of strategy p (T_p^r) is greater than the true duration (T_0^r) are computed. The results are collected in Table 20.1.

Table 20.1 illustrates that, whatever the scenario, the strategy of analysis yields to very good results ensuring its efficiency. Indeed, the mean values of the real duration are very close to the mean duration estimated by the different strategies. This result

Table 20.1 Average duration (in days) as a function of the strategy together with its 95% confidence intervals. Absolute error between expected duration and true duration ($E_{0,p}$) as a function of the strategy together with its 95% confidence interval and the proportion of overestimation ($S_{0,p}$)

		Scenario 1	Scenario 2	Scenario 3
Real duration	Mean	384.37	337.92	369.17
	CI (95%)	[351,415]	[303,373]	[343,398]
Strategy 1	Mean	381.92	337.80	367.95
	CI (95%)	[340,431]	[304,374]	[330,412]
	$E_{0,p}$	13.81	9.78	11.04
	CI (95%)	[2,13]	[0,29]	[1,32]
	$S_{0,p}$	0.41	0.44	0.44
Strategy 2	Mean	374.66	336.41	356.94
	CI (95%)	[336,421]	[303,372]	[321,398]
	$E_{0,p}$	15.42	9.88	14.88
	CI (95%)	[1,40]	[1,29]	[1,38]
	$S_{0,p}$	0.27	0.40	0.16

is confirmed by the values of $E_{0,p}$ and highlights by the width of the confidence intervals of $E_{0,p}$. These results are enriched by Figs. 20.3 and 20.4. Figure 20.3 is the regression plot of the expected duration as a function of the true duration for each scenario and each strategy and allows the evaluation of the predictive efficiency by comparing regression line with $y = x$. Figure 20.4 is the plot of the empirical density curves for each strategy completed by one of the true durations.

Figure 20.3 advocates for predictive efficiency since there are no significant differences between regression line and $y = x$ (F-statistics p values are always lesser than 0.01, and there is no significant auto-correlation, and homoscedasticity and normal distribution for the residuals are observable from ad hoc graphs not presented here).

For any scenario, the three strategies underevaluate the trial duration. This important fact is observed considering the values of $S_{0,p}$ and Fig. 20.4. In [13], histograms of the distributions of the durations of the trial estimated by each strategy are plotted and are unimodal, symmetric and exhibit a shift to the left comparing with the one of the real duration which confirms this phenomenon. The underestimation of the strategies can be observed in Fig. 20.4 (shift of the densities to the left) and in Fig. 20.3 (the regression lines are above $y = x$). The strategies are thus moderately biased.

Whatever the strategy and the scenario, the model involved yields to relevant results. Results are more or less the same for Scenarios 1 and 3 and a bit better for Scenario 2 dealing with the multinomial breaks. Finally, it is easily seen regarding plots of Fig. 20.4 that the histogram which is closest to the real durations is always the one of Strategy 1. That is confirmed by the regression plots for which the corresponding line is closest to line $y = x$.

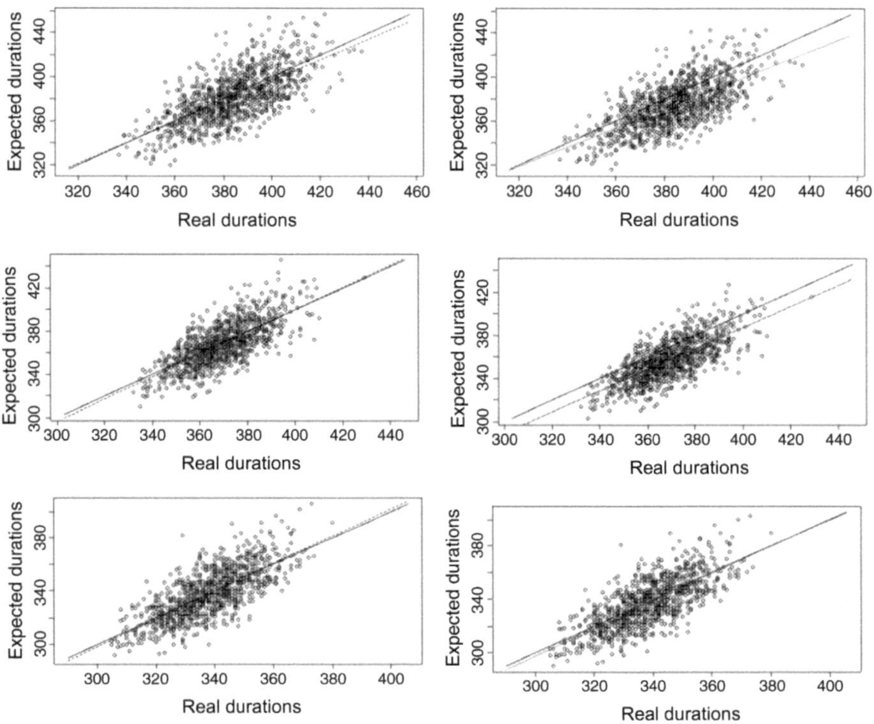

Fig. 20.3 Each row corresponds to a scenario and is the scatter plots of the expected trial duration estimated by Strategy 1 on the left and Strategy 2 on the right as a function of the true trial duration together with the regression line (dotted line) and the line $y = x$ (solid line)

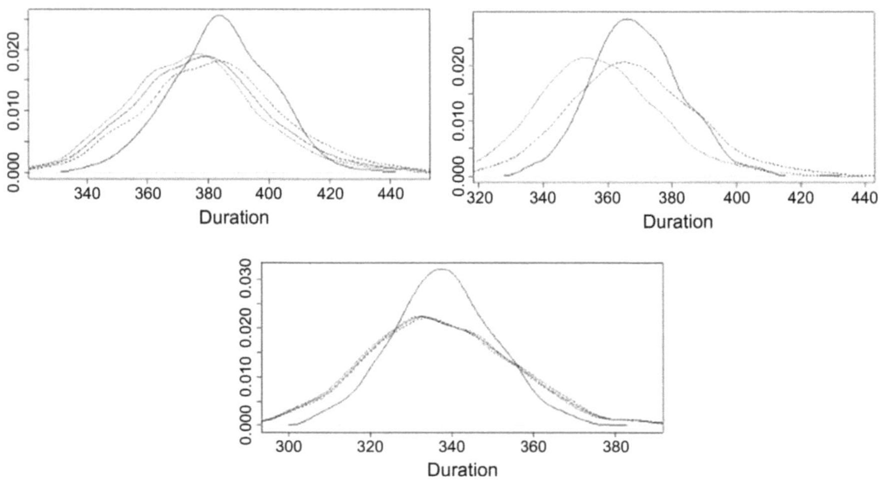

Fig. 20.4 Empirical densities of the distribution of T_0 (solid line), of T_1 (dashed line) and of T_2 (dotted line): on the top, Scenario 1 on the left, Scenario 2 on the right and Scenario 3 on the bottom

20.6 Conclusions

The first simulation study allows us to state that the Poisson–gamma model is sensitive to the parameters of the model, especially C and t_1. The parameters are deeply linked, and for small values of parameters, it is not easy to see if a given configuration may lead to a setting for which Poisson–gamma model performs well.

The second simulation study states that the role of the breaks in recruitment is really moderate. Indeed, first, simulations illustrate that there is a relevant strategy for accounting for the break with a moderate bias, and second, the strategy consisting in not wondering with the breaks and to make use of a standard Poisson–gamma process appears to be the better strategy among these investigated.

To conclude, one suggests to perform simulation study for each recruitment design in order to be sure that the model will perform optimally, and to not collect information on breaks in recruitment. The powerful Poisson–gamma model will balance the delay due to breaks by an underestimation of the rate. These results are deepened in [13]. A third strategy of analysis considering only large breaks is investigated. The strategies are compared, and Strategy 1 (not accounting for breaks) appears to be the best way to deal with the breaks concern.

Acknowledgements This research has received the help from IRESP during the call for proposals launched in 2012 as a part of French "Cancer Plan 2009–2013".

References

1. Anisimov, V.V.: Using mixed Poisson models in patient recruitment in multicentre clinical trials. In: Proceegings of the World Congress on Ingineering, vol. II, pp. 1046–1049. London, United Kingdom (2008)
2. Anisimov, V.V.: Predictive modelling of recruitment and drug supply in multicenter clinical trials. In: Proceedings of the Joint Statistical Meeting, ASA, pp. 1248–1259. Washington, USA (2009)
3. Anisimov, V.V.: Recruitment modeling and predicting in clinical trials. Pharm. Outsourcing **10**, 44–48 (2009)
4. Anisimov, V.V.: Effects of unstratified and centre-stratified randomization in multi-centre clinical trials. Pharm. Stat. **10**, 50–59 (2011)
5. Anisimov, V.V.: Predictive event modelling in multicentre clinical trials with waiting time to response. Pharm. Stat. **10**, 517–522 (2011)
6. Anisimov, V.V.: Statistical modeling of clinical trials (recruitment and randomization). Comm. Statist. Theory Methods **40**, 3684–3699 (2011)
7. Anisimov, V.V., Fedorov, V.V.: Modelling, prediction and adaptive adjustment of recruitment in multicentre trials. Stat. Med. **26**, 4958–4975 (2007)
8. Anisimov, V.V., Downing, D., Fedorov, V.V.: Recruitment in multicentre trials: prediction and adjustment. In: 8th International Workshop in Model-Oriented Design and Analysis, pp. 1–8. Physica-Verlag/Springer, Heidelberg, Almagro, Spain (2007)
9. Barnard, K.D., Dent, L., Cook, A.: A systematic review of models to predict recruitment to multicentre trials. BMC Med. Res. Methodol. **63** (2010)
10. Carter, R.E.: Application of stochastic processes to participant recruitment in clinical trials. Control. Clin. Trials **25**, 429–436 (2004)

11. Lee, Y.J.: Interim recruitment goals in clinical trials. J. Chronic Dis. **36**, 379–389 (1983)
12. Mijoule, G., Savy, S., Savy, N.: Models for patients' recruitment in clinical trials and sensitivity analysis. Stat. Med. **31**(16), 1655–1674 (2012)
13. Minois, N., Savy, S., Lauwers-Cances, V., Andrieu, S., Savy, N.: Poisson-gamma model for patients' recruitment in clinical trials with breaks in recruitment dynamic. Contemp. Clin. Trials Commun. **5**, 144–152 (2017)
14. Morgan, T.M.: Nonparametric estimation of duration of accrual and total study length for clinical trials. Biometrics **43**, 903–912 (1987)
15. Rojavin, M.: Patient recruitment and retention: from art to science. Contemp. Clin. Trials **30**, 387–387 (2009)
16. Senn, S.: Some controversies in planning and analysing multi-centre trials. In: Statistics in Medicine, pp. 1753–1765 (1998)

Chapter 21
Simulated Clinical Trials: Principle, Good Practices, and Focus on Virtual Patients Generation

Nicolas Savy, Stéphanie Savy, Sandrine Andrieu and Sébastien Marque

Abstract It is a well-known fact that clinical trials is a challenging process essentially for financial, ethical, and scientific concern. For twenty years, simulated clinical trials (SCT for short) has been introduced in the drug development. It becomes more and more popular mainly due to pharmaceutical companies which aim to optimize their clinical trials (duration and expenses) and the regulatory agencies which consider simulations as an alternative tool to reduce safety issues. The whole simulation plan is based on virtual patients generation. The natural idea to do so is to perform Monte Carlo simulations from the joined distribution of the covariates. This method is named Discrete Method. This is trivial when the parameters of the distribution are known, but, in practice, data available come from historical databases. A preliminary estimation step is necessary. For Discrete Method that step may be not effective, especially when there are a lot of covariates mixing continuous and categorical ones. In this chapter, simulation studies illustrate that the so-called Continuous Method may be a good alternative to the discrete one, especially when marginal distributions are moderately bi-modal.

Keywords Simulated clinical trials · Database generation
Monte Carlo simulation

N. Savy (✉)
Toulouse Institute of Mathematics, University of Toulouse III,
31062 Toulouse, France
e-mail: Nicolas.Savy@math.univ-toulouse.fr

S. Savy · S. Andrieu
INSERM UMR 1027, University of Toulouse III, 31073 Toulouse, France
e-mail: sm.savy@gmail.com

S. Andrieu
Epidemiology Unit of Toulouse CHU, 31073 Toulouse, France
e-mail: sandrine.andrieu@univ-tlse.fr

S. Marque
Capionis, Paris, France
e-mail: sebastien.marque@capionis.com

S. Marque
Osmose, Bordeaux, France

J. Pilz et al. (eds.), *Statistics and Simulation*, Springer Proceedings
in Mathematics & Statistics 231, https://doi.org/10.1007/978-3-319-76035-3_21

21.1 Introduction

Clinical trials is a challenging process for financial, ethical, and scientific concern. For twenty years, simulated clinical trials (SCT for short) has been introduced in drug development. The main idea is to summarize the available information on the patients, the drug of interest and the trial design in order to build a stochastic model. They are used to model biological systems and pharmacology of treatments' action on those systems. They also allow in silico identification of weaknesses in the design of a trial, adjustment of the procedures before the initiation of a trial while reducing logistics barriers. The aim of simulation strategy is to make rational decisions with regard to optimizing the development plan of a new compound (see [11] and references therein). It has been shown that it leads to increase the likelihood of achieving the objectives of study and patient safety, to reduce the duration of the study and protocol deviations as well as avoiding inconclusive situations [4].

While introducing simulations in clinical research seems to be natural in drug development, the literature reviews actually show small impact and use. This has been pointed out in the state of the art [6] on the period before 2000 and confirmed in the reviews [5] on the period 2000–2010 and the review authors has made on the period 2010–2015. Authors explain that paradox arguing a reporting bias, as such investigations are often performed by pharmaceutical companies and not necessary published for industrial confidentiality concerns. Furthermore, they wonder whether such investigations are done with respect to the good practices stated in [2]. It is important to highlight that regulatory agencies now stimulates the use of simulation in drug development.

The main property of SCT which makes its setting up really versatile is modularity. A SCT is constructed from sub-models which can be developed independently and may be clustered in three main groups: execution models, input/output models, and covariate distribution models. That third module is fundamental. It allocates the covariates values for each (virtual) patient. These values are used to calibrate most of the other modules. The natural idea is to perform Monte Carlo simulation from the joined distribution. When the parameters of the distribution are known, the, usually named, Discrete Method is exact. When these parameters are estimated from a historical database—which is the case in practice—Discrete Method is less effective, especially when there is a large number of covariates mixing continuous and categorical ones. The so-called Continuous Method introduced in [11] to generate database directly from the population parameters may be a good alternative.

The chapter is organized as follows: Sect. 21.2 is devoted to the main steps of the construction of a simulated clinical trial together with the main ideas of the guidelines given in [2]. Section 21.3 focuses on the virtual patients generation. Discrete Method and Continuous Method are detailed. Section 21.4 is devoted to a simulation study which aims to assess and to compare the performances of these two methods to generate data sets preserving the marginal distributions and the correlation structure of the underlying historical database.

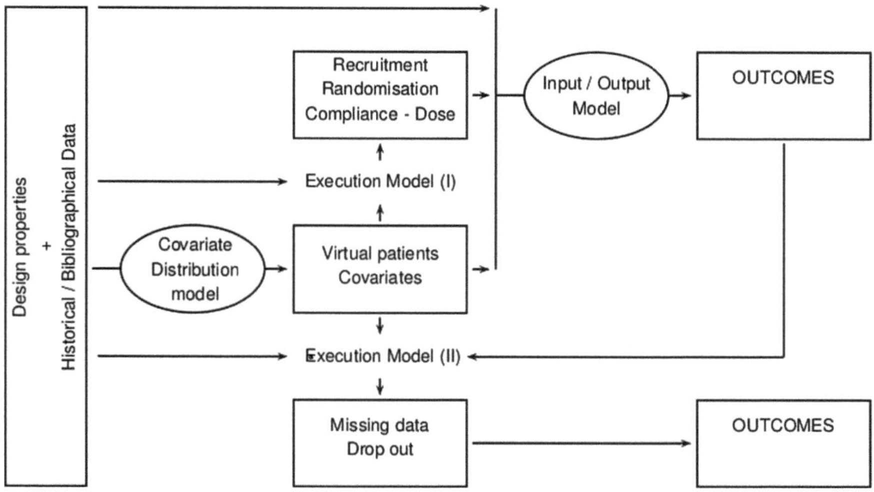

Fig. 21.1 Example of design's scheme for a Simulated Clinical Trial

21.2 Main Steps of the Setting Up of a SCT: Principe - Guidelines

For a rational use of SCT, [2] proposes guidances established on three methodological pillars. **Clarity**: The report of the simulation should be understandable in terms of scope and conclusions by intended users. **Completeness**: Assumptions, methods, and results have to be described with enough details in order to be reproduced by an independent team. **Parsimony**: Complexity of the model and simulations procedure has to be no more numerous that necessary. Figure 21.1 is an example of what may be the simulation design's scheme of a SCT.

A SCT is composed of a sequence of sub-models:

- **Covariate distribution model (Virtual Patients Generator)**. A dataset of virtual patients' covariates is stochastically generated. This database has to be consistent with the protocol we aim to investigate. This step involves essentially Monte Carlo generation (see, for instance, [9, 10] for details) taking into account correlations between the different covariates.
- **Execution models**. The design is modified taking into account adverse events which may happen during the trial. Deviation to protocol, compliance failure, dropout are typical examples of such side effects which can be integrated into models. The model may be enriched for instance including patients recruitment models [1, 8] in order to investigate the duration of the trial. Execution model (II) differs from Execution model (I) because it depends on the outcomes.
- **Input–Output Model**. Virtual patients database and executive models allow to construct the outcome values by means of input/output model (PK–PD techniques [3] or disease progression model [7]).

21.3 Covariate Distribution Modelling

In what follows, C^k denotes the kth covariate (k varies from 1 to K) and c_i^k denotes the values of that covariate of the ith patient (i varies from 1 to n). For a sake of notational simplicity, $\mathbf{c}_i$ denotes the vector of patient i covariates' values. Covariate C may be continuous (denoted ${}^cC$) or categorical (denoted ${}^dC$). Throughout that section, continuous covariates are assumed to be normally distributed but it can be any other distribution up to a change of variable.

If the joint distribution of the covariates, denoted $f_{(C^1,\ldots,C^K)}$ for simplicity, is known, the strategy is nothing but a Monte Carlo generation of data. To be meaningful, the data generation has to rely on available information on the covariates. That information may come from the literature (called bibliographical data) or from an existing database (called historical database). Dealing with bibliographical data, the covariates distributions parameters are parameters of the population while dealing with historical data, these parameters are estimations of population parameters. Bibliographical data are more relevant but, most of the time, only marginal distributions are easy to obtain. The better we can do is often to assume covariates as independent that is not satisfactory. From historical database, whole the correlation structure may be estimated but the question of how to estimate parameters with enough precision raises. In what follows, the question of reconstruction of a database (D) is to be understood in the sense on how to generate a database with marginal distributions and the correlation structure close to the one of (D).

21.3.1 How to Generate Virtual Patients Given Bibliographical Data?

21.3.1.1 Discrete Method

Discrete Method is an exact method to reconstruct a database. The idea is to split continuous variables and discrete variables by conditioning, writing, with notational abuse: $f_{(C^1,\ldots,C^K)} = f_{(({}^cC^1,\ldots,{}^cC^L)|({}^dC^{L+1},\ldots,{}^dC^K))} \times f_{({}^dC^{L+1},\ldots,{}^dC^K)}$. The simulation of a database of size n consists in performing n times the algorithm

- Draw a configuration from the multinomial distribution,
- Given this configuration, draw the remaining values from the multinormal distribution.

This method is obviously the better we can expect. Notice that the problem can be split into groups of independent covariates.

21.3.1.2 Continuous Method

The idea is to consider all the covariates $\mathcal{N}(\boldsymbol{\mu}, \Sigma)$-distributed. The simulation of a database of size n consists in drawing n values $(u_i^1, \ldots, u_i^K)_{i=1,\ldots,n}$ from the multinormal distribution $\mathcal{N}(\boldsymbol{\mu}, \Sigma)$.

- For a continuous covariate ${}^c c^k = u^k$ for $k = 1, \ldots, L$
- For a categorical covariate with M modalities ${}^d C^k$, one makes use of the, so-called, critical values

$$\begin{cases} CrV_m^k = \mu_k + \Sigma_{k,k}\phi^{-1}(\sum_{i=1}^m p_i), & 1 \leq m \leq M-1 \\ CrV_M^k = +\infty \\ CrV_0^k = -\infty \end{cases}$$

where $(p_m;\ 1 \leq m \leq M)$ are the proportions of each modality of the categorical covariate, μ_k and $\Sigma_{k,k}$ are the parameters of the normal distribution, ϕ denotes the cumulative function of standard normal distribution.
Finally, ${}^d c^k = m$ if and only if $CrV_{m-1}^k < u_i^k \leq CrV_m^k$.

21.3.2 *How to Generate Virtual Patients Given a Historical Database?*

Comparison of Discrete and Continuous Methods given bibliographical data has been investigated in [11] assuming continuous covariates normally distributed. Here, attention is paid on the performances of these techniques on a closer to practice setting, when a historical database is given. The aim of the machinery is to generate a realistic copy of this historical database (the marginal distributions coincides and the correlation structure between covariates is preserved). Dealing with a historical database, an additional estimation of the parameters step is needed. For the Discrete Method that step consists in

- Fit the distribution of $({}^d C^{L+1}, \ldots, {}^d C^K)$ by estimating the proportion of each modality,
- Fit the distribution of $f_{(({}^c C^1,\ldots,{}^c C^L)|({}^d C^{L+1},\ldots,{}^d C^K))}$, estimating the mean vector and variance–covariance matrix for each configuration $({}^d C^{L+1}, \ldots, {}^d C^K)$.

For the Continuous Method, the estimation step consists in fitting a multinormal distribution for whole the covariates.

The Discrete Method yields two problems: first, this technique needs a lot of estimations and, for situations where there are a lot of categorical covariates, thus a lot of modalities for the vector of covariates, the estimation of the parameters of the continuous covariates is poor because of a small number of data for several modalities. These questions make the Continuous Method more appealing. Meanwhile, the Continuous Method is not able to catch multi-modal distributions.

Example 21.1 Given a historical database with 500 patients involving 5 continuous covariates of interest and 3 categorical covariates with, respectively, 2, 3, and 4 modalities. Discrete Method necessitates 23 estimations for the proportions of each of the 24 configurations and $24 \times 20 = 480$ estimations to estimate the 24 means vector and variance–covariance matrices of each conditional distribution. Thus, there are 503 parameters to estimate. Moreover, there are, on average, $\frac{500}{23} \simeq 22$ values available to estimate the multinormal distribution parameters.

21.4 Simulation Study

In order to investigate the performances of the Continuous Method as an alternative to the Discrete Method, a simulation study is performed. A "toy model", close to the one used in [11], is considered. The population consists of three variables (X, Y, Z). X is a categorical variable with two modalities (1 and 2) Bernoulli distributed of parameter π, Y is a random variable log-normally distributed conditionally to X and Z a random variable normally distributed conditionally to X. These conditional distributions are correlated. The aim is to investigate the impact on Continuous Method performances of parameters π, μ, and ρ. π is the proportions of each modality of the categorical variable. μ is the conditional to $X = 1$ mean. As the conditional expectation given $X = 2$ is fixed (equal to 90) and as the coefficients of variation are fixed equal to 0.3 whatever the scenario, the difference between conditional means yields to bi-modality in the distribution of Y. Finally, ρ is the coefficient of correlation between the conditional distributions of Y and Z. Note that $\rho_{(Y,Z)|X=1}$ and $\rho_{(Y,Z)|X=2}$ are assumed to be equal.

The algorithm follows the steps:

1. **Fix parameters of the population**. These scenarios differ from parameters π, μ and ρ. 27 scenarios are considered taking $\pi \in \{0.1, 0.25, 0.5\}$, $\mu \in \{10, 50, 90\}$, and $\rho \in \{0, 0.5, 0.9\}$. The values of the parameters for each scenario are presented in Table 21.1.
2. **Build the Historical Database**. To generate a database from this population (Historical database), a Monte Carlo simulation is performed. First generate values x of X and then generate values of (Y, Z) given $X = x$. Details on the procedure to generate these values are relegated to Appendix 1.
3. **Build the Generated Databases**. Make use of the Discrete (resp. Continuous) Method to generate 1000 databases. The choice of 1000 databases is usual, it allows to have a precise idea of the performances of the method and it is not too large for computational issue.
4. **Assess of the performance to reconstruct a parameter**. Consider θ a parameter of interest in the population and denotes $\hat{\theta}_H$ its estimation from the historical database. For each simulation run r ($r = 1, \ldots, 1000$), denote $\hat{\theta}_r^D$ (resp. $\hat{\theta}_r^C$) its estimation from the rth-generated database by means of the Discrete (resp. Continuous) Method. In order to evaluate the performances of method $J = C$ or D,

Table 21.1 Values of the parameters defining the different scenarios investigated. Expectation and variance–covariance matrix of (Y, Z) are computed by means of formulas detailed in Appendix 2

Scenario	Parameters of conditionals			Parameters of marginals				
	π	μ	ρ	μ_Y	CV_Y	μ_Z	CV_Z	$\rho_{Y,Z}$
1	0.10	10	0.0	82	0.43	100	0.30	0.00
2	0.10	10	0.5	82	0.43	100	0.30	0.35
3	0.10	10	0.9	82	0.43	100	0.30	0.63
4	0.10	50	0.0	86	0.33	100	0.30	0.00
5	0.10	50	0.5	86	0.33	100	0.30	0.45
6	0.10	50	0.9	86	0.33	100	0.30	0.81
7	0.10	90	0.0	90	0.30	100	0.30	0.00
8	0.10	90	0.5	90	0.30	100	0.30	0.50
9	0.10	90	0.9	90	0.30	100	0.30	0.90
10	0.25	10	0.0	82	0.43	100	0.30	0.00
11	0.25	10	0.5	82	0.43	100	0.30	0.35
12	0.25	10	0.9	82	0.43	100	0.30	0.63
13	0.25	50	0.0	86	0.33	100	0.30	0.00
14	0.25	50	0.5	86	0.33	100	0.30	0.45
15	0.25	50	0.9	86	0.33	100	0.30	0.81
16	0.25	90	0.0	90	0.30	100	0.30	0.00
17	0.25	90	0.5	90	0.30	100	0.30	0.50
18	0.25	90	0.9	90	0.30	100	0.30	0.90
19	0.50	10	0.0	82	0.43	100	0.30	0.00
20	0.50	10	0.5	82	0.43	100	0.30	0.35
21	0.50	10	0.9	82	0.43	100	0.30	0.63
22	0.50	50	0.0	86	0.33	100	0.30	0.00
23	0.50	50	0.5	86	0.33	100	0.30	0.45
24	0.50	50	0.9	86	0.33	100	0.30	0.81
25	0.50	90	0.0	90	0.30	100	0.30	0.00
26	0.50	90	0.5	90	0.30	100	0.30	0.50
27	0.50	90	0.9	90	0.30	100	0.30	0.90

the error between generated database and population (resp. historical database) denoted $\mathrm{EP}^J(\theta) = \hat{\theta}_r^J - \theta$ and $\mathrm{EH}^J(\theta) = \hat{\theta}_r^J - \hat{\theta}_H$ are computed. As 1000 simulation runs are performed for each scenario, the performance of method $J = C, D$ for strategy $I = H, P$ is thus measured by $\mathrm{EI}^J(\theta) = \frac{1}{1000}\sum_{r=1}^{1000} \mathrm{EI}_r^J(\theta)$, and its 95% confidence interval, denoted $\mathrm{CI}_{95\%}(\mathrm{EI}^J(\theta))$, i.e. the 25th and 975th value of the sorted sample $\{\mathrm{EI}_{(r)}^J(\theta),\ r = 1, \ldots, 1000\}$. The performance of method J to reconstruct parameter θ is thus assessed by verifying if $0 \in \mathrm{CI}_{95\%}(\mathrm{EI}^J(\theta))$.

Remark 21.1 It is usual to measure an error by means of relative error defined as $\frac{\hat{\theta}_G^J - \theta}{\theta}$, but here we prefer to use error defined above because, first, we have not observed difference in the results, second, the confidence intervals are, for a few parameters close to 0, very large and finally the comparisons with several parameters are not possible (for instance correlation coefficient equal to 0).

21.5 Results and Discussion

21.5.1 Comparison with Population Parameters

It is readily seen that for $J = C, D, \text{EP}^J(\theta) = \text{EH}^J(\theta) + (\hat{\theta}_H - \theta)$. The difference between the reconstruction of a parameter of the population and the reconstruction of the estimation of that parameter from data of the historical database is thus nothing but the difference $\hat{\theta}_H - \theta$. This term can be seen as a bias which comes from the sampling of the historical database. $\hat{\theta}_H$ may be far from θ especially when the proportion of $X = 1$ is small and may lead to a poor reconstruction of parameters. This is magnified for settings of highly correlated scenarios. For instance, for Scenario 7, only 68% of the parameters of the population have been reconstructed by Discrete Method and 80% by the Continuous Method. The weakness of the performances comes from the conditional to $X = 2$ expectation of Y which is 90 for the population and estimated to 87.92 from historical database. These artefacts may lead to situation for which the results are better for Population rather than from Historical database. It is thus of none interest to consider $\text{EP}^J(\theta)$ whatever the method.

21.5.2 Comparison with Historical Database Parameters

21.5.2.1 Performances of Discrete Method

For the Discrete Method, all the parameters of the historical database are reconstructed. This is not surprising since reconstructed reduces, in this setting, to verify that the estimation of a parameter is in its 95% confidence interval. The performances of the Discrete Method decreases with the number of covariates. In our simple setting, the Discrete Method will play the role of standard method to assess the performances of the Continuous Method. Indeed the concept of reconstruction ($0 \in \text{CI}_{95\%}$) depends on the width of the $\text{CI}_{95\%}$. Figures 21.2 and 21.3 plot $\text{CI}_{95\%}$ as a function of the scenario and illustrate this phenomenon. The shape of the confidence intervals for Discrete Method (crosses and dotted lines) will serve as reference and will be compared to the one for Continuous Method (dots and plain lines). Moreover, these graphs allow us to conclude if a parameter is considered to be reconstructed because its value is very close to 0 or because the $\text{CI}_{95\%}$ is large. In order to shorten

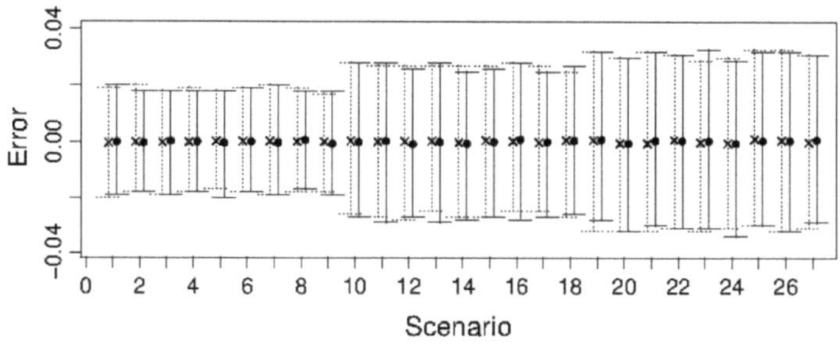

Fig. 21.2 Mean errors and the error bars (95% confidence intervals) in the reconstruction, from the historical database as a function of the scenarios, of the proportion of modality 1. Crosses and dotted lines correspond to Discrete Method and dots and plain lines to Continuous Method

the analysis, these graphs are plotted only for parameters π (Fig. 21.2), the conditional expectations of Y and the expectation of Y and the conditional coefficient of correlation and the coefficient of correlation (Fig. 21.3).

Keeping in mind the construction of confidence intervals for a proportion, for a mean and for a coefficient of correlation the shape of the confidence intervals for Discrete Method are coherent: the width of the confidence interval for the proportion of $X = 1$ depends on the proportion and of the sample size. It is thus natural to observe that the width of the $CI_{95\%}$ increases with the proportion of $X = 1$ the sample size being fixed to 1000. The width of the confidence interval of the conditional to $X = 1$ expectations of Y depends on the conditional to $X = 1$ standard deviation and sample size. The simulation scheme fixed the values of the coefficient of variation and thus this standard deviation depends on the mean. Obviously, the width of the $CI_{95\%}$ increases with the conditional to $X = 1$ expectation and with the proportion of $X = 1$. The width of the confidence interval of the conditional to $X = 1$ coefficient of correlation between Y and Z depends on the parameter itself and of the sample size.

21.5.2.2 Performances of Continuous Method

The results for the Continuous Method are collected in Table 21.2 (the number of scenario for which the parameter is reconstructed as a function of the parameters of interest) and Table 21.3 (the number of parameters reconstructed by the Continuous Method as a function of the scenario).

Table 21.3 indicates that for 48% of the scenarios investigated, more than 75% of the parameters are reconstructed and this proportion increases to 85% considering scenarios where 50% of the parameters are reconstructed. Table 21.2 indicates that only a few parameters are not reconstructed for most of the scenarios. These parameters are the ones of the conditional to $X = 1$ and conditional to $X = 2$ distributions of Y, as a matter of fact, the marginal distribution of Y together with the coefficients of correlation of Y and Z conditional or not.

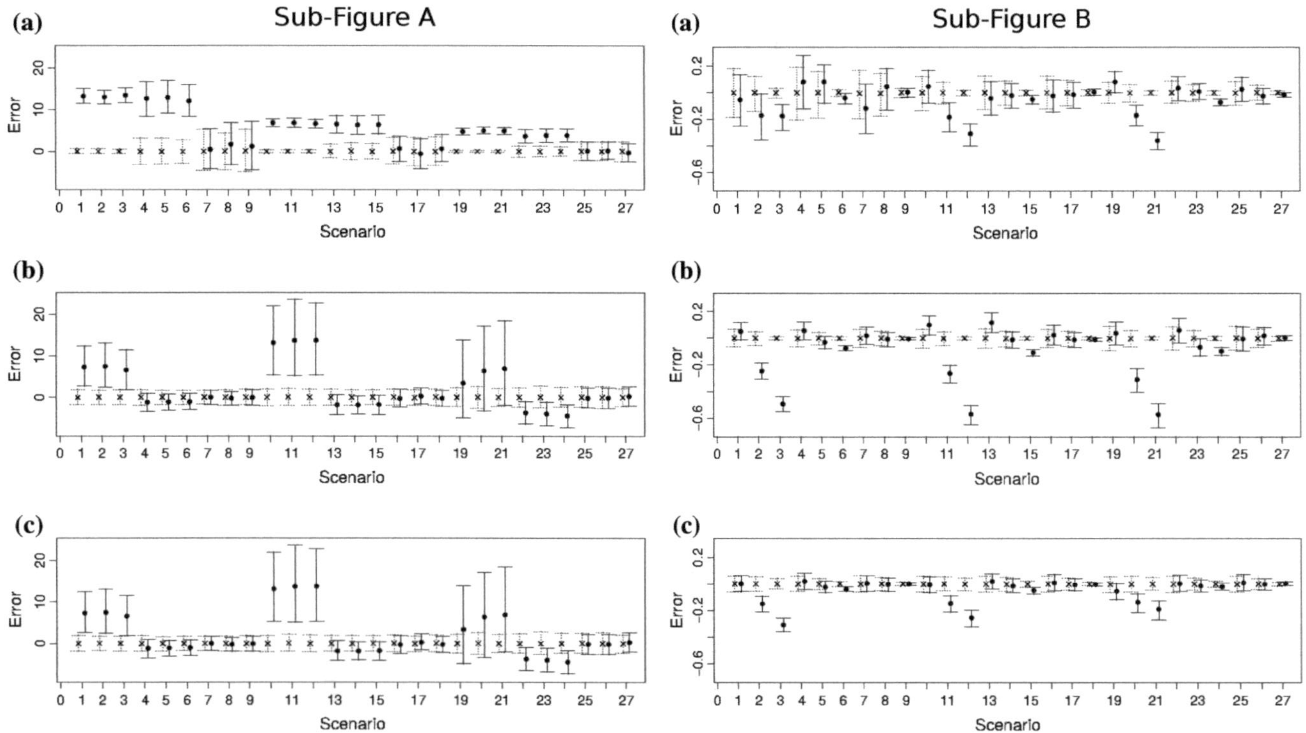

Fig. 21.3 Mean errors and the error bars (95% confidence intervals) in the reconstruction, from the historical database as a function of the scenarios, of **a** $\mu_{Y|X=1}$, **b** $\mu_{Y|X=2}$ and **c** μ_Y on the left hand side (Sub-Figure A) and **a** $\rho_{(Y,Z)|X=1}$, **b** $\rho_{(Y,Z)|X=2}$ and **c** $\rho_{(Y,Z)}$ on the left hand side (Sub-Figure B). Crosses and dotted lines correspond to Discrete Method and dots and plain lines to Continuous Method

Table 21.2 The second row is the number of scenarios (over 27 scenarios) for which the estimations, from data of historical database, of the parameters of the first row are reconstructed

Binomial	π				
	27				
Conditional to $X = 1$	$\mu_{Y\|X=1}$	$CV_{Y\|X=1}$	$\mu_{Z\|X=1}$	$CV_{Z\|X=1}$	$\rho_{Y,Z\|X=1}$
	9	13	26	21	18
Conditional to $X = 2$	$\mu_{Y\|X=2}$	$CV_{Y\|X=2}$	$\mu_{Z\|X=2}$	$CV_{Z\|X=2}$	$\rho_{Y,Z\|X=2}$
	18	9	27	27	15
Marginal	μ_Y	CV_Y	μ_Z	CV_Z	$\rho_{Y,Z}$
	19	14	27	27	19

Table 21.3 The second row is the number of parameters (over 16 parameters investigated) for which the estimations, from data of historical database, of the parameters of scenario of the first row are reconstructed

$\pi = 0.10$	1	2	3	4	5	6	7	8	9
	10	7	6	14	14	10	15	15	16
$\pi = 0.25$	10	11	12	13	14	15	16	17	18
	8	7	7	11	13	10	15	16	16
$\pi = 0.50$	19	20	21	22	23	24	25	26	27
	12	8	8	11	11	9	16	16	15

Table 21.4 Proportion (in %) of parameters reconstructed from Historical Database by Continuous Method as a function of the input parameter of the different scenario

Factor	$\pi =$			$\mu =$			$\rho =$		
	0.10	0.25	0.50	10	50	90	0.0	0.5	0.9
Proportion	74.3	71.5	73.6	50.7	71.5	97.2	77.8	74.3	66.4

In order to investigate which modifications yield to main change, Table 21.4, which presents the cumulated proportions of parameters reconstructed as a function of the level of each parameter varying in the simulation scheme, is constructed and indicates that the parameter of major impact on the reconstruction is the conditional expectation $\mu_{Y|X=1}$. It is not surprising as the difference between $\mu_{Y|X=1}$ and $\mu_{Y|X=2}$ generates bi-modality which is not caught by the Continuous Method. It is important to notice that the proportion π is of low impact on the reconstruction. Finally, the conditional correlation yields to poor reconstruction only when fixed to 0.9, situation of high correlation. These results are confirmed by results of Table 21.3. In fact, the scenarios for which parameters are often reconstructed (greater than 91% of the parameters) are these with no bi-modality ($\mu_{Y|X=1} = \mu_{Y|X=2} = 90$). Scenarios with moderate bi-modality ($\mu_{Y|X=1} = 50$ and $\mu_{Y|X=2} = 90$) appear with more than 50%

of parameters reconstructed and even more than 68% avoiding highly correlated situations. Notice that the results are better when the proportion of $X = 1$ is low.

Considering dots and plain line of Figs. 21.2 and 21.3, the results are deepened accounting for the width of the corresponding $CI_{95\%}$. Notice that the explanations of the shape of the interval of confidence are the same as the ones given for the Discrete Method. However, as, for many scenarios, there are bias in the reconstruction, the observed behaviour may differ. The proportion of $X = 1$ is perfectly reconstructed, there is no difference with the Discrete Method (Fig. 21.2).

For the expectation of Y, the situation is very different for scenarios with high and moderate bi-modality. Figure 21.3A.a illustrates that the reconstruction is biased but the width of the $CI_{95\%}$ are more or less the same as for Discrete Method. Figure 21.3A.b shows that the results for the conditional to $X = 2$ expectation is substantially modified for scenarios with high bi-modality. Most of the time, this parameter is not reconstructed. Finally, Fig. 21.3A.b insures that the behaviour is smoothed considering the marginal and the parameter is reconstructed except for highly bi-modal setting. The coefficients of correlation are well reconstructed. Regarding Fig. 21.3B.a, the scenarios for which these parameters are not reconstructed are those corresponding to high and moderate correlation together with a moderate or high bi-modality. Notice that for scenarios 6-15-24, the error is small but the parameters are not reconstructed because the width of the $CI_{95\%}$ is very small due to very high correlation. Regarding Fig. 21.3B.b, we observe that the width of the $CI_{95\%}$ are smaller than on Fig. 21.3B.a for most settings. This is observed for scenario where the sample size involved for the conditional to $X = 1$ is smaller than for $X = 2$ ($\pi \neq 0.50$). As a consequence, the parameter is not reconstructed for some new scenarios. Finally, Fig. 21.3B.c the bias is less important, the widths of the $CI_{95\%}$ are more or less the same as the ones on Fig. 21.3B.b.

21.6 Conclusions

Discrete Method is an exact reconstruction of the conditional distributions and is the better method to reconstruct a database given historical data. However, the simulation study highlights the role of the proportion of each modality of the categorical variable. This point is of paramount interest because it justifies that Discrete Method will be of little interest in situation where there are a lot of categorical variables.

Simulation study illustrates that Continuous Method yields to really good results, especially when the bi-modality is moderate. What is of paramount interest is that this result remains true even when the proportion of observed values for a modality of a categorical variable is small. In fact, for practical use, Discrete Method is difficult to use when categorical distribution has a large number of modality. The proportion of several modalities become small and the number of observations by modalities may be too small for yielding to relevant reconstruction. In this setting, Continuous Method is a really relevant alternative. Notice that both methods can be used in the same simulation plan. In fact, variables of interest can be split into groups of independent variables and different methods can be used for different groups.

Acknowledgements This research has received the help from IRESP during the call for proposals launched in 2012 as a part of French "Cancer Plan 2009–2013".

Appendix 1

For $i = 1, 2$, μ_i^Y and σ_i^Y (resp. μ_i^Z and σ_i^Z) denote the expectation and the standard deviation of $(Y|X = i)$ (resp. $(Z|X = i)$) distribution, ρ_i denotes the coefficient of correlation between $(Y|X = i)$ and $(Z|X = i)$, and π denotes the probability that $X = 1$. The relationships between conditional and marginal expectations are $\mathbf{E}[Y] = \pi.\mu_1^Y + (1-\pi).\mu_2^Y$ and $\mathbf{E}[Z] = \pi.\mu_1^Z + (1-\pi).\mu_2^Z$. The relationships between conditional and marginal variances are:

$$\mathbf{V}[Y] = \mathbf{E}[\mathbf{V}[Y|X]] + \mathbf{V}[\mathbf{E}[Y|X]],$$
$$\mathbf{V}[Y] = \pi(\sigma_1^Y)^2 + (1-\pi)(\sigma_2^Y)^2 + \left(\pi(\mu_1^Y)^2 + (1-\pi)(\mu_2^Y)^2 - (\pi\mu_1^Y + (1-\pi)\mu_2^Y)^2\right),$$
$$\mathbf{V}[Z] = \pi(\sigma_1^Z)^2 + (1-\pi)(\sigma_2^Z)^2 + \left(\pi(\mu_1^Z)^2 + (1-\pi)(\mu_2^Z)^2 - (\pi\mu_1^Z + (1-\pi)\mu_2^Z)^2\right).$$

The relationships between conditional covariances and covariance are:

$$\mathrm{cov}[Y, Z] = \pi\sigma_1^Y\sigma_1^Z\rho_1 + (1-\pi)\sigma_2^Y\sigma_2^Z\rho_2 + \left(\pi\mu_1^Y\mu_1^Z + (1-\pi)\mu_2^Y\mu_2^Z - \mathbf{E}[Y]\mathbf{E}[Z]\right).$$

Appendix 2

Consider Y a random variable log-normally-distributed with expectation (resp. standard deviation) denoted μ_Y (resp. σ_Y), Z a random variable $\mathcal{N}(\mu_Z, \sigma_Z)$ distributed, and $\rho_{Y,Z}$ the coefficient of correlation. In order to generate the random vector (Y, Z), consider $Y = \exp(U)$ and (U, Z) a Gaussian vector where U is $\mathcal{N}(\mu_U, \sigma_U)$ distributed and $\rho_{U,Z}$ denotes the coefficient of correlation. The parameters of (U, Z) and these of (Y, Z) are linked by the relationships:

$$\mu_Y = \mathbf{E}[Y] = \mathbf{E}\left[\exp(U)\right] = \exp\left(\mu_U + \frac{\sigma_U^2}{2}\right)$$
$$\sigma_Y^2 = \mathbf{V}[Y] = \mathbf{E}\left[\exp(2U)\right] - (\mathbf{E}\left[\exp(U)\right])^2 = \exp(\sigma_U^2 - 1)\exp\left(2\mu^U + \sigma_U^2\right)$$

An application of Stein's Lemma with $g(x) = \exp(x)$ we have:

$$\rho_{Y,Z} = \mathrm{cov}[Y, Z] = \mathrm{cov}\left[e^U, Z\right] = \mathbf{E}\left[\exp(U)\right]\mathrm{cov}[U, Z] = \mu_Y\rho_{U,Z}$$

After some algebra, this yields to the following parametrization:

$$\mu_U = \ln(\mu_Y) - \frac{1}{2}\ln\left(1 + \frac{\sigma_Y^2}{(\mu_Y)^2}\right), \quad \sigma_U^2 = \ln\left(1 + \frac{\sigma_Y^2}{(\mu_Y)^2}\right) \quad \text{and} \quad \rho_{U,Z} = \frac{\rho_{Y,Z}}{\mu_Y}.$$

References

1. Anisimov, V.V., Fedorov, V.V.: Modelling, prediction and adaptive adjustment of recruitment in multicentre trials. Stat. Med. **26**(27), 4958–4975 (2007). https://doi.org/10.1002/sim.2956
2. Bonate, P., Gillespie, W., Ludden, T., Rubin, D., Stanski, D.: Simulation in drug development: Good practices. In: Holford, N., Hale, M., Ko, H., Steimer, J.L., Sheiner, L., Peck, C. (eds.) Published on the CDDS web site. http://holford.fmhs.auckland.ac.nz/docs/simulation-in-drug-development-good-practices.pdf (1999). Accessed 25 April 2017
3. Bonate, P.L.: Pharmacokinetic-Pharmacodynamic Modeling and Simulation. Springer, New York (2011)
4. Brindley, P.G., Dunn, W.F.: Simulation for clinical research trials: a theoretical outline. J. Crit. Care **24**(2), 164–167 (2009)
5. Holford, N., Ma, S.C., Ploeger, B.A.: Clinical trial simulation: a review. Clin. Pharmacol. Ther. **88**(2), 166–182 (2010)
6. Holford, N.H., Kimko, H.C., Monteleone, J.P., Peck, C.C.: Simulation of clinical trials. Annu. Rev. Pharmacol. Toxicol. **40**, 209–234 (2000)
7. Kimko, H.H.C., Peck, C.C.: Clinical Trial Simulations - Applications and Trends. Springer, New York (2011)
8. Mijoule, G., Savy, N., Savy, S.: Models for patients recruitment in clinical trials and sensitivity analysis. Stat. Med. **31**(16), 1655–1674 (2012)
9. Robert, C.P., Casella, G.: Monte Carlo Statistical Methods, 2nd edn. Springer Texts in Statistics. Springer, New York (2004). https://doi.org/10.1007/978-1-4757-4145-2. Accessed 25 April 2017
10. Robert, C.P., Casella, G.: Introducing Monte Carlo Methods With R. Use R! Springer, New York (2010). https://doi.org/10.1007/978-1-4419-1576-4. Accessed 25 April 2017
11. Tannenbaum, S.J., Holford, N.H., Lee, H., Peck, C.C., Mould, D.R.: Simulation of correlated continuous and categorical variables using a single multivariate distribution. J. Pharmacokinet. Pharmacodyn. **33**(6), 773–794 (2006)

Chapter 22
Determination of the Optimal Size of Subsamples for Testing a Correlation Coefficient by a Sequential Triangular Test

Dieter Rasch, Takuya Yanagida, Klaus D. Kubinger and Berthold Schneider

Abstract Schneider, Rasch, Kubinger and Yanagida [8] (Schneider, Rasch, Kubinger and Yanagida [8]. Stat. Pap. 56, 689 600) suggested a sequential triangular test for testing a correlation coefficient (see also Rasch, Yanagida, Kubinger, and Schneider [6]). In contrast to other sequential (triangular) tests, it is not possible to decide after each additional sampled research unit whether

(a) the null-hypothesis is to accept or
(b) to reject or
(c) to sample further units.

For the calculation of the correlation coefficient and to use Fisher's transformation, step-by-step $k \geq 4$ units are needed at once. In the present chapter, we improve the test proposed by Rasch, Yanagida, Kubinger and Schneider (2014) by determining which number k of subsampled research units is minimal (optimal), in order to hold the type-I-risk, given a specific type-II-risk and a specific effect size $\delta = \rho_1 - \rho_0$. Selected results are presented. For parameters not included irrespective tables, the reader may use a R package called seqtest for own simulations.

Keywords Optimal experimental design · Minimum sample size · Simulation Sequential analysis

---

D. Rasch (✉)
University of Natural Resources and Life Sciences, Vienna, Austria
e-mail: d_rasch@t-online.de

T. Yanagida
University of Vienna, Vienna, Austria
e-mail: takuya.yanagida@univie.ac.at

K. D. Kubinger
Division of Psychological Assessment and Applied Psychometrics,
Faculty of Psychology, University of Vienna, Vienna, Austria
e-mail: klaus.kubinger@univie.ac.at

B. Schneider
Institute for Biometry, Hannover Medical School, Hannover, Germany
e-mail: Schneider.Berthold@mh-hannover.de

J. Pilz et al. (eds.), *Statistics and Simulation*, Springer Proceedings in Mathematics & Statistics 231, https://doi.org/10.1007/978-3-319-76035-3_22

22.1 Introduction

The most effective strategy within statistics, that is sequential testing, has not been established for testing the composite null-hypothesis $H_0 : 0 < \rho \leq \rho_0$, before Schneider, Rasch, Kubinger and Yanagida [8]. Beyond the first concepts of sequential testing by Wald [9], a special group of sequential tests with a maximal number of research units needed are the sequential triangular tests. Such tests go back to Whitehead [10] and Schneider [7]. They have a fundamental advantage as their average sample size is quite smaller than that one of the corresponding tests with fixed sample size. Of course, a sequential test is in general appropriate only, if the time of sampling has no effect on the interesting character but the data are actually sampled step by step.

Given the distribution of a two-dimensional quantitative vector of random variables $(\mathbf{x}, \mathbf{y})^1$ is normal, so that the finite second moments σ_x^2, σ_y^2 and σ_{xy}, and the correlation coefficient $\rho = \sigma_{xy}/(\sigma_x\sigma_y)$ exist. Then the null-hypothesis $H_0 : 0 < \rho \leq \rho_0$ should be tested against the alternative hypothesis $H_1 : 0 < \rho_0 \leq \rho \leq \rho_1$ with a type-I-risk α, i.e. the probability of wrongly rejecting H_0 and a type-II-risk β, i.e. the probability of wrongly accepting H_0 (in particular as long as $\delta \geq \rho_1 - \rho_0$ with a ρ_1 to be fixed in advance). The method of the test was first described in Schneider et al [8] and will be only summarized. A more detailed description of sequential testing in general and especially of sequential triangular tests is given in Rasch and Schott [5] and Rasch, Kubinger and Yanagida [3].

In sequential analysis after each single observation or after each group of observations, a decision is made between (a) accept H_0, (b) reject H_0 or (c) continue with the next observation. But in the case of the correlation coefficient, we must have at least two observations and this calculated correlation coefficient is our "observation". The first question is, how many pairs k of values (x, y) we should use to calculate an observed value r (the sample correlation coefficient) to come as soon as possible to an end of the test we call this value of k optimal. Schneider et al [8] gave very rough intervals for the number of pairs, and it is the aim of the present chapter to improve this.

The empirical correlation coefficient $r = \frac{s_{xy}}{(s_x s_y)}$ based on k observations $(x, y)(i = 1, \ldots, k)$, i.e. realizations of $(\mathbf{x}, \mathbf{y})$, allows an estimation of the parameter $\rho(s_{xy}, s_x^2, s_y^2)$ are the empirical covariance and variances, respectively. When using r as a test statistic, we refer to the fact that the distribution of $\boldsymbol{r}$, i.e. the corresponding random variable, was derived by R.A. Fisher [1] under the assumption of a bivariate normal distribution of $(\mathbf{x}, \mathbf{y})$. He showed that the distribution of $\boldsymbol{r}$ then only depends on k and ρ. Later, Fisher [2] suggested the transformed value $z = \ln \frac{1+r}{1-r}$ as a test statistic and showed that the distribution of the corresponding random variable $\boldsymbol{z} = \ln\left(\frac{1+\boldsymbol{r}}{1-\boldsymbol{r}}\right)$ is approximately normal with expectation $E\mathbf{z} = \ln\left(\frac{1+\mathbf{r}}{1-\mathbf{r}}\right)$ even if k is rather small.

The statistic $\mathbf{z}$ can be used to test the hypothesis $H_0 : \rho \leq \rho_0$ against the one-sided (we restrict on this) alternative hypothesis $H_1 : \rho > \rho_0$ (respectively $H_0 : \rho \geq \rho_0$ against $H_1 : \rho < \rho_0$) for data with a fixed sample size k. $H_0 : \rho \leq \rho_0$ is rejected with error probability α, if $z \geq \xi(\rho_0) + z_{1-\alpha} \cdot \frac{2}{\sqrt{k-3}}$ (respectively for $H_0 : \rho \geq \rho_0$, if $z \geq \xi(\rho_0) - z_{1-\alpha} \cdot \frac{2}{\sqrt{k-3}}$); $z_{1-\alpha}$ is the $(1-\alpha)$-quantile of the standard normal distribution).

22.2 Method

The decision in a sequential triangular test is based on some statistic which is calculated at each step of sampling data. The values of this statistic is shown on a Cartesian coordinate system as the ordinate and the steps or sample sizes, respectively, at the abscissa. The result is a sequential path. As presented in the following, there is some continuation area—a triangle, anchored at the origin of the step axis. As long as the statistic's values lie within that triangle, more data have to be sampled. When the path touches or exceeds any borderline of the triangle, data sampling is completed and due to which borderline is concerned, either the null-hypothesis is accepted or rejected. Taken into account that one borderline is determined in such a way that the null-hypothesis is wrongly rejected only with probability α, the type-I-risk; the other borderline is determined so that the null-hypothesis is wrongly accepted only with probability β at most, the type-II-risk.

In details, some cumulative ascertained ancillary values Z_m and V_m are calculated for the actual values y_m. The values Z_m correspond to the ordinate and the values V_m to the abscissa. For a one-sided alternative hypothesis, two straight lines are defined in dependence on type-I and type-II risk (and, of course, in dependence on the practically relevant minimal difference $\delta = \rho_1 - \rho_0$ with respect to the hypothesized parameter). They create the talked about triangle which is open to the left side. Both the lines intersect each other at V_{max} that value corresponds to the maximal sample size n_{max} of the sequential triangular test which will be needed. As long as the sequence of the Z_m values remains within this triangle, sequential testing and data sampling, respectively, must be continued. In the case of a two-sided alternative hypothesis, there are two triangles, one for each of the two sides of the alternative hypothesis. Then the two-sided alternative hypothesis is to reject if the path touches or leaves one of the two triangles and enters the area of the null-hypothesis. For all this, we only have to use $\frac{\alpha}{2}$ instead of α for each side of the two-sided alternative hypothesis. Both triangles are open towards the left side and end at the same point of the abscissa on the right side.

As a triangular test must be based on a statistic with expectation 0, given the null-hypothesis, we transform Fishers statistic $z = \ln\left(\frac{1+r}{1-r}\right)$ into the standardized variable

$$z^* = [z - \xi(\rho_0)]\frac{\sqrt{k-3}}{2} = \left[z - \ln\left(\frac{1+\rho_0}{1-\rho_0}\right) - \frac{\rho_0}{k-1}\right]\frac{\sqrt{k-3}}{2} \tag{22.1}$$

which is (for not too small values of k) approximate normally distributed with variance 1 and the expectation:

$$\theta = E(z^*) = [\xi(\rho) - \xi(\rho_0)]\frac{\sqrt{k-3}}{2} = \left[\ln\frac{1+\rho}{1-\rho} - \ln\frac{1+\rho_0}{1-\rho_0} + \frac{\rho-\rho_0}{k-1}\right]\frac{\sqrt{k-3}}{2} \tag{22.2}$$

$$\theta = \left[\ln\frac{1+\rho_1}{1-\rho_1} - \ln\frac{1+\rho_0}{1-\rho_0} + \frac{\rho_1-\rho_0}{k-1}\right]\frac{\sqrt{k-3}}{2} \tag{22.3}$$

The difference $\delta = \rho_1 - \rho_0$ is the practical relevant difference which should be detected with the power $1 - \beta$.

From each subsample j, we now calculate the sample correlation coefficient $\mathbf{r}_j$ as well as its transformed value $z_j = \ln\frac{1+r_j}{1-r_j}$ and $z_j^* = \left[z_j - \ln\left(\frac{1+\rho_j}{1-\rho_0}\right) - \frac{\rho_0}{k-1}\right]\frac{\sqrt{k-3}}{2}$ $(j = 1, 2, \ldots, m)$.

Now the sequential path is defined by points (V_m, Z_m) for $m = 1, 2, \ldots$ up to the maximum of V below or exactly at the point where a terminal decision can be done. The continuation region is a triangle whose three sides depend on α, β and θ_1 via

$$a = \frac{\left(1 + \frac{z_{1-\beta}}{z_{1-\alpha}}\right)\ln\left(\frac{1}{2\alpha}\right)}{\theta_1} \tag{22.4}$$

and

$$b = \frac{\theta_1}{2\left(1 + \frac{z_{1-\beta}}{z_{1-\alpha}}\right)} \tag{22.5}$$

with the P-quantiles z_p of the standard normal distribution. That is, one side of the triangle lies between $-a$ and a on the ordinate of the (V, Z) plane $(V = 0)$. The two other borderlines are defined by the lines $L_1 : Z = a + cV$ and $L_2 : Z = -a + 3cV$, which intersect at

$$\left(V_{\max} = \frac{a}{c}, Z_{\max} = 2a\right). \tag{22.6}$$

The maximum total sample size is of course $k \cdot V_{\max}$. If $\theta = \theta_1 > \theta$ we get $a > 0$ and $c > 0$, and if $\theta_1 < \theta$ we get $a < 0$ and $c < 0$.

Table 22.1 A typical result from Schneider et al. [8] for $\rho_0 = 0.5$ and $\rho_1 = 0.6$ with $\alpha_{nominal} = 0.05$ and $\beta_{nominal} = 0.2$

k	12	16	20	50
α_{actual}	0.096	0.074	0.064	0.037
β_{actual}	0.082	0.105	0.123	0.147

The decision rule now is: continue sampling as long as $-a + 3cV_m < Z_m < a + cV_m$ if $\theta_1 > \theta$ or $a + 3cV_m > Z_m > a + acV_m$ if $\theta_1 < \theta$. Given $\theta_1 > \theta$, accept H_1 in the case Z_m reaches or exceeds L_1 and accept H_0 in the case Z_m reaches or underruns L_2. If the point $V_{\max} = \frac{a}{c}$, $Z_{\max} = 2a$ is reached, H_1 is to accept.

A typical result of Schneider et al. [8] is given in Table 22.1.

From this table, we can conclude that we have to choose k between 20 and 50 in order to obtain an actual value of α near to 0.05; but we do not know, which k is really optimal.

Furthermore, we now realize that the actual value of the type-II-risk was too small. That is, we have to look for an alternative nominal type-II-risk so that the corresponding actual type-II-risk lies below (nevertheless as near as possible) to the nominal one. In our example in Table 22.1, it should be below 0.2 but as near as possible to 0.2.

22.3 Simulation Study

In a simulation study

(a) we determined the optimal size of subsamples (k_{opt}), where the actual type-I-risk (α_{act}) is below but as close as possible to the nominal type-I-risk (α_{nom}) and
(b) we determined the optimal nominal type-II-risk (β_{opt}), where the corresponding actual type-II-risk ($\beta_{act)}$) is below but as close as possible to the nominal type-II-risk (β_{nom}).

Starting from $k = 4$, the size of the subsample was systematically increased with an increment of 1 for each parameter combination until the actual type-I-risk (α_{act}) fell below the nominal type-I-risk (α_{nom}). This optimal size of subsample (k_{opt}) was found in the next step to determine the optimal nominal type-II-risk (β_{opt}). That is, the nominal type-II-risk (β_{nom}) was systematically increased with an increment of 0.005 until the actual type-II-risk ($\beta_{act)}$) fell below the nominal type-II-risk (α_{nom}).

Paths (Z, V) were generated by bivariate normally distributed random numbers x and y with means $\mu_x = \mu_y = 0$, variances $\sigma_x^2 = \sigma_y^2 = 1$, and a correlation coefficient $\sigma_{xy} = \rho$. By the seqtest package version 0.1-0 [11] simulations can be performed for any α_{nom}, β_{nom} and $\delta = \rho_1 - \rho_0$. We present here results for nominal risks $\alpha_{nom} =$ 0.05 and 0.01, β_{nom} 0.01 and 0.2, values of ρ_0 ranging 0.1 to 0.9 with an increment of 0.1, and $\delta = \rho_1 - \rho_0 = 0.05, 0.10, 0.15,$ and 0.20.

For each parameter combination, 100 000 runs (paths) were generated. As criteria, we calculated

(a) the relative frequency of wrongly accepting H_1, given $\rho = \rho_0$, which is an estimate of the actual type-I-risk (α_{act}),
(b) the relative frequency of keeping H_0, given $\rho = \rho_1$ which is an estimate of the actual type-II-risk (β_{act}).
(c) the average number of sample pairs (x, y), i.e. average sample number (ASN), is the mean number of sample pairs over all 100 000 paths runs of the simulation study.

Results of the simulation study are shown in Table 22.2 (for $\alpha_{nom} = 0.05$) and Table 22.3 (for $\alpha_{nom} = 0.01$). We found that the optimal size of the subsample (k_{opt}) decreases with increasing $\delta = \rho_1 - \rho_0$, that k_{opt} is smaller for $\beta_{nom} = 0.2$ than for $\beta_{nom} = 0.1$ and that k_{opt} is smaller for $\alpha_{nom} = 0.05$ than for $\alpha_{nom} = 0.01$. As for

Table 22.2 Optimal values of k and β_{nom} (use) for $\alpha = 0.05$

Given values of the test problem			Optimal values		
ρ_0	ρ_1	β	k	β_{opt}	$ASN\|\rho_1$
0.1	0.15	0.1	14	0.110	2320
		0.2	10	0.220	1975
	0.20	0.1	7	0.135	683
		0.2	6	0.255	591
	0.25	0.1	5	0.160	373
		0.2	5	0.275	302
	0.30	0.1	5	0.160	211
		0.2	5	0.270	173
0.2	0.25	0.1	16	0.110	2116
		0.2	14	0.220	1719
	0.30	0.1	10	0.120	571
		0.2	8	0.240	483
	0.35	0.1	7	0.135	280
		0.2	6	0.265	239
	0.40	0.1	5	0.175	185
		0.2	5	0.285	153
0.3	0.35	0.1	18	0.115	1840
		0.2	16	0.220	1505
	0.40	0.1	11	0.120	492
		0.2	10	0.230	406
	0.45	0.1	8	0.135	231
		0.2	7	0.255	195
	0.50	0.1	6	0.160	141
		0.2	5	0.300	128

(continued)

Table 22.2 (continued)

Given values of the test problem			Optimal values		
ρ_0	ρ_1	β	k	β_{opt}	$ASN\|\rho_1$
0.4	0.45	0.1	17	0.115	1564
		0.2	16	0.225	1259
	0.50	0.1	11	0.125	408
		0.2	10	0.240	334
	0.55	0.1	8	0.140	190
		0.2	7	0.260	160
	0.60	0.1	7	0.150	107
		0.2	6	0.275	94
0.5	0.55	0.1	17	0.120	1220
		0.2	16	0.230	984
	0.60	0.1	11	0.130	315
		0.2	9	0.250	264
	0.65	0.1	8	0.145	144
		0.2	7	0.265	123
	0.70	0.1	6	0.175	84
		0.2	6	0.285	70
0.6	0.65	0.1	16	0.120	884
		0.2	15	0.230	715
	0.70	0.1	10	0.140	223
		0.2	9	0.255	185
	0.75	0.1	8	0.150	98
		0.2	7	0.270	84
	0.80	0.1	6	0.170	98
		0.2	5	0.325	51
0.7	0.75	0.1	15	0.130	543
		0.2	13	0.240	450
	0.80	0.1	9	0.145	136
		0.2	8	0.265	114
	0.85	0.1	6	0.185	60
		0.2	6	0.295	50
	0.90	0.1	5	0.215	31
		0.2	4	0.320	27
0.8	0.85	0.1	11	0.140	268
		0.2	11	0.250	219
	0.90	0.1	7	0.170	61
		0.2	6	0.305	54
	0.95	0.1	4	0.220	23
		0.2	4	0.325	20
0.9	0.95	0.1	7	0.175	66
		0.2	7	0.285	56

Table 22.3 Optimal values of k and β_{nom} (use) for $\alpha = 0.01$

Given values of the test problem			Optimal values		
ρ_0	ρ_1	β	k	β_{opt}	$ASN\|\rho_1$
0.1	0.15	0.1	14	0.0110	3713
		0.2	12	0.0220	3218
	0.20	0.1	9	0.120	1022
		0.2	8	0.235	896
	0.25	0.1	5	0.175	591
		0.2	5	0.290	507
	0.30	0.1	5	0.170	334
		0.2	5	0.285	287
0.2	0.25	0.1	19	0.110	3380
		0.2	16	0.215	2877
	0.30	0.1	11	0.125	903
		0.2	8	0.245	814
	0.35	0.1	7	0.140	442
		0.2	6	0.275	401
	0.40	0.1	6	0.155	264
		0.2	6	0.265	227
0.3	0.35	0.1	22	0.110	2920
		0.2	17	0.220	2520
	0.40	0.1	11	0.125	778
		0.2	10	0.235	678
	0.45	0.1	10	0.125	349
		0.2	9	0.240	304
	0.50	0.1	7	0.145	211
		0.2	6	0.280	192
0.4	0.45	0.1	20	0.120	2477
		0.2	19	0.225	2083
	0.50	0.1	12	0.130	642
		0.2	11	0.235	552
	0.55	0.1	9	0.135	291
		0.2	8	0.255	255
	0.60	0.1	7	0.150	169
		0.2	6	0.285	155
0.5	0.55	0.1	19	0.115	1947
		0.2	16	0.230	1668
	0.60	0.1	12	0.125	495
		0.2	10	0.245	434
	0.65	0.1	9	0.140	219
		0.2	8	0.255	195
	0.70	0.1	7	0.155	125
		0.2	7	0.270	108

(continued)

Table 22.3 (continued)

Given values of the test problem			Optimal values		
ρ_0	ρ_1	β	k	β_{opt}	$ASN\vert\rho_1$
0.6	0.65	0.1	19	0.120	1382
		0.2	16	0.230	1196
	0.70	0.1	11	0.135	347
		0.2	10	0.250	303
	0.75	0.1	8	0.150	153
		0.2	8	0.260	132
	0.80	0.1	6	0.180	86
		0.2	5	0.340	83
0.7	0.75	0.1	18	0.120	860
		0.2	15	0.235	743
	0.80	0.1	10	0.140	208
		0.2	9	0.260	183
	0.85	0.1	7	0.165	88
		0.2	6	0.30	82
	0.90	0.1	5	0.220	48
		0.2	5	0.330	42
0.8	0.85	0.1	13	0.135	413
		0.2	12	0.245	360
	0.90	0.1	7	0.175	95
		0.2	7	0.285	83
	0.95	0.1	5	0.220	35
		0.2	5	0.330	31
0.9	0.95	0.1	8	0.185	436
		0.2	7	0.340	378

the optimal nominal type-II-risk (β_{opt}), the difference $\beta_{opt} - \beta_{nom}$ is larger with increasing ρ_0 and increasing $\delta = \rho_1 - \rho_0$.

In order to determine the optimal size of subsamples ($k_{opt)}$) and the optimal nominal type-II-risk (β_{opt}) for parameter combination not included in Tables 22.2 and 22.3, the reader may use the R package seqtest for own simulations.

22.4 The R-Program and an Example

The sequential triangular test for testing a correlation coefficient is implemented in the R package seqtest [11], which is available on The Comprehensive R Archive Network (CRAN) [6] and can be installed via command line

```
install.packages("seqtest").
```

This package offers a simulation function to determine the optimal size of subsamples (k_{opt}) and the optimal nominal type-II-risk (β_{opt}) for a user-specified parameter combination. In the following example, we determine k_{opt} and β_{opt} for $H_0 : \rho_0 \leq 0.3$ and $H_1 : \rho_1 > 0.3$ with $\delta = 0.25$ and $\alpha_{nom} = 0.01$ and $\beta_{nom} = 0.05$.
After installing the package, it is loaded using

```
library(seqtest)
```

In the first step, we determine the optimal size of subsamples (k_{opt}). We type

```
sim.seqtest.cor(rho.sim = 0.3, k = seq(4, 10, by = 1), rho = 0.3,
alternative = "greater", delta = 0.25, alpha = 0.05, beta = 0.05,
runs = 10000)
```

That is, we apply the function `sim.seqtest.corr()` using the first argument `rho.sim` to specify the simulated correlation coefficient ρ and the arguments k to specify a sequence for k, i.e. from 4 to 10 by increment of 1, for which the simulation is conducted. With the argument `alternative ="greater"`, we state that the alternative hypothesis is one-sided and the arguments delta, alpha and beta are used to specify ρ, α_{nom} and β_{nom}. Last, we specify 10000 runs using argument `runs` for each simulation condition.
As a results, we obtain:

```
Statistical Simulation for the Sequential Triangular Test

   H0: rho <= 0.3   versus  H1: rho > 0.3

   Nominal type-I-risk (alpha):        0.05
   Nominal type-II-risk (beta):        0.05
   Practical relevant effect (delta):  0.25

   Simulated data based on rho:        0.3
   Simulation runs:                    10000

  Estimated empirical type-I-risk (alpha):
   k = 4:   0.057
   k = 5:   0.054
   k = 6:   0.048
   k = 7:   0.043
   k = 8:   0.042
   k = 9:   0.040
   k = 10:  0.039
```

[output shortend]

Simulation results indicate that $k = 6$ is the optimal value, where α_{act} is below but close to α_{nom}.

In the next step, we determine the optimal nominal type-II-risk β_{opt} based on the optimal size of subsamples $k_{opt} = 6$. We type

```
sim.seqtest.cor(rho.sim = 0.55, k = 6, rho = 0.3,
alternative = "greater",
delta = 0.25, alpha = 0.05,
beta = seq(0.05, 0.10, by = 0.01), runs = 10000)
```

That is, again we apply the function `sim.seqtest.cor()` and specify the argument $k = 6$ for $k_{opt} = 6$, which was determined in the previous step. This time, we specify `rho.sim = 0.55` to simulate the H_1 condition and use the argument `beta` to specify a sequence for β_{nom}, i.e. from 0.05 to 0.10 by increment of 0.01, for which the simulation is conducted. As a result, we obtain:

```
Statistical Simulation for the Sequential Triangular Test

   H0: rho <= 0.3  versus  H1: rho > 0.3

   Nominal type-I-risk (alpha):        0.05
   Practical relevant effect (delta): 0.25
   n in each subsample (k):           6

   Simulated data based on rho:        0.55
   Simulation runs:                    10000

  Estimated empirical type-II-risk (beta):
   Nominal beta = 0.05: 0.022
   Nominal beta = 0.06: 0.029
   Nominal beta = 0.07: 0.038
   Nominal beta = 0.08: 0.046
   Nominal beta = 0.09: 0.044
   Nominal beta = 0.10: 0.057
```

[output shortend]

Simulation results indicate that $\beta_{nom} = 0.10$ is the optimal value, where β_{act} is below but close to β_{nom}.

The optimal values k_{opt} and β_{opt} determined by the simulation function are used for the sequential triangular test for testing a correlation coefficient. Let us assume that the first correlation coefficient calculated from a sample of 6 pairs is $r_1 = 0.75$. We type

```
seq.obj <- seqtest.cor(0.75, k = 6, rho = 0.3,
alternative = "greater",
delta = 0.25, alpha = 0.05, beta = 0.10,
plot = TRUE)
```

That is, we apply the function `seqtest.corr()`, using the first argument to specify the sampled correlation coefficient 0.75. We specify ρ_0, δ and α using arguments `rho`, `delta` and `alpha` and specify k_{opt} and β_{opt} using function `k` and `beta`. With the argument `alternative ="greater"`, we state that the alternative hypothesis is one-sided and with `plot = TRUE`, we request a plot for the results. The result is assigned to the `object seq.obj`. As a result, we obtain:

```
Sequential triangular test for the product-moment  correlation
coefficient

  H0: rho <= 0.3   versus  H1: rho.1 > 0.3
  alpha: 0.05  beta: 0.1  delta: 0.25  k: 6

  Step 1
    V.m:      1.000        Z.m:       1.097
    Continuation range | V.m: [-6.597, 7.247]

  Test not finished, continue by adding data via
update()
  Current sample size for 1 correlation coefficient:
1 x 6 = 6
```

Results show that the test statistic Z_m is within the continuation range conditioned on V_m. Hence, no final decision is achievable and for that reason, we continue our study. Next, let us assume we sampled $r_2 = 0.83, r_3 = 0.86, r_4 = 0.79, r_5 = 0.81$ and $r_6 = 0.80$ from $k = 6$ pairs each.

We type

```
update(seq.obj, x = c(0.83, 0.86, 0.79, 0.81, 0.80))
```

That is, we apply the function `update()` to update results in the seq.obj object. As a result, we obtain:

```
Sequential triangular test for Pearson's correlation coefficient

  H0: rho.0 <= 0.3  versus  H1: rho.1 > 0.3
  alpha: 0.05  beta: 0.10  delta: 0.25  k: 6

  Step 2
    V.m:      2.000        Z.m:       2.567
    Continuation range | V.m: [-6.109, 7.409]

  Step 3
    V.m:      3.000        Z.m:       4.219
    Continuation range | V.m: [-5.622, 7.572]

  Step 4
    V.m:      4.000        Z.m:       5.487
    Continuation range | V.m: [-5.134, 7.734]
```

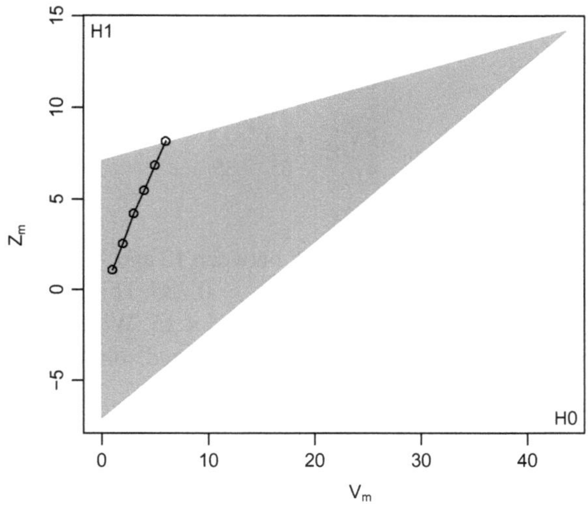

Fig. 22.1 Graph of the triangle of the example with corner points (0; −7.08), (0; 7.08), and (43.60; 14.20), the arbitrarily sampled steps of $k = 6$ data pairs included leading to $r_1 = 0.75$, $r_2 = 0.83$, $r_3 = 0.86$, $r_4 = 0.79$, $r_5 = 0.81$, $r_6 = 0.80$; the point $(V_1 = 1, Z_1 = 1.097)$, $(V_2 = 2, Z_2 = 2.567)$, $(V_3 = 3, Z_3 = 4.219)$, $(V_4 = 4, Z_4 = 5.487)$, $(V_5 = 5, Z_5 = 6.851)$ and $(V_6 = 6, Z_6 = 8.166)$ represented by the circle by six connected circles

```
    Step 5
      V.m:      5.000        Z.m:        6.851
      Continuation range | V.m: [[-4.647, 7.897]


    Step 6
      V.m:      6.000        Z.m:        8.166
      Continuation range | V.m: [-4.159, 8.059]


    Test finished: Accept alternative hypothesis (H1)
    Final sample size for 5 correlation coefficients:
  6 x 6 = 36
```

Results show that the cumulated test statistic Z_m leaves the continuation range conditioned on V_m at Step 6. Hence, the test is finished and the alternative hypothesis is to be accepted (Fig. 22.1).

22.5 Discussion

Let us show by an example how good the improvement with the proposed new approach can be. We consider Table 22.1 in Schneider et al. (2014) and look at the row for $\rho_0 = .5$, $\rho_1 = .0.7$. and $\alpha = 0.05$. We find there the result:

	$\beta_2 = 0.2$	
k	12	16
α_{act}	0.53	0.42
β_{act}	0.114	0.13
$ASN\vert\rho_1$	62.1	62.3
n_{fix}	65	65

From this table, we do not know which k between 12 and 16 we have to choose. In Table 22.2, we find an optimal $k = 13$ and $\beta_{(opt)} = 0.285$. This leads to an $ASN|\rho_1 = 54$ and this means a mean subsample size of $\frac{54}{13} = 4.15$. When the readers uses the R-program given, they are able to determine an optimal solution for any parameter configuration.

References

1. Fisher, R.A.: Frequency distribution of the values of the correlation coefficient in samples from an indefinitely large population. Biometrika **10**, 507–521 (1915)
2. Fisher, R.A.: On the probable error of a coefficient of correlation deduced from a small sample. Metron **1**, 3–32 (1921)
3. Rasch, D., Kubinger, K.D., Yanagida, T.: Statistics in Psychology Using R and SPSS. Wiley, Chichester (2011)
4. Rasch, D., Yanagida, T., Kubinger, K.D., Schneider, B.: Towards sequential statistical testing as some standard: Pearson's correlation coefficient. GMS Med Inform Biom Epidemiol **10**(1):Doc07 (2014028) (2014)
5. Rasch, D., Schott, D.: Mathematical Statistics. Wiley, Oxford (2018)
6. R Core Team: R: A language and environment for statistical computing. R Foundation for Statistical Computing, Vienna, Austria (2013). http://www.R-project.org/. Accessed 19 Aug 2017
7. Schneider, B.: An interactive computer program for design and monotoring of sequential clinical trials. In Proceedings of the XVIth international biometric conference, pp. 237–250. Hamilton, New Zealand (1992)
8. Schneider, B., Rasch, D., Kubinger, K.D., Yanagida, T.: A Sequential Triangular Test of a Correlation Coefficients Null-Hypothesis: $0<\rho \leq \rho_0$. Stat. Pap. **56**, 689 600 (2015)
9. Wald, A.: Sequential Analysis. Wiley, New York (1947)
10. Whitehead, J.: The Design and Analysis of Sequential Clinical Trials, 2nd edn. Ellis Horwood, Chichester (1992)
11. Yanagida, T.: Seqtest: sequential triangular test. R package version 0.1-0 (2016). http://CRAN.R-project.org/package=seqtest. Accessed 19 Aug 2017

Chapter 23
Explicit T-optimal Designs for Trigonometric Regression Models

Viatcheslav B. Melas and Petr V. Shpilev

Abstract This chapter devotes to the problem of constructing T-optimal discriminating designs for Fourier regression models which differ by at most three trigonometric functions. Here we develop the results obtained in a paper (Dette, Melas and Shpilev (2015). T-optimal discriminating designs for Fourier regression models. 1–17) [11] and give a few its generalizations. We consider in detail the case of discriminating between two models where the order of the larger one equals two. For this case, we provide explicit solutions and investigate the dependence of the locally T-optimal discriminating designs on the parameters of the larger model. The results obtained in the chapter can also be applied in classical approximation theory.

Keywords T-optimal design · Model discrimination · Linear optimality criteria Trigonometric models

23.1 Introduction

This chapter addresses the discriminating design problem for regression models when the primary outcome is continuous, and it is not known a priori which model is an appropriate one to use. Such problems are common for applied regression analysis; [see, for example, [2, 4, 6]]. In this situation, one of the possible ways is to consider a class of feasible models to which we believe an adequate model for fitting the data belongs. The focal point is how to design the experiment to choose the most appropriate model from within this class. There are two different approaches to this problem in the literature. The first one [14, 15, 25] consists in considering two nested models, i.e., such as those for which the model with a smaller number of parameters can be obtained from another model by setting specific values for the parameters.

V. B. Melas · P. V. Shpilev (✉)
Department of Mathematics, St. Petersburg State University,
7/9 Universitetskaya nab., St. Petersburg 199034, Russia
e-mail: pitshp@hotmail.com

V. B. Melas
e-mail: vbmelas@post.ru

J. Pilz et al. (eds.), *Statistics and Simulation*, Springer Proceedings
in Mathematics & Statistics 231, https://doi.org/10.1007/978-3-319-76035-3_23

The experimenter is interested in finding efficient design which allows to identify an appropriate model and, at the same time, estimate these parameters most precisely. Since its advent, this approach was developed by numerous authors (see [5, 7–9, 13, 23, 24, 26, 31] among others). The alternative approach was presented in the fundamental paper of [3] who introduced the T-optimality criterion for discriminating between two competing regression models. Since its introduction, the problem of determining T-optimal designs has been considered by numerous authors [see [1, 4, 12, 27, 28] or [29, 30] among others]. T-optimal designs are usually used to discriminate between homoscedastic models with normal errors [2, 4, 6, 14]. For discriminating nonlinear models, only numerical results are possible; [19] investigated optimal designs maximizing the weighted average of two T-criterion functions, and [20] constructed T -optimal designs for Michaelis–Menten-like models. The T-optimal design problem is essentially a minimax problem, and, except for very simple models, the corresponding optimal designs are not easy to find and have to be determined numerically. For this reason, the analytical solutions for models with a large number of parameters are very useful not only in terms of application but also as a tool for testing numerical optimization methods. In recent papers, [10, 11] some explicit solutions of the T-optimal design problem for discriminating between two polynomial regression models [10] and for two Fourier regression models [11] were obtained, but to our best knowledge, no other analytical solutions are available in the literature.

In the present chapter, we consider the problem of constructing T-optimal discrimination designs for Fourier regression models which are widely used in applications to describe periodic phenomena. Typical subject areas include engineering [see, e.g., [21]], medicine [see, e.g., [17]], and biology [18].

Discriminating designs in sense of [14, 15, 25] have been investigated by [5, 31] among others, but only one paper [11] was devoted to the problem of constructing T-optimal designs for Fourier regression models in the literature so far. In the present work, we provide some further results on this issue. In Sect. 23.2, we introduce the problem and present some basic notions. In Sect. 23.3, we give a short review of the main results obtained in the paper [11]. In the last section, we provide a few theoretical results and give some explicit solutions for discriminating between two trigonometric models where the largest one has the order $m = 2$.

23.2 T-optimal Discriminating Designs

Consider the classical regression model

$$y = \eta(x) + \varepsilon \tag{23.2.1}$$

where the explanatory variable x varies in the design space $\mathscr{X}$, and observations at different locations, say x and x', are assumed to be uncorrelated with the same variance. In (23.2.1), the quantity ε denotes a random variable with mean 0 and variance σ^2, and $\eta(x)$ is a function which is called regression function in the literature [see, e.g., [22]].

We assume that the experimenter has two parametric models for this function in mind, that is

$$\eta_1(x, \theta_1) \text{ and } \eta_2(x, \theta_2). \tag{23.2.2}$$

And the first goal of the experiment is to discriminate between these two models. In order to find "good" designs for discriminating between the models η_1 and η_2, we consider approximate designs, as suggested by [16], which are probability measures on the design space $\mathscr{X}$ with finite support. The support points, say $x_1, \dots, x_s$, of an (approximate) design ξ give the locations where observations are taken, while the weights define the corresponding relative proportions of total observations to be taken at these points. If the design ξ has masses $\omega_i > 0$ at the different points x_i $(i = 1, \dots, k)$ and N observations can be made by the experimenter, the quantities $\omega_i N$ are rounded to integers, say n_i, satisfying $\sum_{i=1}^{s} n_i = N$, and the experimenter takes n_i observations at each location x_i $(i = 1, \dots, k)$.

T-optimal design is the design which maximizes the minimal deviation between the model η_2 and the class of models defined by η_1, that is,

$$\xi^* = \arg\max_{\xi} \int_{\chi} \left(\eta_2(x, \theta_2) - \eta_1(x, \widehat{\theta_1})\right)^2 \xi(dx)$$

where the parameter $\widehat{\theta_1}$ minimizes the expression

$$\widehat{\theta_1} = \arg\min_{\theta_1} \int_{\chi} (\eta_2(x, \theta_2) - \eta_1(x, \theta_1))^2 \, \xi(dx)$$

In present work, we consider the regression functions $\eta_1(x, \theta_1)$ and $\eta_2(x, \theta_2)$ given by

$$\eta_1(x, \theta_1) = \overline{q}_0 + \sum_{i=1}^{k_1} \overline{q}_{2i-1} \sin(ix) + \sum_{i=1}^{k_2} \overline{q}_{2i} \cos(ix) \tag{23.2.3}$$

and

$$\begin{aligned} \eta_2(x, \theta_2) = {} & \tilde{q}_0 + \sum_{i=1}^{k_1} \tilde{q}_{2i-1} \sin(ix) + \sum_{i=1}^{k_2} \tilde{q}_{2i} \cos(ix) \\ & + \sum_{i=k_1+1}^{m} b_{2(i-k_1)-1} \sin(ix) + \sum_{i=k_2+1}^{m} b_{2(i-k_2)} \cos(ix), \end{aligned} \tag{23.2.4}$$

where

$$\theta_1 = (\overline{q}_0, \overline{q}_2, \ldots, \overline{q}_{2k_2}, \overline{q}_1, \ldots, \overline{q}_{2k_1-1})$$
$$\theta_2 = (\tilde{q}_0, \ldots, \tilde{q}_{2k_2}, \tilde{q}_1, \ldots, \tilde{q}_{2k-1}, b_2, \ldots, b_{2m}, b_1, \ldots, b_{2m-1})$$

are the parameter vectors in model η_1 and η_2, respectively.

We assume that the design space is given by the interval $\chi = [0, 2\pi]$ and denote the difference $\eta_2(x, \theta_2) - \eta_1(x, \theta_1)$ by

$$\begin{aligned}\overline{\eta}(x, q, \overline{b}) = q_0 + \sum_{i=1}^{k_1} q_{2i-1} \sin(ix) + \sum_{i=1}^{k_2} q_{2i} \cos(ix) + \\ + \sum_{i=k_1+1}^{m} b_{2(i-k_1)-1} \sin(ix) + \sum_{i=k_2+1}^{m} b_{2(i-k_2)} \cos(ix),\end{aligned} \tag{23.2.5}$$

where $q = (q_0, q_1, \ldots, q_{2k_1-1}, q_2, \ldots, q_{2k_2})$, $q_i = \tilde{q}_i - \overline{q}_i$ and $\overline{b} = (b_1, b_3, \ldots, b_{2(m-k_1)-1}, b_2, b_4, \ldots, b_{2(m-k_2)})^T$ denote the vector of "additional" parameters in the model (23.2.4). With these notations, we can rewrite the T-optimality criterion as follows

$$T(\xi, \overline{b}) = \min_q \int_\chi \overline{\eta}(x, q, \overline{b})^2 \xi(dx), \ \chi = [0, 2\pi],$$
$$\xi^* = \arg\max_\xi T(\xi, \overline{b})$$

As pointed out in the introduction, the explicit determination of T-optimal discriminating designs is a very challenging problem. The complexity of the problem depends on the dimension of the vector $\overline{b}$. In the next section, we give a short review of the main results obtained in the paper [11].

23.3 Explicit Solutions

In this section, we consider some explicit T-optimal discriminating designs for Fourier regression models obtained in the paper [11] for the models (23.2.3) and (23.2.4), where

$$k_1 = k_2 = m - 1, \tag{23.3.1}$$
$$k_1 = m - 1, \ k_2 = m - 2, \tag{23.3.2}$$
$$k_1 = m - 2, \ k_2 = m - 1. \tag{23.3.3}$$

23.3.1 Discriminating Designs for $k_1 = k_2 = m - 1$

Theorem 23.1 *Consider the Fourier regression models* (23.2.3) *and* (23.2.4) *with* $k_1 = k_2 = m - 1$. *Let* $b_1, b_2 \neq 0$, *then the design*

$$\xi^* = \begin{pmatrix} \frac{1}{m}\arctan(\frac{1}{b}) & \frac{1}{m}\arctan(\frac{1}{b}) + \frac{\pi}{m} & \dots & \frac{1}{m}\arctan(\frac{1}{b}) + \frac{(2m-1)\pi}{m} \\ \frac{1}{2m} & \frac{1}{2m} & \dots & \frac{1}{2m} \end{pmatrix} \quad (23.3.4)$$

is a T*-optimal discriminating design, where* $b = b_2/b_1$.

Corollary 23.1 *Consider the Fourier regression models* (23.2.3) *and* (23.2.4) *with* $k_1 = k_2 = m - 1$. *If* $b_1 = 0$, *then the design*

$$\xi^* = \begin{pmatrix} 0 & \frac{\pi}{m} & \dots & \frac{(2m-1)\pi}{m} \\ \frac{1}{2m} & \frac{1}{2m} & \dots & \frac{1}{2m} \end{pmatrix}$$

is a T*-optimal discriminating design. If* $b_2 = 0$, *then the design*

$$\xi^* = \begin{pmatrix} \frac{\pi}{2m} & \frac{3\pi}{2m} & \dots & \frac{(4m-1)\pi}{2m} \\ \frac{1}{2m} & \frac{1}{2m} & \dots & \frac{1}{2m} \end{pmatrix}$$

is a T*-optimal discriminating design.*

23.3.2 Discriminating Designs for $k_1 = m - 1$, $k_2 = m - 2$

If $k_1 = m - 1$, $k_2 = m - 2$, the function $\overline{\eta}$ in (23.2.5) has the representation

$$\begin{aligned} \overline{\eta}(x, q, \overline{b}) = q_0 + \sum_{i=1}^{m-1} q_{2i-1}\sin(ix) + \sum_{i=1}^{m-2} q_{2i}\cos(ix) + \\ + b_0\cos((m-1)x) + b_1\sin(mx) + b_2\cos(mx). \end{aligned} \quad (23.3.5)$$

Define support and weights points as follows

$$x_i^*(b) = \arccos\left(-\left(1 + \frac{1}{2m|b|}\right)\cos\left(\frac{(m-i+1)\pi}{m}\right) - \frac{1}{2m|b|}\right), \quad (23.3.6)$$

$$\omega_i^* = \frac{1}{m}\cos^2\left(\frac{(i-1)\pi}{2m}\right), \quad i = 1, \dots, m. \quad (23.3.7)$$

Theorem 23.2 gives an explicit solution of the T-optimal design problem in the case $b_1 = 0,\ b_2 \neq 0$.

Theorem 23.2 *Consider the difference between two Fourier regression models* (23.3.5) *with* $b_0 = 1,\ b_1 = 0,\ b_2 \neq 0.$

(a) If $b_2 \geq \frac{1}{2m}\cot^2\left(\frac{\pi}{2m}\right)$, *then the design*

$$\xi_1^* = \begin{pmatrix} x_1^*(b_2) & \dots & x_m^*(b_2) & 2\pi - x_m^*(b_2) & \dots & 2\pi - x_2^*(b_2) \\ \omega_1^* & \dots & \omega_m^* & \omega_m^* & \dots & \omega_2^* \end{pmatrix} \quad (23.3.8)$$

is a T-discriminating optimal design, where the support points and weights are defined in (23.3.6) and (23.3.7), respectively.

(b) If $b_2 \leq -\frac{1}{2m}\cot^2\left(\frac{\pi}{2m}\right)$, *then the design*

$$\xi_2^* = \begin{pmatrix} \pi - x_m^*(b_2) & \dots & \pi - x_1^*(b_2) & \pi + x_2^*(b_2) & \dots & \pi + x_m^*(b_2) \\ \omega_m^* & \dots & \omega_1^* & \omega_2^* & \dots & \omega_m^* \end{pmatrix} \quad (23.3.9)$$

is a T-discriminating optimal design, where the support points and weights are defined in (23.3.6) and (23.3.7), respectively.

The next theorem considers the case $b_1 \neq 0,\ b_2 = 0$, which is substantially harder. Here, the locally T-optimal discriminating designs are determined explicitly only for the case m is odd, where m is the degree of the Fourier regression model.

Theorem 23.3 *Consider the difference between two Fourier regression models* (23.3.5) *with* $b_0 = 1, b_1 \neq 0, b_2 = 0$, *where* m *is odd. For* $\ell = 1, 2$ *let* $t_i^{(\xi_\ell)}$ *and* $\omega_i^{(\xi_\ell)}$, *denote the support points and weights of the designs* ξ_1 *and* ξ_2 *defined in* (23.3.8) *and* (23.3.9) *of Theorem 23.2, and define*

$$t_i^{(\ell)} = t_i^{(\xi_\ell)} + \frac{\pi}{2}\ mod\ 2\pi;\ \ \ell = 1, 2.$$

(a) If $b_1 \geq \frac{1}{2m}\cot^2\left(\frac{\pi}{2m}\right)$, *then the design*

$$\tilde{\xi}_1^* = \begin{pmatrix} t_1^{(1)} & \dots & t_{2m-1}^{(1)} \\ \omega_1^{(\xi_1)} & \dots & \omega_{2m-1}^{(\xi_1)} \end{pmatrix}$$

is a T-optimal discriminating design.

(b) If $b_1 \leq -\frac{1}{2m}\cot^2\left(\frac{\pi}{2m}\right)$, *then the design*

$$\tilde{\xi}_2^* = \begin{pmatrix} t_1^{(2)} & \dots & t_{2m-1}^{(2)} \\ \omega_1^{(\xi_2)} & \dots & \omega_{2m-1}^{(\xi_2)} \end{pmatrix}$$

is a T-optimal discriminating design.

23.3.3 Discriminating Designs for $k_1 = m - 2, k_2 = m - 1$

If $k_1 = m - 2, k_2 = m - 1$, the function $\overline{\eta}$ in (23.2.5) has the representation

$$\begin{aligned}\overline{\eta}(x, q, \overline{b}) = q_0 + \sum_{i=1}^{m-2} q_{2i-1} \sin(ix) + \sum_{i=1}^{m-1} q_{2i} \cos(ix) + \\ + b_0 \sin((m-1)x) + b_1 \sin(mx) + b_2 \cos(mx).\end{aligned} \quad (23.3.10)$$

Theorem 23.4 *Consider the difference between two Fourier regression models* (23.3.10) *with* $b_0 = 1, b_1 = 0, b_2 \neq 0$, *where* m *is even. For* $\ell = 1, 2$ *let* $t_i^{(\xi_\ell)}$ *and* $\omega_i^{(\xi_\ell)}$, *denote the support points and weights of the designs* ξ_1 *and* ξ_2 *defined in* (23.3.8) *and* (23.3.9) *of Theorem 23.2, and define*

$$t_i^{(\ell)} = t_i^{(\xi_\ell)} + \frac{3\pi}{2} \; mod \; 2\pi; \quad \ell = 1, 2.$$

(a) If $b_2 \geq \frac{1}{2m} \cot^2\left(\frac{\pi}{2m}\right)$, *then the design*

$$\tilde{\xi}_1^* = \begin{pmatrix} t_1^{(1)} & \dots & t_{2m-1}^{(1)} \\ \omega_1^{(\xi_1)} & \dots & \omega_{2m-1}^{(\xi_1)} \end{pmatrix}$$

is a T*-optimal discriminating design.*

(b) If $b_2 \leq -\frac{1}{2m} \cot^2\left(\frac{\pi}{2m}\right)$, *then the design*

$$\tilde{\xi}_2^* = \begin{pmatrix} t_1^{(2)} & \dots & t_{2m-1}^{(2)} \\ \omega_1^{(\xi_2)} & \dots & \omega_{2m-1}^{(\xi_2)} \end{pmatrix}$$

is a T*-optimal discriminating design.*

As was mentioned before, all results in this section were obtained in the paper [11]; see this paper for more details.

In general, the solution of the locally T-optimal design problem depends in a complicated way on the parameters $\overline{b}$, and the number of support points of the T-optimal discriminating design changes if the vector $\overline{b}$ is located in different areas of the space $\mathbb{R}^2$. In the following section, we give some explicit solutions for the Fourier regression model of second order ($m = 2$).

23.4 Explicit Solution. Case M = 2

In this section, we consider the problem of constructing T-optimal designs for special case m=2. The theoretical results obtained in this section follow from the properties of trigonometric functions. If $m = 2$ and $k_1 = 1, k_2 = 0$, the function $\overline{\eta}$ in (23.2.5) has the representation

$$\overline{\eta}(x, q, \overline{b}) = q_0 + q_1 \sin(x) + \cos(x) + b_1 \sin(2x) + b_2 \cos(2x). \quad (23.4.11)$$

The number of T-optimal designs' support points equals 2 or 3 and depends on which area a point (b_1, b_2) belongs to.

Note that according to the equivalence theorem for T-optimality (see, e.g., [11]), support points of any optimal design ξ are extremums of some function ψ^* which is satisfied to certain conditions. Such function is often called an extremal function for the design ξ.

The following theorem provides explicit T-optimal designs for the difference between two models (23.4.11).

Theorem 23.5 *Consider the function $\overline{\eta}(x, q, \overline{b})$ (23.4.11). Let $b_2^*(b_1) : [0, \infty) \to [0, \infty)$ be a function such that for any point (b_1, b_2) the following conditions hold true*

$$\#supp(\xi^*) = \begin{cases} 2, & |b_2| \le b_2^*(|b_1|), \\ 3, & |b_2| > b_2^*(|b_1|), \end{cases} \quad (23.4.12)$$

where $\#supp(\xi^*)$ is the number of support points of a T-optimal design ξ^* for $\overline{\eta}(x, q, \overline{b})$. Then, if $-b_2^*(b_1) < b_2 \le b_2^*(b_1)$

$$\xi^* = \begin{pmatrix} x^* & \pi - x^* \\ \frac{1}{2} & \frac{1}{2} \end{pmatrix}, \quad x^* = \arcsin\left(\frac{-1 + \sqrt{32 b_1^2 + 1}}{8 b_1}\right), \quad b_1 \in [0, \infty)$$

is the T-optimal design for $\overline{\eta}(x, q, \overline{b})$.

Proof The optimality of the design ξ^* follows from the equivalence theorem and can be checked by direct construction of the corresponding extremal function. According to this theorem, the design ξ is a T-optimal if and only if there exists a vector θ^* and a positive constant h such that the function $\psi^*(x) = \overline{\eta}(x, \theta^*, \overline{b})$ (see (23.2.5)) satisfies the following conditions

(i) $|\psi^*(x)| \le h, \quad$ for all $\quad x \in [0, 2\pi]$,
(ii) $|\psi^*(x_i)| = h, \quad$ for all $\quad i = 1, 2, \ldots, n$,
(iii) The support points and weights satisfy the conditions

$$\sum_{i=1}^{n} \psi^*(x_i) \frac{\partial \overline{\eta}(x_i, \theta, \overline{b})}{\partial \theta_j} \omega_i \bigg|_{\theta = \theta^*} = 0, \quad j = 0, \ldots, k_1 + k_2. \quad (23.4.13)$$

Let us consider as an extremal function $\psi^*(x)$ for the design ξ^* the following one

$$\psi^*(x) = \frac{b_2(-32b_1^2 + \sqrt{32b_1^2+1} - 1)}{(16b_1^2)} + \\ + \frac{b_2(-1+\sqrt{32b_1^2+1})\sin(x)}{2b_1} + \cos(t) + b_1\sin(2x) + b_2\cos(2x)$$

Direct calculations show that this function satisfies the conditions $(i) - (iii)$ with

$$h = \frac{3+\sqrt{32b_1^2+1}}{32}\sqrt{\frac{32b_1^2 + 2\sqrt{32b_1^2+1} - 2}{b_1^2}}$$

□

Example 23.1 Suppose that $m = 2, b_1 = 1, b_2 = 0.2$ and k_1=1, k_2=0, then it follows from Theorem 23.5 that the design

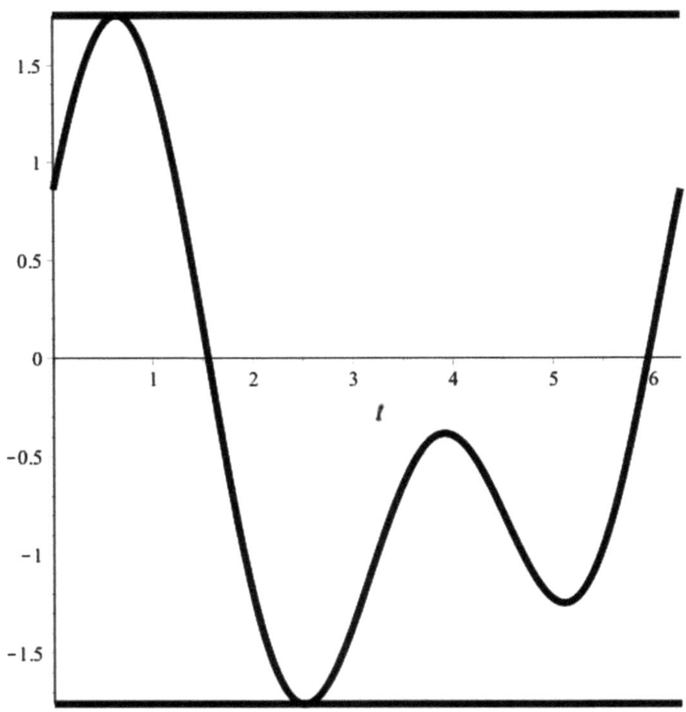

Fig. 23.1 *Extremal function ψ^* for the T-optimal discriminating design for the difference between two models* (23.4.11) ($b_1 = 1,\ b_2 = 0.2$)

$$\xi^* = \begin{pmatrix} 0.635 & 2.507 \\ \frac{1}{2} & \frac{1}{2} \end{pmatrix}$$

is a T-optimal discriminating design for the difference between two models (23.4.11).

The extremal function ψ^* for this design is depicted in Fig. 23.1.

Theorem 23.6 *Let $b_1 \in [0, \infty]$. The function $b_2^*(b_1)$ defined in the previous theorem can be represented in explicit form*

$$b_2^*(b_1) = \frac{2b_1(-2b_1\cos(2t) + \sin(t))}{\cos(t)\sqrt{32b_1^2 + 1} - 4b_1\sin(2t) - \cos(t)}, \quad t = 2\pi + \arctan(z),$$

where

$$z = \frac{64b_1^3\sqrt{8192b_1^6 + 12288b_1^4 + 576b_1^2 + (96b_1^2 - 3)\sqrt{(32b_1^2+1)^3} + (576b_1^2+3)\sqrt{32b_1^2+1}}}{\left(\sqrt{(32b_1^2+1)^3} + 96b_1^2 + 3\sqrt{32b_1^2+1} + 4\right)\sqrt{16b_1^2 + \sqrt{32b_1^2+1} - 1}\left(-8b_1^2 + \sqrt{32b_1^2+1} - 1\right)}$$

The statement of the Theorem 23.6 can be checked by direct calculations.

Remark 23.1 It follows from the Theorems 23.5 and 23.6 that

$$\lim_{b_1=\infty} b_2^*(b_1) = \frac{\sqrt{2}}{4}, \quad \lim_{b_1=0} \xi^* = \begin{pmatrix} 0 & \pi \\ \frac{1}{2} & \frac{1}{2} \end{pmatrix} \text{ and } \lim_{b_1=\infty} \xi^* = \begin{pmatrix} \frac{\pi}{4} & \frac{3\pi}{4} \\ \frac{1}{2} & \frac{1}{2} \end{pmatrix}.$$

For our next result, we need to define the notion of equivalence between two models.

Definition 23.1 We say that a function $\overline{\eta}_1(x, \widehat{q}, \overline{b}_1)$ (see (23.2.5)) is equivalent to a function $\overline{\eta}_2(x, q, \overline{b}_2)$ $\left(\overline{\eta}_1(x, \widehat{q}, \overline{b}_1) \sim \overline{\eta}_2(x, q, \overline{b}_2)\right)$ if for any fixed vectors $\widehat{q}$ and $\overline{b}_1$ there exist vectors q^* and $\overline{b}_2^*$ such that $\overline{\eta}_1(x, \widehat{q}, \overline{b}_1) - \overline{\eta}_2(x, q^*, \overline{b}_2^*) \equiv 0$.

Theorem 23.7 *For any m and $k_1 = m - 1, k_2 = m - 2$ suppose that a design*

$$\widetilde{\xi} = \begin{pmatrix} x_1 & \dots & x_n \\ \omega_1 & \dots & \omega_n \end{pmatrix}$$

is a T-optimal for the difference between two models (23.2.5):

$$\overline{\eta}_1(x, \widehat{q}, |\overline{b}|) = \widehat{q}_0 + \sum_{i=1}^{m-1} \widehat{q}_{2i-1}\sin(ix) + \sum_{i=1}^{m-2} \widehat{q}_{2i}\cos(ix) + \\ + |b_0|\cos((m-1)x) + |b_1|\sin(mx) + |b_2|\cos(mx)$$

then any design ζ which is a T-optimal for

$$\overline{\eta}_2(x,q,\overline{b}) = q_0 + \sum_{i=1}^{m-1} q_{2i-1}\sin(ix) + \sum_{i=1}^{m-2} q_{2i}\cos(ix) + \\ +b_0\cos((m-1)x) + b_1\sin(mx) + b_2\cos(mx)$$

can be obtained from the design $\widetilde{\xi}$ *by one of 3 transformation* $x_i \to -x_i,\ x_i \to \pi + x_i$ *or* $x_i \to \pi - x_i,\ i = 1,\dots,n$.

Proof Note that without loss of generality, we can assume that $b_0 \equiv 1$ or 0. Indeed, if $b_0 \neq 0$, the T-optimal design ζ depends only on values of the parameters b_1, b_2, since we can divide all coefficients by b_0. Suppose that $b_1 = p_1|b_1|$ and $b_2 = p_2|b_2|$, $p_1, p_2 = \pm 1$. Then it follows from the properties of trigonometric functions that

$$\begin{cases} \text{if } p_1 = -1,\ p_2 = \ \ 1 \text{ then } \overline{\eta}_1(-x,\widehat{q},|\overline{b}|) \sim \overline{\eta}_2(x,q,\overline{b}), \\ \text{if } p_1 = \ \ 1,\ p_2 = -1 \text{ then } (-1)^{m-1}\overline{\eta}_1(\pi - x,\widehat{q},|\overline{b}|) \sim \overline{\eta}_2(x,q,\overline{b}), \\ \text{if } p_1 = -1,\ p_2 = -1 \text{ then } (-1)^{m-1}\overline{\eta}_1(\pi + x,\widehat{q},|\overline{b}|) \sim \overline{\eta}_2(x,q,\overline{b}). \end{cases}$$

□

Corollary 23.2 *If* $k_1 = m-2, k_2 = m-1$ *and a design* $\widetilde{\xi}$ *is a T-optimal for the function* $\overline{\eta}_1(x,\widehat{q},|\overline{b}|)$ *(23.2.5) then any design* ζ *which is a T-optimal for* $\overline{\eta}_2(x,q,\overline{b})$ *can be obtained from the design* $\widetilde{\xi}$ *one of 3 transformation* $x_i \to -x_i,\ x_i \to \pi + x_i$ *or* $x_i \to \pi - x_i,\ i = 1,\dots,n$ *where* x_i*-th are the support points of the design* $\widetilde{\xi}$.

Theorem 23.8 *Let m is even. Denote by* $\overline{\eta}_1(x,q,\overline{b})$ *the difference between two models (23.2.5) for* $k_1 = m-1, k_2 = m-2$:

$$\overline{\eta}_1(x,\widehat{q},\overline{b}) = \widehat{q}_0 + \sum_{i=1}^{m-1} \widehat{q}_{2i-1}\sin(ix) + \sum_{i=1}^{m-2} \widehat{q}_{2i}\cos(ix) + \\ +b_0\cos((m-1)x) + b_1\sin(mx) + b_2\cos(mx)$$

and by $\overline{\eta}_2(x,q,\overline{b})$ *the difference between two models (23.2.5) for* $k_1 = m-2, k_2 = m-1$:

$$\overline{\eta}_2(x,q,\overline{b}) = q_0 + \sum_{i=1}^{m-2} q_{2i-1}\sin(ix) + \sum_{i=1}^{m-1} q_{2i}\cos(ix) + \\ +b_0\sin((m-1)x) + b_1\sin(mx) + b_2\cos(mx).$$

Suppose that a design

$$\widetilde{\xi}_1 = \begin{pmatrix} x_1 & \dots & x_n \\ \omega_1 & \dots & \omega_n \end{pmatrix}$$

is a T-optimal for $\overline{\eta}_1(x,q,\overline{b})$ *Then a design*

$$\widetilde{\xi}_2 = \begin{pmatrix} x_1 - \pi/2 & \dots & x_n - \pi/2 \\ \omega_1 & \dots & \omega_n \end{pmatrix}$$

is a T-optimal for $\overline{\eta}_2(x, q, \overline{b})$.

Proof It follows from the properties of trigonometric functions that $(-1)^{m-1}\overline{\eta}_2(x - \pi/2, q, \overline{b}) \sim \overline{\eta}_1(x, \widehat{q}, \overline{b})$. □

Theorem 23.9 *Let m is odd. Denote by* $\overline{\eta}_1(x, q, \overline{b}_1)$ *the difference between two models (23.2.5) for* $k_1 = m - 1, k_2 = m - 2$:

$$\overline{\eta}_1(x, \widehat{q}, \overline{b}_1) = \widehat{q}_0 + \sum_{i=1}^{m-1} \widehat{q}_{2i-1} \sin(ix) + \sum_{i=1}^{m-2} \widehat{q}_{2i} \cos(ix) + \\ +b_0 \cos((m-1)x) + b_1 \sin(mx) + b_2 \cos(mx)$$

and by $\overline{\eta}_2(x, q, \overline{b}_2)$ *the difference between two models (23.2.5) for* $k_1 = m - 1, k_2 = m - 2$:

$$\overline{\eta}_2(x, q, \overline{b}_2) = q_0 + \sum_{i=1}^{m-1} q_{2i-1} \sin(ix) + \sum_{i=1}^{m-2} q_{2i} \cos(ix) + \\ +b_0 \cos((m-1)x) + b_2 \sin(mx) + b_1 \cos(mx).$$

Suppose that a design

$$\widetilde{\xi}_1 = \begin{pmatrix} x_1 & \dots & x_n \\ \omega_1 & \dots & \omega_n \end{pmatrix}$$

is a T-optimal for $\overline{\eta}_1(x, q, \overline{b}_1)$ *Then a design*

$$\widetilde{\xi}_2 = \begin{pmatrix} \pi/2 - x_1 & \dots & \pi/2 - x_n \\ \omega_1 & \dots & \omega_n \end{pmatrix}$$

is a T-optimal for $\overline{\eta}_2(x, q, \overline{b}_2)$.

Proof It follows from the properties of trigonometric functions that $(-1)^{\frac{m-1}{2}}\overline{\eta}_2 (\pi/2 - x, q, \overline{b}_2) \sim \overline{\eta}_1(x, \widehat{q}, \overline{b}_1)$. □

Corollary 23.3 *The Theorems 23.3 and 23.4 directly follow from the Theorems 23.7, 23.8 and 23.9.*

Corollary 23.4 *For* $m = 2, k_1 = 1, \; k_2 = 0$ *and* $-b_2^*(b_1) < b_2 \le b_2^*(b_1)$ *a design*

$$\xi^* = \begin{pmatrix} \pi + x_1^* & 2\pi - x_1^* \\ \frac{1}{2} & \frac{1}{2} \end{pmatrix}, \; x_1^* = \arcsin\left(\frac{-1 + \sqrt{32b_1^2 + 1}}{8|b_1|}\right), \; b_1 \in (-\infty, 0]$$

is a T-optimal design for the function $\overline{\eta}(x, q, \overline{b})$ *(23.2.5).*

Corollary 23.5 *Suppose that* $m = 2,\ k_1 = 0,\ k_2 = 1$ *and* $b_1 \in (-\infty, \infty)$. *Then*

- *if* $0 \le b_2 \le b_2^*(b_1)$ *a design*

$$\xi_1^* = \begin{pmatrix} \pi/2 - x_1^* & 3\pi/2 + x_1^* \\ \frac{1}{2} & \frac{1}{2} \end{pmatrix},\ x_1^* = \arcsin\left(\frac{-1 + \sqrt{32b_1^2 + 1}}{8|b_1|}\right)$$

  is a T-optimal design for the function $\overline{\eta}(x, q, \overline{b})$ *(23.2.5);*
- *if* $-b_2^*(b_1) \le b_2 \le 0$ *a design*

$$\xi_2^* = \begin{pmatrix} \pi/2 + x_1^* & 3\pi/2 - x_1^* \\ \frac{1}{2} & \frac{1}{2} \end{pmatrix},\ x_1^* = \arcsin\left(\frac{-1 + \sqrt{32b_1^2 + 1}}{8|b_1|}\right)$$

  is a T-optimal design for the function $\overline{\eta}(x, q, \overline{b})$ *(23.2.5).*

For $m = 2$, the Theorem 23.5 and the Corollaries 23.4 and 23.5 provide a complete solution of the problem of constructing T-optimal designs with two support points. Note that T-optimal designs with 3 support points can also be found explicitly, but the corresponding expressions are too large to be represented here. For the particular cases: $k_1 = 1,\ k_2 = 0,\ b_1 = 0,\ b_2 \neq 0$ and $k_1 = 0,\ k_2 = 1,\ b_1 = 0,\ b_2 \neq 0$, T-optimal designs with 3 support points are constructed in the Theorems 23.2 and 23.4.

Acknowledgements The authors would like to thank Lyudmila Kuznetsova, who helped improving the text of this manuscript with considerable language expertise. This work has been supported by St. Petersburg State University (project "Actual problems of design and analysis for regression models," 6.38.435.2015) and by Russian Foundation for Basic Research (project no. 17-01-00161-a).

References

1. Atkinson, A.C.: The Non-Uniqueness of Some Designs for Discriminating Between Two Polynomial Models in One Variablel. MODA 9, Advances in model-oriented design and analysis, pp. 9–16 (2010)
2. Atkinson, A.C., Donev, A.N., Tobias, R.D.: Optimum Experimental Designs. Oxford Univ. Press, Oxford (2007)
3. Atkinson, A.C., Fedorov, V.V.: The designs of experiments for discriminating between two rival models. Biometrika **62**, 57–70 (1975)
4. Atkinson, A.C., Fedorov, V.V.: Optimal design: experiments for discriminating between several models. Biometrika **62**, 289–303 (1975)
5. Biedermann, S., Dette, H., Hoffmann, P.: Constrained optimal discrimination designs for Fourier regression models. Ann. Inst. Stat. Math. **61**(1), 143–157 (2009)

6. Box, G.E.P., Hill, W.J.: Discrimination among mechanistic models. Technometrics **9**, 57–71 (1967)
7. Dette, H.: Discrimination designs for polynomial regression on a compact interval. Ann.Stat. **22**, 890–904 (1994)
8. Dette, H.: Optimal designs for identifying the degree of a polynomial regression. Ann. Stat. **23**, 1248–1267 (1995)
9. Dette, H., Haller, G.: Optimal designs for the identification of the order of a Fourier regression. Ann. Stat. **26**, 1496–1521 (1998)
10. Dette, H., Melas, V.B., Shpilev, P.: T-optimal designs for discrimination between two polynomial models. Ann. Stat. **40**(1), 188–205 (2012)
11. Dette, H., Melas, V.B., Shpilev, P.: T-optimal discriminating designs for fourier regression models. Comput. Stat. Data Anal. **113**, 196–206 (2017)
12. Dette, H., Titoff, S.: Optimal discrimination designs. Ann. Stat. **37**(4), 2056–2082 (2009)
13. Hill, P.D.: A review of experimental design procedures for regression model discrimination. Technometrics **20**(1), 15–21 (1978)
14. Hill, W.J., Hunter, W.G., Wichern, W.D.: A joint design criterion for the dual problem of model discrimination and parameter estimation. Technometrics **10**, 145–160 (1968)
15. Hunter, W.G., Reiner, A.M.: Designs for discriminating between two rival models. Technometrics **7**(3), 307–323 (1965)
16. Kiefer, J.: General equivalence theory for optimum designs (approximate theory). Ann. Stat. **2**, 849–879 (1974)
17. Kitsos, C.P., Titterington, D.M., Torsney, B.: An optimal design problem in rhythmometry. Biometrics **44**, 657–671 (1988)
18. Lestrel, P.E.: Fourier Descriptors and Their Applications in Biology. Cambridge University Press, New York (1997)
19. López-Fidalgo, J., Tommasi, C., Trandafir, P.: An optimal experimental design criterion for discriminating between non-normal models. J. R. Stat. Soc. B **69**, 1–12 (2007)
20. López-Fidalgo, J., Tommasi, C., Trandafir, P.: Optimal designs for discriminating between some extensions of the Michaelis-Menten model. J. Stat. Plan. Inference **138**, 3797–3804 (2008)
21. McCool, J.I.: Systematic and random errors in least squares estimation for circular contours. Precis. Eng. **1**, 215–220 (1979)
22. Pukelsheim, F.: Optimal Design of Experiments. SIAM, Philadelphia (2006)
23. Song, D., Wong, W.K.: On the construction of g_{rm}-optimal designs. Stat. Sinica **9**, 263–272 (1999)
24. Spruill, M.C.: Good designs for testing the degree of a polynomial mean. Sankhya, Ser. B **52**(1), 67–74 (1990)
25. Stigler, S.: Optimal experimental design for polynomial regression. J. Am. Stat. Assoc. **66**, 311–318 (1971)
26. Studden, W.J.: Some robust-type D-optimal designs in polynomial regression. J. Am. Stat. Assoc. **77**(380), 916–921 (1982)
27. Tommasi, C., López-Fidalgo, J.: Bayesian optimum designs for discriminating between models with any distribution. Comput. Stat. Data Anal. **54**(1), 143–150 (2010)
28. Ucinski, D., Bogacka, B.: T-optimum designs for discrimination between two multiresponse dynamic models. J. R. Stat. Soc. Ser. B **67**, 3–18 (2005)
29. Wiens, D.P.: Robust discrimination designs, with Matlab code. J. R. Stat. Soc. Ser. B **71**, 805–829 (2009)
30. Wiens, D.P.: Robustness of design for the testing of lack of fit and for estimation in binary response models. Comput. Stat. Data Anal. **54**, 3371–3378 (2010)
31. Zen, M.M., Tsai, M.H.: Criterion-robust optimal designs for model discrimination and parameter estimation in Fourier regression models. J. Stat. Plan. Inference **124**(2), 475–487 (2004)

Chapter 24
Simulations on the Combinatorial Structure of D-Optimal Designs

Roberto Fontana and Fabio Rapallo

Abstract In this work, we present the results of several simulations on main-effect factorial designs. The goal of such simulations is to investigate the connections between the D-optimality of a design and its geometric structure. By means of a combinatorial object, namely the circuit basis of the model matrix, we show that it is possible to define a simple index that exhibits strong connections with the D-optimality.

Keywords Algebraic statistics · Circuits · Design of experiments
Fractional factorial designs · Optimal designs

24.1 Introduction

Many experimental situations call for standard designs, such as fractional factorials. However in many situations, standard designs are not available, for example, when not all combinations of the factor levels are feasible or resource limitations restrict the number of experiments that can be performed. In these nonstandard situations, D-optimal designs are often used [8].

In the recent work [3], saturated fractions, which are designs where the number of points is equal to the number of estimable parameters of the model, have been characterized through the circuits of the model matrix. The key point of such theory is the identification of a fraction with a $\{0, 1\}$-valued multiway contingency table where the points belonging to the fraction are denoted with 1 and the points outside the fraction are denoted with 0. Under this kind of representations, it is possible to study some properties of the design by using combinatorial objects derived from the model matrix. In particular, a circuit is a special element of the kernel of an

R. Fontana (✉)
Department DISMA, Politecnico di Torino, Corso Duca degli Abruzzi 24, 10127 Torino, Italy
e-mail: roberto.fontana@polito.it

F. Rapallo
Department DISIT, Università del Piemonte Orientale, Viale Teresa Michel 11, 15121 Alessandria, Italy
e-mail: fabio.rapallo@uniupo.it

J. Pilz et al. (eds.), *Statistics and Simulation*, Springer Proceedings in Mathematics & Statistics 231, https://doi.org/10.1007/978-3-319-76035-3_24

integer-valued matrix. We will recall the definition and the basic properties of circuits in the next section. The structure of saturated D-optimal designs in connection with the circuits has been studied in [4].

Since the circuits yield major information on the D-optimality of saturated fractions, in this work we perform a simulation study for investigating the geometric structure of non-saturated D-optimal designs in connection with their circuits. We limit our analysis to main-effect models, and we present some test cases dealing with both symmetric and asymmetric designs. From these examples, we argue that there are strong connections between the D-optimality and the circuits. We use `Proc Optex` of `SAS/QC` [13] for generating D-optimal designs and `4ti2` [1] for generating circuits.

`Proc Optex` searches for optimal experimental designs in the following way. The user specifies an efficiency criterion, a set of candidate design points, a model and the size of the design to be found, and the procedure generates a subset of the candidate set so that the terms in the model can be estimated as efficiently as possible. There are several algorithms for searching for D-optimal designs. They have a common structure. They start from an initial design, randomly generated or user specified, and move, in a finite number of steps, to a better design. All of the search algorithms are based on adding points to the growing design and deleting points from a design that is too big. Main references to optimal designs include [2, 5, 10, 12, 14, 16].

`4ti2` is a symbolic software which computes the circuits of a given integer-valued matrix. The use of software for Combinatorics and Computer Algebra inside statistical simulations usually leads to limitations in the size of the problems. The algorithms become actually unfeasible when the number of the design points grows, and our problem does not make exception. Therefore, we will restrict to small-sized examples.

It is worth noting that despite these computational limitations, we are able to consider a variety of examples, including both binary and multilevel designs, with an example of mixed-level design.

The chapter is organized as follows. In Sect. 27.1, we briefly describe the results of [3] and, in particular, how saturated designs can be characterized in terms of the circuits of the relevant model matrix. In Sect. 27.2, we recall some major results on the D-optimality of saturated fractions and we introduce our simulation study for main-effect models. In Sect. 27.3, we present and discuss the results of our simulations, while in Sect. 24.5, we give some concluding remarks and some pointers to future work.

24.2 Circuits, Saturated Designs, and D-optimality

In this section, we recall the definition of circuits and we review their applications to Design of Experiments. A full account on circuits including some applications to Statistics is available in [9].

Given a model matrix X on a full factorial design $\mathcal{D}$ with K design points, an integer vector f is in the kernel of X^t if and only if $X^t f = 0$. We denote by A the transpose of X. Moreover, we denote by $\mathrm{supp}(f)$ the support of the integer vector f, i.e., the set of indices j such that $f_j \neq 0$. Finally, the indicator vector of f is the binary vector $(f_j \neq 0)$, where $(\cdot)$ is the indicator function. An integer vector f is a circuit of A if and only if:

(a) $f \in \ker(A)$;
(b) there is no other integer vector $g \in \ker(A)$ such that $\mathrm{supp}(g) \subset \mathrm{supp}(f)$ and $\mathrm{supp}(g) \neq \mathrm{supp}(f)$.

The set of all circuits of A is denoted by $\mathcal{C}_A = \{f_1, \ldots, f_L\}$ and is named as the circuit basis of A. It is known that $\mathcal{C}_A$ is always finite. The set $\mathcal{C}_A$ can be computed through specific software. In our examples, we have used `4ti2` [1]. Notice that $\mathcal{C}_A$ is a special basis of $\ker(A)$ as vector space, and therefore, the circuit basis is computed from the model matrix on the full factorial design $\mathcal{D}$. Thus, the circuit basis $\mathcal{C}_A$ depends only on the model, but not on the fraction. This remark is particularly useful when we use this theory in the definition of algorithms for finding optimal designs, since the computation of the circuit basis can be performed once for each model matrix, independently of the particular fraction.

To show explicitly the circuits on a practical example, consider the 2^4 design with main effects. The matrix $A = X^t$ for the full factorial design is

$$A = \begin{pmatrix} 1 & 1 & 1 & 1 & 1 & 1 & 1 & 1 & 1 & 1 & 1 & 1 & 1 & 1 & 1 & 1 \\ 1 & 1 & 1 & 1 & 1 & 1 & 1 & 1 & 0 & 0 & 0 & 0 & 0 & 0 & 0 & 0 \\ 1 & 1 & 1 & 1 & 0 & 0 & 0 & 0 & 1 & 1 & 1 & 1 & 0 & 0 & 0 & 0 \\ 1 & 1 & 0 & 0 & 1 & 1 & 0 & 0 & 1 & 1 & 0 & 0 & 1 & 1 & 0 & 0 \\ 1 & 0 & 1 & 0 & 1 & 0 & 1 & 0 & 1 & 0 & 1 & 0 & 1 & 0 & 1 & 0 \end{pmatrix},$$

where each column represents a design point (indexed lexically from left to right) and each row represents a model parameter. Note that other choices of the model matrix are possible, but they lead to the same $\ker(A)$ as vector space, and therefore, they generate the same set of circuits. Running the function `circuits` on `4ti2`, we obtain 1, 348 circuits that can be grouped into the following 8 types:

- 100 circuits (with support on 4 points) of the form:

$$f_1 = (0, 0, 0, 0, 0, 0, 0, 0, 0, 0, 1, -1, -1, 1, 0, 0);$$

- 160 circuits (with support on 5 points) of the form:

$$f_2 = (0, 0, 0, 0, 1, 0, -2, 1, 0, -1, 1, 0, 0, 0, 0, 0);$$

- 432 circuits (with support on 6 points) of the form:

$$f_3 = (0, 0, 0, 0, 0, 0, 1, -1, -1, 0, 0, 1, 0, 1, 0, -1);$$

- 384 circuits (with support on 6 points) of the form:

$$f_4 = (0, 0, 0, 0, 0, 0, 2, -2, -1, 0, 0, 1, 0, 1, -1, 0)\,;$$

- 96 circuits (with support on 6 points) of the form:

$$f_5 = (0, 0, 0, 1, -2, 0, 1, 0, 1, 0, 0, -2, 0, 1, 0, 0)\,;$$

- 96 circuits (with support on 6 points) of the form:

$$f_6 = (0, 0, 0, 1, -1, 0, 0, 0, -1, 0, 0, 0, 0, 2, 2, -3)\,;$$

- 16 circuits (with support on 6 points) of the form:

$$f_7 = (0, 0, 0, 1, -1, 0, 0, 0, -1, 0, 0, 0, 3, -1, -1, 0)\,;$$

- 64 circuits (with support on 6 points) of the form:

$$f_8 = (0, 0, 0, 1, 0, -2, 1, 0, 2, 0, -3, 0, 0, 0, 0, 1)\,.$$

Note that the situation is a bit less complicated if we consider only the cardinality of the supports and we discard the values of each entry. In fact, we have 100 circuits with support on 4 points, 160 circuits with support on 5 points, and $1,088$ circuits with support on 6 points.

The connection between saturated fractions and circuits is given in the following theorem, to be found in [3]. Remember that saturated fractions are fractions with the minimal number of points $p = \text{rank}(A)$ such that all the p independent parameters are estimable.

Theorem 24.1 *A fraction $\mathcal{F} \subset \mathcal{D}$ with p design points is a saturated fraction if and only if it does not contain any of the supports $\{\text{supp}(f_1), \ldots, \text{supp}(f_L)\}$ of the circuits of $A = X^t$.*

In light of the theorem above, it is natural to investigate how the geometry of a fraction determines its optimality. For saturated fractions, some experiments have been presented in [4], where the problem of finding D-optimal saturated fractions is translated into an optimization problem using two different objective functions. In words, such objective functions consider the cardinality of the intersection between a fraction and each circuit, and for each circuit, they count how many points are needed to complete the circuit. We will recall some results in that direction in the next section.

24.3 Design of the Simulation Study

In this section, we show how fractions generated by the procedure `Proc Optex` can be classified according to their geometrical structure and their D-optimality.

To measure the D-optimality of a fraction $\mathcal{F}$, we use the D-efficiency; see [13]. The determinant of the information matrix is $D_{\mathcal{F}} = \det(X_{\mathcal{F}}^T X_{\mathcal{F}})$, where $X_{\mathcal{F}}$ is the model matrix restricted to the fraction points. The D-efficiency of $\mathcal{F}$ is then defined as

$$E_{\mathcal{F}} = 100 \left(\frac{1}{\#\mathcal{F}} D_{\mathcal{F}}^{1/\#\mathcal{F}} \right)$$

where $\#\mathcal{F}$ is the number of points of $\mathcal{F}$.

To analyze the position of the design points with respect to the supports of the circuits, let us give some definitions. Let $C_A = (c_{ij}, i = 1, \ldots, L, j = 1, \ldots, K)$ be the matrix, whose rows contain the values of the indicator functions of the circuits $f_1, \ldots, f_L$, $c_{ij} = (f_{ij} \neq 0), i = 1, \ldots, L, j = 1, \ldots, K$ and $Y_{\mathcal{F}} = ((y_{\mathcal{F}})_1, \ldots, (y_{\mathcal{F}})_K)$ be the K-dimensional column vector that contains the unknown values of the indicator function of the points of $\mathcal{F}$, and let $b = (b_1, \ldots, b_L)$ be the column vector defined by $b_i = \#\text{supp}(f_i), i = 1, \ldots, L$.

For each circuit $f_i, i = 1, \ldots, L$, we consider the cardinality $(b_{\mathcal{F}})_i$ of the intersection between its support $\text{supp}(f_i)$ and the fraction $\mathcal{F}$:

$$(b_{\mathcal{F}})_i = \langle \text{supp}(f_i), Y_{\mathcal{F}} \rangle .$$

For each fraction $\mathcal{F}$, these value form the vector $b_{\mathcal{F}} = ((b_{\mathcal{F}})_1, \ldots, (b_{\mathcal{F}})_L))$.

In the case of saturated fractions, in [4] the geometry of a fraction $\mathcal{F}$ has been summarized through its indicator function Y by means of the objective functions

$$g_2(\mathcal{F}) = \sum_{i=1}^{L} (b - b_{\mathcal{F}})_i^2 \quad \text{and} \quad g_3(\mathcal{F}) = \max(b_{\mathcal{F}}) .$$

In the examples illustrated in [4] concerning saturated fractions, the D-optimality is reached when the values of g_2 and g_3 are maximal. This seems to suggest that D-optimal fractions correspond to fractions as close as possible to the circuits.

When analyzing fractions with an arbitrary number of points (not necessarily saturated), the objective functions g_2 and g_3 defined above have a less clear meaning. In fact, for saturated fractions the vector $(b - b_{\mathcal{F}})$ is strictly positive in view of Theorem 24.1, while this property does not hold in general. Another issue which makes the interpretation of g_2 and g_3 not easy to understand is the fact that there are circuits with different cardinalities.

To overcome the difficulties mentioned above, we have considered here only a subset of the circuits, namely the circuits with support on 4 points. It is known, see [6], that 4 is the minimal cardinality of the circuits for the main-effect models. In the combinatorial theory of contingency tables, such simple circuits are known as *basic moves* and have several interesting properties; see [6, 11]. In particular, under mild conditions, the basic moves preserve the connectivity of the fiber of a contingency table without the use of a Markov basis, and nevertheless their number is dramatically smaller than the cardinality of the whole circuit basis. For instance, in the 2^5 design with main effects there are $353,616$ circuits, but only 720 of them are basic moves. We denote with $\overline{\mathscr{C}}_A$ the set of the basic moves in $\mathscr{C}_A$ and with $\overline{L}$ its cardinality.

When considering only the basic moves in $\overline{\mathscr{C}}_A$, we can consider only a sub-vector $\overline{b}_{\mathscr{F}} = ((\overline{b}_{\mathscr{F}})_1, \ldots, (\overline{b}_{\mathscr{F}})_{\overline{L}})$ of $b_{\mathscr{F}}$ using only the basic moves in $\overline{\mathscr{C}}_A$. Note that by construction, the vector $\overline{b}_{\mathscr{F}}$ has elements in $\{0, 1, 2, 3, 4\}$. To analyze a fraction, we then consider:

- the table of counts of $\overline{b}_{\mathscr{F}}$;
- the mean and the variance of $\overline{b}_{\mathscr{F}}$:

$$\mathrm{m}(\overline{b}_{\mathscr{F}}) = \frac{1}{\overline{L}} \sum_{i=1}^{\overline{L}} (\overline{b}_{\mathscr{F}})_i \qquad \text{and} \qquad \mathrm{var}(\overline{b}_{\mathscr{F}}) = \frac{1}{\overline{L}} \sum_{i=1}^{\overline{L}} (\overline{b}_{\mathscr{F}})_i^2 - \mathrm{m}(\overline{b}_{\mathscr{F}})^2 .$$

We have considered the main-effect model for 4 different designs and with different numbers of design points. More precisely, we have considered the 2^4 design, the 2^5 design, the 3^3 design, and the $2 \times 3 \times 4$ design. For each design, we have considered fractions with $k = p, p+1, p+2, p+3$ design points, where p is the cardinality of a saturated design or, equivalently, the number of parameters of the model. In all cases, we have analyzed 500 fractions generated by the `Proc Optex`.

24.4 Results

24.4.1 First Scenario. Design 2^4

Let us consider first the 2^4 design. The model matrix X of the full design has 16 rows and 5 columns, the number of estimable parameters. The matrix X has rank 5; and therefore, we analyze fractions with $k = 5, 6, 7, 8$ points. For this design, the circuit basis has been presented in Sect. 24.2, and it consists of $1,348$ elements with 100 basic moves. The remaining $1,248$ circuits have support on 5 or 6 points.

We generated 500 fractions with `Proc Optex` for each of the design sizes $k = 5, 6, 7, 8$, and for each fraction $\mathscr{F}$, we computed the intersections with the 100 basic moves in $\overline{\mathscr{C}}_A$, obtaining the vectors $\overline{b}_{\mathscr{F}}$. We have classified the table of counts of $\overline{b}_{\mathscr{F}}$, together with its mean and variance, with respect to the D-optimality, and the results are reported in Table 24.1.

The first row of Table 24.1 says that all the 500 fractions with 5 points generated by `Proc Optex` have a common behavior in terms of intersections with the circuits, namely each fraction has null intersection with 15 circuits and intersection on 1 point

Table 24.1 Tables of counts of $\overline{b}_{\mathscr{F}}$, the means $\mathrm{m}(\overline{b}_{\mathscr{F}})$, the variances $var(\overline{b}_{\mathscr{F}})$, and the D-optimality for the 2^4 design

$\#\mathscr{F}$	Table($\overline{b}_{\mathscr{F}}$)					$\mathrm{m}(\overline{b}_{\mathscr{F}})$	$\mathrm{var}(\overline{b}_{\mathscr{F}})$	$E_{\mathscr{F}}$	n
	0	1	2	3	4				
$k = 5$	15	45	40	0	0	1.25	0.49	94.09	500
$k = 6$	9	39	45	7	0	1.5	0.57	91.98	500
$k = 7$	6	22	66	3	3	1.75	0.55	93.93	500
$k = 8$	3	18	58	18	3	2	0.60	94.41	117
	6	0	88	0	6	2	0.48	100.00	383

with 45 circuits, on 2 points with 40 circuits, while no intersection on 3 and 4 points occurs.

In particular, for all the fractions sizes we see that for a given value of $E_{\mathscr{F}}$, all the fractions have exactly the same vector $\overline{b}_{\mathscr{F}}$. In all the remaining scenarios, we will observe that, for a given value of $E_{\mathscr{F}}$ all the fractions have just few possible values of $\overline{b}_{\mathscr{F}}$. This confirms once more the connection between D-optimality and circuits.

For $k = 8$ points, `Proc Optex` provides 117 fractions with $E_{\mathscr{F}} = 94.41$ and 387 fractions with $E_{\mathscr{F}} = 100$ (these latter ones are resolution III orthogonal designs). Both groups of designs have the same mean value of $\overline{b}_{\mathscr{F}}$ (equal to 2) but different variances (0.60 and 0.48). The designs with the highest value of $E_{\mathscr{F}}$ have the lowest variance, that is, 0.48.

24.4.2 Second Scenario. Design 2^5

We analyze now the 2^5 design. The model matrix X of the full design has 32 rows and 6 columns, the number of estimable parameters. The matrix X has rank 6, and therefore, we analyze fractions with $k = 6, 7, 8, 9$ points. For this design, the circuit basis has 353, 616 elements, but there are only 720 basic moves.

We generated 500 fractions with `Proc Optex` for each of the sample sizes $k = 6, 7, 8, 9$, and the results of the simulation study are reported in Table 24.2.

For all the fraction sizes that we have considered in this scenario, `Proc Optex` provides groups of designs with different values of the D-optimality criterion. We observe that for each fraction size the mean of $\overline{b}_{\mathscr{F}}$ is constant while the variances of $\overline{b}_{\mathscr{F}}$ decrease as $E_{\mathscr{F}}$ increase. For $k = 6$ (i.e., for saturated fractions), the minimum variance corresponds to two different values of D-efficiency, but in any case the maximal D-efficiency is attained when the variance reaches the minimum. Moreover, note that often the D-optimal fractions contain the support of some basic move, while the fractions not containing the support of basic moves have smaller values of D-efficiency. In this scenario, this holds for $k = 7$ and 8 points.

Table 24.2 Tables of counts of $\overline{b}_{\mathscr{F}}$, the means $m(\overline{b}_{\mathscr{F}})$, the variances $var(\overline{b}_{\mathscr{F}})$, and the D-optimality for the 2^5 design

$\#\mathscr{F}$	Table($\overline{b}_{\mathscr{F}}$)					$m(\overline{b}_{\mathscr{F}})$	$var(\overline{b}_{\mathscr{F}})$	$E_{\mathscr{F}}$	n
	0	1	2	3	4				
$k=6$	300	300	120	0	0	0.75	0.52	83.99	13
	289	342	96	2	0	0.75	0.47	83.99	97
	282	336	102	0	0	0.75	0.47	90.48	390
$k=7$	249	321	141	9	0	0.88	0.58	83.87	12
	238	342	132	8	0	0.88	0.54	88.18	20
	230	353	135	1	1	0.88	0.51	90.71	468
$k=8$	194	348	162	16	0	1	0.58	90.86	35
	191	344	182	0	3	1	0.56	95.32	182
	186	352	180	0	2	1	0.53	100.00	283
$k=9$	157	335	212	13	3	1.12	0.61	95.10	82
	155	339	209	15	2	1.12	0.60	97.58	418

Remark 24.1 Notice that the mean $m(\overline{b}_{\mathscr{F}})$ is constant for a fixed design and a fixed number of design points, due to the properties of the circuit basis. In fact, with a symmetry argument it is easy to show that each point of the full factorial design $\mathscr{D}$ belongs to the same number of basic moves, i.e., to $4\overline{L}/\#\mathscr{D}$. Thus, when computing the mean $m(\overline{b}_{\mathscr{F}})$, each design point in $\mathscr{F}$ appears $4\overline{L}/\#\mathscr{D}$ times, and therefore, the following formula holds:

$$m(\overline{b}_{\mathscr{F}}) = \frac{4\#\mathscr{F}}{\#\mathscr{D}}.$$

This result suggests that the algorithm for searching for D-optimal designs could be improved if also the variances were taken into account.

24.4.3 Third Scenario. Design 3^3

We consider a multilevel design, namely the 3^3 design. The model matrix X of the full design has 27 rows and 7 columns, the number of estimable parameters. The matrix X has rank 7, and therefore, we analyze fractions with $k = 7, 8, 9, 10$ points. For this design, the circuit basis has 73, 071 elements, 243 of which are basic moves.

We generated 500 fractions with `Proc Optex` for each of the sample sizes $k = 7, 8, 9, 10$, and the results of the simulation study are reported in Table 24.3.

As in the previous scenarios for each fraction size, all the designs have the same mean of $\overline{b}_{\mathscr{F}}$ while the best designs have the lowest variances of $\overline{b}_{\mathscr{F}}$.

Table 24.3 Tables of counts of $\overline{b}_{\mathcal{F}}$, the means $m(\overline{b}_{\mathcal{F}})$, the variances $var(\overline{b}_{\mathcal{F}})$, and the D-optimality for the 3^3 design

$\#\mathcal{F}$	Table($\overline{b}_{\mathcal{F}}$)					$m(\overline{b}_{\mathcal{F}})$	$var(\overline{b}_{\mathcal{F}})$	$E_{\mathcal{F}}$	n
	0	1	2	3	4				
$k = 7$	54	126	63	0	0	1.04	0.48	54.44	500
$k = 8$	48	108	81	6	0	1.19	0.60	52.59	19
	40	122	77	4	0	1.19	0.51	55.72	185
	39	120	84	0	0	1.19	0.47	56.67	296
$k = 9$	29	112	94	8	0	1.33	0.53	57.95	192
	27	108	108	0	0	1.33	0.44	62.45	308
$k = 10$	21	96	114	12	0	1.48	0.52	61.02	500

Table 24.4 Tables of counts of $\overline{b}_{\mathcal{F}}$, the means $m(\overline{b}_{\mathcal{F}})$, the variances $var(\overline{b}_{\mathcal{F}})$, and the D-optimality for the $2 \times 3 \times 4$ design

$\#\mathcal{F}$	Table($\overline{b}_{\mathcal{F}}$)					$m(\overline{b}_{\mathcal{F}})$	$var(\overline{b}_{\mathcal{F}})$	$E_{\mathcal{F}}$	n
	0	1	2	3	4				
$k = 7$	30	86	57	1	0	1.17	0.50	48.48	500
$k = 8$	20	80	70	4	0	1.33	0.50	51.71	332
	21	76	76	0	1	1.33	0.50	51.71	168
$k = 9$	14	68	84	7	1	1.50	0.53	52.80	246
	14	69	81	10	0	1.50	0.53	52.80	254
$k = 10$	8	60	88	18	0	1.67	0.52	54.25	157
	9	56	94	14	1	1.67	0.52	54.25	286
	11	48	106	6	3	1.67	0.52	54.25	57

24.4.4 Fourth Scenario. Design 2 × 3 × 4

The last scenario concerns an asymmetric design, the $2 \times 3 \times 4$ design. The model matrix X of the full design has 24 rows and 7 columns, the number of estimable parameters. The matrix X has rank 7, and therefore, we analyze fractions with $k = 7, 8, 9, 10$ points. For this design, the circuit basis has $13,470$ elements, 174 of which are basic moves.

The results of this scenario, displayed in Table 24.4, reinforce the connection between D-optimality and the variance of $\overline{b}_{\mathcal{F}}$. Except for the case of saturated fractions, for each fraction size we obtain several groups of designs with different $\overline{b}_{\mathcal{F}}$ but equal means $m(\overline{b}_{\mathcal{F}})$, equal variances $var(\overline{b}_{\mathcal{F}})$, and equal D-efficiencies $E_{\mathcal{F}}$.

24.5 Concluding Remarks

The simulations discussed in the previous sections for various designs show that the cardinalities of the intersections between a fraction and the basic moves are able to predict the D-optimality of the fraction. In particular, as low is the variance of such cardinalities as high is the D-efficiency of the fraction, at least for the simple-effect models analyzed here.

These results are encouraging and suggest to analyze such connection in a more general framework, in order to characterize D-optimal fractions following three main directions: First, to study the behavior of the D-optimality in terms of the intersection with the basic moves also for models with interactions and to find connections with other known notions in the model-free context, such as uniformity and discrepancy; see [7, 15]; second, to characterize the basic moves in order to extend our study to large-sized designs; finally, to implement the criterion based on the basic moves in statistical software to improve the existing algorithm for finding D-optimal designs.

References

1. 4ti2 team: 4ti2—a software package for algebraic, geometric and combinatorial problems on linear spaces (2008). www.4ti2.de. Accessed 10 Feb 2017
2. Atkinson, A.C., Donev, A.N., Tobias, R.D.: Optimum Experimental Designs, with SAS. Oxford University Press, New York (2007)
3. Fontana, R., Rapallo, F., Rogantin, M.P.: A characterization of saturated designs for factorial experiments. J. Stat. Plan. Inference **147**, 204–211 (2014)
4. Fontana, R., Rapallo, F., Rogantin, M.P.: D-optimal saturated designs: a simulation study. In: Melas, V., Mignani, S., Monari, P., Salmaso, L. (eds.) Topics in Statistical Simulation, pp. 183–190. Springer, Berlin (2014)
5. Goos, P., Jones, B.: Optimal Design of Experiments: A Case Study Approach. Wiley, UK (2011)
6. Hara, H., Takemura, A., Yoshida, R.: Markov bases for two-way subtable sum problems. J. Pure Appl. Algebra **213**(8), 1507–1521 (2009)
7. Liu, M.Q.: Using discrepancy to evaluate fractional factorial designs. In: Fang, K.T., Niederreiter, H., Hickernell, F.J. (eds.) Monte Carlo and Quasi-Monte Carlo Methods 2000, pp. 357–368. Springer, Heidelberg (2002)
8. Mitchell, T.J.: Computer construction of D-optimal first-order designs. Technometrics **16**(2), 211–220 (1974)
9. Ohsugi, H.: A dictionary of Gröbner bases of toric ideals. In: Hibi, T. (ed.) Harmony of Gröbner bases and the modern industrial society, pp. 253–281. World Scientific, Hackensack, NJ (2012)
10. Pukelsheim, F.: Optimal Design of Experiments, Classics in Applied Mathematics, vol. 50. Society for Industrial and Applied Mathematics, Philadelphia, PA (2006)
11. Rapallo, F., Yoshida, R.: Markov bases and subbases for bounded contingency tables. Ann. Inst. Stat. Math. **62**(4), 785–805 (2010)
12. Rasch, D., Pilz, J., Verdooren, L., Gebhardt, A.: Optimal Experimental Design with R. CRC Press, FL (2011)
13. SAS Institute: SAS/QC 9.2 User's Guide, 2 edn. Cary, NC (2010)
14. Shah, K.R., Sinha, B.K.: Theory of Optimal Designs. Lecture notes in statistics, vol. 54. Springer, Berlin (1989)

15. Tang, Y., Xu, H., Lin, D.K.: Uniform fractional factorial designs. Ann. Stat. **40**(2), 891–907 (2012)
16. Wynn, H.P.: The sequential generation of D-optimum experimental designs. Ann. Math. Stat. **41**(5), 1655–1664 (1970)

Part VI
Simulations for Reliability and Queueing Models

Chapter 25
On the Consequences of Model Misspecification for Biased Samples from the Weibull Distribution

George Tzavelas and Polychronis Economou

Abstract Model misspecification is common in practice specially when the sampling mechanism is not known. A sized-biased sample arises in case where the probability of a unit of the population to be chosen in a sample is proportional to some nonnegative weight function $w(x)$ of its size x. In this chapter, we study the model misspecification results when a sized-biased sample from the Weibull distribution is treated as a random one as well as when a random sample is treated as biased. Special attention is paid on the misspecification effects on the parameter estimation and on some of the most important characteristics of the distribution, such as the mean, the median, and the variance. It is proven that when we treat a biased sample as a random one, the parameters are overestimated and in the opposite case are underestimated. Simulation results verify the theoretical findings for small as well as for large samples.

Keywords Weighted distributions · Misspecification · r-size biased sampling Parameter estimation

25.1 Introduction

A biased sample arises when the individuals of a population do not have the same probability of being selected during the sampling process. If the probability of a population unit to be selected in a sample is proportional to some nonnegative weight function $w(x)$ of its size x, the observed sample is refereed as a size-biased sample. Under such a biased sampling scheme, the observed size-biased sample from a random variable X with probability density function (pdf) $f(x;\theta)$ ($\theta \in \Theta$ where Θ

G. Tzavelas
Department of Statistics and Insurance Sciences, University of Piraeus,
80 Karaoli & Dimitriou str., 185 34 Piraeus, Greece
e-mail: tzafor@unipi.gr

P. Economou (✉)
Department of Civil Engineering, University of Patras,
26504 Rio Achaia, Greece
e-mail: peconom@upatras.gr

J. Pilz et al. (eds.), *Statistics and Simulation*, Springer Proceedings
in Mathematics & Statistics 231, https://doi.org/10.1007/978-3-319-76035-3_25

is an open interval in $\mathbb{R}^s$ with $s \geq 1$) can be interpreted as a random sample from a population with pdf given by

$$f_w(x;\theta) = \frac{w(x)}{E\left[w(X)\right]} f(x;\theta). \tag{25.1}$$

The above weighted pdf is well defined provided that $E\left[w(X)\right] < \infty$.

The most common weight function is the power function $w(x) = x^r$ where $r \geq 0$ is known, which results to a size-biased sample. In this case, the $f_w(x;\theta)$ is also denoted as $f_r(x;\theta)$. For $r = 1, 2$, we obtain a length and an area-biased sample, respectively. Biased sampling is a common phenomenon in practice. Reference [7] gives many examples from various areas where weighted sampling appears rather naturally. Reference [1] considers biased sampling in his study concerning the life length of electron tubes in a system. Reference [6] detects biasness in their sample concerning the strength of SiC fiber and [2] studies and applies the weighted Weibull distribution to forestry data.

If the weight function $w(x)$ is known, the pdf (25.1) can be used in order to estimate the parameter θ of the parent distribution. Unfortunately, in several cases, the used sampling mechanism is not known or even ignored and as a result there is an eminent danger of handling a biased sample as a random one and vice versa. This model misspecification problem may have serious influence not only on the parametric inference but also on the estimation of the characteristic of the distribution such as the mean, the variance, and the median.

In order to clarify the previous statement, let us examine the model misspecification effects of the biasness on various statistical features such as the mean, the variance, and the median in a data set concerning the duration of strikes occurring in USA.

Reference [4] quoted a sample (Table 25.1) of strike lengths (in days) occurring on expiration or reopening of a contract with major issue the wage changes. All strikes reported by [4] began in June of each year for a 9 year period (1968–1976) in US large manufacturing industries (with 1,000 or more workers). Reference [4] reported that sampling only the strikes beginning in June (or in any other time frame) will produce a length-biased sample and analyzed these data assuming a Weibull distribution. To our view, this is not true. The probability of a strike starting in June to be observed is 30/365, which is independent and obviously not proportional to their duration. Of course, one may expect some biasness in the sample under the additional assumption of homogeneity of occurrence of strikes through the year. In order to clarify this statement, let us assume for a moment that we sample only the

Table 25.1 Strike duration (in days)

1	2	2	2	3	3	3	3	4	5	7	8	9	9	10	11	12	12	13	14	15	17	19
21	21	22	23	25	26	27	27	28	29	32	33	35	37	38	41	42	43	44	49	52	61	72

Plus twelve observations censored at duration 80 days

Table 25.2 The estimated parameters and the corresponding statistical features for the strikes duration using a Weibull (first row) and a length biased Weibull distribution (second row)

	Log-likelihood	Shape	Scale	Mean	St.Dev.	Median
$w(x) = 1$	−218.178	0.86713	42.2940	45.4571	52.5925	27.715
$w(x) = x$	−217.787	0.35358	1.00430	4.87697	19.0095	0.3562

strikes that include at least one day in June. Then, the probability P of a strike of k days of duration to be observed is

$$P = \begin{cases} \frac{30+(k-1)}{365} = \frac{29}{365} + \frac{1}{365}k, & 1 \leq k \leq 365 - 29 \\ 1, & k > 336. \end{cases} \tag{25.2}$$

which is a linear function of k and not proportional to that. In any case, this sampling mechanism clearly raises some serious questions on the nature of the data.

In order to examine the significance of the sampling scheme at the parametric inference, we will treat the sample of Table 25.1 as a length biased as [4] suggested, and as a random one, as the actually used method suggests, under the assumption that the parent distribution of the strike duration is a Weibull distribution. The estimates and the corresponding estimated statistical features of the estimated distributions are reported in Table 25.2. From the results, it is clear that adopting the two different assumptions for the used sampling mechanism results in two different estimated distributions for the duration of the strikes with significantly different statistical features. For example, assuming that the data consists a random sample, we get an estimation of the mean duration of the strikes about 45.46 days, while under the assumption of a length-biased sample, we get an estimation of the mean duration of only 4.88 days. These differences are so large that potentially can lead to policy changes or even to changes in business plans.

From the above discussion on the way, the sample was obtained, and from the results of Table 25.2, it is clear that the study of the model misspecification effects on the parameter estimation as well as on the main statistical features of the population is of major importance. In the present chapter, the aforementioned misspecification effects are studied when the population distribution is the Weibull and the data is complete (data without censoring).

In what follows the next set up is adopted: A sample $\underline{X} = (X_1, X_2, \ldots, X_n)$ is drawn from a population with pdf $f_0(x; \beta, \gamma) = \frac{\gamma}{\beta}\left(\frac{x}{\beta}\right)^{\gamma-1} \exp\left[-\left(\frac{x}{\beta}\right)^{\gamma}\right]$, $x > 0$, i.e., from a Weibull distribution where γ and β are the shape and the scale parameter, respectively. If the sample is random, then $X_i \sim f_0(x_i; \theta)$, and if it is biased with weight $w(x) = x^r$, $r > 0$, then $X_i \sim f_r(x_i; \theta)$ with

$$f_r(x, \beta, \gamma) = \frac{x^r}{E_0(X^r)} \frac{\gamma}{\beta}\left(\frac{x}{\beta}\right)^{\gamma-1} \exp\left[-\left(\frac{x}{\beta}\right)^{\gamma}\right] \tag{25.3}$$

where $E_0(X^r)$ is the expectation of X^r with respect to f_0. We assume ignorance of the true underline sampling method, and we study the consequences on the estimation of θ and on the main statistical features such as the mean, the variance, and the median.

In terms of the notation, we write $E_r(\cdot)$ and $E_0(\cdot)$ for the expectation with respect to f_r and f_0, respectively, $\Psi(x)$ is the logarithmic derivative of the Gamma function $\Gamma(x)$. Additionally, the notation $0/r$ is used for the case in which the f_0 is adopted for analyzing the data of a biased sample (i.e., $X_i \sim f_r(x_i;\theta)$). Conversely, the notation $r/0$ model is used for the case in which a random data is analyzed using falsely the f_r distribution instead the f_0.

The rest of the chapter is organized as follows. In Sect. 25.2, we give some preliminary results. In Sect. 25.3, we study the misspecification effects on the parametric estimation of the model, and in Sect. 25.4, the effects on estimation of some characteristics of the distribution. In Sect. 25.5, we support our findings with a simulation study, and we conclude with a discussion in Sect. 25.6.

25.2 Preliminary Results

The mth moment of the Weibull distribution is given by $E_0(X^m) = \beta^m \Gamma(1+\frac{m}{\gamma})$, while the mth moment with respect to f_r is given by $E_r\,(X^m) = \beta^m \frac{\Gamma\left(\frac{r+m}{\gamma}+1\right)}{\Gamma\left(\frac{r}{\gamma}+1\right)},\ r \geq 0.$ The major difference in the shape of f_0 and f_r is that while the f_0 is positively skewed for $\gamma > 1$ and it has the shape of reversed J for $\gamma \leq 1$, the f_r is always positively skewed if $r+\gamma \geq 1$ which implies that if $r \geq 1$ (which holds almost always in practice) the f_r is always positively skewed for every γ.

Using the transformation $u = (x/\beta)^\gamma$, the following two useful relations can be proved

$$E_r\left[\log\left(\frac{X}{\beta}\right)\right] = \frac{1}{\gamma}\Psi\left(\frac{r}{\gamma}+1\right) \tag{25.4}$$

$$E_r\left[\left(\frac{X}{\beta}\right)^\gamma \log\left(\frac{X}{\beta}\right)\right] = \frac{1}{\gamma}\left(\frac{r}{\gamma}+1\right)\Psi\left(\frac{r}{\gamma}+1\right)+\frac{1}{\gamma}. \tag{25.5}$$

The maximum likelihood estimators (MLEs) $\hat{\beta}_n$ and $\hat{\gamma}_n$ of β and γ are obtained from the following system of equations

$$\frac{\partial \log f_r\,(x;\beta,\gamma,r)}{\partial\beta} = 0 \tag{25.6}$$

$$\frac{\partial \log f_r\,(x;\beta,\gamma,r)}{\partial\gamma} = 0 \tag{25.7}$$

where $r \geq 0$. The aforementioned equations can be expressed equivalently as

$$-\frac{r}{\beta} - \frac{\gamma}{\beta} + \frac{\gamma}{\beta}\frac{1}{n}\sum_{i=1}^{n}\left(\frac{x_i}{\beta}\right)^{\gamma} = 0 \quad (25.8)$$

$$\frac{r}{\gamma^2}\Psi\left(\frac{r}{\gamma}+1\right) + \frac{1}{\gamma} + \frac{1}{n}\sum_{i=1}^{n}\log\left(\frac{x_i}{\beta}\right) - \frac{1}{n}\sum_{i=1}^{n}\left(\frac{x_i}{\beta}\right)^{\gamma}\log\left(\frac{x_i}{\beta}\right) = 0. \quad (25.9)$$

25.3 Model Misspecification Effects on the Parameter Estimation

25.3.1 The $0/r$ Case

In this section, the case in which the f_0 is adopted for analyzing the data of a biased sample with weight function $w(x) = x^r,\ r > 0$ is considered. Under this scenario, the estimations of the parameters (β, γ) are obtained using the system of equations (25.8) and (25.9) for $r = 0$.

In other words, the estimators $(\hat{\beta}_n, \hat{\gamma}_n)$ of (β, γ) are obtained as a solution of the system

$$-\frac{\gamma}{\beta} + \frac{\gamma}{\beta}\frac{1}{n}\sum_{i=1}^{n}\left(\frac{x}{\beta}\right)^{\gamma} = 0 \quad (25.10)$$

$$\frac{1}{\gamma} + \frac{1}{n}\sum_{i=1}^{n}\log\left(\frac{x_i}{\beta}\right) - \frac{1}{n}\sum_{i=1}^{n}\left(\frac{x}{\beta}\right)^{\gamma}\log\left(\frac{x_i}{\beta}\right) = 0. \quad (25.11)$$

Such estimators based on a wrong log-likelihood (because the sample follows the f_r pdf and not the f_0) are called quasi–maximum–likelihood estimator (QMLE) [9] and are not always consistent estimators of (β, γ). In order to prove that the QMLE $(\hat{\beta}_n, \hat{\gamma}_n)$ is not a consistent estimator for $r > 0$, let us assume that $(\hat{\beta}_n, \hat{\gamma}_n)$ converges in probability to (β, γ) with respect to the true model f_r. By letting $n \to \infty$, the system of equations (25.10) and (25.11) is written as follows

$$\frac{\gamma}{\beta} + \frac{\gamma}{\beta}E_r\left[\left(\frac{X}{\beta}\right)^{\gamma}\right] = 0 \quad (25.12)$$

$$\frac{1}{\gamma} + E_r\left[\log\left(\frac{x}{\beta}\right)\right] - E_r\left[\left(\frac{X}{\beta}\right)^{\gamma}\log\left(\frac{X}{\beta}\right)\right] = 0. \quad (25.13)$$

By using relations (25.4) and (25.5), the above equations can be written as $-\frac{r}{\beta} = 0$ and $\frac{r}{\gamma^2}\Psi\left(\frac{r}{\gamma}+1\right) = 0$, respectively, which are satisfied only for $r = 0$.

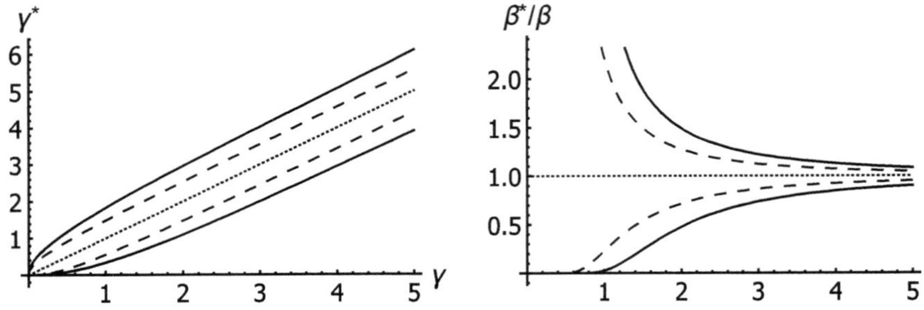

Fig. 25.1 The γ^* against γ plot (left graph) and β^*/β against γ plot (right graph) for different values of r ($r = 1$ dashed lines, $r = 2$ solid lines) for the $0/r$ and $r/0$ cases

So, the QMLEs $(\hat{\beta}_n, \hat{\gamma}_n)$ do not converge (under the correct model f_r) in probability to the true parameters but rather to another set of values denoted as (β^*, γ^*). For a proof that such a limit exists see [3] and [10]. Here, we presented the relation between (β^*, γ^*) and the true parameters (β, γ).

The values (β^*, γ^*) satisfy the system (25.12), (25.13) from which the following equations are obtained

$$\beta^* = \left(\frac{\Gamma(\frac{r+\gamma^*}{\gamma} + 1)}{\Gamma(\frac{r}{\gamma} + 1)} \right)^{\frac{1}{\gamma^*}} \beta \tag{25.14}$$

$$\frac{\gamma^*}{\gamma} \left(\Psi \left(\frac{r + \gamma^*}{\gamma} + 1 \right) - \Psi \left(\frac{r}{\gamma} + 1 \right) \right) = 1. \tag{25.15}$$

Unfortunately, Eq. (25.15) can be solved with respect to γ^* only numerically. However, some interesting conclusions can be conducted by plotting the γ^* against γ for different values of r. Dashed and solid lines above the diagonal line in the left graph of Fig. 25.1 show the relation between the γ^* and γ for $r = 1$ and $r = 2$, respectively, for the $0/r$ model. It is also worth noticing that the relation between γ^* and γ is almost linear for $\gamma > 1$.

Regarding the relation between β^* and β, relation (25.14) can be written as $\beta^*/\beta = \lambda_r(\gamma)$ where $\lambda_r(\gamma) = \left(\frac{\Gamma(\frac{r+\gamma^*}{\gamma}+1)}{\Gamma(\frac{r}{\gamma}+1)} \right)^{\frac{1}{\gamma^*}}$ and γ^* is obtained from (25.15).

Dashed and solid lines above the horizontal dotted line in the right graph of Fig. 25.1 present the graphs of β^*/β in terms of γ for $r = 1$ and $r = 2$, respectively, for the $0/r$ model. It is worth mentioning that for large values of γ, the difference between β^* and β is not significant. In fact from (25.14) and (25.15), we can prove that $\lim \beta^*/\beta \to 1$ and $\lim \gamma^*/\gamma \to 1$, respectively, for $\gamma \to \infty$.

25.3.2 The $r/0$ case

In this scenario, the QMLEs of the parameters (β, γ) are obtained using the system of equations (25.8) and (25.9) for some known fixed $r > 0$ instead of the correct $r = 0$.

Following similar arguments with the previous case, it can be proved that the QMLEs $(\hat{\beta}_n, \hat{\gamma}_n)$ converge in probability to (β^*, γ^*) under the correct model f_0. These values satisfy the following relations

$$\frac{\beta^*}{\beta} = \left(\frac{\Gamma\left(\frac{\gamma^*}{\gamma} + 1\right)}{\frac{r}{\gamma^*} + 1} \right)^{\frac{1}{\gamma^*}} = \Lambda_{\gamma^*, r}(\gamma) \tag{25.16}$$

$$\frac{r}{\gamma^{*2}} \Psi \left(\frac{r}{\gamma^*} + 1 \right) + \frac{1}{\gamma^*} - \frac{r}{\gamma^{*2}} \left\{ \log\left(\frac{r}{\gamma^*} + 1 \right) - \log \Gamma \left(\frac{\gamma^*}{\gamma} + 1 \right) - \right\} \\ - \frac{C}{\gamma} - \frac{1}{\gamma} \Psi \left(\frac{\gamma^*}{\gamma} + 1 \right) \left(\frac{r}{\gamma^*} + 1 \right) = 0 \tag{25.17}$$

where C is the Euler's constant. Dashed and solid lines below the diagonal line in the left graph of Fig. 25.1 show the relation between the γ^* and γ for $r = 1$ and $r = 2$ respectively for the $r/0$ model. Dashed and solid lines below the horizontal dotted line in the right graph of Fig. 25.1 present the graphs of β^*/β in terms of γ for $r = 1$ and $r = 2$, respectively, for the $r/0$ model. From the plots, it is clear that in this case, both the parameters tent to be underestimated by the corresponding QMLEs. The underestimation is more severe for γ close to zero and increases as r increases. Again, as in the $0/r$ case, the effect on the shape parameter vanishes as its value increases.

25.4 Model Misspecification Effects on the Characteristics of the Distribution

The misspecification effects on the estimation of the characteristics of the Weibull distribution such as the mean, the variance, and the median are studied in terms of the ratio

$$\frac{\text{Characteristic of the Weibull distribution based on the limit of the QMLEs}}{\text{Characteristic of the true Weibull distribution.}}$$

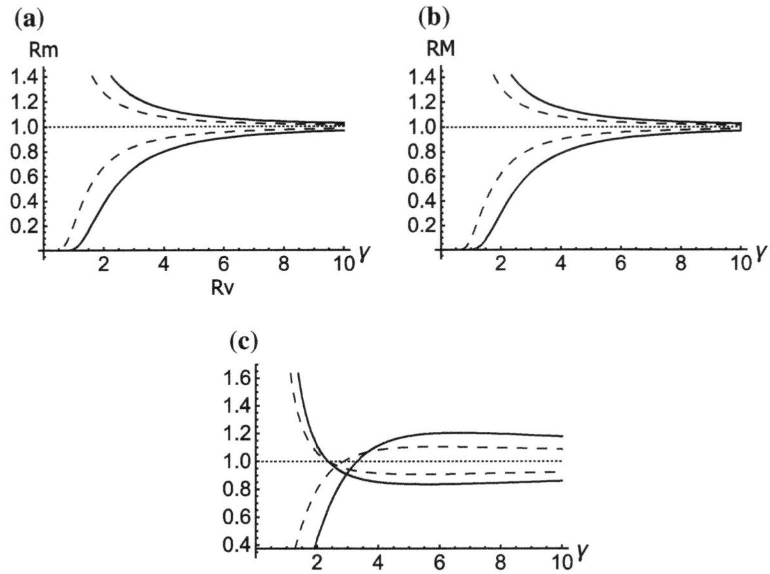

Fig. 25.2 The plots for the ratio of **a** the mean, **b** the median, and **c** the variance against γ ($r = 1$ dashed lines, $r = 2$ solid lines) for the $0/r$ and $r/0$ cases

25.4.1 For the Mean

For the mean, we rely on the ratio $Rm(\gamma, r) = \frac{E_0(X|\gamma^*, \beta^*)}{E_0(X|\gamma, \beta)}$ which is given by

$$Rm(\gamma, r) = \frac{E_0(X|\gamma^*, \beta^*)}{E_0(X|\gamma, \beta)} = \ell_{\gamma^*,r}(\gamma)\frac{\Gamma(\frac{1}{\gamma^*}+1)}{\Gamma(\frac{1}{\gamma}+1)}, \quad r > 0 \tag{25.18}$$

where $\ell_{\gamma^*,r}(\gamma)$ equals to $\lambda_{\gamma^*,r}(\gamma)$ for the $0/r$ case and to $\Lambda_{\gamma^*,r}$ for the $r/0$ case.

Concerning the misspecification effects on the mean, we can see from the plot in Fig. 25.2a that for the 0/r case, the mean is overestimated (lines above the horizontal dotted line), while for the r/0 case is underestimated (lines below the horizontal dotted line). We can prove in either case that the ratio of the means converges to 1 as $\gamma \to \infty$. Also, the misspecification effects increase as r increases.

25.4.2 For the Median

The median of the Weibull distribution is given by the relation $M_0(\beta, \gamma) = \beta^*(\log 2)^{1/\gamma}$. Thus, for the study of the misspecification effects on the median, we rely on the ratios

$$RM(\gamma, r) = \frac{M_0(\gamma^*, \beta^*)}{M_0(\gamma, \beta)} = \ell_{\gamma^*,r}(\gamma)(\log 2)^{\frac{1}{\gamma^*}-\frac{1}{\gamma}}, \quad r > 0. \tag{25.19}$$

The misspecification effects on the median are similar to that on the mean (see Fig. 25.2b). In other words, for the 0/r case, the mean is overestimated, while for the r/0 case is underestimated. In either case, the ratio of the means converges to 1 as $\gamma \to \infty$. Also, the misspecification effects increase as r increases.

25.4.3 For the Variance

For the variance, we consider the ratios

$$Rv(\gamma, r) = \frac{Var_0(X|\gamma^*, \beta^*)}{Var_0(X|\gamma, \beta)} = \lambda^2_{\gamma^*,r}(\gamma)\frac{\Gamma(\frac{1}{\gamma^*}+1) - \Gamma^2(\frac{1}{\gamma^*}+1)}{\Gamma(\frac{2}{\gamma}+1) - \Gamma^2(\frac{1}{\gamma}+1)}, \quad r > 0 \tag{25.20}$$

Compared to the mean and the median, the behavior of the ratio of the variances is different (see Fig. 25.2c). For the 0/r case, the variance is overestimated for small values of γ and underestimated for large γ while for the r/0 case, it behaves in the opposite direction.

25.5 Simulation Study

A simulation study was carried out in order to investigate firstly how quickly the QMLEs converge to their limit and secondly what are the model misspecification effects on the estimation of the distribution's characteristics for finite sample sizes. More specifically, initially, the $0/r$ case was studied by generating 1,000 biased samples from the Weibull distribution using the weight function $w(x) = x^r$ for $r = 1$ and $r = 2$, for each combination of sample size $n = 50, 100, 200, 500$ and value of the parameters $\gamma = 0.5, 1, 2$ and $\beta = 0.25, 1, 4$. For each sample, the QMLE of (β, γ) was obtained and the ratio

$$\frac{\text{Characteristic of the Weibull distribution based on the QMLEs (with finite sample)}}{\text{Characteristic of the correct Weibull distribution}}$$

was calculated for the mean, the median, and the variance.

The results from the simulation study for $r = 1$ and $r = 2$ are presented in Tables 25.3 and 25.4. At the second column, the sample size is given. At the next two columns, under the term "correct mode," the means (based on the 10,000 biased samples) of the MLEs of the parameters using the correct model are given. At the next two columns, under the term "incorrect model" the means of the QMLEs of

Table 25.3 Misspecification results with the help of simulated samples for the $0/r$ case with r =1

	Sample size	True model		Incorrect model		Ratios		
		γ	β	QMLE γ	QMLE β	$Rm(\gamma, r)$	$RM(\gamma, r)$	$Rv(\gamma, r)$
$r = 1$	50	0.52322	0.31186	0.94864	2.88383	5.97415	16.25720	8.71987
	100	0.51114	0.28012	0.93210	2.87611	5.97690	16.13130	8.63727
	200	0.50611	0.26628	0.92504	2.87293	5.97585	16.07980	8.55800
	500	0.50147	0.25484	0.91896	2.87154	5.98301	16.03850	8.57581
	∞	0.50000	0.25000	0.91639	2.86886	5.97913	16.01110	8.53428
	50	0.52554	1.25883	0.95149	11.46920	5.93201	16.18180	8.55198
	100	0.51124	1.12230	0.93230	11.52370	5.98525	16.16050	8.64771
	200	0.50558	1.06295	0.92454	11.51040	5.98760	16.10220	8.60627
	500	0.50236	1.02529	0.91997	11.48150	5.97697	16.03890	8.53796
	∞	0.50000	1.00000	0.91639	11.47550	5.97913	16.01110	8.53428
	50	0.52136	4.92823	0.94644	46.13760	5.98179	16.24000	8.79691
	100	0.51018	4.44521	0.93116	45.95070	5.97053	16.10240	8.62590
	200	0.50554	4.23705	0.92451	45.92150	5.97154	16.06040	8.55675
	500	0.50235	4.10483	0.91989	45.97730	5.98437	16.05570	8.56479
	∞	0.50000	4.00000	0.91639	45.90180	5.97913	16.01110	8.53428
	50	1.04095	0.25915	1.53143	0.55425	2.00326	2.51235	1.85697
	100	1.02034	0.25491	1.50690	0.55490	2.00602	2.50826	1.87699
	200	1.00896	0.25188	1.49374	0.55453	2.00519	2.50239	1.88834
	500	1.00407	0.25094	1.48754	0.55471	2.00581	2.50148	1.89154
	∞	1.00000	0.25000	1.48245	0.55478	2.00621	2.50023	1.89618
	50	1.03547	1.03015	1.52581	2.21814	2.00511	2.51140	1.87299
	100	1.01850	1.01787	1.50546	2.22119	2.00774	2.50941	1.88501
	200	1.00958	1.00824	1.49440	2.21789	2.00486	2.50243	1.88583
	500	1.00338	1.00323	1.48658	2.21962	2.00669	2.50199	1.89536
	∞	1.00000	1.00000	1.48245	2.21910	2.00621	2.50023	1.89618
	50	1.03896	4.14331	1.52921	8.88442	2.00738	2.51603	1.87092
	100	1.02021	4.07044	1.50696	8.86822	2.00385	2.50518	1.87577
	200	1.00818	4.02556	1.49283	8.86981	2.00470	2.50134	1.88863
	500	1.00321	4.00893	1.48634	8.87201	2.00527	2.50006	1.89330
	∞	1.00000	4.00000	1.48245	8.87641	2.00621	2.50023	1.89618
	50	2.06734	0.25108	2.60678	0.31749	1.27367	1.32346	1.03683
	100	2.03581	0.25085	2.57240	0.31791	1.27449	1.32369	1.04804
	200	2.01551	0.25014	2.54997	0.31776	1.27339	1.32185	1.05569
	500	2.00743	0.25009	2.54110	0.31788	1.27361	1.32193	1.05857
	∞	2.00000	0.25000	2.53295	0.31802	1.27398	1.32208	1.06244
	50	2.06501	1.00326	2.60471	1.26908	1.27278	1.32243	1.03667
	100	2.03225	1.00086	2.56867	1.26963	1.27244	1.32128	1.04781
	200	2.01699	1.00182	2.55182	1.27232	1.27470	1.32330	1.05669

(continued)

Table 25.3 (continued)

	Sample size	True model		Incorrect model		Ratios		
		γ	β	QMLE γ	QMLE β	$Rm(\gamma, r)$	$RM(\gamma, r)$	$Rv(\gamma, r)$
	500	2.00582	1.00015	2.53958	1.27169	1.27378	1.32200	1.06001
	∞	2.00000	1.00000	2.53295	1.27207	1.27398	1.32208	1.06244
	50	2.07562	4.02485	2.61538	5.08174	1.27429	1.32453	1.03252
	100	2.03237	4.00874	2.56876	5.08487	1.27403	1.32294	1.05047
	200	2.01629	4.00633	2.55100	5.08892	1.27460	1.32314	1.05723
	500	2.00779	4.00253	2.54148	5.08702	1.27387	1.32221	1.05871
	∞	2.00000	4.00000	2.53295	5.08829	1.27398	1.32208	1.06244

Table 25.4 Misspecification results with the help of simulated samples for the $0/r$ case with r = 2

	Sample size	True model		Incorrect model		Ratios		
		γ	β	QMLE γ	QMLE β	$Rm(\gamma, r)$	$RM(\gamma, r)$	$Rv(\gamma, r)$
$r = 2$	50	0.52364	0.36217	1.22749	7.99282	15.05510	49.19440	32.64330
	100	0.51236	0.30632	1.20789	7.98389	15.04710	48.98880	32.44280
	200	0.50581	0.27730	1.19601	7.99064	15.07150	48.92660	32.56740
	500	0.50327	0.26343	1.19049	7.98358	15.06190	48.83680	32.49770
	∞	0.50000	0.25000	1.18502	7.98352	15.06910	48.78450	32.58330
	50	0.52534	1.47027	1.22914	31.94050	15.03000	49.18260	32.28410
	100	0.51314	1.23603	1.20872	31.95260	15.05310	49.02450	32.42670
	200	0.50816	1.13267	1.19894	31.89720	15.03260	48.86050	32.27910
	500	0.50226	1.04336	1.18978	31.93270	15.06350	48.82520	32.54370
	∞	0.50000	1.00000	1.18502	31.93410	15.06910	48.78450	32.58330
	50	0.52579	5.91667	1.23000	128.46300	15.10930	49.46120	32.59830
	100	0.51200	4.90082	1.20679	128.02000	15.08400	49.08000	32.66070
	200	0.50610	4.45930	1.19661	127.83700	15.06910	48.92740	32.54830
	500	0.50275	4.19070	1.19032	127.68200	15.05600	48.81300	32.48530
	∞	0.50000	4.00000	1.18502	127.73600	15.06910	48.78450	32.58330
	50	1.04889	0.26901	1.90018	0.84758	3.01446	4.02463	2.83288
	100	1.02045	0.25795	1.86198	0.84704	3.01181	4.01046	2.87551
	200	1.01139	0.25469	1.84887	0.84727	3.01184	4.00814	2.88308
	500	1.00439	0.25176	1.83924	0.84691	3.01028	4.00347	2.89103
	∞	1.00000	0.25000	1.83277	0.84689	3.01002	4.00138	2.89802
	50	1.04262	1.06350	1.89299	3.38339	3.00842	4.01392	2.83525
	100	1.02332	1.03636	1.86488	3.38579	3.00935	4.00903	2.86063
	200	1.01214	1.01982	1.84986	3.38767	3.01051	4.00694	2.87725
	500	1.00525	1.00836	1.84028	3.38677	3.00945	4.00288	2.88677

(continued)

Table 25.4 (continued)

Sample size	True model		Incorrect model		Ratios		
	γ	β	QMLE γ	QMLE β	$Rm(\gamma, r)$	$RM(\gamma, r)$	$Rv(\gamma, r)$
∞	1.00000	1.00000	1.83277	3.38754	3.01002	4.00138	2.89802
50	1.05086	4.31406	1.90317	13.53610	3.00852	4.01884	2.80812
100	1.02193	4.14178	1.86427	13.56300	3.01376	4.01472	2.87064
200	1.01121	4.06533	1.84860	13.52660	3.00523	3.99928	2.87066
500	1.00429	4.02760	1.83910	13.55190	3.01061	4.00382	2.89226
∞	1.00000	4.00000	1.83277	13.55020	3.01002	4.00138	2.89802
50	2.07618	0.25247	3.05663	0.37173	1.49983	1.58221	1.08032
100	2.03589	0.25121	3.00937	0.37218	1.50044	1.58212	1.09676
200	2.01758	0.25066	2.98684	0.37245	1.50095	1.58228	1.10530
500	2.00490	0.25000	2.97126	0.37229	1.49992	1.58090	1.10955
∞	2.00000	0.25000	2.96490	0.37242	1.50025	1.58121	1.11128
50	2.08226	1.01127	3.06330	1.48686	1.49993	1.58248	1.07782
100	2.03895	1.00583	3.01247	1.48903	1.50083	1.58263	1.09570
200	2.02102	1.00394	2.99023	1.49001	1.50124	1.58273	1.10338
500	2.00792	1.00152	2.97464	1.48997	1.50080	1.58197	1.10860
∞	2.00000	1.00000	2.96490	1.48966	1.50025	1.58121	1.11128
50	2.07759	4.04607	3.05911	5.95738	1.50235	1.58485	1.08388
100	2.03652	4.01918	3.00974	5.95405	1.50025	1.58192	1.09654
200	2.01594	4.00721	2.98466	5.95732	1.50043	1.58165	1.10596
500	2.00795	4.00515	2.97460	5.95874	1.50052	1.58166	1.10839
∞	2.00000	4.00000	2.96490	5.95866	1.50025	1.58121	1.11128

γ and β and at the next three columns under the term "Ratios" the ratios $Rm(\gamma, r)$, $RM(\gamma, r)$ and $Rv(\gamma, r)$ are presented. For comparison purposes, for every combination of the parameters, there is a line indicated with "∞," in which the true values of the parameters β and γ of the Weibull distribution and the limits of QMLEs, $Rm(\gamma, r)$, $RM(\gamma, r)$, and $Rv(\gamma, r)$ are presented. Simulation results verify that also for small samples, the QMLEs overestimate the parameters. The same holds also for the mean, the median, and the variance. We observe that the QMLEs converge slower to the limit compared to the the MLEs. The misspecification effects on the mean, the median, and the variance decrease as γ increases, and they are not affected by the β. The effects are more severe as r increases.

A similar procedure was carried out and for the $r/0$ case. The results were similar with those of the $0/r$. More specifically, the QMLEs underestimates the parameters as well as the mean and the median. The misspecification effects on the mean, the median, and the variance decrease as γ increases. The effects are more severe as r increases. The tables are not presented here, but they are available from the authors upon request.

25.6 Conclusions

As [5] claim, model misspecification is unavoidable in practice. Therefore, this phenomenon must be studied extensively. Reference [8] examines condition under which the QMLE is a consistent estimator. In this chapter, the inconsistency of the QMLEs was proved and the model misspecification effects on the estimation of the population mean, median, and variance were studied when a biased sample is treated as a random one and vice-versa. We have focused on the length (r = 1) and area (r = 2) biased sampling cases. It turns out that for the $0/r$, $r = 1, 2$ case, i.e., when a length or an area-biased sample is treated as a random one, then all the parameters are overestimated. For the $r/0$, $r = 1, 2$ case, the population parameters are underestimated. In both cases, the misspecification results are more severe for the area-biased sampling ($r = 2$) compared to the length-biased sampling ($r = 1$).

References

1. Blumenthal, S.: Proportional sampling in life length studies. Technometrics **9**(2), 205–218 (1966)
2. Gove, J.H.: Moment and maximum likelihood estimators for weibull distributions under length- and area biased sampling. Environ. Ecol. Stat. **10**, 455–467 (2003)
3. Keith, K.: Mathematical Statistics. Chapman & Hall, Boca Raton (2000)
4. Kiefer, N.M.: Economic duration data and hazard functions. J. Econ. Lit. **26**(2), 646–79 (1988)
5. Lv, J., Liu, J.S.: Model selection principles in misspecified models. J. R. Stat. Soc. Ser. B **76**(1), 141–167 (2014)
6. Morimoto, T., Nakagawa, S., Shinji, S.: Bias in the weibull strength estimation of a sic fiber for the small gauge length case. JSME Int. J. Ser. A **48**(4), 194–198 (2005)
7. Patil, G.: Weighted distributions. Encyclopedia of Environmetrics, pp. 2369–2377. Wiley, Chichester (2002)
8. Tzavelas, G., Douli, M., Economou, P.: Model misspecification effects for biased samples. Metrika **80**(2), 171–185 (2017)
9. White, H.: Maximum likelihood estimation in misspecified models. Econometrica **50**(1), 1–25 (1982)
10. Yi, Y.G., Reid, N.: A note on misspecified estimating functions. Statistica Sinica **20**, 1749–1769 (2010)

Chapter 26
An Overview on Recent Advances in Statistical Burn-In Modeling for Semiconductor Devices

Daniel Kurz, Horst Lewitschnig and Jürgen Pilz

Abstract In semiconductor manufacturing, the early life of the produced devices can be simulated by means of burn-in. In this way, early failures are screened out before delivery. To reduce the efforts associated with burn-in, the failure probability p in the early life of the devices is evaluated using a burn-in study. Classically, this is done by computing the exact Clopper–Pearson upper bound for p. In this chapter, we provide an overview on a series of new statistical models, which are capable of considering further available information (e.g., differently reliable chip areas) within the Clopper–Pearson estimator for p. These models help semiconductor manufacturers to more efficiently evaluate the early life failure probabilities of their products and therefore reduce the efforts associated with burn-in studies of new technologies.

Keywords Area scaling · Binomial distribution · Burn-in
Power semiconductors · Sampling

26.1 Introduction

Power semiconductors are used in many safety-critical applications like cars, planes, trains. For that reason, it is of particular importance to ensure high reliability of semiconductor devices by screening out weak devices before delivery.

The failure rate λ of semiconductor devices (over time) can be described by the bathtub curve, see Fig. 26.1 [22]. In other words, at the beginning of the lifetime, the

D. Kurz (✉) · J. Pilz
Department of Statistics, Alpen-Adria University of Klagenfurt,
Universitätsstrasse 65-67, 9020 Klagenfurt, Austria
e-mail: daniel.kurz@aau.at

J. Pilz
e-mail: juergen.pilz@aau.at

H. Lewitschnig
Infineon Technologies Austria AG, Siemensstrasse 2, 9500 Villach, Austria
e-mail: horst.lewitschnig@infineon.com

J. Pilz et al. (eds.), *Statistics and Simulation*, Springer Proceedings
in Mathematics & Statistics 231, https://doi.org/10.1007/978-3-319-76035-3_26

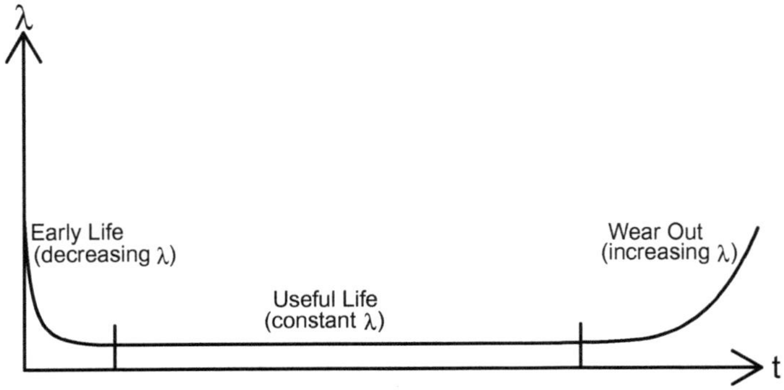

Fig. 26.1 Bathtub curve describing the failure rate λ of semiconductor devices over time

devices are assumed to have an increased failure rate, which decreases over time. This life phase is typically referred to as the early life.

Semiconductor manufacturers aim at reducing the failure rate of the devices before delivery. One efficient method to do so is burn-in (BI), see, e.g., [1, 6–10]. The purpose of BI is to simulate the early life of the produced devices before delivery. This is done by operating the devices under accelerated voltage and temperature stress conditions for a certain period of time (BI time). In this way, early failures (i.e., devices, which fail in the early life) can be detected and weeded out.

In general, one can distinguish between two concepts of performing BI: 100% BI and BI study. 100% BI means that always all produced devices are burnt. In this case, the efforts of BI are lowered by successively reducing the BI time, typically, based on the lifetime distribution of early failures, see, e.g., [18, 19, 23].

In contrast to that, in a BI study, only a random sample of produced devices is burnt. Furthermore, the burnt devices are physically investigated for BI relevant failures (e.g., metalization residues, particles in oxide, random defects). Based on the number of failures, the failure probability of the devices in the early life can be assessed at a certain confidence level (CL). If the early life failure probability can be shown to be below the predefined ppm-target, BI can be released for the current product under test. In this chapter, we focus on BI studies.

From a statistical point of view, the random number of early failures X observed in a BI study can be modeled using a binomial distribution, i.e., $X \sim Bi(n, p)$ with n denoting the number of burnt devices and p being the early life failure probability of a single device. Given k failures out of n devices ("k/n"), an $(1-\alpha)$-upper bound for p can then be derived using the classical Clopper–Pearson (CP) approach [5], which is still widely in use, see, e.g., [2, 20, 21]. More precisely, the CP upper bound $\widehat{p}$ is the solution of

$$F_X(k; n, \widehat{p}) = \alpha, \tag{26.1}$$

where F_X denotes the cumulative distribution function of X. Notice that the CP upper bound is exact, i.e., has coverage probability $P(\widehat{p} > p) \geq 1-\alpha$ for all n,

p and α. Moreover, it holds that $F_X(k; n, \widehat{p}) = 1 - F_Z(\widehat{p}; k+1, n-k)$ with $Z \sim Be(k+1, n-k)$ and thus $\widehat{p} = F_Z^{-1}(1-\alpha; k+1, n-k)$, see, e.g., [12].

In semiconductor manufacturing, however, one typically has further available information to be considered with regard to the estimation of p. These information can result from

- countermeasures implemented in the production process,
- synergies between different chip technologies,
- multiple reference products with different chip sizes, or
- differently reliable chip areas, like logic and DMOS.

For each of these cases, we built an estimation model for p, see [12–16]. These models extend (26.1) in order to take into account the additional information.

In this chapter, we provide an overview on the basic steps for running the new models. Moreover, we illustrate how these models can help semiconductor manufacturers to reduce the efforts associated with BI studies and, therefore to speed up the release of BI. Last but not least, we discuss combinations of the models, which are of practical relevance whenever several additional information are available.

26.2 Countermeasure Model

In general, a BI study with zero failures out of n devices is required to release the BI. In this way, the required sample size can be derived by solving $F_X(0; n, p_{target}) = \alpha$ with respect to n, where p_{target} denotes the ppm-target.

Whenever failures occur in the BI study, countermeasures (CMs) (e.g., ink out, optical inspections, process and design measures) are implemented in the production process in order to avoid these failures. Subsequently, the BI study is restarted. In general, this procedure is repeated as long as zero failures are observed, which, clearly, involves increased BI efforts.

Semiconductor manufacturers, however, typically have prior knowledge on the effectivenesses of the implemented CMs regarding the avoidance of early failures. These prior knowledge can now be considered within the assessment of an upper bound for p using the CM model as covered in [12, 17]. In particular, we

1. infer lower bounds from the prior distributions of the CM effectivenesses (in order to avoid an overestimation of the effectivenesses with a high certainty),
2. assess probabilities ξ_j that j failures would have occurred if the CMs would have been introduced already before the BI study on the basis of the Poisson binomial distribution and
3. compute the $(1-\alpha)$-upper bound for p after the introduction of the CMs solving

$$\sum_{j=0}^{k} \xi_j \cdot F_X(j; n, \widehat{p}) = \alpha \tag{26.2}$$

Table 26.1 90%-upper bounds for p and additional sample sizes according to CM model for BI study with $k = 1$ failure out of $n = 100$k devices and different CM effectivenesses

CM	0%	25%	50%	75%	100%
$\widehat{p}$ at 90% CL	38.90 ppm	36.14 ppm	32.72 ppm	28.39 ppm	23.03 ppm
n_{add}	69 k	57 k	42.2 k	23.4 k	0 k

with respect to $\widehat{p}$, see [12].

In this way, the (reduced) early life failure probability of the devices after the implementation of CMs can be assessed without restarting the BI study. Moreover, the additional sample size n_{add} (with zero failures) for reaching the ppm-target can be essentially lower than n. This is illustrated in Table 26.1 showing $\widehat{p}$ at 90% CL and n_{add} for a BI study with $k = 1$ failure out of $n = 100$k devices and different CM effectivenesses. The computations were done using [17].

26.3 Synergies Model

In semiconductor manufacturing, there are several chip technologies. Classically, BI studies for different technologies are treated separately from each other with regard to the estimation of early life failure probabilities.

Nevertheless, it often occurs that different chip technologies exhibit synergies among each other, basically due to technology variants and further developments of technologies. In the context of BI studies, this means that certain subsets of the current technology under test (e.g., logic, DMOS, package) might have been already investigated in the course of BI studies of related technologies. These additional information can now be considered with regard to the estimation of p using the model presented in [16]. More precisely, we

1. collect all available information for the subsets of the current product under test (i.e., k_i failures out of n_i items on subset i),
2. derive probabilities ϕ_j that n devices with j failures are randomly assembled from n_i items with k_i failures of subset i ($n = \min_i n_i$) and
3. obtain the $(1 - \alpha)$-upper bound for p using (26.2) with ϕ_j instead of ξ_j, see [16].

In this way, we are led to a more efficient estimation of the failure probability of the devices in their early life. Moreover, in the case of failures, this model can help us to avoid a restart of BI studies.

To illustrate this, let us again assume $k = 1$ failure out of $n = 100$k devices in a BI study. Further suppose that the failure is on a subset, which has already been tested n_1^{add} times with zero failures in a former BI study. For the remaining subsets, however, we do not have additional data. Thus, in total, we have $1/(n + n_1^{add})$ for the failed subset and $0/n$ for the "rest." In Table 26.2, we then summarize 90%-upper bounds for p for different values of n_1^{add}. Moreover, we report the additionally

Table 26.2 90%-upper bounds for p and additional sample sizes according to synergies model for BI study with $k = 1$ failure out of $n = 100\,\text{k}$ devices and different values for n_1^{add}

n_1^{add}	0 k	100 k	200 k	300 k	400 k
$\widehat{p}$ at 90% CL	38.90 ppm	32.72 ppm	29.95 ppm	28.39 ppm	27.39 ppm
n_{add}	69 k	48.3 k	35.4 k	27.3 k	22 k

required sample sizes n_{add} (with zero failures) in the BI study, which have been computed using [11]. One can see that for larger n_1^{add}, n_{add} is essentially lower than $n = 100\,\text{k}$ and, therefore, a restart of the BI study is not necessary anymore.

26.4 Model for Multiple Reference Products

For each chip technology, there are several products, which typically only differ with respect to their chip sizes. In general, a BI study is performed for only one of these products. The failure probability p' of some follower product is then obtained by means of area scaling. Classically, this is done assuming a serial system of equally reliable areas for a chip. Hence,

$$\widehat{p'} = 1 - (1 - \widehat{p})^{A'/A}, \tag{26.3}$$

where A [mm^2] and A' [mm^2] refer to the sizes of the reference and follower product. Clearly, $\widehat{p'} > \widehat{p}$ if $A' > A$ and vice versa. Thus, if $A' > A$ ($A' < A$) more (less) than n devices with zero failures have to be burnt in order to reach the ppm-target for the follower product.

Nevertheless, it can also happen that BI studies are performed on multiple reference products. In this case, the information from all reference products can be taken into account with regard to the estimation of the early life failure probabilities of follower products, see [14]. To be more concrete, we

1. scale the number of failures for each reference product down to the greatest common size (GCS) of the reference products (this leads to probabilities $\phi_{j_{GCS}}$ to have j_{GCS} failures out of n_{GCS} items of size A_{GCS} [mm^2]),
2. estimate the $(1 - \alpha)$-upper bound for p_{GCS} using [14]

$$\sum_{j_{GCS}} \phi_{j_{GCS}} \cdot F_{X_{GCS}}\big(j_{GCS}; n_{GCS}, \widehat{p}_{GCS}\big) = \alpha \tag{26.4}$$

   with $X_{GCS} \sim Bi(n_{GCS}, p_{GCS})$ and
3. compute $\widehat{p'}$ using $\widehat{p}_{GCS}$ and A_{GCS} instead of $\widehat{p}$ and A in (26.3).

This model contributes to an earlier release of BI for follower products. This can be seen from the following example. Let us assume two reference products with chip

Table 26.3 90%-upper bounds for p' and additional sample sizes in BI study of the second reference product ($n_{add,2}$) according to the model for multiple reference products

A'	6 mm^2	8 mm^2	10 mm^2	12 mm^2	14 mm^2
$\widehat{p}'$ at 90% CL	15.56 ppm	20.75 ppm	25.93 ppm	31.12 ppm	36.31 ppm
$n_{add,2}$	0 k	0 k	19 k	52.8 k	86.6 k

sizes $A_1 = 5$ mm^2 and $A_2 = 10$ mm^2. Let us further suppose that the BI study of the first reference product has been successful, i.e., zero failures out of 100 k devices, while in the BI study of the second, larger reference product a failure has occurred. Table 26.3 then shows the 90%-upper bounds for p' for different follower products, which have been computed using [11]. Moreover, the additionally required sample sizes (with zero failures) in the BI study of the larger reference product to reach the ppm-target for the follower products are provided. One can see that, although there is a failure in the BI study of the second reference product, BI can be released for the first two follower products. Furthermore, even in case of equally sized or slightly larger follower products, just a reduced number of additional devices in BI (with zero failures) are necessary to prove the ppm-target.

26.5 Separate Area Scaling Model

In the classical area scaling (CAS), see (26.3), one assumes that each chip area (e.g., logic, DMOS, chip edge) has an equal failure probability per mm^2. Nevertheless, for reasons of different production and testing conditions (e.g., different test coverage), this assumption must not necessarily be confirmed by the numbers of failures on the subsets. For instance, when considering two subsets, it might happen that the larger number of failures occur on the smaller subset, which provides evidence against the validity of the CAS. In such cases, the failure probabilities of the subsets have to be scaled separately from each other using the separate area scaling (SAS) model as introduced in [15]. In this model, we

1. check for a significant evidence of differently reliable subsets taking into account the numbers of subset failures as well as the sizes of the subsets,
2. in case that we find a significant evidence, we then adapt the failure probabilities of the subsets according to the observed failures without changing $\widehat{p}$ and
3. scale the subset failure probabilities separately from each other, i.e., compute the failure probability of follower products using [15]

$$\widehat{p}' = 1 - \prod_{i=1}^{m} (1 - \widehat{p}_i)^{A_i'/A_i}, \tag{26.5}$$

Table 26.4 90%-upper bounds for p' for different sizes of second subset on follower product according to CAS and SAS

A'_2	2 mm^2	4 mm^2	6 mm^2	8 mm^2	10 mm^2
$\widehat{p}'_{CAS}$ at 90% CL	23.34 ppm	33.71 ppm	44.08 ppm	54.46 ppm	64.83 ppm
$\widehat{p}'_{SAS}$ at 90% CL	31.06 ppm	36.28 ppm	41.51 ppm	46.74 ppm	51.96 ppm

where $\widehat{p}_i$ denotes the estimated failure probability of subset i and A_i and A'_i are the sizes of the i-th subset on the reference and follower product, $i = 1, \ldots, m$.

In this way, we are led to a more accurate estimation of early life failure probabilities of follower products. To illustrate this, let us again assume a BI study with $k = 1$ failure out of $n = 100$k devices. Furthermore, we suppose that the reference product can be partitioned into two subsets (e.g. logic and DMOS) with sizes $A_1 = 2.5$ mm^2 and $A_2 = 5$ mm^2, while the failure is located on subset one (i.e., the smaller subset). This provides significant evidence against an equal failure probability per mm^2 for the subsets. When now considering a follower product, which only differs from the reference product with respect to the size of the second subset, we can compute $\widehat{p}'$ at 90% CL according to the CAS and the SAS for different sizes A'_2 [mm^2]. Using [11], we obtain the results in Table 26.4. One can see that for $A'_2 > A_2$ ($A'_2 < A_2$), the SAS correctly provides lower (larger) ppm-values than the CAS, which is basically because the CAS overestimates (underestimates) p' in case of differently reliable subsets, see [15].

26.6 Model Combinations

Basically, several combinations of the models discussed in Sects. 26.2–26.5 are possible, see Fig. 26.2. From a practical point of view, however, the most important combinations are

- the CM model with the synergies model whenever we have failures on different subsets and the failures are tackled by CMs,
- the CM model with the model for multiple reference products whenever we have failures on differently sized reference products, which are tackled by CMs, and
- the CM model with the SAS model in order to accurately handle failures on differently reliable chip subsets after the introduction of CMs.

The first two combinations just require an adaption of the probabilities ϕ_j in Sect. 26.3 and ϕ_{JGCS} in Sect. 26.4 to ϕ_j^{CM} and ϕ_{JGCS}^{CM}, see [14, 16]. For the third combination, however, we have to adapt the "check" for differently reliable subsets as well as the estimation of the subset failure probabilities to consider the effectivenesses of the CMs, see [15].

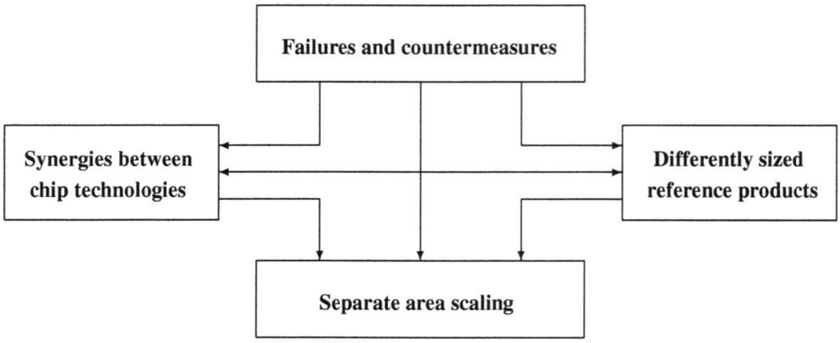

Fig. 26.2 Illustration of possible model combinations

Table 26.5 90%-upper bounds for p and additional sample sizes according to CM model in combination with synergies model for BI study with $k = 1$ failure out of $n = 100$ k devices

CM \ n_1^{add}	0 k	100 k	200 k	300 k	400 k
0%	38.90 ppm	32.72 ppm	29.95 ppm	28.39 ppm	27.39 ppm
	69 k	48.3 k	35.4 k	27.3 k	22 k
25%	36.14 ppm	30.68 ppm	28.39 ppm	27.14 ppm	26.36 ppm
	57 k	37.7 k	26.8 k	20.3 k	16.3 k
50%	32.72 ppm	28.39 ppm	26.71 ppm	25.82 ppm	25.28 ppm
	42.2 k	25.7 k	17.7 k	13.4 k	10.7 k
75%	28.39 ppm	25.82 ppm	24.91 ppm	24.45 ppm	24.17 ppm
	23.4 k	12.9 k	8.7 k	6.5 k	5.2 k
100%	23.03 ppm	23.03 ppm	23.03 ppm	23.03 ppm	23.03 ppm
	0 k	0 k	0 k	0 k	0 k

To illustrate the benefit of combining the CM model with the remaining models, let us again consider the example in Sect. 26.3, in which we assumed a BI study with $k = 1$ failure on a subset that has been already tested with zero failures in the BI study of a related technology. However, let us now additionally suppose that the observed failure is tackled by a CM. In this way, we can update the results in Table 26.2 considering the CM's effectiveness. The updated results (which can again be computed using [11]) are shown in Table 26.5. One can see that by considering synergies in combination with CMs the additionally required sample size in the BI study can be further reduced.

26.7 Summary and Outlook

In this chapter, an overview on a series of new statistical models for calculating early life failure probabilities of semiconductor devices has been provided. These models are capable of considering further available information within the classical Clopper–Pearson estimator for a binomial proportion. In particular, we reported on

- a model for estimating the failure probability of semiconductor devices in their early life after the introduction of countermeasures in the production process (countermeasure model),
- a model that takes advantage of synergies between different chip technologies with regard to the failure probability estimation (synergies model),
- a model which accurately combines burn-in studies on differently sized reference products with regard to the assessment of early life failure probabilities of follower products (model for multiple reference products) and
- a model which allows us to scale differently reliable chip subsets separately from each other (separate area scaling model).

These models (and combinations among them) were shown to provide improved estimates of early life failure probabilities of reference and follower products. In this way, the proposed models help semiconductor manufacturers to reduce the efforts associated with the demonstration of ppm-targets for new products or technologies.

To provide a look into the future, we aim at further taking into account the lifetime of early failures when calculating ppm-values of semiconductor devices. This will further improve the estimation of early life failure probabilities. In particular, however, this will essentially increase the flexibility with regard to the practical application of burn-in studies for new products and technologies.

Acknowledgements The work has been performed in the project EPT300, co-funded by grants from Austria, Germany, Italy, The Netherlands and the ENIAC Joint Undertaking. This project is co-funded within the programme "Forschung, Innovation und Technologie für Informationstechnologie" by the Austrian Ministry for Transport, Innovation and Technology.

References

1. Barlow, R., Proschan, F.: Statistical Theory of Reliability and Life Testing. Holt, Renerhart & Winston, New York (1975)
2. Berg, B.A.: Clopper-Pearson bounds from HEP data cuts. AIP Conf. Proc. **583**, 104–106 (2001)
3. Brown, L.D., Cai, T.T., DasGupta, A.: Interval estimation for a binomial proportion. Stat. Sci. **16**, 101–133 (2001)
4. Brown, L.D., Cai, T.T., DasGupta, A.: Confidence intervals for a binomial proportion and asymptotic expansions. Ann. Stat. **30**, 160–201 (2002)
5. Clopper, C.J., Pearson, E.S.: The use of confidence or fiducial limits illustrated in the case of the binomial. Biometrika **26**, 404–413 (1934)
6. Gerstle, D., Lee, P.: Impact of burn-in on power supply reliability. Power Electron. Technol. 20–25 (2005)
7. Jensen, F., Petersen, N.E.: Burn-In. Wiley, New York (1982)
8. Kececioglu, D., Sun, F.: Burn-in Testing - Its Quantification and Optimization. Prentice Hall, New Jersey (1997)
9. Kuo, W., Kuo, Y.: Facing the headaches of early failures: a state-of-the-art review of burn-in decisions. Proc. IEEE. **71**, 1257–1266 (1983)

10. Kuo, W., Chien, W.T.K., Kim, T.: Reliability, Yield, and Stress Burn-in. Kluwer Academic Publishers, Norwell, MA (1998)
11. Kurz, D., Lewitschnig, H.: AdvBinomApps. R-package. http://cran.r-project.org/web/packages/AdvBinomApps. (Cited 3 May 2016)
12. Kurz, D., Lewitschnig, H., Pilz, J.: Decision-theoretical model for failures tackled by countermeasures. IEEE Trans. Reliab. **63**, 583–592 (2014)
13. Kurz, D., Lewitschnig, H., Pilz, J.: Survey of recent advanced statistical models for early life failure probability assessment in semiconductor manufacturing. Proc. Winter Sim. Conf. 2600–2608 (2014)
14. Kurz, D., Lewitschnig, H., Pilz, J.: Failure probability estimation with differently sized reference products for semiconductor burn-in studies. Appl. Stoch. Model. Bus. **31**, 732–744 (2015)
15. Kurz, D., Lewitschnig, H., Pilz, J.: An advanced area scaling approach for semiconductor burn-in. Microelectron. Reliab. **55**, 129–137 (2015)
16. Kurz, D., Lewitschnig, H., Pilz, J.: Failure probability estimation under additional subsystem information with application to semiconductor burn-in. J. Appl. Stat. **44**, 955–967 (2017)
17. Lewitschnig, H., Lenzi, D.: GenBinomApps. R-package. http://cran.r-project.org/web/packages/GenBinomApps. (Cited 3 May 2016)
18. Ooi, M.P.-L., Kassim, Z.A., Demidenko, S.N.: Shortening burn-in test: application of HVST and Weibull statistical analysis. IEEE Trans. Instrum. Meas. **56**, 990–999 (2007)
19. Reliability Edge: Guidelines for burn-in justification and burn-in time determination. ReliaSoft. **7** (2007). http://reliasoft.com/newsletter/v7i2/burn_in.htm. (Cited 4 May 2016)
20. Sullivan, A.K., Raben, D., Reekie, J., Rayment, M., Mocroft, A., et. al.: Feasibility and Effectiveness of Indicator Condition-Guided Testing for HIV: Results from HIDES I (HIV Indicator Diseases across Europe Study). PLoS ONE. **8**, e52845 (2013)
21. Ward, L.G., Heckman, M.G., Warren, A.I., Tran, K.: Dosing accuracy of insulin aspart flexpens after transport through the pneumatic tube system. Hosp. Pharm. **48**, 33–38 (2013)
22. Wilkins, D.J.: The Bathtub curve and product failure behavior. HotWire. **21** (2002). http://weibull.com/hotwire/issue21/hottopics21.htm. (Cited 3 May 2016)
23. Zakaria, F., Kassim, Z.A., Ooi, M.P.L., Demidenko, S.: Reducing burn-in time through high-voltage stress test and Weibull statistical analysis. IEEE Des. Test. Comput. **23**, 88–98 (2006)

Chapter 27
Simplified Analysis of Queueing Systems with Random Requirements

Konstantin E. Samouylov, Yuliya V. Gaidamaka and Eduard S. Sopin

Abstract In this work, a simplification approach for analysis of queueing systems with random requirements is proposed. The main point of the approach is to keep track of only total amount of occupied system resources. Therefore, we cannot know the exact amount of resources released by the departure of a customer, so we assume it a random variable with conditional cumulative distribution function depending on only number of customers in the system and total occupied resources at the moment just before the departure. In the chapter, we briefly describe the queuing system with random requirements, the simplification method and show that in case of Poisson arrival process simplified system has exactly the same stationary probability distribution as the original one.

Keywords Queuing system · Limited resources · Probabilistic characteristics Insensitivity

27.1 Introduction

We consider the queuing systems, in which resources are required to serve customers. Random variables related to the resource requirements can follow either discrete or continuous distribution. Arriving customers are lost if the system does not have free resources needed for their service. As at the end of the service held resources should be released, such systems can be called as occupy-and-release systems. The random

---

K. E. Samouylov · Y. V. Gaidamaka (✉) · E. S. Sopin
Peoples' Friendship University of Russia (RUDN University), 117198 Miklukho-Maklaya str. 6, Moscow, Russia
e-mail: gaydamaka_yuv@rudn.university

K. E. Samouylov
e-mail: samuylov_ke@rudn.university

K. E. Samouylov · Y. V. Gaidamaka · E. S. Sopin
Institute of Informatics Problems, FRC CSC RAS, 119333 Vavilova Str. 44-2, Moscow, Russia
e-mail: sopin_es@rudn.university

J. Pilz et al. (eds.), *Statistics and Simulation*, Springer Proceedings in Mathematics & Statistics 231, https://doi.org/10.1007/978-3-319-76035-3_27

process that describes their behavior has to keep track of the amount of resources occupied by each customer. This differs occupy-and-release systems from classical supply-and-demand inventories [1, 2] and significantly complicates the stochastic processes describing its behavior.

In [3], a simplification for the occupy-and-release queueing systems with general arrival and service processes has been proposed. Instead of tracking the amount of resources occupied by each customer, the simplified model considers only the number of customers and the total amount of occupied resources. Simplified system functions similarly to the original, except that the amounts of resources, released at the end of the service, may be different from those which have been occupied at the beginning of the service. Amount of resources released at the customer departure is random and has specially selected probability distribution.

First results obtained by simulations indicated that the stationary characteristics of the original and simplified models are very close to each other [3, 4]. So, the study was carried out to obtain the characteristics of the simplified systems in analytical form and compare it with the results for the initial systems. Multi-server queueing system with Poisson arrival process, exponential service times, and random requirements was studied in [5]. In [6], the expressions for the stationary probability distribution have been obtained for the simplified version of the system. It was established that the simplification of the said systems offers exact results for stationary distribution of the total amount of occupied resources. It follows from results on multi-server loss system with random requirements and generally distributed service times that stationary joint distribution of the number of customers and the amount of occupied resources is independent of the service time distribution function, but only on its first moment [7, 8]. In [9], it was proved also for the simplified system.

In this chapter, we study stationary joint distribution of the number of customers and the amount of occupied resources in the simplified multi-server loss system with general service-time and multi-item resource requirements. This work is an extension of the development in [6, 9].

27.2 Original Queueing System M/M/N with Random Requirements

Consider a multi-server queuing system with $N \leq \infty$ servers and $M \leq \infty$ types of resources. Arrival process is Poisson with the rate λ. The service times are independent of each other, independent of the arrival process, and exponentially distributed with the rate μ (Fig. 27.1).

The system operates as follows.

1. Each customer requires a certain amount of resources of several types.
2. If upon the arrival of a customer, the remaining free resources are insufficient to serve it, and the customer is considered lost.
3. As soon as the service of a customer begins, the total amount of occupied resources is increased by the amount of resources allocated to this customer.

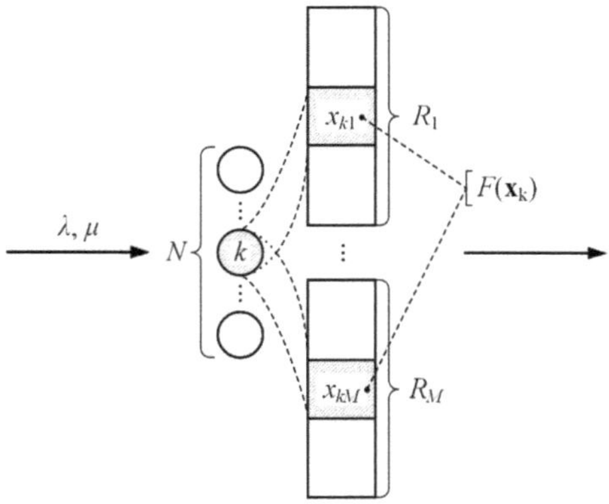

Fig. 27.1 N-server queuing system with losses with total amount of resources given by the vector **R**

4. Upon the departure of a customer, the total amount of occupied resources is decreased by the amount of resources allocated to this customer.

Denote by $\mathbf{R} = (R_1, \ldots, R_M)$ the total amount of resources and by $\mathbf{r}_j$ the amount of resources required for customer j. We assume that the random vectors $\mathbf{r}_j$ are independent of the arrival and service processes, mutually independent, and identically distributed with a cumulative distribution function (CDF) $F(\mathbf{x})$.

The system state at the time instant t can be described by a semi-Markov process $X(t) = (\xi(t), \boldsymbol{\gamma}(t))$ [10], where $\xi(t)$ is the number of customers in the system, and $\boldsymbol{\gamma}(t) = (\boldsymbol{\gamma}_1(t), \boldsymbol{\gamma}_2(t), \ldots, \boldsymbol{\gamma}_{\xi(t)}(t))$, where $\boldsymbol{\gamma}_i(t)$ is the vector of resources occupied by ith customer. Customers at service are assigned a number according to their residual service time in the decreasing order; that is, a customer with the longest residual service time is assigned the number 1. Upon the arrival of a new customer, all the customers are renumbered.

The process $X(t)$ is the jump process with transitions at time instants t_i of arrivals and departures. Consider an interval (t_{i-1}, t_i), when it is in a state $X(t) = (k, \mathbf{c}_1, \ldots, \mathbf{c}_k)$. The length of this interval is exponentially distributed with parameter $\lambda + k\mu$. At the end of this interval, with probability $\frac{\lambda}{\lambda+k\mu}$, new customer arrives, and with probability $\frac{k\mu}{\lambda+k\mu}$, a customer leaves the system. Hence, if t_i is a departure time, then at this instant the random process $X(t)$ jumps from the state $(k, \mathbf{c}_1, \ldots, \mathbf{c}_k)$ to the state $(k-1, \mathbf{c}_1, \ldots, \mathbf{c}_{k-1})$.

If t_i is the arrival time, then the process $X(t)$ can move to several different states. Let us denote $\mathbf{c}$ as the amount of resources required by the customer arriving at the time t_i and $\mathbf{d}$ as the total amount of occupied resources just before customer's arriving at time t_i, i.e., $\mathbf{d} = \mathbf{c}_1 + \mathbf{c}_2 + \cdots + \mathbf{c}_k$. Since residual service times and service time of arriving customer are independent and equally distributed arriving customer can get any of $k+1$ internal numbers. If upon arrival there are less than N customers in the system and $\mathbf{c} + \mathbf{d} \leq \mathbf{R}$, then a customer is accepted and the process $X(t)$ with equal probabilities will jump from the state $(k, \mathbf{c}_1, \mathbf{c}_2, \ldots, \mathbf{c}_k)$ to one of the state $(k+1, \mathbf{c}, \mathbf{c}_1, \mathbf{c}_2, \ldots, \mathbf{c}_k)$, $(k+1, \mathbf{c}_1, \mathbf{c}, \mathbf{c}_2, \ldots, \mathbf{c}_k)$, $(k+1, \mathbf{c}_1, \mathbf{c}_2, \ldots, \mathbf{c}_k, \mathbf{c})$. Otherwise state of the process $X(t)$ at time t_i does not changes.

Consider the stationary probability distribution of the process $X(t)$,

$$p_0 = \lim_{t\to\infty} P\{\xi(t) = 0\},$$

$$P_k(\mathbf{x}_1, \mathbf{x}_2, \dots, \mathbf{x}_k) = \lim_{t\to\infty} P\{\xi(t) = k; \boldsymbol{\gamma}_1(t) \le \mathbf{x}_1, \boldsymbol{\gamma}_2(t) \le \mathbf{x}_2, \dots, \boldsymbol{\gamma}_k(t) \le \mathbf{x}_k\}.$$

The above state transitions for our system unambiguously define the transition kernel of the process $X(t)$ [10] and lead to the system of equations for the stationary distribution:

$$\lambda F(\mathbf{R}) p_0 = \mu P_1(\mathbf{R}); \tag{27.1}$$

$$\lambda \int\limits_{\mathbf{0}\le \mathbf{y}_1 \le \mathbf{x}_1} F(\mathbf{R} - \mathbf{y}_1) P_1(d\mathbf{y}_1) + \mu P_1(\mathbf{x}_1) = \lambda F(\mathbf{x}_1) p_0 +$$
$$+2\mu \int\limits_{\substack{\mathbf{0}\le \mathbf{y}_1 \le \mathbf{x}_1 \\ \mathbf{0}\le \mathbf{y}_2 \le \mathbf{R} - \mathbf{y}_1}} P_2(d\mathbf{y}_1, d\mathbf{y}_2), \mathbf{0} \le \mathbf{x}_1 \le \mathbf{R}; \tag{27.2}$$

$$\lambda \int\limits_{\substack{\mathbf{0}\le \mathbf{y}_i \le \mathbf{x}_i, i=1,2,\dots,k \\ \mathbf{y}_1 + \dots + \mathbf{y}_k \le \mathbf{R}}} F(\mathbf{R} - \mathbf{y}_1 - \mathbf{y}_2 - \dots - \mathbf{y}_k) P_k(d\mathbf{y}_1, d\mathbf{y}_2, \dots, d\mathbf{y}_k) +$$
$$+ k\mu P_k(\mathbf{x}_1, \mathbf{x}_2, \dots, \mathbf{x}_k) = \frac{\lambda}{k} \sum_{i=1}^{k} P_{k-1}(\mathbf{x}_1, \dots, \mathbf{x}_{i-1}, \mathbf{x}_{i+1}, \dots, \mathbf{x}_k) F(\mathbf{x}_i) +$$
$$+ (k+1)\mu \int\limits_{\substack{\mathbf{0}\le \mathbf{y}_i \le \mathbf{x}_i, i=1,2,\dots,k \\ \mathbf{0}\le \mathbf{y}_{k+1} \le \mathbf{R} - \mathbf{y}_1 - \dots - \mathbf{y}_k}} P_{k+1}(d\mathbf{y}_1, \dots, d\mathbf{y}_k, d\mathbf{y}_{k+1}), \mathbf{x}_1, \mathbf{x}_2, \dots, \mathbf{x}_k \ge \mathbf{0},$$
$$\sum\nolimits_{i=1}^{k} \mathbf{x}_i \le \mathbf{R}, 1 < k < N; \tag{27.3}$$

$$N\mu P_N(\mathbf{x}_1, \mathbf{x}_2, \dots, \mathbf{x}_N) = \frac{\lambda}{N} \sum_{i=1}^{N} P_{N-1}(\mathbf{x}_1, \dots, \mathbf{x}_{i-1}, \mathbf{x}_{i+1}, \dots, \mathbf{x}_N) F(\mathbf{x}_i),$$
$$\mathbf{x}_1, \mathbf{x}_2, \dots, \mathbf{x}_N \ge \mathbf{0}, \quad \sum\nolimits_{i=1}^{N} \mathbf{x}_i \le \mathbf{R}. \tag{27.4}$$

It can be easily verified by substitution that solution to the system of Eqs. (27.1)–(27.4) with a normalization condition

$$p_0 + \sum_{k=1}^{N} \int\limits_{\substack{\mathbf{x}_1, \mathbf{x}_2, \dots, \mathbf{x}_k \ge \mathbf{0} \\ \mathbf{x}_1 + \mathbf{x}_2 + \dots + \mathbf{x}_k \le \mathbf{R}}} P_k(d\mathbf{x}_1, d\mathbf{x}_2, \dots, d\mathbf{x}_k) = 1,$$

can be written as

$$p_0 = \left(1 + \sum_{k=1}^{N} F^{(k)}(\mathbf{R})\frac{\rho^k}{k!}\right)^{-1}, \tag{27.5}$$

$$P_k(\mathbf{x}_1, \mathbf{x}_2, \ldots, \mathbf{x}_k) = p_0 F(\mathbf{x}_1) F(\mathbf{x}_2) \ldots F(\mathbf{x}_k)\frac{\rho^k}{k!}, \tag{27.6}$$
$$\mathbf{x}_1, \mathbf{x}_2, \ldots, \mathbf{x}_k \geq \mathbf{0}, \sum_{i=1}^{k} \mathbf{x}_i \leq \mathbf{R}, 1 \leq k \leq N.$$

Here, $\rho = \lambda/\mu$, and $F^{(k)}(\mathbf{x})$ is the k-fold convolution of the CDF $F(\mathbf{x})$.

Let $\boldsymbol{\delta}(t) = \sum_{i=1}^{\xi(t)} \boldsymbol{\gamma}_i(t)$ be the vector of total amount of resources occupied at time t. It follows from (27.6) the following expression for the stationary distribution of the process $Y(t) = (\xi(t); \boldsymbol{\delta}(t))$,

$$Q_k(\mathbf{x}) = \lim_{t\to\infty} P\{\xi(t) = k; \boldsymbol{\delta}(t) \leq \mathbf{x}\} = p_0 F^{(k)}(\mathbf{x})\frac{\rho^k}{k!}, \mathbf{0} \leq \mathbf{x} \leq \mathbf{R}, 1 \leq k \leq N. \tag{27.7}$$

Therefore, blocking probability can be calculated by

$$B = 1 - p_0 \sum_{k=0}^{N-1} F^{(k+1)}(\mathbf{R})\frac{\rho^k}{k!}, \tag{27.8}$$

and the vector of the mean volume of occupied resources is given by

$$b = p_0 \sum_{k=1}^{N} b_k \frac{\rho^k}{k!}, \quad b_k = \int\limits_{\mathbf{0}\leq\mathbf{x}\leq\mathbf{R}} x F^{(k)}(d\mathbf{x}). \tag{27.9}$$

There are two important particular cases, namely continuous and discrete. If the CDF $F(\mathbf{x})$ has the probability density function (PDF) $f(\mathbf{x})$, then the CDF $F^{(k)}(\mathbf{x})$ also has the PDF $f^{(k)}(\mathbf{x})$, and therefore, there exist PDF $p_k(\mathbf{x}_1, \mathbf{x}_2, \ldots, \mathbf{x}_k)$ and PDF $q_k(\mathbf{x})$ of stationary distributions $P_k(\mathbf{x}_1, \mathbf{x}_2, \ldots, \mathbf{x}_k)$ and $Q_k(\mathbf{x})$.

Let resources required by a customer be discrete random vectors with probability distribution $\pi(\mathbf{x})$ and values from the set $\mathrm{Z} = \{\mathbf{z}_1, \mathbf{z}_2, \ldots, \mathbf{z}_K\}$, i.e.,

$$\pi(\mathbf{x}) = \begin{cases} \pi_i, & \mathbf{x} = \mathbf{z}_i, \\ 0, & \mathbf{x} \notin \mathrm{Z}. \end{cases} \tag{27.10}$$

Then, k-fold convolution of $\pi(\mathbf{x})$ is given by

$$\pi^{(k)}(\mathbf{x}) = \sum_{\substack{n_1, \ldots, n_K \in \mathrm{N} \\ n_1 + \cdots + n_K = k \\ n_1\mathbf{z}_1 + \cdots + n_K\mathbf{z}_K = \mathbf{x}}} \prod_{i=1}^{K} \pi_i^{n_i}, \tag{27.11}$$

where N is the set of integers.

27.3 Simplified Queueing System M/M/N with Random Requirements

Generally speaking, the process $Y(t) = (\xi(t), \boldsymbol{\delta}(t))$ is not Markov process, because at the departure time resources occupied by the customer should be released in amounts equal to the amount of resources occupied upon arrival. The simplified system is similar to the original system in all aspects, except for the rule 4 stated previously. The release of the occupied resources upon a customer departure follows next rule.

4*. At departure time t_i, the vector of occupied resources is decreased by a random vector $\boldsymbol{\nu}_i$. Given the number of customers k and the amount of occupied resources $\mathbf{y}$, the random vector $\boldsymbol{\nu}_i$ is independent of the previous system behavior and has the CDF $F_k(\mathbf{x}|\mathbf{y})$ given by

$$F_k(\mathbf{x}|\mathbf{y}) = P(\mathbf{r}_k \leq \mathbf{x}|\mathbf{r}_1 + \mathbf{r}_2 + \ldots + \mathbf{r}_k = \mathbf{y}).$$

Here, $\mathbf{r}_i$, $i = 1, 2, \ldots$, are mutually independent random vectors with CDF $F(\mathbf{x})$. Note that in the case of the fixed amount of the required resources, i.e., when $\mathbf{r}_i = \mathbf{c}$ are the same constant vector for all $i = 1, 2, \ldots$, the simplified model is identical to the original one.

Note that $F_1(\mathbf{x}|\mathbf{y})$ is CDF of constant vector $\mathbf{y}$ and for $k > 1$ conditional probability $F_k(\mathbf{x}|\mathbf{y})$ is a solution of Eq. (27.12), in which left and right sides are equal to the probability $P\{\mathbf{r}_1 + \ldots + \mathbf{r}_{k-1} \leq \mathbf{x}, \mathbf{r}_1 + \ldots + \mathbf{r}_k \leq \mathbf{R}\}$:

$$\int\limits_{\substack{\mathbf{0} \leq \mathbf{z} \leq \mathbf{y} \leq \mathbf{R} \\ \mathbf{y} - \mathbf{z} \leq \mathbf{x}}} F_k(d\mathbf{z}|\mathbf{y}) F^{(k)}(d\mathbf{y}) = \int\limits_{\mathbf{0} \leq \mathbf{y} \leq \mathbf{x}} F(\mathbf{R} - \mathbf{y}) F^{(k-1)}(d\mathbf{y}), \mathbf{0} \leq \mathbf{x} \leq \mathbf{R}. \tag{27.12}$$

Let $\xi^*(t)$ be the number of customers and $\boldsymbol{\delta}^*(t)$ be the vector of occupied resources in the simplified system. Process $Y^*(t) = (\xi^*(t), \boldsymbol{\delta}^*(t))$ is semi-Markov process [10], and its stationary distribution

$$q_0^* = \lim_{t\to\infty} P\{\xi^*(t) = 0\}, \quad Q_k^*(x) = \lim_{t\to\infty} P\{\xi^*(t) = k; \boldsymbol{\delta}^*(t) \leq \mathbf{x}\}, 1 \leq k \leq N,$$

satisfies the following equilibrium equations:

$$\lambda F(\mathbf{R}) q_0^* = \mu Q_1^*(\mathbf{R}); \tag{27.13}$$

$$\lambda \int\limits_{\mathbf{0} \leq \mathbf{y} \leq \mathbf{x}} F(\mathbf{R} - \mathbf{y}) Q_1^*(d\mathbf{y}) + \mu Q_1^*(\mathbf{x}) = \lambda F(\mathbf{x}) q_0^* +$$
$$+2\mu \int\limits_{\substack{\mathbf{0} \leq \mathbf{z} \leq \mathbf{y} \leq \mathbf{R} \\ \mathbf{y} - \mathbf{z} \leq \mathbf{x}}} (F_2(d\mathbf{z}|\mathbf{y}) Q_2^*(d\mathbf{y})), \quad \mathbf{0} \leq \mathbf{x} \leq \mathbf{R}; \tag{27.14}$$

$$\lambda \int\limits_{0 \le \mathbf{y} \le \mathbf{x}} F(\mathbf{R}-\mathbf{y})Q_k^*(d\mathbf{y}) + k\mu Q_k^*(\mathbf{x}) = \lambda \int\limits_{0 \le \mathbf{y} \le \mathbf{x}} F(\mathbf{x}-\mathbf{y})Q_{k-1}^*(d\mathbf{y}) +$$
$$+(k+1)\mu \int\limits_{\substack{\mathbf{0} \le \mathbf{z} \le \mathbf{y} \le \mathbf{R} \\ \mathbf{y}-\mathbf{z} \le \mathbf{x}}} F_{k+1}(d\mathbf{z}|\mathbf{y})Q_{k+1}^*(d\mathbf{y})), \quad \mathbf{0} \le \mathbf{x} \le \mathbf{R}, 1 < k < N; \tag{27.15}$$

$$\lambda \int\limits_{0 \le \mathbf{y} \le \mathbf{x}} F(\mathbf{R}-\mathbf{y})Q_N^*(d\mathbf{y}) = \lambda \int\limits_{0 \le \mathbf{y} \le \mathbf{x}} F(\mathbf{x}-\mathbf{y})Q_{N-1}^*(d\mathbf{y}), \mathbf{0} \le \mathbf{x} \le \mathbf{R}. \tag{27.16}$$

By substituting $q_0^* = p_0$ and $Q_k^*(\mathbf{x}) = Q_k(\mathbf{x})$, given by (27.5) and (27.7), and using equality (27.12), it easy to check that p_0 and $Q_k(\mathbf{x})$ are solutions of Eqs. (27.13)–(27.16). In other words, stationary distributions of total amount of occupied resources in the original and simplified systems are the same.

27.4 Insensitivity Property of the Simplified Queueing System

Now, we consider simplified queueing system with general CDF $B(x)$ of the service times with finite mean and show that formulas (27.5) and (27.7) still valid. We follow the idea of the proof in [11] and show that the joint stationary distribution of the number of customers and the amount of occupied resources in simplified system depends on the service time distribution only through its mean. Behavior of the system can be described by Markov process $(\xi(t), \boldsymbol{\delta}(t), \boldsymbol{\beta}(t))$, where $\boldsymbol{\beta}(t) = \big(\beta_1(t), \beta_2(t), \ldots, \beta_{\xi(t)}(t)\big)$ is vector of elapsed service times of each customer. Let us denote P_t probability distribution at time t and P_0 initial distribution at $t = 0$. Assume that distribution P_0 is symmetric on subspace $\{\xi(t) = k, \boldsymbol{\delta}(t) \le \mathbf{x}\}$ about variables $\tau_1, \tau_2, \ldots \tau_k$, then P_t is also symmetric on $\{\xi(t) = k, \boldsymbol{\delta}(t) \le \mathbf{x}\}$.

Lemma. For any distribution P_0, distribution P_t has k-dimensional PDF $Q_k(\mathbf{x}, \tau_1, ..., \tau_k; t)$ at $(\xi(t) = k, \boldsymbol{\delta}(t) < \mathbf{x}, \tau_1, \tau_2, \ldots \tau_k; t)$ if $t > \max(\tau_1, \tau_2, \ldots \tau_k)$, and

$$Q_k(\mathbf{x}, \tau_1, \tau_2, \ldots \tau_k; t) \le \lambda^k F^{(k)}(\mathbf{x}) \prod_{i=1}^{k} [1 - B(\tau_i)], \quad 1 \le k \le N. \tag{27.17}$$

Proof Following inequalities hold true

$$P\{\xi(t) = k, \boldsymbol{\delta}(t) < \mathbf{x}, \tau_i < \beta_i(t) < \tau_i + \Delta_i, 1 \le i \le k\} = P(A) \le$$
$$\le F^{(k)}(\mathbf{x}) \prod_{i=1}^{k} [1 - B(\tau_i)][1 - e^{-\lambda\Delta_i}] \le \lambda^k F^{(k)}(\mathbf{x}) \prod_{i=1}^{k} [1 - B(\tau_i)]\Delta_i,$$

since $1 - e^{-\lambda\Delta_i} \le \lambda\Delta_i$, and for occurrence of the event A, customers have to arrive at time intervals $(t - (\tau_i + \Delta_i), t - \tau_i)$, $i = 1, 2, \ldots, k$, with service times at least τ_i, $i = 1, 2, \ldots, k$, and total amount of occupied resources by arrived customers does not exceed $\mathbf{x}$. Thus, PDF existence and inequality (27.17) are proved. □

Transition probabilities in time interval Δt have the following form:

$$Q_0(\mathbf{0}; t + \Delta t) = Q_0(\mathbf{0}; t)(1 - \lambda F(\mathbf{R})\Delta t) + \int_{\mathbf{0}}^{\mathbf{R}} \int_0^{\infty} Q_1(d\mathbf{x}, \tau_1; t) \frac{B(\tau_1 + \Delta t) - B(\tau_1)}{1 - B(\tau_1)} d\tau_1 + o(\Delta t); \tag{27.18}$$

$$Q_k(\mathbf{x}, \tau_1, \ldots, \tau_k; t + \Delta t) = (k+1) \prod_{j=1}^{k} \frac{1 - B(\tau_j)}{1 - B(\tau_j - \Delta t)} \cdot \int_{\mathbf{x} \le \mathbf{y} \le \mathbf{R}} (1 - F_k(\mathbf{y} - \mathbf{x}|\mathbf{y})) \int_0^{\infty} \left[Q_{k+1}(d\mathbf{y}, \tau_1 - \Delta t, \ldots, \tau_k - \Delta t, \tau_{k+1}; t) \frac{B(\tau_{k+1} + \Delta t) - B(\tau_{k+1})}{1 - B(\tau_{k+1})} \right] d\tau_{k+1} + \tag{27.19}$$

$$+ \int_{\mathbf{0} \le \mathbf{y} \le \mathbf{x}} Q_k(d\mathbf{y}, \tau_1 - \Delta t, \ldots, \tau_k - \Delta t; t)(1 - \lambda F(\mathbf{R} - \mathbf{y})\Delta t) \cdot \prod_{j=1}^{k} \frac{1 - B(\tau_j)}{1 - B(\tau_j - \Delta t)};$$

$$Q_N(\mathbf{x}, \tau_1, \ldots, \tau_k; t + \Delta t) = Q_N(\mathbf{x}, \tau_1 - \Delta t, \ldots, \tau_k - \Delta t; t) \prod_{j=1}^{N} \frac{1 - B(\tau_j)}{1 - B(\tau_j - \Delta t)}. \tag{27.20}$$

Let us denote $Q_k^*(\mathbf{x}, \tau_1, \tau_2, \ldots \tau_k; t) = \frac{Q_k(\mathbf{x}, \tau_1, \tau_2, \ldots \tau_k; t)}{[1 - B(\tau_1)][1 - B(\tau_2)] \ldots [1 - B(\tau_k)]}$. Assume existence of partial derivatives $\frac{\partial Q_k^*}{\partial t}$, $\frac{\partial Q_k^*}{\partial \tau_i}$, $1 \le i \le k$, $0 \le k \le N$, then using (27.18)–(27.20) we obtain following differential equations:

$$\frac{\partial Q_0^*(\mathbf{0})}{\partial t} + \lambda Q_0^*(\mathbf{0}) F(\mathbf{R}) = \int_{\mathbf{0} \le \mathbf{x} \le \mathbf{R}} \int_0^{\infty} Q_1^*(d\mathbf{x}, \tau_1; t) dB(\tau_1), \tag{27.21}$$

$$\frac{\partial Q_k^*(\mathbf{x})}{\partial t} + \frac{\partial Q_k^*(\mathbf{x})}{\partial \tau_1} + \ldots + \frac{\partial Q_k^*(\mathbf{x})}{\partial \tau_k} + \lambda \int_{\mathbf{0} \le \mathbf{y} \le \mathbf{x}} Q_k^*(d\mathbf{y}, \tau_1, \ldots, \tau_k; t) F(\mathbf{R} - \mathbf{y}) =$$

$$= (k+1) \int_{\mathbf{x} \le \mathbf{y} \le \mathbf{R}} (1 - F_k(\mathbf{y} - \mathbf{x}|\mathbf{y})) \int_0^{\infty} Q_{k+1}^*(d\mathbf{y}, \tau_1, \ldots, \tau_{k+1}; t) dB(\tau_{k+1}), \tag{27.22}$$

$$\frac{\partial Q_N^*(\mathbf{x})}{\partial t} + \frac{\partial Q_N^*(\mathbf{x})}{\partial \tau_1} + \ldots + \frac{\partial Q_N^*(\mathbf{x})}{\partial \tau_k} = 0, \tag{27.23}$$

with boundary condition

$$\lambda \int\limits_{\mathbf{0}\le\mathbf{y}\le\mathbf{x}} F(\mathbf{x}-\mathbf{y})Q_k^*(d\mathbf{y},\tau_1,\tau_2,\dots,\tau_k;t) = (k+1)Q_{k+1}^*(\mathbf{x},\tau_1,\dots,\tau_k,0;t),$$
$$0 \le k \le N-1. \tag{27.24}$$

We can make sure by substitution that stationary solution of system of Eqs. (27.21)–(27.23) with boundary condition (27.24) is

$$Q_k^*(\mathbf{x},\tau_1,\tau_2,\dots,\tau_k) = Q_0^*(\mathbf{0})\frac{\lambda^k}{k!}F^{(k)}(\mathbf{x}), \tag{27.25}$$

$$Q_0^*(\mathbf{0}) = \left(1+\sum_{k=1}^{N}\frac{\lambda^k}{k!}F^{(k)}(\mathbf{R})\right)^{-1}. \tag{27.26}$$

Thus, we proved the following theorem.

Theorem 1 *If service time distribution with CDF $B(x)$ have finite mean $b > 0$, then stationary probability distribution of random process $(\xi(t),\ \boldsymbol{\delta}(t),\ \boldsymbol{\beta}(t))$ is given by*

$$Q_k(\mathbf{x},\tau_1,\tau_2,\dots,\tau_k) = \lim_{t\to\infty} P\{\xi(t)=k;\ \boldsymbol{\delta}(t)\le\mathbf{x};\ \beta_1(t)<\tau_1,\dots,\ \beta_k(t)<\tau_k\} =$$
$$= q_0 F^{(k)}(\mathbf{x})\frac{\rho^k}{k!}[1-B(\tau_1)]\dots[1-B(\tau_k)],\quad \mathbf{0}\le\mathbf{x}\le\mathbf{R},\ 0<k\le N,$$

where $\rho = \lambda b$ and q_0 is given by formula (27.26).

In particular, it follows that stationary probability distribution of random process $(\xi(t), \delta(t))$ is also determined by formulas (27.5) and (27.7) as in case of exponential service time distribution. Hence, it is insensitive to service-time CDF.

27.5 Conclusion

Method of simplification was proposed as an easy to use approximate method and its scope is not clear yet. In this chapter, we presented results on the stationary distribution of the multi-server loss system with generally distributed service times and multi-item resource requirements. It was proved that stationary joint distribution of the number of customers and the amount of occupied resources depends on the service time distribution only through its mean. It would be interesting to analyze applicability of the simplification method to the analysis of complex queueing systems with random requirements.

Acknowledgements The reported study was supported by the Russian Science Foundation, research project No. 16-11-10227. We thank Prof. Valeriy Naumov for the methodic assistance and scientific guidance in the preparation of this chapter, as well as for the constant and invaluable attention to our scientific work.

References

1. Prabhu, N.U.: Queues and Inventories: A Study of their Basic Stochastic Processes. Wiley, New York (1965)
2. Afanas'eva, L.G., Bulinskaya, E.V.: Stochastic Processes in the Theory of Queues and Inventory Control. Moscow State University, Moscow (1980)
3. Naumov, V.A., Samouylov, K.E.: On the modeling of queuing systems with multiple resources. Bull. Peoples Friendsh. Univ. Rus. Math. Inf. Sci. Phys. **1**(3), 58–62 (2014)
4. Naumov, V., Samuoylov, K., Sopin, E., Andreev, S.: Two approaches to analysis of queuing systems with limited resources. In: Proceedings of 7th international congress on ultra modern telecommunications and control systems and workshops, 585–588 (2014)
5. Romm, E.L., Skitovich, V.V.: On certain generalization of problem of erlang. Autom. Remote Control **32**(6), 1000–1003 (1971)
6. Naumov, V., Samuoylov, K., Sopin, E., Yarkina, N., Andreev, S., Samuylov, A.: LTE performance analysis using queuing systems with finite resources and random requirements. In: Proceedings of 8th international congress on ultra modern telecommunications and control systems and workshops, 100–103 (2015)
7. Tikhonenko, O.M., Klimovich, K.G.: Analysis of queuing systems for random-length arrivals with limited cumulative volume. Probl. Inf. Transm. **37**(1), 77–79 (2001)
8. Tikhonenko, O.M.: Generalized erlang problem for service systems with finite total capacity. Probl. Inf. Transm. **41**(3), 77–79 (2005)
9. Naumov, V., Samuoylov, K., Sopin, E.: On the insensitivity of stationary characteristics to the service time distribution in queuing system with limited resources. In: Proceedings of 9th international workshop on applied problems in theory of probabilities and mathematical statistics, 36–40 (2015)
10. Korolyuk, V.S., Turbin, A.F.: Renewal processes in system reliability problems. Naukova Dumka, Kiev (1982)
11. Sevastyanov, B.A.: An ergodic theorem for markov processes and its application to telephone systems with refusals. Probab. Theory Appl. **2**(1), 106–116 (1957)

Chapter 28
On Sensitivity of Steady-State Probabilities of a Cold Redundant System to the Shapes of Life and Repair Time Distributions of Its Elements

Vladimir Rykov and Dmitry Kozyrev

Abstract The problem of sensitivity of a redundant system's reliability characteristics to shapes of their input distributions is considered. In Efrosinin and Rykov, Information Technologies and Mathematical Modelling, 2014, [1] an analytical form for dependence of a two-unit cold standby redundant system reliability characteristics on life and repair time input distributions was obtained and investigated for the case of exponential distribution of one of the time lengths. In the current chapter this study is extended with the help of simulation method to a general case of both non-exponential distributions. Comparison of analytic and simulation results was carried out.

Keywords System reliability · Steady state probabilities · Sensitivity Mathematical modeling and simulation · Redundant systems

28.1 Introduction

Stability of behavior of different systems and sensitivity of their characteristics to the changes in initial states or exterior factors are among the key problems in all natural sciences. For stochastic systems stability often means insensitivity or low sensitivity of their output characteristics to the shape of some input distributions. One of the

V. Rykov (✉) · D. Kozyrev
Peoples' Friendship University of Russia (RUDN University),
6 Miklukho-Maklaya St, Moscow, Russian Federation 117198
e-mail: vladimir_rykov@mail.ru

V. Rykov
Gubkin Russian State Oil and Gas University, Moscow, Russia

D. Kozyrev
V.A. Trapeznikov Institute of Control Sciences of Russian Academy of Sciences,
Moscow, Russia
e-mail: kozyrev_dv@rudn.university

J. Pilz et al. (eds.), *Statistics and Simulation*, Springer Proceedings
in Mathematics & Statistics 231, https://doi.org/10.1007/978-3-319-76035-3_28

earliest results concerning insensitivity of systems' characteristics to the shape of service time distribution has been obtained by B. Sevast'yanov [2], who proved the insensitivity of Erlang formulas to the shape of service time distribution with fixed mean value for loss queueing systems with Poisson input flow.

In [3] I. Kovalenko found the necessary and sufficient condition for insensitivity of stationary reliability characteristics of redundant restorable systems with exponential life time distribution and general repair time distribution to the shape of the latter. This condition consists in sufficient amount of repairing units, i.e. in possibility of immediate start of repair for any failed element. The sufficiency of this condition for the case of general life and repair time distributions has been found in [4] with the help of multi-dimensional alternative processes theory. However, in the case of limited possibilities for restoration these results do not hold, as it was shown, for example, in [5] with the help of additional variable method.

On the other hand, as it follows from investigations by B.V. Gnedenko and A.D. Solov'ev [6–8] under "quick" restoration the sensitivity of reliability characteristics to the shape of distributions of life and repair times of their elements will be vanishingly small. In papers [1, 9] the problem of sensitivity of system's steady state reliability characteristics to the shape of life and repair time distributions of its elements has been considered for the simple case of a cold double redundant system when one of the input distributions (either of life or repair time lengths) is exponential. For these models explicit expressions for both stationary and non-stationary probabilities have been obtained which show their evident dependence on the non-exponential distributions in the form of their Laplace–Stiltjes transforms. However the numerical investigations show that this dependence becomes vanishingly small under "quick" restoration.

In the chapter we extend these studies with the help of simulation method to a general case of cold double redundant system with general distributions of both life and repair time lengths of elements.

The chapter is organized as follows. In Sect. 28.2 we set the problem and introduce the notations. In Sect. 28.3 we work out the closed-form analytical expressions for the steady-state probabilities of a cold standby redundant system with one repair server in two major particular cases when one of the input distributions is non-exponential. These explicit formulas are used in subsequent section for numerical analysis. In the last section the general discrete-event simulation model is described by the means of the flowchart and the pseudocode with comments, the results of simulation modeling are presented and comparison of analytic and simulation results is carried out. The chapter ends with conclusion and some problems description.

28.2 Problem Set and Notations

Consider a cold standby restorable system with one repair unit and generally distributed life and repair time lengths. Throughout the chapter we will use a generalization of Kendall's notation [10] for queueing systems. In this notation the symbols

$\langle GI_n|GI|m\rangle$ stand for a closed system, i.e. a system where the flow of customers is generated by a finite number n of sources that is shown by index in the first position. Symbol GI means "General Independent" and in the first position of this notation it denotes the general distribution of independent life times of the elements of the system and in the second one — the general distribution of their independent repair times. These symbols can be substituted by M for exponential ($exp(\cdot)$), Erlang $E(\cdot,\cdot)$, Gnedenko-Weibull ($GW(\cdot,\cdot)$) with appropriate parameters or any other symbol describing the distribution of life and/or repair time. Finally, the last factor m denotes the number of repair units in the system. In the current chapter we consider a simple cold double redundant model, namely $\langle GI_2|GI|1\rangle$ and compare its steady state probabilities (SSP) under different distributions.

The cumulative distribution functions (CDF) of the random life time A and random repair time B are denoted respectively by $A(x)$ and $B(x)$. We suppose the existence of the corresponding probability density functions (PDF), which are denoted by $a(x) = A'(x)$ and $b(x) = B'(x)$. The mean time between failures, the mean service (repair) time, the failure and repair hazard functions are denoted as follows:

$$a = \int_0^\infty (1 - A(x))dx, \quad \text{and} \quad b = \int_0^\infty (1 - B(x))dx.$$

and

$$\alpha(x) = \frac{a(x)}{1 - A(x)}, \quad \text{and} \quad \beta(x) = \frac{b(x)}{1 - B(x)}.$$

Define also the moment-generating functions (m.g.f.) of life A and repair B times, the Laplace–Stiltjes transforms (LST) of their distributions by the following expressions:

$$\tilde{a}(s) = \int_0^\infty e^{-sx} a(x)dx \quad \text{and} \quad \tilde{b}(s) = \int_0^\infty e^{-sx} b(x)dx, \ Re[s] \geq 0.$$

In order to compare the simulation results with the numerical results obtained analytically, we first recall the analytical results for models $\langle M_2|GI|1\rangle$ and $\langle GI_2|M|1\rangle$ from [1, 9, 11].

28.3 Analytical Results for the Models $\langle M_2|GI|1\langle$ and $\langle GI_2|M|1\rangle$

28.3.1 Two-Unit Cold Standby $\langle M_2|GI|1\rangle$ System

Consider a two-unit cold standby redundant system $\langle M_2|GI|1\rangle$ with one repair server. The elements of the system (units) have exponentially distributed times to failure with parameter α and general repair time distribution $B(t)$. Denote by

$$\{Z(t)\}_{t\geq 0} = \{N(t),\ X(t)\}_{t\geq 0} \tag{28.1}$$

a two-dimensional stochastic process, where the first component $N(t)$ stands for the number of failed elements at time t and the second one stands for the elapsed repair time of the unit at time t. The process $\{Z(t)\}_{t\geq 0}$ is obviously Markovian one with the state space $E = \{0, (n, x) : n \in \{1, 2\},\ x \in \mathbb{R}_+\}$. Define the following state probability density functions (p.d.f'.s):

(1) $\pi_0(t) = \mathbf{P}\{N(t) = 0\}$ — the probability of a "good" (non-failure) state of both units at time t.
(2) $\pi_n(t; x)dx = \mathbf{P}\{N(t) = n;\ x < X(t) \leq x + dx\}$ — the joint probability that at time t there are n failed units and the elapsed repair time of the failed unit (that is being repaired) takes a value between x and $x + dx, n = 1, 2$.

By considering transitions of the process $\{Z(t)\}_{t\geq 0}$ between time t and $t + \Delta t$ and letting $\Delta t \to 0$, in [1, 9] the system of Kolmogorov forward partial differential equations for probability $\pi_0(t)$ and p.d.f'.s $\pi_n(t; x)$ in domain $n = 0, 1, 2$ and $x > 0$ has been obtained. Because the process $\{Z(t)\}_{t\geq 0}$ is a Harris one with a positive atom in zero state, the steady state probabilities

$$\pi_0 = \lim_{t\to\infty} \pi_)(t), \quad \pi_n(x) = \lim_{t\to\infty} \pi_n(t; x) \quad (n = 1, 2)$$

exist and satisfy to the appropriate system of ordinary differential equations (see also [1, 9]). Moreover, the closed form solution that has been obtained in these papers are presented in the theorem below, where $\rho = \frac{E[A]}{E[B]}$.

Theorem 28.1 *Steady state probabilities of the system $\langle M_2|GI|1\rangle$ are:*

$$\begin{aligned}
\pi_0 &= \frac{\rho\tilde{b}(\alpha)}{1 + \rho\tilde{b}(\alpha)}, \\
\pi_1(x) &= \frac{\rho\alpha}{1 + \rho\tilde{b}(\alpha)} e^{-\alpha x}(1 - B(x)), \\
\pi_2(x) &= \frac{\rho\alpha}{1 + \rho\tilde{b}(\alpha)} \left(1 - e^{-\alpha x}\right)(1 - B(x)).
\end{aligned}$$

The macro-state probabilities $\pi_0,\ \pi_n = \int \pi_i(x)dx\ (n = 1, 2)$ are obtained by integration.

Corollary 28.1 *Macro-state probabilities are:*

$$\pi_0 = \frac{\rho\tilde{b}(\alpha)}{1 + \rho\tilde{b}(\alpha)}, \quad \pi_1 = \frac{\rho(1 - \tilde{b}(\alpha))}{1 + \rho\tilde{b}(\alpha)}, \quad \pi_2 = \frac{1 - \rho(1 - \tilde{b}(\alpha))}{1 + \rho\tilde{b}(\alpha)}. \tag{28.2}$$

28.3.2 Two-Unit Cold Standby $\langle GI_2|M|1\rangle$ System

Consider now a similar system with generally distributed life time of the unit and exponentially distributed repair time. Denote by $\{Z(t)\}_{t\geq 0}$ the analogous stochastic process (28.1), where the first component is the same as before, and the second one denotes the elapsed operating time of the working unit. Define the state probabilities as follows:

(1) $\pi_n(t;\, x)dx = \mathbf{P}\{N(t) = n,\ x < X(t) \leq x + dx\}$ — the joint probability that at time t there are n failed units and the elapsed operating time of the functioning one takes a value between x and $x + dx, n = 0, 1$.
(2) $\pi_2(t) = \mathbf{P}\{N(t) = 2\}$ — the probability of the "bad" state (complete system failure state) at time t.

Also as before in [1, 9] a system of Kolmogorov forward partial differential equations for these probabilities in domain $n = 0, 1, 2$ and $x > 0$ together with boundary, normalizing and initial conditions has been found. Moreover, using Harris property of the process and the presence of a positive atom in state zero for the steady state probabilities appropriate system of usual differential equations has been done in these previous papers.

These equations admit an analytical solution, presented in the following Theorem 28.2, which after integration over variable x gives the solution for macro-state probabilities, given in Corollary 28.2.

Theorem 28.2 *Steady state probabilities of the system $\langle GI_2|M|1\rangle$ are:*

$$\pi_0(x) = \frac{\beta}{\rho + \tilde{a}(\beta)}(1 - e^{-\beta x})(1 - A(x)),$$
$$\pi_1(x) = \frac{\beta}{\rho + \tilde{a}(\beta)}e^{-\beta x}(1 - A(x)),$$
$$\pi_2 = \frac{\tilde{a}(\beta)}{\rho + \tilde{a}(\beta)}.$$

Corollary 28.2 *In steady-state mode the macro-state probabilities $\pi_n = \lim_{t\to\infty} \mathbf{P}\{N(t) = n\}$ are given by*

$$\pi_0 = \frac{\rho - (1 - \tilde{a}(\beta))}{\rho + \tilde{a}(\beta)}, \quad \pi_1 = \frac{1 - \tilde{a}(\beta)}{\rho + \tilde{a}(\beta)}, \quad \pi_2 = \frac{\tilde{a}(\beta)}{\rho + \tilde{a}(\beta)}. \tag{28.3}$$

28.4 Simulation Results

In this section we consider a two-unit cold standby restorable system $\langle GI_2|GI|1\rangle$ with one repair server and general distributions of both life and repair times. Define the states of the system as follows:

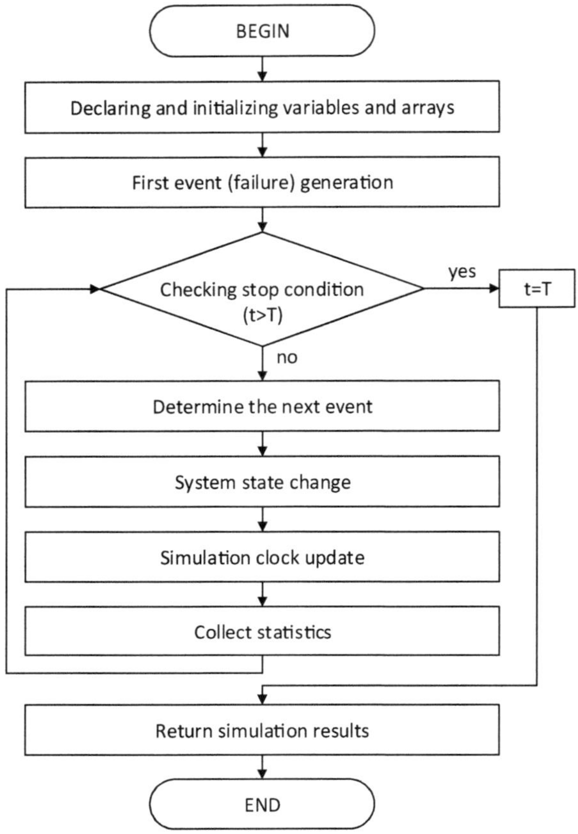

Fig. 28.1 Flowchart of the discrete-event simulation model

- state 0: one (main) unit is working, the other (duplicating) one is in reserve;
- state 1: one unit has failed and is being repaired, the other one is working;
- state 2: both units have failed (one is being repaired and the other one is waiting for his turn to be repaired).

28.4.1 General Simulation Model

We perform the simulation using the discrete event modeling method. We consider the functioning of the system being modeled as a sequence of operations being performed across entities (events). The simulation model is specified graphically as a process flowchart (see Fig. 28.1).

In order to ensure the precise understanding and reproducibility of the simulation model, we present an algorithm for a simulation process which is represented in the form of pseudocode (see Fig. 28.2). For those readers who are interested in reproducing the simulation results the source code of the simulation model is available free of charge upon request via e-mail: kozyrevdv@gmail.com.

In the algorithm according to ergodic theorem the estimates $\hat{\pi}_n$ of SSP π_n are calculated as

$$\hat{\pi}_n = \frac{\text{time spent by process in state } n \text{ during modeling time } T}{\text{modeling time } T}. \tag{28.4}$$

28.4.2 Comparison of Analytical Solution and Simulation Results for $\langle GI_2|GI|1\rangle$

In this section we show that under 'quick' restoration the steady-state probabilities become insensitive to the shape of distributions of life and repair time of system's elements. As a model parameter we consider the value $\rho = \frac{\mathbf{E}[A]}{\mathbf{E}[B]} = \frac{\text{restoration rate}}{\text{failure rate}}$, which can be interpreted as a relative rate of system recovery [12, 13]. It will be shown that as $\rho \to \infty$ the sensitivity of the model to shapes of input distributions becomes negligible. Distributions that we've used in our experiments include, but are not limited to the following ones: Exponential (Exp(α)), Erlang (E(k, α)), Gnedenko-Weibull (GW) and Pareto (P). The simulation time has been chosen equal to $T = 10000$.

Table 28.1 contains both the analytical and simulation values of the steady-state probability π_2 of system failure for different cases of life time CDF ($GI^{(1)}$) and repair time CDF ($GI^{(2)}$).

It can be seen from the table that the results of exact analytical calculation (where possible) and simulation results have close agreement. For illustrative purposes we

Table 28.1 System steady-state failure probability π_2 for the $\langle GI_2|GI|1\rangle$ model

$GI^{(1)}$	$GI^{(2)}$	$Exp(\frac{1}{EB})$		$E(\frac{2}{EB})$		$GW(\frac{2}{EB}, \frac{1}{2})$		$P\ (k, \frac{k}{(k-1)EB})$	
		Simul.	Theor.	Simul.	Theor.	Simul.	Theor.	Simul.	Theor.
$Exp(\frac{1}{EA})$	$\rho = 1$	0.33021	0.33333	0.30742	0.30769	0.39018	0.39602	0.26981	0.26985
	$\rho = 10$	0.00921	0.00901	0.00684	0.00698	0.01966	0.02036	0.00479	0.00486
	$\rho = 100$	0.00013	0.0001	0.00011	0.00007	0.00025	0.00029	0.00005	0.00005
$E(\frac{2}{EA})$	$\rho = 1$	0.30443	0.30769	0.27304	–	0.37735	–	0.21328	–
	$\rho = 10$	0.00256	0.00277	0.00149	–	0.01224	–	0.00062	–
	$\rho = 100$	0	0	0.00001	–	0.00001	–	0	–
$GW(\frac{2}{EA}, \frac{1}{2})$	$\rho = 1$	0.39613	0.39602	0.38346	–	0.42290	–	0.37061	–
	$\rho = 10$	0.03335	0.03037	0.03092	–	0.04222	–	0.02772	–
	$\rho = 100$	0.00195	0.00116	0.00157	–	0.00269	–	0.00140	–
$P\ (k, \frac{k}{(k-1)EA})$	$\rho = 1$	0.26532	0.26985	0.21292	–	0.35937	–	0.04505	–
	$\rho = 10$	0	0.00001	0	–	0.00487	–	0	–
	$\rho = 100$	0	0	0	–	0	–	0	–

```
Input: a, b, T, 'GI(1)', 'GI(2)'
a – mean life time of an element, b – mean repair time, T – maximum simulation time,
'GI(1,2)' denote CDFs of life and repair time lengths, respectively.
Output: steady state probabilities π0, π1, π2
begin
    double t := 0.0 ;            /* simulation clock initialization */
    int i := 0; j := 0 ;                  /* process state variables */
    double t_nextfail:= 0.0 ;    /* variable that holds time till next
    failure */
    double t_nextrepair:= 0.0 ;  /* variable that holds time till next
    end of repair */
    int k := 1 ;    /* counter of number of replications before T is
    reached */
    array r[] := [0,0,0] ;    /* declare a multidimensional array that
    holds results of the k-th step of the main loop */
    s := df_Exp(1/a) ;          /* generate a random real number s with
    exponential CDF which is a time until first event
    (failure) */
    t_nextfail := t + s;
    while t < T do
        if i = 0 then
            t_nextrepair := ∞;
            j := j + 1; t := t_nextfail;
        else if i = 1 then
            s1 := df_GI1(..) ;    /* generate a random time s1 with GI(1)
            CDF */
            s2 := df_GI2(..) ;    /* generate a random time s2 with GI(2)
            CDF */
            t_nextfail := t + s1; t_nextrepair := t + s2;
            if t_nextfail < t_nextrepair then
                j := j + 1; t := t_nextfail;
                else
                |  j := j − 1; t := t_nextrepair
                end
            end
        else
            i = 2; t_nextfail := ∞;
            j := j − 1; t := t_nextrepair;
        end
        if t > T then
        |  t := T
        end
        r[k] := [t, i, j];
        i := j; k := k + 1;
    end
    Evaluate duration of time spent in each state n, n = 0,1,2;
    Calculate estimates of steady state probabilities according to formula4.
end
```

Fig. 28.2 Pseudocode for the simulation process of $\langle GI_2|GI|1\rangle$ model

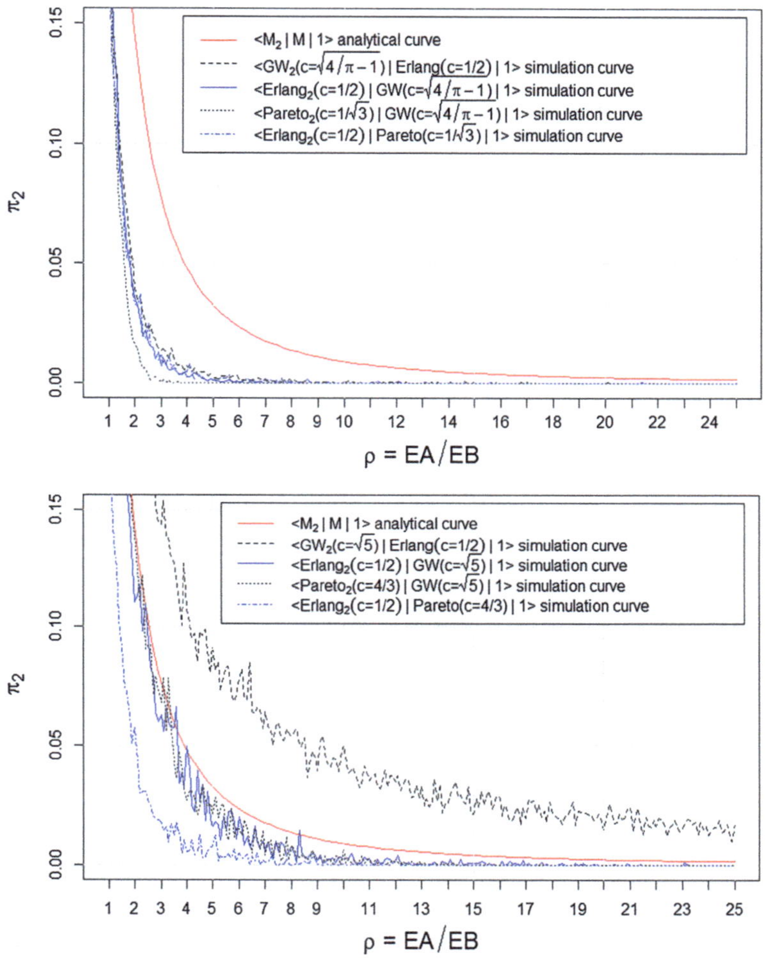

Fig. 28.3 Simulation values of π_2 versus ρ (averaged values based on 200 replications)

conduct this comparison graphically at Fig. 28.3, where results of simulation are represented for different distributions $GI^{(1)}$, $GI^{(2)}$ and different values of ρ. In all cases the parameters of distributions have been chosen so that the value of $\mathbf{E}[B]$ remained fixed ($\mathbf{E}[B] = 5$) and the mean time to failure of an element would ascend $\mathbf{E}[A] = \rho\mathbf{E}[B]$ according to the values of ρ which are indicated on the horizontal axis of both figures. Instead of parameters of distributions the coefficient of variation c (the ratio of the standard deviation to the mean) is indicated in parentheses in the legends of Fig. 28.3. All simulation plots of the upper figure have been built for the case of distributions with $c < 1$ (except for Erlang) and the lower figure contains plots for the case $c > 1$.

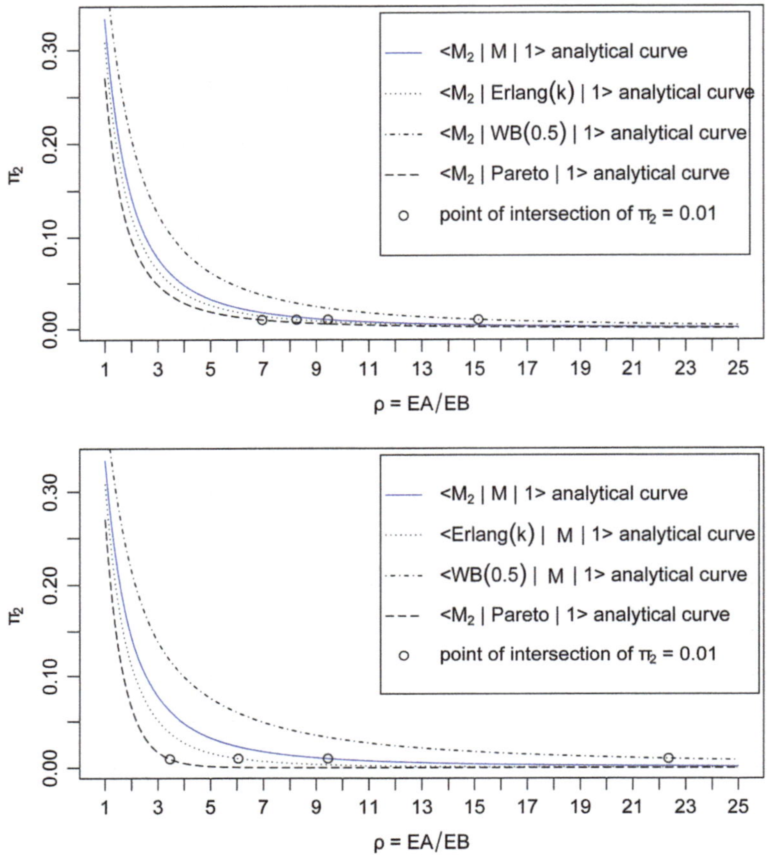

Fig. 28.4 Analytical values of π_2 versus ρ

Figure 28.3 depicts the plots of the steady-state probability π_2 of system failure versus the model parameter ρ for 5 different special cases of the $\langle GI_2|GI|1\rangle$ model. As it can be seen from the figure, the differences between both simulation and analytical curves become indistinguishable very quickly. Even at relatively small values of ρ the probability of system failure π_2 is already very close to zero for all cases. The observed behavior is fairly expected, as it was proved by B.V. Gnedenko and A.D. Solov'ev [7, 8]. What is more important and interesting — is that we can assess the rate of convergence of π_2 with the means of quantiles for the given probability level. For this reason we've plotted the analytical curves of the steady-state probability π_2 of system failure versus the model parameter ρ for all considered particular cases (see Fig. 28.4).

The upper of the two figures of Fig. 28.4 represents the analytical results of calculation of π_2 for models with different (see the legend) distributions of repair time and with exponentially distributed life time of system's elements. The displayed results show very good asymptotic insensitivity of the probability of system failure π_2 under $\rho \to \infty$ to the shapes of repair time distributions.

The lower figure represents analogous results, where analytical curves of π_2 are drawn for models with exponentially distributed repair time and non-exponential life time distributions of system's elements. The displayed results also show very good asymptotic insensitivity of the probability of system failure, what can be clearly seen from the proximity of the corresponding curves. For instance near $\rho = 20$ all the curves are almost indistinguishable.

The represented above results of experiments show that the sensitivity of the steady-state probabilities of the model gets vanishingly small as ρ increases.

28.5 Conclusion

The sensitivity problem of the steady-state probabilities of a cold standby redundant system $\langle GI_2|GI|1\rangle$ to the shape of distributions of life and repair times of its elements is considered. In spite of the fact that the obtained closed-form expressions for these probabilities show evident dependence of these probabilities on the shape of input distributions, the simulation experiments prove that this sensitivity becomes negligible under "quick" recovery. Nevertheless, as may be inferred from Fig. 28.4, the same given probability level ($\pi_2 = 0.01$) for different distributions is reached at quite different values of ρ.

Acknowledgements The publication was prepared with the support of the "RUDN University Program 5-100", and was financially supported by the Russian Foundation for Basic Research according to the research projects No. 17-07-00142 and No. 17-01-00633.

References

1. Efrosinin, D., Rykov, V.: Sensitivity analysis of reliability characteristics to the shape of the life and repair time distributions. In: Dudin, A., Nazarov, A., Yakupov, R., Gortsev, A. (eds.) Information Technologies and Mathematical Modelling. (Proceedings of 13th International Scientific Conference ITMM 2014 named after A.F. Terpugov, Anzhero-Sudzhensk, Russia, 20–22 Nov 2014.) Communication in Computer and Information Science, vol. 487, pp. 101–112
2. Sevast'yanov, B.A.: An ergodic theorem for Markov processes and its application to telephone systems with refusals. Theory Prob. Appl. **2**(1), 104 (1957)
3. Kovalenko, I.N.: Investigations on Analysis of Complex Systems Reliability. Kiev, Naukova Dumka (1976) 210 p. (In Russian)
4. Rykov, V.: Multidimensional alternative processes as reliability models. In: Dudin, A., Klimenok, V., Tsarenkov, G., Dudin, S. (eds.) Modern Probabilistic Methods for Analysis of Telecommunication Networks. (BWWQT 2013) Proceedings. Series: CCIS 356, p. 147-157. Springer (2013)
5. Koenig, D., Rykov, V., Schtoyn, D.: Queueing Theory. - M.: Gubkin University Press (1979), 115 p. (In Russian)

6. Gnedenko, B.V.: On cold double redundant system. Izv. AN SSSR. Texn. Cybern. **4**, 312 (1964). (In Russian)
7. Gnedenko, B.V.: On cold double redundant system with restoration. Izv. AN SSSR. Texn. Cybern. **5**, 111118 (1964). (In Russian)
8. Solov'ev, A.D.: On reservation with quick restoration. Izv. AN SSSR. Texn. Cybern. **1**, 5671 (1970). (In Russian)
9. Rykov, V., Ngia, T.A.: On sensitivity of systems reliability characteristics to the shape of their elements life and repair time distributions. Vestnik PFUR. Ser. Math. Inf. Phys. **3**, 65–77 (2014). (In Russian)
10. Kendall, D.G.: Stochastic processes occurring in the theory of queues and their analysis by the method of embedded Markov chains. Ann. Math. Stat. **24**, 338–354 (1953)
11. Efrosinin, D., Rykov, V., Vishnevskiy, V.: Sensitivity of Reliability Models to the Shape of Life and Repair Time Distributions. (9-th International Conference on Availability, Reliability and Security (ARES 2014), pp. 430–437 (2014) IEEE. https://doi.org/10.1109/ARES2014.65
12. Kozyrev, D.V.: Analysis of Asymptotic Behavior of Reliability Properties of Redundant Systems under the Fast Recovery. Bulletin of Peoples Friendship University of Russia. Series "Mathematics Information Sciences Physics" No.3 (2011), pp.49–57. (In Russian)
13. Rykov, V.V., Kozyrev, D.V.: Reliability model for hierarchical systems: regenerative approach. Automat. Rem. Control **71**(7), 1325–1336 (2010). https://doi.org/10.1134/S0005117910070064

Chapter 29
Reliability Analysis of an Aging Unit with a Controllable Repair Facility Activation

Dmitry Efrosinin, Janos Sztrik, Mais Farkhadov and Natalia Stepanova

Abstract The chapter utilizes the continuous-time Markov chain for modeling the processes of the gradual aging with maintenance on a finite discrete set of an intermediate failure states. The transitions occur according to the birth-and-death process, and the unit fails completely after visiting the last available state. The unit of a multiple and single use is studied. The switching of the repair facility is performed by a hysteresis control policy with two threshold levels for switching on/off the repair server. We provide the expressions for the stationary and non-stationary performance and reliability characteristics, solution of optimization problems, and sensitivity analysis of the reliability function.

Keywords Reliability function · Aging unit · Sensitivity analysis
Markov chain · Average reward

29.1 Introduction

The most technical units are continuously in operation and are subject to the gradual aging, degradation, or deterioration. These processes always lead to the reduction in performance and reliability and hence must be exhaustively analyzed. Markov chains are widely adopted for modeling of aging processes with maintenance repair.

D. Efrosinin (✉)
Johannes Kepler University Linz, Altenbergerstrasse 69, 4040 Linz, Austria
e-mail: dmitry.efrosinin@jku.at

D. Efrosinin · M. Farkhadov
Institute of Control Sciences, Profsoyuznaya street 65, 117997 Moscow, Russia
e-mail: mais.farhadov@gmail.com

J. Sztrik
University of Debrecen, Egyetem ter, Debrecen 4032, Hungary
e-mail: sztrik.janos@inf.unideb.hu

N. Stepanova
Altai Economics and Law Institute, Krasnoarmejskiy per 108, 656015 Barnaul, Russia
e-mail: natalia0410@rambler.ru

J. Pilz et al. (eds.), *Statistics and Simulation*, Springer Proceedings
in Mathematics & Statistics 231, https://doi.org/10.1007/978-3-319-76035-3_29

An excellent review and contribution of the earlier papers can be found in [3, 5, 8]. The multi-state reliability models were elaborated for the aging and degradation models with gradual failures; see, for example, [2, 6, 7].

The aging process is assumed to be observable or some measure parameter can be associated with a process, for example, signal of acoustic emission, measures of the gravimetric analysis, and electromagnetic flaw detection. The hysteresis policy (N_1, N_2) specifies the switching rule for the repair facility. This policy is well known in the production–inventory problems and can find also applications in maintenance of an aging unit. Here, thresholds stand for the number of the passed aging states. The defined control policy can be used in a corrosion process of a unit with protective covering, in a damage process due to the fatigue crack growth, in a wear process of a tool of machine tools, in a wear of plane bearing, in a process of discharge of an external load, and so on. Two types of mathematical models are of interest. In first case, the aging unit is assumed to be of a multiple use when in a complete failure state the unit can be repaired and becomes so good as a new one. In this case, stationary characteristics are evaluated and the cost function is derived as the average reward per unit of time. In second case, the aging unit operates till the first visit of the complete failure state. The expressions for the time-dependent performance and reliability characteristics are derived in terms of the Laplace transform. The cost function can be represented in this case as a total average reward during a life time.

The accumulation process of the aging states can be treated as an arrival stream of the customers at the finite-population queueing system with removable server and increasing arrival rate. The Markov type models are of interest. Although the system is Markovian one, only few papers deal with a removable server under (N_1, N_2)-policy in queues with finite population, so in contrast, performance and reliability analysis of the system with hysteresis policy combined with the finite-population queues is a new task. We derive the useful formula for computing the stationary probabilities, time-dependent state probabilities, the probability density function of the remaining life time, the reliability function, the mean time to failure. Additionally, a new reliability metric such as the number of switching of the repair facility is introduced as well. A cost model is derived to determine the optimal threshold policy at the average cost per unit of time for the multiple usage case and the total average cost per life time for the single usage model. Hence, the results obtained in this chapter differ from those presented in other research and they can be adopted for a wide variety of the Markov models with threshold-based control policies.

29.2 The Model Description

Assume that the aging process starts from some initial state and ends in a complete failure state. Before this process comes to the complete failure state, it goes through a number $L > 0$ of discrete intermediate failure states where the unit remains capable to work although with a lower efficiency. The intermediate aging states will be divided into two groups: the states, where the repair facility is deactivated and the transition to the previous aging state (recovering) is not possible, and the states with operational repair facility, where the transitions to the neighboring states take place in both directions. The switching between the groups occurs according to the hysteresis control policy $f = (N_1, N_2)$, where $0 \le N_1 < N_2 < L < \infty$. The control principle can be easily explained as follows. The first group of states includes a starting state up to the aging state $N_2 - 1$, where the transitions will be associated with a pure birth process. The further aging is accompanied by the transition to another group of states associated with a birth-and-death process. The aging process can either stay in this group until the unit will be repaired up to the state $N_1 + 1$ or reach the complete failure state, where the unit can be completely repaired or not.

Let $D(t) \in \{0, 1\}$ denote the state of the server at time t, 0 and 1 means that the server is switched off and on, and $N(t)$ denote the number of customers in the system at time t. The system states at time t are described by the continuous-time Markov chain which will refer to as Markov process,

$$\{X(t)\}_{t\ge 0} = \{D(t), N(t)\}_{t\ge 0} \tag{29.1}$$

with a state space

$$E = \{x = (0, n);\ 0 \le n \le N_2 - 1,\ (1, n);\ N_1 + 1 \le n \le L\} \tag{29.2}$$

and infinitesimal matrix $\Lambda = [\lambda_{xy}]_{x,y\in E}, \lambda_x = -\lambda_{xx} = \sum_{y\ne x} \lambda_{xy}$, where $\lambda_{xy} = \lambda_{xy}(f)$ depends on the switching hysteresis policy $f = (N_1, N_2)$.

29.3 Stationary Probabilities and Average Reward

According to above description, $\{X(t)\}_{t\ge 0}$ is an irreducible Markov process where

$$\pi = (\pi_{(0,0)}, \pi_{(0,1)} \ldots, \pi_{(0,N_2-1)}, \pi_{(1,N_1+1)}, \pi_{(1,N_1+2)}, \ldots, \pi_{(1,L)})$$

is a stationary probability row vector for the policy $f = (N_1, N_2)$. The system of balance equations is of the form,

$$\begin{aligned}
(n+1)\lambda\pi_{(0,n)} &= n\lambda\pi_{(0,n-1)},\ 0 \le n \le N_2 - 1,\ n \ne N_1, \\
(N_1+1)\lambda\pi_{(0,N_1)} &= N_1\lambda\pi_{(0,N_1-1)} + \mu\pi_{(1,N_1+1)}, \\
((N_2+1)\lambda + \mu)\pi_{(1,N_1+1)} &= \mu\pi_{(1,N_1+2)}, \\
((n+1)\lambda + \mu)\pi_{(1,n)} &= n\lambda\pi_{(1,n-1)} + \mu\pi_{(1,n+1)},\ N_1 + 2 \le n \le L - 1,\ n \ne N_2, \\
((N_2+1)\lambda + \mu)\pi_{(1,N_2)} &= N_2\lambda(\pi_{(1,N_2-1)} + \pi_{(0,N_2-1)}) + \mu\pi_{(1,N_2+1)}, \\
\mu\pi_{(1,L)} &= (L-1)\lambda\pi_{(1,L-1)}.
\end{aligned} \tag{29.3}$$

Since the set E is finite, $\boldsymbol{\pi}$ exists and satisfies the system $\boldsymbol{\pi}\Lambda = \mathbf{0}$, $\boldsymbol{\pi}\mathbf{e} = 1$. Define the following cost structure:

c_1—the reward per unit of time for each remaining failure state if server is off,
c_2—the reward per unit of time for each remaining failure state if server is on,
$(n+1)\,c_3$—fixed costs per switching on of the repair facility at aging state n,
$n\,c_4$—fixed costs per switching off of the repair facility at aging state n,
c_5—the repair costs per unit of time in a complete failure state $x = (1, L)$.

Now we can formulate optimization problem: Find an optimal policy $f^* = (N_1^*, N_2^*)$ to maximize the average reward per unit of time

$$g^f = \sum_{x \in E} c(x, f)\pi_x^f, \quad \text{where}$$

$c(x, f) = c(x) - \sum_{y \neq x} \lambda_{xy}(f) c_{xy}(f)$ – *immediate cost* in state x under policy f,

$c(x) = c_1 \sum_{n=0}^{N_2-1} (L-n)1_{\{x=(0,n)\}} + c_2 \sum_{n=N_1+1}^{L-1} (L-n)1_{\{x=(1,n)\}}$ –

reward per unit of time when the process is in state $x \in E$,

$\sum_{y \neq x} \lambda_{xy}(f) c_{xy}(f) = (N_1+1)c_3\mu 1_{\{x=(1,N_1+1)\}} + N_2^2 c_4 \lambda 1_{\{x=(0,N_2-1)\}} + c_5 1_{\{x=(1,L)\}}$ –

fixed cost incurred each time when the process jumps from x to y.

Denote by

$$C_n^l = \prod_{k=n}^{l} \tau_k, \; \tau_{N_1+1} = \frac{\mu}{(N_1+2)\lambda + \mu},$$

$$\tau_k = \frac{\mu}{(k+1)\lambda + \mu - k\lambda\tau_{k-1}}, \; N_1 + 2 \le k \le L-1, \; k \neq N_2,$$

$$\tau_{N_2} = \frac{\mu}{(N_2+1)\lambda + \mu - N_2\lambda\tau_{N_2-1} - \mu C_{N_1+1}^{N_2-1}}.$$

Theorem 1 *The average reward per unit of time has the form*

$$g(N_1, N_2) = c_1 \sum_{n=0}^{N_2-1} (L-n)\pi_{(0,n)} + c_2 \sum_{n=N_1+1}^{L-1} (L-n)\pi_{(1,n)} \qquad (29.4)$$
$$- \left((N_1+1)c_3\mu\pi_{(1,N_1+1)} + (N_2-1)N_2 c_4\lambda\pi_{(0,N_2-1)} + c_5\pi_{(1,L)}\right),$$

where $\pi_x, x \in E$, satisfy the explicit expressions,

$$\pi_{(1,L)} = \left[1 + \frac{\mu}{\lambda} C_{N_1+1}^{L-1} \sum_{n=N_1}^{N_2-1} \prod_{i=N_1}^{n} \frac{1}{i+1} + \sum_{n=N_1+1}^{L-1} C_n^{L-1}\right]^{-1},$$

$$\pi_{(0,n)} = \frac{\mu}{\lambda} C_{N_1+1}^{L-1} \prod_{i=N_1}^{n} \frac{1}{i+1} \pi_{(1,L)}, \; N_1 \le n \le N_2 - 1,$$

$$\pi_{(1,n)} = C_n^{L-1} \pi_{(1,L)}, \; N_1 + 1 \le n \le L - 1.$$

Proof The statement follows by solving recursively the system of balance equations for the stationary state probabilities taking into account that for transient states $\pi_{(0,n)} = 0, 0 \le n \le N_1 - 1$.

Our aim is to find the optimal policy $f^* = (N_1^*, N_2^*)$ such that

$$g(f^*) = \min_f g(f), \tag{29.5}$$
$$\text{subject to } f = (N_1, N_2), \; 0 \le N_1 < N_2 < L.$$

It is also possible to formulate an optimization problem with the aim to find the joint optimal value (f^*, μ^*). Mathematically, it can be described by

$$g(f^*, \mu^*) = \min_{f,\mu} g(f, \mu) \tag{29.6}$$
$$\text{subject to } 0 \le N_1 < N_2 < L, \; 0 < \mu < \mu^U,$$

where μ^U is predefined upper bound. The function g is nonlinear and quite complex in order to solve the optimization problem analytically. To find a discrete optimal vector f^* for the fixed parameters, a direct search method can be applied. For the joint values (f^*, μ^*), a method for numerical solution of the cost optimization problem can be used. It uses the principles of the a quasi-Newton method; see, for example, [1].

29.4 Reliability Analysis During the Life Time

Assume that at time $t = 0$, the system starts from initial state $x = (0, 0)$ and the complete failure state $(1, L)$ will be the absorbing one. Denote by T the life time of the system or the time to absorption, i.e., $T = \inf\{t : X(t) = (1, L)\}$. Here we analyze the system during the time T. The transient Markov process $\hat{X}(t)$, which describes the system states at time t, has the same state space E and almost the same infinitesimal matrix Λ as (29.1) with one exception that in latter case there is no transition from $(1, L)$ to $(1, L - 1)$. For the time-dependent state probabilities

$$\pi_{(0,n)}(t) = \mathbb{P}[X(t) = (0, n), t < T], \; 0 \le n \le N_2 - 1$$
$$\pi_{(1,n)}(t) = \mathbb{P}[X(t) = (1, n), t < T], \; N_1 + 1 \le n \le L,$$

referring the state transition rate diagram we can write down the corresponding Kolmogorov differential equations (KDEs), $\boldsymbol{\pi}'(t) = \boldsymbol{\pi}(t)\Lambda$ with initial condition $\pi_{(0,0)}(0) = 1, \pi_x(0) = 0, x \neq (0,0)$. Applying the Laplace transforms (LT) $\tilde{\pi}_{(d,n)}(s) = \int_0^\infty e^{-st}\pi_{(d,n)}(t)dt, Re[s] > 0$, we get the system of equations, which can be rewritten in matrix form

$$\tilde{\boldsymbol{\pi}}(s)\Lambda(s) = \boldsymbol{\pi}(0), \tag{29.7}$$

where $\tilde{\boldsymbol{\pi}}(s) = (\tilde{\pi}_{(0,0)}(s), \ldots, \tilde{\pi}_{(0,N_2-1)}(s), \tilde{\pi}_{(1,N_1+1)}(s), \ldots, \tilde{\pi}_{(1,L)}(s))$, $\Lambda(s) = sI - \Lambda$ is a $(L + N_2 - N_1) \times (L + N_2 - N_1)$ matrix, I is the identity matrix of the appropriate size, $\boldsymbol{\pi}(0) = (1, 0, \ldots, 0)$—initial probability vector. It can be shown that for the Markov process $\{\hat{X}(t)\}_{t\geq 0}$ with an absorption the total average reward is equal to

$$g^f = \sum_{x\in E} c(x, f) \int_0^T \pi_x(u)du = \sum_{x\in E} c(x, f)\tilde{\pi}_x(0).$$

Denote by

$$B_n^l(s) = \prod_{k=n}^{l} \rho_k(s),\ \rho_0(s) = \frac{1}{s+\lambda},\ \rho_k(s) = \frac{k\lambda}{s+(k+1)\lambda},$$

$$C_n^l(s) = \prod_{k=n}^{l} \tau_k(s),\ \tau_{N_1}(s) = \frac{\mu}{s+(N_1+1)\lambda},\ \tau_{N_1+1}(s) = \frac{\mu}{s+(N_1+2)\lambda+\mu},$$

$$\tau_{N_2}(s) = \frac{\mu}{s+(N_2+1)\lambda+\mu-N_2\lambda\tau_{N_2-1}(s)-N_2\lambda B_{N_1+1}^{N_2-1}(s)C_{N_1}^{N_2-1}(s)},$$

$$\tau_k(s) = \frac{\mu}{s+(k+1)\lambda+\mu-k\lambda\tau_{k-1}(s)},\ N_1+2\leq k\leq L-1,\ k\neq N_2,$$

$$\nu_{N_2}(s) = \frac{N_2\lambda B_0^{N_2-1}(s)}{s+(N_2+1)\lambda+\mu-N_2\lambda\tau_{N_2-1}(s)-N_2\lambda B_{N_1+1}^{N_2-1}(s)C_{N_1}^{N_2-1}(s)},$$

$$\nu_k(s) = \frac{k\lambda\nu_{k-1}(s)}{s+(k+1)\lambda+\mu-k\lambda\tau_{k-1}(s)},\ N_2+1\leq k\leq L-1,$$

$$\nu_L(s) = \frac{L\lambda\nu_{L-1}(s)}{s-L\lambda\tau_{L-1}(s)}.$$

Theorem 2 *The total average reward during the time T has the form*

$$g(N_1, N_2) = c_1\sum_{n=0}^{N_2-1}(L-n)\tilde{\pi}_{(0,n)}(0) + c_2\sum_{n=N_1+1}^{L-1}(L-n)\tilde{\pi}_{(1,n)}(0) \tag{29.8}$$
$$-(c_3\mu\tilde{\pi}_{(1,N_1+1)}(0) + c_4N_2\lambda\tilde{\pi}_{(0,N_2-1)}(0)),\ \textit{where}$$

$$\tilde{\pi}_{(0,n)}(s) = B_0^n(s),\ 0 \le n \le N_1 - 1,$$
$$\tilde{\pi}_{(0,n)}(s) = B_0^n(s) + \tau_{N_1}(s) B_{N_1+1}^n(s) \tilde{\pi}_{(1,N_1+1)}(s),\ N_1 \le n \le N_2 - 1,$$
$$\tilde{\pi}_{(1,n)}(s) = \sum_{i=0}^{L-N_2} C_n^{N_2+i-1}(s) \nu_{N_2+i}(s),\ N_1 + 1 \le n \le N_2 - 1,$$

$$\tilde{\pi}_{(1,n)}(s) = \sum_{i=0}^{L-n} C_n^{n+i-1}(s) \nu_{n+i}(s),\ N_2 \le n \le L$$

is a solution of the system of KDEs in terms of the LT.

Proof The statement follows by solving recursively the system of KDEs in terms of the LT.

Denote by
T_{yx}—time spent in $x \in E$ starting from y,
$T_y = \sum_{x \in E} T_{yx}$—time to absorption from y (residual life time).
For the initial distribution $\boldsymbol{\pi}(0)$ over E, define a *ratio of means* distribution by

$$p_x = \frac{\sum_{y \in E} \pi_y(0) \mathbb{E}[T_{yx}]}{\sum_{y \in E} \pi_y(0) \mathbb{E}[T_y]} = \frac{\sum_{y \in E} \int_0^\infty \pi_y(0) p_{yx}(t) dt}{\sum_{y \in E} \int_0^\infty \pi_y(0)(1 - p_{y(1,L)}(t)) dt},$$

where $p_{yx}(t)$ is a transition probability from state y to state x in time t of the absorbing Markov chain $\{\hat{X}(t)\}_{t \ge 0}$.

Remark 1 The reward function $g(N_1, N_2)$ can be evaluated with respect to the ratio of means distribution $p_{(d,n)}$ depending on $\boldsymbol{\pi}(0)$,

$$p_{(d,n)} = \frac{\tilde{\pi}_{(d,n)}(0)}{\sum_{n=0}^{N_2-1} \tilde{\pi}_{(0,n)}(0) + \sum_{n=N_1+1}^{L-1} \tilde{\pi}_{(1,n)}(0)}.$$

In this case, the optimal policy (N_1, N_2) can differ from that which minimizes the total reward.

29.5 Reliability Function and Evaluation Methods

The system reliability function is defined by

$$R(t) = \mathbb{P}[T > t] = 1 - \pi_{(1,L)}(t),\ t \ge 0. \tag{29.9}$$

If $\tilde{R}(s) = \int_0^\infty e^{-st} R(t)dt$, $Re[s] > 0$, then it follows

$$\tilde{R}(s) = \frac{1}{s} - \tilde{\pi}_{(1,L)}(s). \tag{29.10}$$

Method 1—Direct Solution of the KDE.

The LT $\tilde{\pi}_{(1,L)}(s)$ can be calculated from the system of KDE,

$$\tilde{\pi}_{(1,L)}(s) = \nu_L(s).$$

The inversion of the Laplace transform completes the evaluation.

Method 2—Solution of the System of KDE Using Cramer's Rule.
The LT $\tilde{\pi}_{(1,L)}(s)$ can be evaluated also by solving the system

$$\tilde{\boldsymbol{\pi}}(s)(sI - \Lambda) = \boldsymbol{\pi}(0),$$
$$\boldsymbol{\pi}(0) = (1, 0, \ldots, 0)$$

using the Cramer's rule

$$\tilde{\pi}_{(1,L)}(s) = \frac{|\Lambda_{L+N_2-N_1}(s)|}{|\Lambda(s)|}, \quad \text{where}$$

$|\Lambda(s)|$—the determinant of the matrix $\Lambda(s)$,
$|\Lambda_{L+N_2-N_1}(s)|$—the determinant obtained by replacing the $(L + N_2 - N_1)$th raw of $\Lambda(s)$ by the initial vector $\boldsymbol{\pi}(0)$.

Theorem 3 *The determinants* $|\Lambda_{L+N_2-N_1}(s)|$ *and* $|\Lambda(s)|$ *are of the form*

$$|\Lambda_{L+N_2-N_1}(s)| = (-1)^L \lambda^L L! |\Delta_{N_1+2,N_2+1}(s)|, \tag{29.11}$$

$$|\Lambda(s)| = s \prod_{i=1}^{N_1} (s + i\lambda) \Big[\prod_{i=N_1+1}^{N_2} (s + i\lambda) |\Delta_{N_1+2,L}(s)| \tag{29.12}$$

$$+ \frac{N_2!(\lambda\,\mu)^{N_2-N_1}}{N_1!} |\Delta_{N_2+2,L}(s)| \Big], \ \textit{where}$$

$$|\Delta_{k,l}(s)| = \prod_{i=k}^{l} a_i \Big[1 + \sum_{r=1}^{\lfloor \frac{l-k+1}{2} \rfloor} \sum_{i_0,\ldots,i_{r-1} \in S_r(2,l-k+1)} \prod_{j=0}^{r} \frac{\mu b_{k+i_j-2}}{a_{k+i_j-2} a_{k+i_j-1}} \Big],$$

$$S_r(2, n) = \begin{cases} \{2, \ldots, n\} & n \ge 2,\ r = 1, \\ \{(i_1, \ldots, i_r) : i_j \in \{2, \ldots, n\}, i_j - i_{j-1} \ge 2\}, & n \ge 4,\ 2 \le r \le \lfloor \frac{n}{2} \rfloor, \end{cases}$$

$a_l = (s + l\lambda + \mu)$, $b_l = -l\lambda$, $\Delta_{k,l}(s)$*—tridiagonal matrix with upper, main and lower diagonals given by* $(b_k, \ldots, b_{l-1}), (a_k, \ldots, a_l), (-\mu, \ldots, -\mu)$.

Proof The result can be easily obtained using the definition of the tridiagonal matrix and its properties, $|\Delta_{k,l}(s)| = a_l|\Delta_{k,l-1}(s)| + b_{l-1}\mu|\Delta_{k,l-2}(s)|, |\Delta_{k,k-1}(s)| = 1$, $|\Delta_{k,k-2}(s)| = 0$. Solving this difference equation as proposed in [4], we get the explicit expression for the determinant $|\Delta_{k,l}(s)|$.

Theorem 4 *The reliability function* $R(t)$ *satisfies the relation*

$$R(t) = -\sum_{k=1}^{l} A_l e^{-s_k t} + \sum_{k=1}^{m} e^{-Re[s_{l+k}]t}\Big[B_k \cos(Im[s_{l+k}]t) + \frac{C_k - B_k Re[s_{l+k}]}{Im[s_{l+k}]} \sin(Im[s_{l+k}]t)\Big],\ t \geq 0,\ where \tag{29.13}$$

$$\begin{aligned} A_0 &= \frac{s|\Lambda_{L+N_2-N_1}(0)|}{|\Lambda(s)|}\Big|_{s=0} = 1, \\ A_n &= \frac{(s+s_n)|\Lambda_{L+N_2-N_1}(-s_n)|}{|\Lambda(s)|}\Big|_{s=-s_n},\ 1 \leq n \leq l, \\ B_n s_{l+n} + C_n &= \\ &\frac{(s + (s_{l+n} + \bar{s}_{l+n})s + s_{l+n}\bar{s}_{l+n})|\Lambda_{L+N_2-N_1}(-s_{l+n})|}{|\Lambda(s)|}\Big|_{s=-s_{l+n}},\ 1 \leq n \leq m, \end{aligned} \tag{29.14}$$

$s_n = n\lambda, 1 \leq n \leq N_1, s_n = n\lambda + \mu, N_2 + 2 \leq n \leq L$ *and other eigenvalues are the solutions of* $|\Delta(s)| = 0$.

Proof The determinant $|\Lambda(s)|$ can be factorized,

$$|\Lambda(s)| = s\prod_{k=1}^{l}(s+s_k)\prod_{k=1}^{m}(s^2 + (s_{l+k} + \bar{s}_{l+k})s + s_{l+k}\bar{s}_{l+k}),$$

where $s_0 = 0$ and $s_1, s_2, \ldots, s_l$ are the possible l real distinct eigenvalues, and $(s_{l+1}, \bar{s}_{l+1})$,$(s_{l+2}, \bar{s}_{l+2})$,…, $(s_{l+m}, \bar{s}_{l+m})$ are the m pairs of distinct conjugate complex eigenvalues obtained from

$$|\Lambda(s)| = |\Lambda - sI| = 0$$

Due to the partial fraction expansion,

$$\tilde{\pi}_{(1,L)}(s) = \sum_{k=0}^{l} \frac{A_k}{s+s_k} + \sum_{k=1}^{m} \frac{B_k s + C_k}{s^2 + (s_{l+k} + \bar{s}_{l+k})s + s_{l+k}\bar{s}_{l+k}}.$$

The constants $A_k, 0 \leq k \leq l$, are the real numbers, which by equating the coefficients can be obtained in form (29.14). Note that $A_0 = \lim_{t\to\infty} \pi_{(1,L)}(t) = 1$. Together with (29.9), the inverse LT implies the explicit relation (29.13).

Method 3—The Remaining Life Time.
Denote by
$T_{(d,n)} = T|X(0) = (d,n)$—the remaining life time given $(d,n) \in E$,
$r_x(t) = \frac{\mathbb{P}[T_x \in [t,t+dt)]}{dt}$—probability density function,
$\tilde{r}_x(s) = \int_0^\infty e^{-st} r_x(t)dt$—LT of the density function $r_x(t)$.

The LT $\tilde{R}(s)$ can be evaluated by

$$\tilde{R}(s) = \frac{1}{s}\Big[1 - \tilde{r}_{(0,0)}(s)\Big]. \tag{29.15}$$

Note that $\tilde{\pi}_{(1,L)}(s) = \frac{L\lambda}{s}\tilde{\pi}_{(1,L-1)}(s)$. It follows then that

$$\tilde{r}_{(0,0)}(s) = L\lambda\tilde{\pi}_{(1,L-1)}(s).$$

The conditional LT $\tilde{r}_x(s)$ can be evaluated directly as well. Define

$$B_n^l(s) = \prod_{k=n}^{l} \rho_k(s),\ \rho_k(s) = \frac{k\lambda}{s + k\lambda},$$
$$C_n^l(s) = \prod_{k=n}^{l} \tau_k(s),\ \tau_{N_1+1}(s) = \frac{(N_1+2)\lambda}{s + (N_1+2)\lambda + \mu},\ \nu_{N_1+1}(s) = \frac{\mu B_{N_1+1}^{N_2}(s)}{s + (N_1+2)\lambda + \mu},$$
$$\tau_k(s) = \frac{(k+1)\lambda}{s + (k+1)\lambda + \mu - \mu\tau_{k-1}(s)},\ N_1 + 2 \le k \le L-1,\ k \ne N_2 - 1,$$
$$\nu_k(s) = \frac{\mu\nu_{k-1}(s)}{s + (k+1)\lambda + \mu - \mu\tau_{k-1}(s)},\ N_1 + 2 \le k \le N_2 - 2,$$
$$\tau_{N_2-1}(s) = \frac{N_2\lambda + \mu\nu_{N_2-2}(s)}{s + N_2\lambda + \mu - \mu\tau_{N_2-2}(s)}.$$

Theorem 5 *The LTs $\tilde{r}_x(s), x \in E$, are obtained by*

$$\tilde{r}_{(0,n)}(s) = B_{n+1}^{N_2}(s)C_{N_2}^{L-1}(s),\ 0 \le n \le N_2 - 1, \tag{29.16}$$
$$\tilde{r}_{(1,n)}(s) = C_{N_2}^{L-1}(s)\sum_{i=0}^{N_2-n-1} C_n^{n+i-1}(s)\nu_{n+i}(s),\ N_1 + 1 \le n \le N_2 - 2,$$
$$\tilde{r}_{(1,n)}(s) = C_n^{L-1}(s),\ N_2 - 1 \le n \le L - 1.$$

Proof Due to the Markov property $r_x(t) = \sum_{y \ne x} \lambda_{xy} e^{-\lambda_x t} * r_y(t)$, hence

$$\tilde{r}_x(s) = \sum_{y \ne x} \frac{\lambda_{xy}}{s + \lambda_x}\tilde{r}_y(s),\ x \in E \setminus \{(1, L)\},$$
$$\tilde{r}_{(1,L)}(s) = 1.$$

Recursively solving the last system, we get the statement.

Corollary 1 *The mean time to failure (MTTF) is obtained as*

$$\mathbb{E}[T] = \int_0^\infty R(t)dt = \lim_{s\to 0} \tilde{R}(s) = -\frac{d}{ds} s\tilde{\pi}_{(1,L)}(s)\Big|_{s=0} = -\frac{d}{ds}\tilde{r}_{(0,0)}(s)\Big|_{s=0}$$
$$= \sum_{k=1}^{l} \frac{A_k}{s_k} + \sum_{k=1}^{m} \frac{C_k}{s_{l+k}\bar{s}_{l+k}}.$$

Theorem 6 *The mean time to failure (MTTF) is obtained as*

$$\mathbb{E}[T] = \frac{1}{\lambda}\sum_{i=1}^{N_2}\frac{1}{i} + \sum_{i=0}^{L-N_2-1} C_{N_2}^{N_2+i-1}\nu_{N_2+i}, \text{ where} \tag{29.17}$$

$$C_n^l = \prod_{k=n}^{l}\tau_k,\ \tau_{N_1+1} = \frac{(N_1+2)\lambda}{(N_1+2)\lambda+\mu},\ \nu_{N_1+1} = \frac{\mu}{(N_1+2)\lambda+\mu},\ \xi_{N_1+1} = \nu_{N_1+1}\sum_{i=N_1+1}^{N_2}\frac{1}{i},$$

$$\begin{aligned}
\tau_k &= \frac{(k+1)\lambda}{(k+1)\lambda+\mu-\mu\tau_{k-1}},\ \nu_k = \frac{\mu\nu_{k-1}}{(k+1)\lambda+\mu-\mu\tau_{k-1}},\ N_1+2\le k\le L-2,\ k\ne N_2,\\
\xi_k &= \frac{\mu\xi_{k-1}}{(k+1)\lambda+\mu-\mu\tau_{k-1}},\ N_1+1\le k\le N_2-1,\\
\tau_{N_2} &= \frac{(N_2+1)\lambda}{(N_2+1)\lambda+\mu-\mu(\tau_{N_2-1}+\nu_{N_2-1})},\ \nu_{N_2} = \frac{\mu\xi_{N_2-1}}{(N_2+1)\lambda+\mu-\mu(\tau_{N_2-1}+\nu_{N_2-1})},\\
\nu_{L-1} &= \frac{1+\mu\nu_{L-2}}{L\lambda+\mu-\mu\tau_{L-2}}.
\end{aligned} \tag{29.18}$$

Proof $\bar{r}_x = \mathbb{E}[T_x]$ can be calculated by

$$\bar{r}_x = \frac{1}{\lambda_x}\Big[1 + \sum_{y\ne x}\frac{\lambda_{xy}}{\lambda_x}\bar{r}_y\Big], \tag{29.19}$$

which follows by differentiating the expressions for $\tilde{r}_x(s)$ in point $s = 0$.

Now we derive the distribution of the number of switches of the repair facility during the life time. Denote by
K—the number of switches (loops) of the repair facility left up to absorption time T,
$\psi_{(d,n)}(k) = \mathbb{P}[K = k | X(0) = (d,n)]$—the probability density function (PDF),
$\tilde{\psi}_{(d,n)}(z) = \sum_{k=1}^{\infty} z^k \psi_{(d,n)}(k), |z| < 1$—the generating function (GF).
The study of this descriptor complements the reliability analysis providing a type of a discrete counterpart of the length of T.

Theorem 7 *The GF $\tilde{\psi}_x(z), x \in E$, satisfies the system for $\tilde{r}_x(s)$ for $s = 0$, but the service rate μ in numerator of $\nu_{N_1+1}(s)$ is replaced by $z\mu$.*

$$\tilde{\psi}_{(0,n)}(z) = zC_{N_2}^{L-1}(z),\ 0 \le n \le N_2 - 1, \tag{29.20}$$

$$\tilde{\psi}_{(1,n)}(z) = C_{N_2}^{L-1}(z) \sum_{i=0}^{N_2-n-1} C_n^{n+i-1}(z)\nu_{n+i}(z),\ N_1 + 1 \le n \le N_2 - 2,$$

$$\tilde{\psi}_{(1,n)}(z) = C_n^{L-1}(z),\ N_2 - 1 \le n \le L - 1,\ \textit{where}$$

$$C_n^l(z) = \prod_{k=n}^{N_2-1} \tau_k 1_{\{l \le N_2-2\}} \prod_{k=i+1}^{l} \tau_k(z) 1_{\{i > N_2-2\}}, \tag{29.21}$$

$$\tau_{N_1+1} = \frac{(N_1+2)\lambda}{(N_1+2)\lambda + \mu},\ \nu_{N_1+1}(z) = \frac{z\mu}{(N_1+2)\lambda + \mu},$$

$$\tau_k = \frac{(k+1)\lambda}{(k+1)\lambda + \mu - \mu\tau_{k-1}},\ \nu_k(z) = \frac{\mu\nu_{k-1}(z)}{(k+1)\lambda + \mu - \mu\tau_{k-1}},\ N_1 + 2 \le k \le N_2 - 2,$$

$$\tau_{N_2-1}(z) = \frac{N_2\lambda + \mu\nu_{N_2-2}(z)}{N_2\lambda + \mu - \mu\tau_{N_2-2}(z)},\ \tau_k(z) = \frac{(k+1)\lambda}{(k+1)\lambda + \mu - \mu\tau_{k-1}(z)},\ N_2 \le k \le L - 1.$$

Proof Due to the Markov property

$$\psi_x(k) = \sum_{\substack{y \ne x \\ y \ne (1,N_2)}} \frac{\lambda_{xy}}{\lambda_x} \psi_y(k) 1_{\{x \ne (0,N_2-1)\}} + \frac{N_2\lambda}{\lambda_x} \psi_{(1,N_2)}(k-1) 1_{\{x=(0,N_2-1)\}},$$

or in terms of the generating function

$$\tilde{\psi}_x(z) = \sum_{\substack{y \ne x \\ y \ne (1,N_2)}} \frac{\lambda_{xy}}{\lambda_x} \tilde{\psi}_y(z) 1_{\{x \ne (0,N_2-1)\}} + \frac{zN_2\lambda}{\lambda_x} \tilde{\psi}_{(1,N_2)}(z) 1_{\{x=(0,N_2-1)\}}. \tag{29.22}$$

Recursively solving the last system leads to the required result.

The distribution $\psi_x(k)$ is then determined by differentiation of the GF,

$$\psi_x(k) = \frac{1}{k!} \frac{d^k}{dz^k} \tilde{\psi}_x(z) \bigg|_{z=0}.$$

Theorem 8 *The mean number of switches $\mathbb{E}[K]$ of the repair facility can be calculated by*

$$\mathbb{E}[K] = 1 + \sum_{i=0}^{L-N_2-1} C_{N_2}^{N_2+i-1} \nu_{N_2+i},\ \textit{where} \tag{29.23}$$

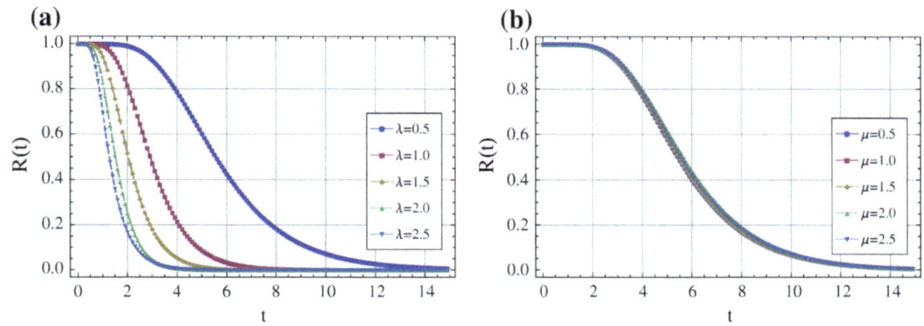

Fig. 29.1 Function $R(t)$ versus λ (**a**) and μ (**b**)

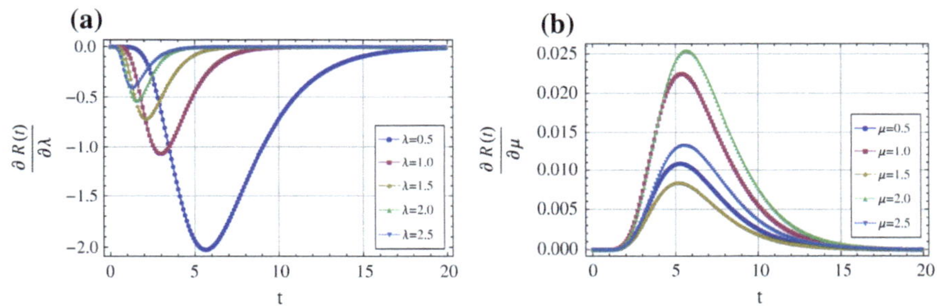

Fig. 29.2 Sensitivity of $R(t)$ versus λ (**a**) and μ (**b**)

$$C_n^l = \prod_{k=n}^{l} \tau_k, \; \tau_{N_1+1} = \frac{(N_1+2)\lambda}{(N_1+2)\lambda+\mu}, \; \nu_{N_1+1} = \frac{\mu}{(N_1+2)\lambda+\mu}, \tag{29.24}$$

$$\tau_k = \frac{(k+1)\lambda}{(k+1)\lambda+\mu-\mu\tau_{k-1}}, \; \nu_k = \frac{\mu\nu_{k-1}}{(k+1)\lambda+\mu-\mu\tau_{k-1}}, \; N_1+2 \le k \le L-1, \; k \ne N_2,$$

$$\tau_{N_2} = \frac{(N_2+1)\lambda}{(N_2+1)\lambda+\mu-\mu\tau_{N_2-1}-\nu_{N_2-1}}, \; \nu_{N_2} = \frac{\mu\nu_{N_2-1}}{(N_2+1)\lambda+\mu-\mu\tau_{N_2-1}-\nu_{N_2-1}},$$

Proof The conditional moments of the number of switches are calculated by

$$\bar{\psi}_x = \frac{d}{dz}\tilde{\psi}_x(z)\Big|_{z=1}.$$

Obviously $\mathbb{E}[K] = \bar{\psi}_{(0,0)}$. The last value can be obtained from the system

$$\bar{\psi}_x = \sum_{\substack{y\ne x \\ y\ne(1,N_2)}} \frac{\lambda_{xy}}{\lambda_x}\bar{\psi}_y 1_{\{x\ne(0,N_2-1)\}} + \frac{N_2\lambda}{\lambda_x}(\bar{\psi}_{(1,N_2)}+1)1_{\{x=(0,N_2-1)\}}$$

obtained by differentiating of (29.22) over z at point $z=1$.

29.6 Sensitivity Analysis

Here we perform a sensitivity analysis for changes in the reliability function $R(t)$ together with changes of specific values of system parameters, for example, failure intensity λ and repair intensities μ. We differentiate the expression (29.13) and get

$$\frac{\partial R(t)}{\partial \lambda} = -\frac{\partial \pi_{(1,L)}(t)}{\partial \lambda}, \ \frac{\partial R(t)}{\partial \mu} = -\frac{\partial \pi_{(1,L)}(t)}{\partial \mu}.$$

All examples are calculated for the optimal hysteresis policy (N_1, N_2), which maximizes the total average reward g during the life time. For the inversion of the LPs, a numerical method is used. Further we fix $L = 10$, $c_1 = 0.5$, $c_2 = 0.1$, $c_3 = c_4 = 1.5$, and consider two cases:

1. λ is varied from 0.5 to 2.5 with a lag 0.5 and $\mu = 2.5$,

$$\mathbb{E}[T] = \{6.01; 3.14; 2.22; 1.64; 1.42\},$$
$$(N_1, N_2) = \{(7, 9); (5, 6); (1, 4); (2, 3); (0, 2)\}$$

2. μ is varied from 0.5 to 2.5 with lag 0.5 and $\lambda = 0.5$,

$$\mathbb{E}[T] = \{5.88; 5.97; 5.92; 6.10; 6.01\},$$
$$(N_1, N_2) = \{(3, 9); (7, 8); (8, 9); (7, 8); (7, 9)\}.$$

Figures 29.1, 29.2 and 29.3 illustrate the function $R(t)$ with derivatives as well as the discrete distribution function $\Psi(k) = \sum_{i=1}^{k} \psi(i)$. It is observed that the reliability function is more sensitive to parameter changing in case $\lambda < \mu$, otherwise the sensitivity almost vanishes. Interesting observations have been made also for the distribution function $\Psi(k)$ of the number of switches K (Fig. 29.3).

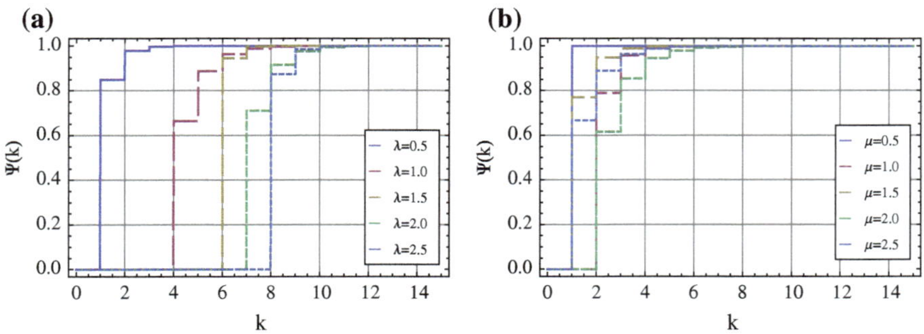

Fig. 29.3 Function $\Psi(k)$ versus λ (**a**) and μ (**b**)

Acknowledgements This work was funded by the Russian Foundation for Basic Research, Project No. 16-37-60072 mol_a_dk, supported by the Austro-Hungarian Cooperation Grant No. 96öu8, OMAA 2017, Stiftung Aktion Österreich-Ungarn.

References

1. Wu, C.-H., Ke, J.-C.: Computational algorithm and parameter optimization for a multi-server system with unreliable servers and impatient customers. J. comput. Appl. Math. **235**, 547–562 (2010)
2. Efrosinin, D.: Optimal parameters of the degrading unit with state-dependent repair time. In: Proceedings of the MMR2013, Stellenbosch (2013)
3. Kopnov, V.A.: Optimal degradation processes control by two-level policies. Reliab. Eng. Syst. Saf. **66**, 1–11 (1999)
4. Mallik, R.K.: On the solution of a second order linear homogeneous difference equation with variable coefficients. J. Math. Anal. Appl. **215**, 32–47 (1997)
5. Murphy, D.N.P., Iskandar, B.P.: A new shock damage model: Part II - optimal maintenance policies. Reliab. Eng. Syst. Saf. **31**, 211–231 (1991)
6. Rykov, V., Efrosinin, D.: Degradation models with random life resources. Commun. Stat. Theory Methods **39**, 398–407 (2010)
7. Rykov, V., Efrosinin, D.: On optimal control of systems on their life time. Recent Advances in System Reliability, pp. 307–319. Springer, Berlin (2011)
8. Welte, T.M., Vatn, J., Heggset, J.: Markov state model for optimization of maintenance and renewal of hydro power components. In: Proceedings of the 9th international conference PMAPS, Stockholm (2006)

MIX
Papier aus verantwortungsvollen Quellen
Paper from responsible sources
FSC® C105338

If you have any concerns about our products,
you can contact us on
ProductSafety@springernature.com

In case Publisher is established outside the EU,
the EU authorized representative is:
Springer Nature Customer Service Center GmbH
Europaplatz 3, 69115 Heidelberg, Germany

Printed by Libri Plureos GmbH
in Hamburg, Germany